Chronic Diseases: Clinical Aspects

Chronic Diseases: Clinical Aspects

Editor: Simon Bishop

FOSTER ACADEMICS

www.fosteracademics.com

www.fosteracademics.com

FOSTER ACADEMICS

Cataloging-in-Publication Data

Chronic diseases : clinical aspects / edited by Simon Bishop.
p. cm.
Includes bibliographical references and index.
ISBN 978-1-63242-634-5
1. Chronic diseases. 2. Diseases. 3. Chronically ill. I. Bishop, Simon.
RC108 .C47 2019
616.044--dc23

Foster Academics,
118-35 Queens Blvd., Suite 400,
Forest Hills, NY 11375, USA

ISBN 978-1-63242-634-5 (Hardback)

Printed and bound in China.

Contents

Preface

A chronic disease is a human condition characterized by a long-lasting and persistent detrimental effect on the human body. It constitutes a major cause of mortality in the world today. Some common chronic diseases in humans are asthma, arthritis, diabetes, cancer, hepatitis C, etc. Chronic conditions can be classified clinically into acute and recurrent conditions. Further, chronic diseases can be categorized as non-communicable or infectious. Various clinical preventive services are available for the detection and diagnosis of chronic diseases. Screening for the presence of a disease or the detection of any predisposition to it, and immunization against infectious agents are some of such preventive measures. Due to the improvement in medical science, there has been considerable extension in the life expectancy, increase in survival rates and provision of better quality of care to people with such diseases. But there can be far simpler and economical solutions for the prevention of chronic diseases. While the risks of developing chronic conditions vary with age and gender, many such conditions are caused due to lifestyle, dietary and metabolic risk factors. Choosing a simple lifestyle can significantly reduce the likelihood of developing chronic diseases. This book contains some path-breaking studies in the area of chronic diseases. It provides significant information of the clinical aspects of chronic diseases to help develop a good understanding of the diagnosis and treatment of these diseases. Those with an interest in this field would find this book helpful.

This book is a result of research of several months to collate the most relevant data in the field.

When I was approached with the idea of this book and the proposal to edit it, I was overwhelmed. It gave me an opportunity to reach out to all those who share a common interest with me in this field. I had 3 main parameters for editing this text:

1. Accuracy - The data and information provided in this book should be up-to-date and valuable to the readers.

2. Structure - The data must be presented in a structured format for easy understanding and better grasping of the readers.

3. Universal Approach - This book not only targets students but also experts and innovators in the field, thus my aim was to present topics which are of use to all.

Thus, it took me a couple of months to finish the editing of this book.

I would like to make a special mention of my publisher who considered me worthy of this opportunity and also supported me throughout the editing process. I would also like to thank the editing team at the back-end who extended their help whenever required.

Editor

1

Mean Platelet Volume and Splenomegaly as Useful Markers of Subclinical Activity in Egyptian Children with Familial Mediterranean Fever: A Cross-Sectional Study

Huda Marzouk,[1] Hala M. Lotfy,[1] Yomna Farag,[1] L. A. Rashed,[2] and Kamal El-Garf[3]

[1]*Department of Pediatrics, Faculty of Medicine, Cairo University, Cairo 11562, Egypt*
[2]*Department of Medical Biochemistry, Faculty of Medicine, Cairo University, Cairo 11562, Egypt*
[3]*Department of Rheumatology, Faculty of Medicine, Cairo University, Cairo 11562, Egypt*

Correspondence should be addressed to Huda Marzouk; nourelhudaahmedyousef@yahoo.com

Academic Editor: Sulaiman M. Al-Mayouf

Objective. To study whether mean platelet volume (MPV) and splenomegaly could be used as subclinical inflammatory markers in children with familial Mediterranean fever (FMF) at the attack-free period. *Patients and Methods.* The study included ninety-seven children with FMF. MPV was carried out within 4 hours of blood sampling according to standard laboratory practice. Splenomegaly was determined by abdominal ultrasound (USG). *Results.* High MPV was detected in 84.45% of our studied patients and was significantly higher in FMF patients with splenomegaly than in patients without splenomegaly. There was a statistically significant correlation between MPV and splenic span ($P = 0.045$). *Conclusion.* Elevated MPV and its significant correlation with splenic span in FMF children during the attack-free periods support the use of MPV and splenomegaly as useful markers of the subclinical inflammation in FMF patients at the attack-free period.

1. Introduction

Familial Mediterranean fever (FMF) is an autosomal recessive disorder characterized by recurrent attacks of peritonitis, arthritis, pleuritis, and erysipelas-like erythema [1]. The disease most commonly occurs in Turks, Armenians, Jews, and Arabs [2]. FMF is caused by Mediterranean fever gene mutation (MEFV); this gene was mapped to the short arm of chromosome 16 [3, 4].

The clinical attacks of FMF are associated with increased erythrocyte sedimentation rate (ESR), C-reactive protein (CRP), serum amyloid A (SAA), and fibrinogen [5]. All these laboratory parameters usually return to normal values in attack-free periods [5, 6]. In some FMF patients, subclinical inflammation is known to continue during the attack-free periods [7].

The spleen is a platelet reservoir; the splenomegaly may be related to increase in hemolysis or may be caused by vascular, infectious, infiltrative, or inflammatory disorders [8]. Affection of reticuloendothelial system in FMF was mentioned in few studies [8–10]; Dursun et al. [8] reported splenomegaly in 27.9% of studied FMF children during attack-free period and Aharoni et al. [9] found splenomegaly in 27.5% and 13.3% of FMF patients at attack and at attack-free period, respectively. In addition, Rimon et al. [10] were the first who diagnosed retroperitoneal lymphadenopathy in FMF patients during life, by means of abdominal ultrasound and computerized tomography (CT).

MPV is the volume of average circulating platelet in femtoliters (fL) and is correlated with platelet function and activation [11]. In recent years, MPV was studied as a simple inflammatory marker in many diseases. Increased MPV was reported in cerebrovascular diseases and myocardial infarction, while decreased MPV was detected in active rheumatoid arthritis [11–17]. In addition, MPV is proposed to be an indicator of possibility of atherosclerosis [18]. The measurement of MPV in FMF has been investigated in few studies [8, 17, 19–21].

The aim of the present study is to study whether MPV and splenomegaly could be used as markers of the subclinical inflammation in children with FMF at the attack-free periods.

2. Patients and Methods

The study enrolled 97 patients with FMF at the attack-free periods, diagnosed according to the new pediatric FMF criteria [22, 23]. The attack-free period was defined as at least 2 weeks from the end of the latest FMF attack according to physical examination and clinical symptoms. All patients included were followed up at the Pediatric Rheumatology Clinic of Cairo University Specialized Pediatric Hospital during the period from June 2011 to December 2013. The samples for MPV measurement were extracted from the patients at the same day of the evaluation of splenomegaly. Inclusion criteria for the included patients were age of disease onset before 18 years and all patients receiving colchicine. Patients who had hepatitis C virus, recent thrombotic episode, diabetes mellitus, uncontrolled hypertension, or abnormal urine analysis for proteinuria were excluded from the present study. Also, patients who had received anticoagulant therapy or nonsteroidal anti-inflammatory drugs (NSAIDs) for 2 weeks before the study were excluded.

For all patients, thorough history taking was performed, including demographic data, age at disease onset and diagnosis, the duration between disease onset and diagnosis, first presenting symptoms, and frequency and duration of attacks. Colchicine duration, adherence to colchicine (adherence was defined as no colchicine dose was missed in at least the last 6 months before the time of study), and the MEFV gene mutations of the patients were recorded from patients' files, together with full physical examination. Complete blood count (CBC), CRP, ESR, and urine analysis were measured by standard laboratory methods at the time of study.

Splenomegaly was determined by abdominal ultrasound (USG). In USG, splenic span was reported according to age and height standards for splenomegaly in children [24]. Patients had been classified according to the presence of splenomegaly or not into 2 groups, group 1 (patients with splenomegaly, $n = 43$) and group 2 (patients without splenomegaly, $n = 54$).

The study was approved by the Cairo University Clinical Research Ethics Committee, and informed consents were taken from the parents of all participants.

MPV Measurement. For MPV measurement, the blood samples were anticoagulated by ethylenediamine tetraacetic acid (EDTA) [25] and then treated with rapid processing within <4 hours. The measurement was done according the standard laboratory technique [25]. CBC was measured using a Coulter blood cell counter (Cell-Dyn 3700; Abbott), CRP was done using latex agglutination test, and the ordinary manual method of ESR measurement was used [26].

3. Statistical Analysis

Data analysis was performed through Statistical Package of Social Sciences (SPSS) software program for Windows version 21. Data was expressed as mean and standard deviation (if parametric) or median and percentiles (if nonparametric) for quantitative variables and number and percentage for qualitative one. Comparison was performed through Chi square or Fisher exact test for qualitative and independent sample t-test (if parametric) or Mann-Whitney test (if nonparametric) for quantitative variables. Pearson or Spearman correlation coefficients were calculated for association of different quantitative variables. P value less than 0.05 was considered significant.

4. Results

The study included 97 patients with FMF, 50 males and 47 females. Their mean age at disease onset was 4.7 ± 2.7 years. Family history of FMF was detected in 14.4% of patients and the parents of 32% of patients were consanguineous.

Demographic data were outlined in Table 1.

Clinical and laboratory characteristics of the studied patients were summarized in Table 2.

The most frequent symptom was abdominal pain, occurring in 96 patients (99%), followed by fever in 87 (89.7%), arthralgia in 77 (79.4%), chest pain in 67 (69.1%), myalgia in 38 (39.2%), arthritis in 32 (33%), and convulsion in 7 (7.2%).

Splenomegaly was detected in 43 patients (44.3%) and the mean of splenic span was 8.8 ± 1.6. MPV was higher than normal value in 82 patients (84.5%). Only 57.7% of the studied patients were adherent to colchicine. All patients had MEFV gene mutation.

Comparison between FMF patients with splenomegaly (group 1) and those without splenomegaly (group 2) was outlined in Table 2.

The duration between the onset of symptoms and diagnosis was prolonged in group 1 compared to in group 2 with significant difference between the 2 groups ($P = 0.04$); however, there was no significant difference between the 2 groups as regards mean age at disease onset ($P = 0.4$) and the mean at diagnosis ($P = 0.7$). The mean duration of attacks in group 1 and group 2 was 2.14 ± 2.07 and 1.43 ± 1.50 days, respectively, with significant difference ($P = 0.02$), while there was no significant difference between both as regards frequency of attacks/month ($P = 0.7$). There were no significant differences between group 1 and group 2 as regards mean duration of colchicine administration and the adherence to colchicine ($P = 0.6$ and 0.1, resp.). There was no statistically significant difference between the 2 groups as regards the type of gene mutation.

The MPV values were statistically significantly higher in group 1 (9.01 ± 2.37) than in group 2 (7.48 ± 1.94), $P = 0.001$. There was no significant difference between the 2 groups as regards platelet count, CRP titer, and ESR.

Convulsion was significantly frequent in group 1 compared to in group 2 (14% and 1.9%, resp., $P = 0.04$), while chest pain was significantly frequent in group 2 compared to in group 1 (45% and 22%, resp., $P = 0.001$).

Statistical correlations between MPV and variable parameters were summarized in Table 3.

Table 1: Characteristics of studied FMF patients ($n = 97$).

Variables	Frequency (%)/ mean ± SD
Male/female	50/47 (51.5/48.5)
Age at time of study (years)	8.7 ± 3.4
Age at disease onset (years)	4.7 ± 2.7
Age at disease diagnosis (years)	6.7 ± 3.2
Duration between the disease onset and diagnosis (years)	1.9 ± 2.0
Frequency of attacks/month	3.3 ± 2.9
Duration of attacks (days)	1.7 ± 1.8
Colchicine duration (years)	2.0 ± 1.9
Adherence to colchicine	56 (57.7)
MPV (fL)	8.2 ± 2.3
Splenic span (cm)	8.8 ± 1.6

Quantitative data are represented as mean ± standard deviation, while qualitative data are represented as frequency (%).

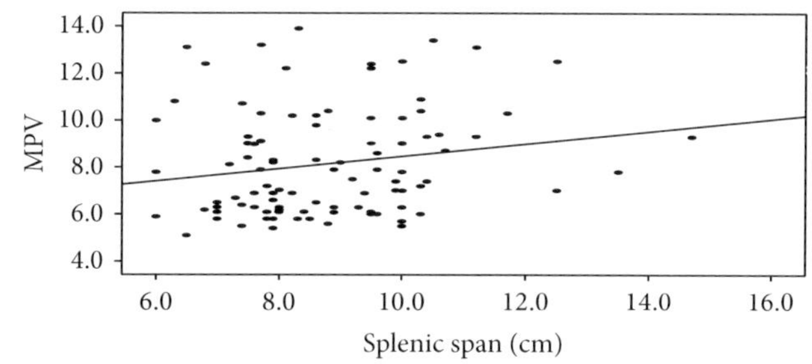

Figure 1: Correlation between MPV and splenomegaly.

Positive significant correlation was found between MPV and splenic span ($r = 0.204$, $P = 0.045$) (Figure 1). There was no significant correlation between MPV, CRP titer, ESR, platelet count, type of MEFV gene mutations, and colchicine treatment duration.

5. Discussion

Few studies investigated the involvement of reticuloendothelial system in FMF patients [8–10]. In the present study, 43 of the patients (44.3%) had splenomegaly at time of study. This was found to be more frequent than that reported by Dursun et al. [8] and Aharoni et al. [9] who reported splenomegaly in 27.9% and 13.3%, respectively, of FMF patients at attack-free periods. Discrepancy between the results may be related to variation in the study design, which also may be related to low adherence of our patients to colchicine treatment (only 57.7% were adherent).

In the present study, we did not find a correlation between splenomegaly and the type of gene mutation in FMF patients which is consistent with the result of Dursun et al. [8] and Inal et al. [27]. On the other hand, Paut et al. [28] found a significant correlation between splenomegaly and homozygosity for M694V mutation. The differences between the results may be related to ethnic difference and variation in the type of genetic mutation between Egyptian FMF patients and patients from other countries.

Recent studies showed that MPV may be used as a marker of inflammation and efficacy of treatment in several chronic inflammatory diseases [11–15, 29, 30]. In the present study, high MPV was detected in 84.5% of the FMF patients during the attack-free periods, similar to the results reported by Arica et al. [20] and Coban and Adanir [21]. On the contrary, Sahin et al. [17] reported that MPV levels were significantly low in FMF patients during either attack or attack-free periods. Many studies reported that some proinflammatory cytokines (one example to these cytokines is IL-6), which are elevated in FMF patients, might affect platelet volume by inducing thrombocytosis [31–33]. These cytokines may be even elevated during the subclinical inflammation at the attack-free periods in FMF patients, resulting in increased MPV and increased risk of atherosclerosis, as many authors reported that high MPV in FMF patients may result in the development of atherosclerosis [19, 34, 35].

Significant correlation between splenomegaly and MPV was found in the present work ($r = 0.204$, $P = 0.045$). To our current knowledge, there is only one study documenting this significant correlation in FMF children [8]. These results suggest the role of splenomegaly and MPV as a subclinical inflammatory marker in FMF children in between the attacks.

In the present study, no correlation was found between MPV and platelet count, which was similar to the result of Arica et al.'s [20] study in FMF patients during the attack-free periods. On the contrary, Makay et al. [19] reported correlation between MPV and platelet count. Also, we did not find correlation between MPV, ESR, and CRP titer similar to the results of Makay et al. [19]. These findings confirm the benefit of MPV as a marker of subclinical inflammation even in patients with normal ESR and CRP titer to allow early management and protect the FMF patients from the risk of developing complications especially amyloidosis and atherosclerosis.

We did not find a correlation between MPV and the duration of colchicine administration similar to what was reported by Arica et al. [20].

6. Conclusion

The present study demonstrated high MPV in 84.5% of studied FMF patients at the attack-free period. FMF children are susceptible to increased platelet activation and increased MPV values due to systemic inflammatory response of the disease even in attack-free periods due to subclinical inflammatory response.

The present study detected significant correlation between MPV and splenomegaly as a subclinical inflammatory marker in FMF children in attack-free periods. High percentage of FMF children with subclinical activity may be related to the low adherence of the studied children to colchicine.

Monitoring the FMF patients at the attack-free period using MPV together with splenomegaly enables us to detect subclinical inflammation and to adjust the lines of treatment in the FMF patients to avoid the possible complications. We

TABLE 2: Characteristics, clinical findings, and laboratory investigations of FMF patients stratified by the presence of splenomegaly ($n = 97$).

Variable	Patients with splenomegaly ($n = 43$)	Patients without splenomegaly ($n = 54$)	P value*
Male/female	21/22	29/25	0.7
Positive consanguinity	16 (37.2%)	15 (27.8%)	0.4
Family history of FMF	7 (16.3%)	7 (13%)	0.8
Age at time of study	8.74 ± 3.59	8.68 ± 3.29	0.9
Age at disease onset	4.42 ± 2.81	4.92 ± 2.68	0.4
Age at diagnosis	6.81 ± 3.33	6.58 ± 3.03	0.7
Duration between the disease onset and diagnosis	2.25 ± 1.93	1.63 ± 2.07	**0.04**
Frequency of attacks/month	3.44 ± 3.00	3.18 ± 2.90	0.7
Duration of attacks/day	2.14 ± 2.07	1.43 ± 1.50	**0.02**
Colchicine duration (years)	2.06 ± 1.86	1.93 ± 1.96	0.6
Adherence to colchicine	21 (48.8%)	35 (64.8%)	0.1
Abdominal pain	42 (97.7%)	54 (100%)	0.4
Fever	37 (86%)	50 (92.6%)	0.3
Arthralgia	34 (79.1%)	43 (79.6)	1
Chest pain	22 (51.2%)	45 (83.3%)	**0.001**
Myalgia	18 (41.9%)	20 (37%)	0.7
Arthritis	17 (39.5%)	15 (27.8%)	0.3
Convulsion	6 (14%)	1 (1.9%)	**0.04**
MPV[a] (fL)	9.01 ± 2.37	7.48 ± 1.94	**0.001**
ESR[b] (mm/h)	29.37 ± 20.19	32.32 ± 19.59	0.4
CRP[c] titer (mg/L)	13.77 ± 11.37	14.89 ± 13.28	0.5
Platelet count ($\times 10^3/\text{mm}^3$)	312.58 ± 75.34	327.32 ± 83.01	0.4
TLC[d] ($\times 10^3/\text{mm}^3$)	7.37 ± 3.23	7.79 ± 3.11	0.5
V726A allelic	16 (18.6%)	16 (14.8%)	0.5
M694I allelic	10 (11.6%)	16 (14.8%)	0.5
E148Q allelic	8 (9.3%)	14 (12.9%)	0.5
M694V allelic	8 (9.3%)	13 (12%)	0.6
M680I allelic	7 (8.1%)	9 (8.3%)	1
P369S allelic	0	1 (0.9%)	1

Quantitative data are represented as mean ± standard deviation, while qualitative data are represented as frequency (%).
*P value < 0.05 is significant. [a]MPV: mean platelet volume; [b]ESR: erythrocyte sedimentation rate; [c]CRP: C-reactive protein; [d]TLC: total leucocytic count.

TABLE 3: Statistical correlations between MPV and variable parameters.

Variables	MPV[a] r	P value*
Age at time of study	0.001	0.995
Age at disease onset	−0.038	0.714
Age at disease diagnosis	−0.015	0.887
Duration between the disease onset and diagnosis	0.067	0.513
Disease duration (time from onset of symptom till now)	0.048	0.643
Frequency of attacks/month	−0.132	0.208
Duration of attack/day	−0.045	0.669
Colchicine duration (years)	0.144	0.163
Splenic span	**0.204**	**0.045**
ESR[b]	−0.009	0.932
CRP[c] titer	0.163	0.427
Platelet count	0.107	0.296
TLC[d]	0.029	0.780

*P value < 0.05 is significant. [a]MPV: mean platelet volume; [b]ESR: erythrocyte sedimentation rate; [c]CRP: C-reactive protein; [d]TLC: total leucocytic count.

recommend further studies with larger number of patients to compare MPV during and in between FMF attacks.

Authors' Contribution

Huda Marzouk carried out data collection, revision of the statistical analysis of the results, writing and revising the results, writing the paper, and corresponding for publication. Hala Mohammed Lotfy was responsible for supervision of data collection, revision of the statistical analysis of the results, and revision of the paper. Yomna Mohammed Farag carried out data collection, revision of the statistical analysis of the results, and revision of the paper. Laila Ahmed Rashed was in charge of performance and supervision of laboratory investigations and revision of the paper. Kamal Ayman El-Garf was responsible for data collection, revision of the statistical analysis of the results, and revision of the paper.

References

[1] J. T. Cassidy and R. E. Petty, "Periodic fever syndromes in children," in *Textbook of Pediatric Rheumatology*, J. T. Cassidy and R. E. Petty, Eds., pp. 657–690, Elsevier, Philadelphia, Pa, USA, 5th edition, 2005.

[2] C. Fonnesu, C. Cerquaglia, M. Giovinale et al., "Familial Mediterranean fever: a review for clinical management," *Joint Bone Spine*, vol. 76, no. 3, pp. 227–233, 2009.

[3] I. Ben-Zvi and A. Livneh, "Chronic inflammation in FMF: markers, risk factors, outcomes and therapy," *Nature Reviews Rheumatology*, vol. 7, no. 2, pp. 105–112, 2011.

[4] R. Gershoni-Baruch, M. Shinawi, K. Leah, K. Badarnah, and R. Brik, "Familial mediterranean fever: prevalence, penetrance and genetic drift," *European Journal of Human Genetics*, vol. 9, no. 8, pp. 634–637, 2001.

[5] H. J. Lachmann, B. Şengül, T. U. Yavuzşen et al., "Clinical and subclinical inflammation in patients with familial Mediterranean fever and in heterozygous carriers of MEFV mutations," *Rheumatology*, vol. 45, no. 6, pp. 746–750, 2006.

[6] C. Notarnicola, M. N. Didelot, F. Seguret, J. Demaille, and I. Touitou, "Enhanced cytokine mRNA levels in attack-free patients with familial Mediterranean fever," *Genes and Immunity*, vol. 3, no. 1, pp. 43–45, 2002.

[7] B. Colak, B. Gurlek, Z. A. Yegin et al., "The relationship between the MEFV genotype, clinical features, and cytokine-inflammatory activities in patients with familial Mediterranean fever," *Renal Failure*, vol. 30, no. 2, pp. 187–191, 2008.

[8] I. Dursun, F. Gok, O. Babacan et al., "Are mean platelet volume and splenomegaly subclinical inflammatory marker in children with familial Mediterranean fever?" *Health*, vol. 2, no. 7, pp. 692–695, 2010.

[9] D. Aharoni, N. Hiller, and I. Hadas-Halpern, "Familial Mediterranean fever: abdominal imaging findings in 139 patients and review of the literature," *Abdominal Imaging*, vol. 25, no. 3, pp. 297–300, 2000.

[10] D. Rimon, Y. Meir, and L. Cohen, "Retroperitoneal lymphadenopathy in familial Mediterranean fever," *Postgraduate Medical Journal*, vol. 65, no. 768, pp. 776–778, 1989.

[11] A. Y. Gasparyan, L. Ayvazyan, D. P. Mikhailidis, and G. D. Kitas, "Mean platelet volume: a link between thrombosis and inflammation?" *Current Pharmaceutical Design*, vol. 17, no. 1, pp. 47–58, 2011.

[12] G. Endler, A. Klimesch, H. Sunder-Plassmann et al., "Mean platelet volume is an independent risk factor for myocardial infarction but not for coronary artery disease," *British Journal of Haematology*, vol. 117, no. 2, pp. 399–404, 2002.

[13] P. Bath, C. Algert, N. Chapman, and B. Neal, "Association of mean platelet volume with risk of stroke among 3134 individuals with history of cerebrovascular disease," *Stroke*, vol. 35, no. 3, pp. 622–626, 2004.

[14] A. Y. Gasparyan, A. Sandoo, A. Stavropoulos-Kalinoglou, and G. D. Kitas, "Mean platelet volume in patients with rheumatoid arthritis: the effect of anti-TNF-alpha therapy," *Rheumatology International*, vol. 30, no. 8, pp. 1125–1129, 2010.

[15] B. Kisacik, A. Tufan, U. Kalyoncu et al., "Mean platelet volume (MPV) as an inflammatory marker in ankylosing spondylitis and rheumatoid arthritis," *Joint Bone Spine*, vol. 75, no. 3, pp. 291–294, 2008.

[16] O. Yüksel, K. Helvacı, Ö. BaŞar et al., "An overlooked indicator of disease activity in ulcerative colitis: mean platelet volume," *Platelets*, vol. 20, no. 4, pp. 277–281, 2009.

[17] S. Sahin, S. Senel, H. Ataseven, and I. Yalcin, "Does mean platelet volume influence the attack or attack-free period in patients with familial Mediterranean fever?" *Platelets*, vol. 24, no. 4, pp. 320–323, 2013.

[18] Y. Bilginer, F. Ozaltin, C. Basaran et al., "Evaluation of intima media thickness of the common and internal carotid arteries with inflammatory markers in familial Mediterranean fever as possible predictors for atherosclerosis," *Rheumatology International*, vol. 28, no. 12, pp. 1211–1216, 2008.

[19] B. Makay, Z. Türkyilmaz, and E. Ünsal, "Mean platelet volume in children with familial Mediterranean fever," *Clinical Rheumatology*, vol. 28, no. 8, pp. 975–978, 2009.

[20] S. Arica, C. Özer, V. Arica, A. Karakuş, T. Çelık, and R. Güneşaçar, "Evaluation of the mean platelet volume in children with familial Mediterranean fever," *Rheumatology International*, vol. 32, no. 11, pp. 3559–3563, 2012.

[21] E. Coban and H. Adanir, "Platelet activation in patients with Familial Mediterranean fever," *Platelets*, vol. 19, no. 6, pp. 405–408, 2008.

[22] A. Livneh, P. Langevitz, D. Zemer et al., "Criteria for the diagnosis of familial Mediterranean fever," *Arthritis & Rheumatism*, vol. 40, no. 10, pp. 1879–1885, 1997.

[23] F. Yalçinkaya, S. Özen, Z. B. Özçakar et al., "A new set of criteria for the diagnosis of familial Mediterranean fever in childhood," *Rheumatology*, vol. 48, no. 4, pp. 395–398, 2009.

[24] Ö. L. Konuş, A. Özdemir, A. Akkaya, G. Erbaş, H. Çelik, and S. Işik, "Normal liver, spleen, and kidney dimensions in neonates, infants, and children: evaluation with sonography," *The American Journal of Roentgenology*, vol. 171, no. 6, pp. 1693–1698, 1998.

[25] M. Diaz-Ricart, L. Brunso, M. Pino et al., "Preanalytical treatment of EDTA-anticoagulated blood to ensure stabilization of the mean platelet volume and component measured with the ADVIA counters," *Thrombosis Research*, vol. 126, no. 1, pp. e30–e35, 2010.

[26] A. Bimpong and J. Burthem, "Supplementary techniques including blood parasite diagnosis," in *Dacie and Lewis Practical Haematology*, B. J. Bain, I. Bates, M. A. Laffan, and S. M. Lewis, Eds., p. 102, Elsevier, 11th edition, 2012.

[27] A. Inal, M. Yilmaz, S. G. Kendirli, D. U. Altintas, and G. B. Karakoc, "The clinical and genetical features of 124 children with Familial Mediterranean fever: experience of a single tertiary center," *Rheumatology International*, vol. 29, no. 11, pp. 1279–1285, 2009.

[28] I. K. Paut, M. Dubuc, J. Sportouch, P. Minodier, J. M. Garnier, and I. Touitou, "Phenotype-genotype correlation in 91 patients with familial Mediterranean fever reveals a high frequency of cutaneomucou features," *Rheumatology*, vol. 39, no. 11, pp. 1275–1279, 2000.

[29] S. Yazici, M. Yazici, B. Erer et al., "The platelet indices in patients with rheumatoid arthritis: mean platelet volume reflects disease activity," *Platelets*, vol. 21, no. 2, pp. 122–125, 2010.

[30] S. Yazici, M. Yazici, B. Erer et al., "The platelet functions in patients with ankylosing spondylitis: anti-TNF-α therapy decreases the mean platelet volume and platelet mass," *Platelets*, vol. 21, no. 2, pp. 126–131, 2010.

[31] A. Kaser, G. Brandacher, W. Steurer et al., "Interleukin-6 stimulates thrombopoiesis through thrombopoietin: role in inflammatory thrombocytosis," *Blood*, vol. 98, no. 9, pp. 2720–2725, 2001.

[32] D. Clarke, P. W. M. Johnson, R. E. Banks et al., "Effects of interleukin 6 administration on platelets and haemopoietic progenitor cells in peripheral blood," *Cytokine*, vol. 8, no. 9, pp. 717–723, 1996.

[33] M. M. Van Gameren, P. H. B. Willemse, N. H. Mulder et al., "Effects of recombinant human interleukin-6 in cancer patients: a phase I-II study," *Blood*, vol. 84, no. 5, pp. 1434–1441, 1994.

[34] A. Akdogan, M. Calguneri, B. Yavuz et al., "Are Familial Mediterranean Fever (FMF) patients at increased risk for atherosclerosis? Impaired endothelial function and increased intima media thickness are found in FMF," *Journal of the American College of Cardiology*, vol. 48, no. 11, pp. 2351–2353, 2006.

[35] M. Caliskan, H. Gullu, S. Yilmaz et al., "Impaired coronary microvascular function in familial Mediterranean fever," *Atherosclerosis*, vol. 195, no. 2, pp. e161–e167, 2007.

2

Efficacy and Safety of Daikenchuto for Constipation and Dose-Dependent Differences in Clinical Effects

Tatsuya Hirose,[1] Yasutaka Shinoda,[1,2] Ayaka Kuroda,[1] Aya Yoshida,[1] Machiko Mitsuoka,[1] Kouki Mori,[1] Yuki Kawachi,[1] Akihiro Moriya,[1] Kouji Tanaka,[1] Atsuko Takeda,[1] Tomoaki Yoshimura,[1,2] and Tadashi Sugiyama[2]

[1]*Department of Pharmacy, Ogaki Municipal Hospital, 4-86 Minaminokawa-cho, Ogaki-shi, Gifu 503-8502, Japan*
[2]*Laboratory of Pharmacy Practice and Social Science, Gifu Pharmaceutical University, 1-25-4 Daigagu-nishi, Gifu-shi 501-1196, Japan*

Correspondence should be addressed to Tatsuya Hirose; h.kanon0827@gmail.com

Academic Editor: Katarzyna Zorena

Background. Daikenchuto (DKT) is a Kampo medicine used for the treatment of constipation. In this study, we evaluated the effectiveness of DKT against constipation. *Patients and Methods.* Thirty-three patients administered DKT for constipation were selected and divided into low-dose (7.5 g DKT; $n = 22$) and high-dose (15 g DKT; $n = 11$) groups. We retrospectively evaluated weekly defaecation frequency, side effects, and clinical laboratory data. *Results.* Median defaecation frequencies after DKT administration (5, 5.5, 5, and 8 for the first, second, third, and fourth weeks, resp.) were significantly higher than that before DKT administration (2) in all 33 cases ($P < 0.01$). One case (3%) of watery stool, one case of loose stools (3%), and no cases of abdominal pain (0%) were observed. Median defaecation frequencies in the high-dose group (7 and 9) were significantly higher than those in the low-dose group (4 and 3) in the first ($P = 0.0133$) and second ($P = 0.0101$) weeks, respectively. There was no significant change in clinical laboratory values. *Conclusion.* We suggest that DKT increases defaecation frequency and is safe for treating constipation.

1. Introduction

The prevalence of chronic constipation in the Japanese population is 28% [1]. The global prevalence of chronic constipation is around 14% [2], of which functional constipation accounts for approximately 4.6% [3]. A characteristic symptom of functional constipation is low defaecation frequency and difficulty with bowel movements. Lifestyle habits, bowel habits, and medicine use may induce functional constipation [4]. Functional constipation is caused by neurological or psychological conditions and may be correlated with intestinal inflammation [5, 6].

Lactulose, bisacodyl, polyethylene glycols (PEGs), dietary fiber, and lubiprostone are recommended as treatments for chronic constipation according to the guidelines of World Gastroenterology Organization prepared by Lindberg et al. [7]. However, there is an opinion that the clinical effect of current conventional western medicine, which has a simplified action mechanism, on constipation is limited [8]. These shortcomings can be overcome by using herbal medicines that exert holistic effects to improve functional constipation [9].

Kampo medicine is a Japanese traditional medicine system employing unified herbal combinations [10]. Although there is no description of Kampo medicine in the treatment guidelines for chronic constipation, the use of Kampo medicine in Japan is not uncommon. Daikenchuto (DKT) is the most frequently prescribed Kampo medicine in Japan. It improves blood circulation and enhances peristalsis [11, 12]. It is used for the prevention of postoperative ileus and the treatment of functional constipation [12, 13]. In addition, DKT is used for improving Qi-deficiency and cold; Qi supplied from food and air is one of the several parameters for diagnosis in Kampo medicine. The mechanism underlying these effects of DKT is not found in western medicine, enabling a holistic approach [14]. According to a previous report, DKT improved the self-assessment scale for constipation [15]. However, the examination was conducted only in 10 cases, and stool frequency did not increase.

In addition, there are reports that the quality-of-life (QOL) of constipated patients can be improved by increasing defaecation frequency [16]. The objective of this study was to evaluate the effectiveness of DKT for constipation, with focus on defaecation frequency and dose-related differences in effectiveness.

2. Patients and Methods

This study was conducted between January 1, 2013, and December 31, 2015. Thirty-three patients were administered DKT to treat constipation upon admission to Ogaki municipal hospital. Constipation was diagnosed by physicians in the hospital based on ROME III criteria and a defaecation frequency of less than three before DKT administration. DKT was manufactured by Tsumura & Co. (Tokyo, Japan). DKT granules (15 g) contained 10 g of maltose and 1.25 g of a dried extract prepared using 2.0 g of Japanese pepper, 5.0 g of dry processed ginger, and 3.0 g of ginseng radix.

2.1. Patients. The exclusion criteria were as follows: cases where the defaecation frequency was four or more one week prior to administration; cases with abnormalities in the gastrointestinal tract; cases in which laxatives were additionally prescribed after DKT administration; cases involving less than seven days of hospitalization before DKT administration; and paediatric cases. There were 33 cases in total during the target period. These cases were divided into low- and high-dose groups. The determination of the therapeutic dose was left at the discretion of the physician. The usual daily dose of DKT is 15 g (6 packs); however, 7.5 g (3 packs) is often used traditionally. There were 22 cases in the low-dose group (7.5 g DKT) and 11 cases in the high-dose group (15 g DKT). Baseline characteristics of all patients enrolled in the study are presented in Table 1.

There were more male patients than female patients among the cases registered. There was no significant difference in patient baseline characteristics between the low- and high-dose groups (Table 1). Data pertaining to cases satisfying the above criteria were extracted from the electronic medical records. Data on aspartate transaminase (AST) and alanine transaminase (ALT) levels, total bilirubin (T-Bil), serum creatinine (Cre), blood urea nitrogen (BUN), Na, K, CL, albumin (Alb), blood sugar (BS), and dietary intake were retrospectively obtained from the electronic medical records.

2.2. Effect of DKT on Defaecation Frequency. From the electronic medical records, defaecation frequencies one week before DKT administration (−7 to −1 day) and in the first week of administration (1 to 7 days), second week of administration (8 to 14 days), third week of administration (15 to 21 days), and fourth week of administration (22 to 28 days) were determined and compared before and after DKT administration in the target patients.

2.3. Adverse Events Associated with DKT. We investigated side effects of DKT treatment, such as watery stools, abdominal pain, and loose stools, using the electronic medical records of the patients. In addition, changes in clinical laboratory values one week before DKT administration, three days after DKT administration, and one week after DKT administration were compared.

2.4. Comparison between Low- and High-Dose Groups. Cases where the daily dose of DKT was 7.5 and 15 g were classified as low-dose and high-dose groups, respectively. From the electronic medical records, defaecation frequencies of the target patients before DKT administration (−7 to −1 day) and in the first week of DKT administration (1 to 7 days), second week of administration (8 to 14 days), third week of administration (15 to 21 days), and fourth week of administration (22 to 28 days) were evaluated and compared between the low- and high-dose groups.

Watery stools, abdominal pain, and loose stools were compared between the low- and high-dose groups. In addition, clinical laboratory values were compared between the low- and high-dose groups before DKT administration and in the first, second, and third weeks of DKT administration.

2.5. Sample Size Assessment and Statistical Analysis. We established the following clinically meaningful criteria for sample size calculation: average difference of 3, standard deviation of 4, the probability of α error as 0.05, and the probability of β error as 0.8. The required number of cases calculated by EZR under these conditions was 28 or more. Statistical analysis was performed using EZR version 1.26. The comparison of median values between the two groups was performed using Mann–Whitney U test. For comparing the ratio between the two groups, Fisher's exact probability test was used. In addition, Friedman's test was conducted to compare the median values among the three groups, and the significance level was set to 5%.

2.6. Ethical Consideration. The present study was conducted with the approval of the Ethics Committee of the Ogaki municipal hospital [20170727-4].

3. Results

3.1. Effect of DKT. In all 33 cases, the median number of defaecations one week (−7 to −1 day) before DKT administration was 2 (interquartile range 1-2). The median number of defaecations in the first (1 to 7 days) and second weeks (8 to 14 days) of DKT administration was 5 (interquartile range 4–7) and 5.5 (interquartile range 3–10), respectively. The median number of defaecations in the third (15 to 21 days) and fourth weeks of DKT administration (22 to 28 days) was 5 (interquartile range 2.25–8.5) and 8 (interquartile range 6–8), respectively, both of which increased significantly ($P < 0.01$) (Figure 1).

The defaecation frequency increased continuously after DKT administration compared with that before DKT administration (Figure 1). In this study, there were no cases using PEG or dietary intervention before DKT administration.

3.2. Side Effects of DKT. One case (3%) of watery stool, one case of loose stools (3%), and no cases of abdominal

TABLE 1: Baseline characteristics of patients.

Characteristics	Total (n = 33)	Subgroups Low-dose group (n = 22)	High-dose group (n = 11)	P value
Male	24 (72.7%)	16 (72.7%)	8 (72.7%)	1
Age, years	74 (68–80)	75 (63–80)	74 (72–80)	0.154
Height, cm	161 (155–166)	162 (155–165)	161 (153–166)	0.924
Weight, kg	57 (50–63)	58 (52–64)	52 (44–61)	0.194
BMI, kg/m^2	22 (18–25)	22 (19–25)	20 (17–24)	0.154
Duration of DKT administration, days	12 (7–20)	8 (5–15)	18 (10–24)	0.075
Percentage of dietary intake eaten to fed before DKT administration, %	60 (50–90)	60 (50–85)	70 (50–85)	0.671
Time since last bowel movement, days	4 (2–6)	4 (2–6)	5 (3–6)	0.714
Concomitant drugs				
Heavy magnesium oxide	21 (63.6%)	14 (63.6%)	7 (63.6%)	1
Senna	17 (51.5%)	10 (45.5%)	7 (36.6%)	0.3245
Opioids	4 (12.1%)	3 (13.6%)	1 (9.0%)	0.7061
Chemotherapy	4 (12.1%)	2 (9.0%)	2 (18.2%)	0.4507
Complications				
Parkinson's disease	0 (0%)	0 (0%)	0 (0%)	1
Cerebral vascular disease	5 (15.2%)	5 (22.7%)	0 (0%)	0.0861
Diabetes	8 (24.2%)	5 (22.7%)	3 (27.3%)	0.7739
Laboratory data				
Na (mEq/L)	139 (136–141)	139 (136–141)	141 (138–142)	0.273
K (mEq/L)	4.2 (4.0–4.5)	4.2 (3.9–4.4)	4.4 (4.1–4.5)	0.893
Cl (mEq/L)	102 (100–105)	103 (99–105)	102 (101–104)	0.863
AST (IU/L)	20 (18–24)	20 (18–24)	20 (18–25)	0.968
ALT (IU/L)	16 (12–23)	18 (12–26)	14 (10–18)	0.0874
T-Bil (mg/dL)	0.6 (0.4–0.7)	0.5 (0.4–0.8)	0.6 (0.41–0.7)	0.809
BUN (mg/dL)	16 (14–20)	17 (14–22)	15 (13–16)	0.231
Cre (mg/dL)	0.8 (0.6–1.0)	0.8 (0.6–1.0)	0.9 (0.6–1.0)	0.633
Alb (g/dL)	3.4 (3.3–3.7)	3.4 (3.3–3.8)	3.4 (3.2–3.7)	0.901
BS (mg/dL)	112 (97–137)	115 (102–137)	109 (97–141)	1

AST, aspartate aminotransferase; ALT, alanine aminotransferase; T-Bil, total bilirubin; Cre, serum creatinine; BUN, blood urea nitrogen; Alb, albumin; BS, blood sugar; DKT, Daikenchuto.

pain (0%) were observed (Table 2). All these side effects improved with continuous DKT administration. There were no significant differences in clinical laboratory values before DKT administration, three days after administration, and one week after DKT administration (Table 3).

3.3. Comparison between Low- and High-Dose Groups. There was no difference in the number of defaecations before the administration of DKT in the low- and high-dose groups (P = 0.364) (Figure 2). In the first week (1 to 7 days) of DKT administration, the median defaecation frequencies in the high- and low-dose groups were 7 (interquartile range 5.5–9) and 4 (interquartile range 3–6), respectively. The defaecation frequency significantly increased in the high-dose group compared to the low-dose group (P = 0.0133) (Figure 2). In the second week (8 to 14 days) of DKT administration, median defaecation frequencies in the high- and low-dose groups were 9 (interquartile range 6–10.25) and 3 (interquartile range 2–5), respectively. The defaecation frequency increased significantly in the high-dose group compared to the low-dose group (P = 0.0101) (Figure 2).

TABLE 2: Side effects of Daikenchuto administration.

Adverse event	Total (n = 33)	Subgroups Low-dose group (n = 22)	High-dose group (n = 11)	P value
Watery stools	1 (3%)	1 (4.5%)	0	1
Abdominal pain	0	0	0	1
Loose stools	1 (3%)	0	1 (9%)	0.33

One case of watery stools was observed in the low-dose group, but there was no difference in side effects between the

TABLE 3: Clinical laboratory data of patients.

	Prior to DKT administration	Three days after DKT administration	One week after DKT administration	P value
Na (mEq/L)	139 (136–141)	137 (134–140)	139 (137–140)	0.318
K (mEq/L)	4.2 (4.0–4.5)	4.2 (3.8–4.6)	4.4 (3.9–4.7)	0.0657
Cl (mEq/L)	102 (100–105)	101 (99–105)	102 (99–105)	0.123
AST (IU/L)	20 (18–24)	18 (13–28)	21 (16–27)	0.927
ALT (IU/L)	16 (12–23)	13 (11–23)	18 (11–25)	0.513
T-Bil (mg/dL)	0.6 (0.4–0.7)	0.5 (0.3–0.7)	0.5 (0.4–0.7)	0.284
BUN (mg/dL)	16 (14–21)	19 (15–26)	15 (10–24)	0.368
Cre (mg/dL)	0.82 (0.62–1.0)	0.7 (0.6–1.0)	0.7 (0.6–0.9)	0.744
Alb (g/dL)	3.4 (3.3–3.7)	3.2 (2.7–3.8)	3.2 (2.9–3.5)	0.135
BS (mg/dL)	112 (97–137)	101 (91–134)	105 (98–119)	0.607

AST, aspartate aminotransferase; ALT, alanine aminotransferase; T-Bil, total bilirubin; Cre, serum creatinine; BUN, blood urea nitrogen; Alb, albumin; BS, blood sugar; DKT, Daikenchuto.

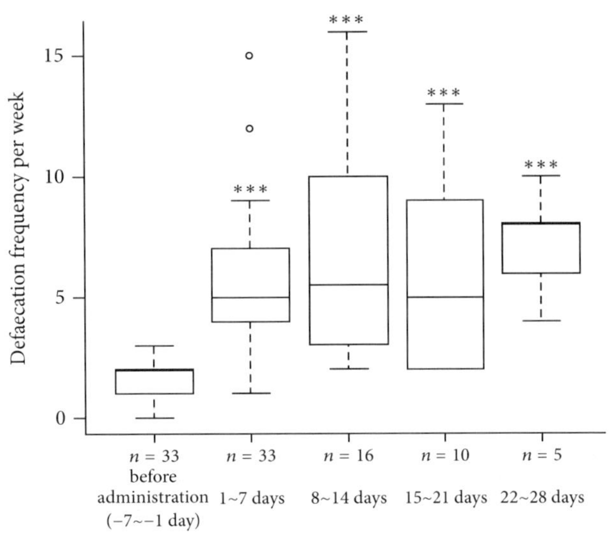

FIGURE 1: Box plot of defaecation frequency per week before and after Daikenchuto (DKT) administration. The box includes observations from the 25th to 75th percentile, and the horizontal line within the box represents the median value. ∗∗∗ indicates significance compared to values before DKT administration.

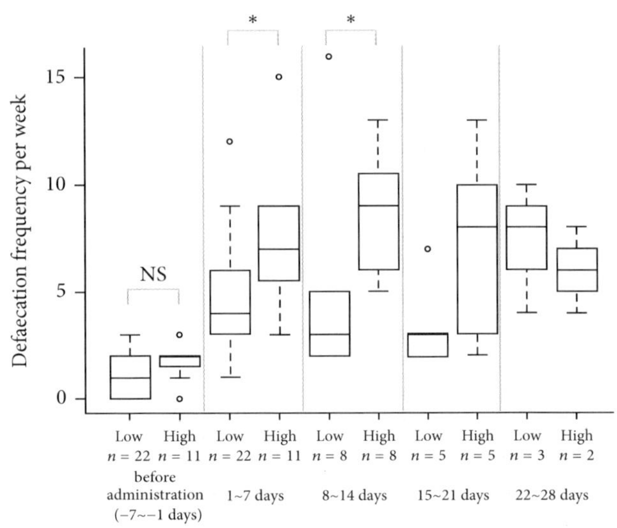

FIGURE 2: Defaecation frequency per week was compared between the high- and low-dose groups at each week. ∗ indicates significance compared to values between the high- and low-dose groups. NS, not significant.

low- and high-dose groups ($P = 1$) (Table 2). One case of loose stools was found in the high-dose group, but there was no difference in side effects between the low- and high-dose groups ($P = 0.33$) (Table 2).

In the second week of DKT administration (8 to 14 days), Alb values in the low- and high-dose groups was 3.0 (interquartile range 2.6–3.4) and 4.0 (interquartile range 3.8–4.2), respectively. The high-dose group exhibited significantly higher Alb values than the low-dose group ($P = 0.0317$) (Table 4).

4. Discussion

Chronic constipation increases the risk of colorectal cancer [17], decreases QOL, and increases medical expenses (US $1,912 to US $7,522 per year) [18]. In this study, we aimed to evaluate the efficacy of DKT in the treatment of constipation and found that DKT can be used as an effective therapeutic agent for constipation.

DKT has been reported to be effective against constipation in specific cases, such as Parkinson's disease, pregnant women, and stroke patients [19–21]. Yuki et al. reported that DKT significantly improves constipation and indigestion in chronic constipation based on the Gastrointestinal Symptom Rating Scale [15]. Thus, it can be suggested that DKT significantly improves constipation and self-evaluated indigestion. This previous study reported that there was no increase in the number of defaecations; moreover, only 10 patients were included in the study. Another study reported that DKT had no effect on functional constipation in women [22]. However, our results contradict these previous reports. This could be because 72.7% of the patients in our study were males.

TABLE 4: Clinical laboratory data in the high- and low-dose groups.

	First week of DKT administration			Second week of DKT administration			Third week of DKT administration		
	Low-dose group ($n = 22$)	High-dose group ($n = 11$)	P-value	Low-dose group ($n = 8$)	High-dose group ($n = 8$)	P value	Low-dose group ($n = 5$)	High-dose group ($n = 5$)	P value
Na (mEq/L)	139 (137–140)	139 (137–141)	0.938	139 (133–141)	137 (134–142)	0.792	136 (132–137)	138 (137–139)	0.291
K (mEq/L)	4.3 (4.0–4.5)	4.5 (3.9–4.9)	0.615	4.3 (3.8–4.6)	4.6 (4.3–4.8)	0.269	4.7 (4.2–4.9)	4.6 (4–5.5)	1
Cl (mEq/L)	103 (98–105)	101 (100–105)	0.938	103 (99–105)	104 (102–105)	0.792	100 (98–102)	102 (96–105)	0.786
AST (IU/L)	23 (18–35)	17 (15–21)	0.153	24 (19–34)	17 (15–23)	0.131	21 (20–25)	15 (14–18)	0.0668
ALT (IU/L)	21 (13–27)	13 (11–21)	0.315	17 (13–26)	16 (10–18)	0.487	12 (12–18)	12 (12–18)	1
T-Bil (mg/dL)	0.6 (0.4–0.8)	0.5 (0.4–0.5)	0.326	0.5 (0.4–0.5)	0.4 (0.3–0.5)	0.283	0.6 (0.6–0.6)	0.7 (0.5–0.8)	1
BUN (mg/dL)	21 (13–24)	11 (10–14)	0.142	17 (15–26)	18 (14–24)	0.779	12 (10–13)	18 (12–26)	0.25
Cre (mg/dL)	0.7 (0.6–1.0)	0.8 (0.6–0.9)	0.91	0.6 (0.5–0.7)	0.7 (0.6–0.9)	0.461	0.5 (0.4–0.6)	0.7 (0.6–0.9)	0.393
Alb (g/dL)	3.2 (2.5–3.3)	3.3 (3.0–4.0)	0.443	3.0 (2.6–3.4)	4 (3.8–4.2)	0.0317	3.0 (3.0–3.2)	3.8 (3.8–4.4)	0.0722
BS (mg/dL)	108 (101–121)	99 (98–114)	0.69	133 (125–140)	106 (99–111)	0.2	89 (89-89)	100 (97–102)	0.667

AST, aspartate aminotransferase; ALT, alanine aminotransferase; T-Bil, total bilirubin; Cre, serum creatinine; BUN, blood urea nitrogen; Alb, albumin; BS, blood sugar; DKT, Daikenchuto.

The increase in defaecation frequency relative to functional constipation has not been confirmed in previous studies. In the present study, DKT increased defaecation frequency, and the effect was sustained up to four weeks after administration.

To our knowledge, this is the first study to report the increase in defaecation frequency following DKT administration in patients with functional constipation. DKT acts on the intestinal smooth muscle cells and accelerates motilin secretion, activates transient receptor potential cation channel subfamily V member 1 and transient receptor potential cation channel subfamily A member 1, and inhibits potassium two-pore domain channel subfamily K member 9 channel, thereby promoting intestinal motility [23–26]. In addition, it has been reported that DKT enhances intestinal motility and promotes the transport of intestinal contents in both animals and healthy adults [27, 28]. In this study, there were no cases of PEG or dietary fiber intake before DKT administration, and the influence of other drugs on defaecation frequency was considered to be small.

It was thought that DKT promoted peristalsis in the intestine to increase defaecation frequency via the action mechanisms described above. Moreover, the subjects in this study were elderly, and they may show reduced intestinal peristalsis. This suggests that DKT may increase defaecation frequency by promoting peristaltic movement in the intestinal tract.

DKT promotes the secretion of calcitonin gene-related peptide and adrenomedullin via the transient receptor potassium channels [11, 25]. In addition, it increases intestinal blood flow [11]. These mechanisms have not been described in western medicine, and it is considered that these mechanisms contribute to holistic effects of DKT and enhances constipation treatment. The high-dose group showed increased defaecation frequency compared to the low-dose group. Moreover, the side effects observed in the high-dose group were comparable to those observed in the low-dose group. These findings suggest that a high dose of DKT is more effective than a low dose. Therefore, a high dose could be recommended if an enhanced effect is desired. Nevertheless, treatment of constipation is possible at low doses.

From the electronic medical records, side effects associated with DKT administration were watery stool (one case; 3%) and loose stools (one case; 3%); no case of abdominal pain was reported. Because these side effects improved upon the continuous administration of DKT, they were considered minor side effects. Senna (sennoside) is used as a medicine for various purposes worldwide, including the treatment of constipation. However, it has been reported to cause diarrhoea (82.8%) and abdominal pain (70.4%) [29, 30].

Therefore, the long-term use of laxatives, including sennoside, might increase the frequency of abdominal pain and diarrhoea and impair the QOL of patients. Nevertheless, as DKT did not cause abdominal pain or diarrhoea, it may be considered safe without affecting the QOL of patients.

The high-dose group exhibited significantly higher Alb values than the low-dose group in the second week of DKT administration. This is an important difference as some drugs are transported in the Alb-bound form. However, this cannot be directly considered as the effect of drugs. The fluctuation in clinical laboratory values following DKT administration was small and this change had no clinical significance. On the other hand, it may be due to the improvement in nutritional status with the alleviation of constipation. DKT may be considered as a safe and effective treatment for constipation.

The present study has several limitations. First, this was a retrospective study and QOL evaluation was not performed. Second, owing to the small sample size, the risk of bias is high, and results are not conclusive. Third, the effects of DKT were not compared with other medications for constipation. Fourth, since cases in which laxatives were additionally prescribed after DKT administration were excluded, there is a possibility that more severe cases were treated with two or more medications and therefore not included in the analysed group. Fifth, we could not investigate the lot number of DKT. Therefore, there is a possibility that the effects and safety differed depending on the lot number of DKT administered. Based on these results, with great cautiousness, we suggest that DKT may be effective and safe to treat constipation. In the future, it is necessary to confirm the benefits of DKT for treating constipation by conducting a prospective randomised placebo comparison study.

References

[1] A. Tamura, T. Tomita, T. Oshima et al., "Prevalence and self-recognition of chronic constipation: Results of an internet survey," *Journal of Neurogastroenterology and Motility*, vol. 22, no. 4, pp. 677–685, 2016.

[2] N. C. Suares and A. C. Ford, "Prevalence of, and risk factors for, chronic idiopathic constipation in the community: systematic review and meta-analysis," *American Journal of Gastroenterology*, vol. 106, no. 9, pp. 1582–1591, 2011.

[3] W. F. Stewart, J. N. Liberman, R. S. Sandler et al., "Epidemiology of constipation (EPOC) study in the United States: relation of clinical subtypes to sociodemographic features," *American Journal of Gastroenterology*, vol. 94, no. 12, pp. 3530–3540, 1999.

[4] D. Nellesen, K. Yee, A. Chawla, B. E. Lewis, and R. T. Carson, "A systematic review of the economic and humanistic burden of illness in irritable bowel syndrome and chronic constipation," *Journal of Managed Care Pharmacy*, vol. 19, no. 9, pp. 755–764, 2013.

[5] K. Winge, D. Rasmussen, and L. M. Werdelin, "Constipation in neurological diseases," *Journal of Neurology, Neurosurgery & Psychiatry*, vol. 74, no. 1, pp. 13–19, 2003.

[6] M. A. Daulatzai, "Chronic functional bowel syndrome enhances gut-brain axis dysfunction, neuroinflammation, cognitive impairment, and vulnerability to dementia," *Neurochemical Research*, vol. 39, no. 4, pp. 624–644, 2014.

[7] G. Lindberg, S. S. Hamid, P. Malfertheiner et al., "World Gastroenterology Organisation global guideline: constipation—a global perspective," *Journal of Clinical Gastroenterology*, vol. 45, no. 6, pp. 483–487, 2011.

[8] P. Gallagher and D. O'Mahony, "Constipation in old age," *Best Practice & Research Clinical Gastroenterology*, vol. 23, no. 6, pp. 875–887, 2009.

[9] H. Suzuki, J. M. Inadomi, and T. Hibi, "Japanese herbal medicine in functional gastrointestinal disorders," *Neurogastroenterology & Motility*, vol. 21, no. 7, pp. 688–696, 2009.

[10] S. Yakubo, M. Ito, Y. Ueda et al., "Pattern classification in Kampo medicine," *Evidence-Based Complementary and Alternative Medicine*, vol. 2014, Article ID 535146, 5 pages, 2014.

[11] Y. Sato, F. Katagiri, S. Inoue, H. Itoh, and M. Takeyama, "Dai-kenchu-to raises levels of calcitonin gene-related peptide and substance P in human plasma," *Biological & Pharmaceutical Bulletin*, vol. 27, no. 11, pp. 1875–1877, 2004.

[12] E. Mochiki, M. Yanai, T. Ohno, and H. Kuwano, "The effect of traditional Japanese medicine (Kampo) on gastrointestinal function," *Surgery Today*, vol. 40, no. 12, pp. 1105–1111, 2010.

[13] T. Kono, M. Shimada, M. Yamamoto et al., "Complementary and synergistic therapeutic effects of compounds found in Kampo medicine: Analysis of daikenchuto," *Frontiers in Pharmacology*, vol. 6, article no. 159, 2015.

[14] N. Iizuka and Y. Hamamoto, "Constipation and herbal medicine," *Frontiers in Pharmacology*, vol. 6, article 73, 2015.

[15] M. Yuki, Y. Komazawa, Y. Kobayashi et al., "Effects of Daikenchuto on Abdominal Bloating Accompanied by Chronic Constipation: A Prospective, Single-Center Randomized Open Trial," *Current Therapeutic Research - Clinical and Experimental*, vol. 77, pp. 58–62, 2015.

[16] K. S. Coyne, J.-L. Poon, C. Thompson, Y. Hu, C. J. Datto, and M. Sostek, "Translating Clinical Findings into the Patient's Perspective: Post-hoc Pooled Analysis of Bowel Movement Changes as a Predictor of Improvement in Patients' Opioid-induced Constipation Symptoms and Outcomes," *Clinical Therapeutics*, vol. 39, no. 1, pp. 75–88, 2017.

[17] A. Guérin, R. Mody, B. Fok et al., "Risk of developing colorectal cancer and benign colorectal neoplasm in patients with chronic constipation," *Alimentary Pharmacology & Therapeutics*, vol. 40, no. 1, pp. 83–92, 2014.

[18] B. R. Collins and L. O'Brien, "Prevention and management of constipation in adults," *Nursing standard*, vol. 29, no. 32, pp. 49–58, 2015.

[19] R. Sakakibara, T. Odaka, Z. Lui et al., "Dietary herb extract dai-kenchu-to ameliorates constipation in parkinsonian patients (Parkinson's disease and multiple system atrophy) [3]," *Movement Disorders*, vol. 20, no. 2, pp. 261-262, 2005.

[20] H. Tsuda, T. Kotani, S. Sumigama, Y. Mano, H. Hayakawa, and F. Kikkawa, "Efficacy and safety of daikenchuto (TJ-100) in pregnant women with constipation," *Taiwanese Journal of Obstetrics and Gynecology*, vol. 55, no. 1, pp. 26–29, 2016.

[21] T. Numata, S. Takayama, M. Tobita et al., "Traditional Japanese medicine Daikenchuto improves functional constipation in poststroke patients," *Evidence-Based Complementary and Alternative Medicine*, vol. 2014, Article ID 231258, 8 pages, 2014.

[22] J. Iturrino, M. Camilleri, B. S. Wong, S. J. Linker Nord, D. Burton, and A. R. Zinsmeister, "Randomised clinical trial: The effects of daikenchuto, TU-100, on gastrointestinal and colonic transit, anorectal and bowel function in female patients with functional constipation," *Alimentary Pharmacology & Therapeutics*, vol. 37, no. 8, pp. 776–785, 2013.

[23] T. Nagano, H. Itoh, and M. Takeyama, "Effect of Dai-kenchu-to on levels of 3 brain-gut peptides (motilin, gastrin and somatostatin) in human plasma," *Biological and Pharmaceutical Bulletin*, vol. 22, pp. 1131–1133, 1999.

[24] D. Kikuchi, C. Shibata, H. Imoto, T. Naitoh, K. Miura, and M. Unno, "Intragastric Dai-Kenchu-To, a Japanese herbal medicine, stimulates colonic motility via transient receptor potential cation channel subfamily V member 1 in dogs," *The Tohoku Journal of Experimental Medicine*, vol. 230, no. 4, pp. 197–204, 2013.

[25] T. Kono, A. Kaneko, Y. Omiya, K. Ohbuchi, N. Ohno, and M. Yamamoto, "Epithelial transient receptor potential ankyrin 1 (TRPA1)-dependent adrenomedullin upregulates blood flow in rat small intestine," *American Journal of Physiology-Gastrointestinal and Liver Physiology*, vol. 304, no. 4, pp. G428–G436, 2013.

[26] K. Kubota, N. Ohtake, K. Ohbuchi et al., "Hydroxy-α sanshool induces colonic motor activity in rat proximal colon: A possible involvement of KCNK9," *American Journal of Physiology-Gastrointestinal and Liver Physiology*, vol. 308, no. 7, pp. G579–G590, 2015.

[27] K. Satoh, K. Hashimoto, T. Hayakawa et al., "Mechanism of atropine-resistant contraction induced by Dai-kenchu-to in guinea pig ileum," *Japanese Journal of Pharmacology*, vol. 86, no. 1, pp. 32–37, 2001.

[28] N. Manabe, M. Camilleri, A. Rao et al., "Effect of daikenchuto (TU-100) on gastrointestinal and colonic transit in humans," *American Journal of Physiology-Gastrointestinal and Liver Physiology*, vol. 298, no. 6, pp. G970–G975, 2010.

[29] A. Shavakhi, M. Kianinia, G. Torabi et al., "High dose Senna or poly ethylene glycol (PEG) for elective colonoscopy preparation: A prospective randomized investigator-blinded clinical trial," *Journal of Research in Medical Sciences*, vol. 16, no. 2, pp. 149–155, 2011.

[30] H. A. Spiller, M. L. Winter, J. A. Weber, E. P. Krenzelok, D. L. Anderson, and M. L. Ryan, "Skin breakdown and blisters from senna-containing laxatives in young children," *Annals of Pharmacotherapy*, vol. 37, no. 5, pp. 636–639, 2003.

3

Untreated Isolated Sytolic Hypertension among Middle-Aged and Old Adults in the United States: Trends in the Prevalence by Demographic Factors During 1999–2010

Xuefeng Liu,[1,2] Van Minh Hoang,[3,4] Yali Liu,[2,5] and Rachel L.W. Brown[6]

[1]*Department of Systems Leadership and Effective Science, University of Michigan, Ann Arbor, MI 48109, USA*
[2]*Institute for Quantitative Biology, East Tennessee State University, Johnson City, TN 37614, USA*
[3]*Department of Health Economics and Center for Health System Research, Hanoi Medical University, Hanoi, Vietnam*
[4]*Institute for Preventive Medicine and Public Health, Hanoi Medical University, Hanoi, Vietnam*
[5]*Department of Mathematics and Statistics, East Tennessee State University, Johnson City, TN 37614, USA*
[6]*Department of Pharmaceutical Practice, East Tennessee State University, Johnson City, TN 37614, USA*

Correspondence should be addressed to Xuefeng Liu; liuxf@umich.edu

Academic Editor: Albert Mellick

Isolated systolic hypertension (ISH) predominates hemodynamic hypertension subtypes and becomes a significant factor for cardiovascular and renal outcomes in middle-aged and old adults. The prevalence and changes of untreated ISH have not been fully investigated in this population. A total of 12,097 participants aged ≥40 years were selected from the National Health and Nutrition Examination Survey 1999–2010. The overall prevalence of untreated ISH was 15.2%. The prevalence decreased significantly from 16.8% in 1999–2004 to 13.5% in 2005–2010. Females, non-Hispanic blacks, and adults with low education had higher prevalence of untreated ISH than males, non-Hispanic whites, and adults with high education, respectively. Compared with 1999–2004, the prevalence of untreated ISH in 2005–2010 reduced in old adults (28.0% versus 37.7%), females (14.3% versus 19.5%), and non-Hispanic whites (12.7% versus 16.2%). The stratified prevalence of untreated ISH decreased in 2005–2010 in non-Hispanic white females (12.8% versus 18.6%) and females who did not attend college (16.9% versus 21.8%). Untreated ISH is more prevalent in old and female subjects, and significant improvements in these groups suggest that public health measures or changes are in the right direction.

1. Introduction

Hypertension includes three hemodynamic subtypes: isolated systolic hypertension (ISH), systolic-diastolic hypertension, and isolated diastolic hypertension. ISH has been defined as a systolic blood pressure (SBP) of at least 140 mm Hg and a diastolic blood pressure (DBP) of less than 90 mm Hg [1]. Typically, ISH predominates as the major form of hypertension for older people after the age of 50 years as SBP continues to rise and DBP tends to fall [2]. It is often characterized as a phenomenon of aging [3, 4]. Risk factors for ISH include being older, being overweight, smoking, and having diabetes. The main cause of ISH may be related to age-associated changes in the blood vessels [5]. If ISH is left uncontrolled, it can lead to heart attack, stroke, and incident heart failure [6–8].

ISH is a growing concern in older adults, and a large percentage of adults are not appropriately managed [9]. Although the prevalence of ISH has been reported in several international studies [10–12], inconsistent age selections between studies limit available results on ISH prevalence in middle-aged and old adults. Several existing studies of ISH in the US adult population focus on the percentage distribution of hypertension subtypes with age among uncontrolled hypertensive subjects, and the prevalence of untreated ISH in the general population of middle-aged and old people has not been investigated [13, 14]. In addition, the studies are based on the third National Health and Nutrition Examination in the prevalence or distribution of related risk factors (e.g., obesity) that occurred during the last decade. Another recent study of ISH examines the prevalence of ISH in the US black population and has not reported the prevalence in the general middle-aged or old population [15].

In this study, sociodemographic factors (including age, gender, race, and education) and blood pressure (BP) measurements were collected from NHANES 1999–2010 and then analyzed to estimate the prevalence of untreated ISH in middle-aged and old people in the Unites States (US). We followed the advisory guidelines from the National High Blood Pressure Education Program with the expressed purpose of further characterizing systolic hypertension. Specific attention was directed toward estimating the prevalence of untreated ISH in the population of adults aged 40 years or older and in the subpopulations of these adults stratified by demographic factors (age, gender, race/ethnicity, and education). As the population in the US is aging and ISH is more prevalent in middle-aged and old people, estimating the prevalence of untreated ISH, particularly the stratified prevalence in different subpopulation, would be critical for identifying the distribution of untreated ISH among people with differential demographic background and reducing the risks of adverse cardiovascular and renal events in adults at higher hypertension risk.

2. Methods

2.1. Study Design and Population. The NHANES program was conducted by the National Center for Health Statistics, the US Centers for Disease Control and Prevention (CDC). Beginning in 1999, the continuous NHANES included a series of two-year cross sectional surveys designed to assess the health and nutrition status among children and adults in the US [16]. In each cycle of the survey, a nationally representative sample of the US civilian noninstitutionalized population was selected across the country through a stratified multistage probability clustered sampling design. All surveys consisted of interviews and examination. Interviews were performed in the participants' home to obtain information regarding sociodemographic characteristics and history of diseases. Examination was conducted in the Mobile Examination Center to obtain measurements about examination and clinical/laboratory factors. All adults provided written informed consent and the data were approved by the CDC Institutional/Ehtics Review Board to ensure confidentiality.

Demographic and examinational data used in the present study were collected from the six cycles of NHANES from 1999 to 2010 to increase sample sizes and improve power for subgroup analyses. The sample from each survey was weighted to the US population corresponding to the respective time periods during which the surveys were performed. The stratified multistage probability clustered sampling design was similar from NHANES 1999-2000 to NHANES 2009-2010. We compared the 6-year prevalence of untreated ISH between 1999–2004 and 2005–2010. For the prevalence estimate of untreated ISH in NHANES 1999–2004, a 6-year weight was created by assigning two thirds of the 2-year weight for NHANES 2003-2004; for the prevalence estimate in NHANES 2005–2010, a 6-year weight was created by assigning one third of the 2-year weight for NHANES 2005-2006, 2007-2008, and 2009-2010, respectively.

Since the goal of this study was to estimate the prevalence and changes of untreated ISH in middle-aged and old adults by demographic factors, the participants aged <40 years were excluded from the study. We also excluded those persons who only participated in the interview or examination but not in both, who had incomplete SBP or DBP measurements, or who were taking antihypertensive medications for hypertension when being interviewed. Finally, a total of 12,097 participants were included in the present study, among which 5,757 persons were from NHANES 1999–2004 and 6,340 persons from NHANES 2005–2010.

2.2. Isolated Systolic Hypertension Assessment. Blood pressure in NHANES 1999–2010 was measured by trained physicians in a standardized procedure using mercury sphygmomanometer and appropriate-size arm cuffs [17]. Participants were recorded up to four SBP and DBP readings after resting for 5 minutes quietly in a sitting position. The average SBP and DBP were calculated based on individual readings according to the NHANES specifications. A participant was determined to have isolated systolic hypertension if his/her average SBP was ≥140 mm Hg and average DBP was <90 mm Hg.

2.3. Demographic Factors of Interest. Four characteristics (age, gender, race, and education) were selected to see differences in the prevalence of untreated ISH across the factors. Sociodemographic information on age, gender, race, and education was assessed through questionnaire files of NHANES. Participants were divided into two groups in terms of age: middle-aged adults if ages are greater than or equal to 40 years and less than 65 years and old adults if ages are 65 years or above. The survey population includes four races of people: Hispanics (including non-Mexican Hispanics and Mexican Americans), non-Hispanic whites, non-Hispanic blacks, and other races. The participant's level of education was classified as receiving education of high school or below and college or above, based on the number of years in school.

2.4. Statistical Analysis. NHANES Analytic and Reporting Guidelines were followed [18]. The study sample with a stratified multistage sampling design was obtained by combining six two-year cycles of continuous NHANES data to estimate overall prevalence of untreated ISH during 1999–2010. The 6-year prevalence of untreated ISH was estimated to examine differences/changes in the prevalence between 1999–2004 and 2005–2010. To reflect unequal probabilities of selection, nonresponse adjustments and poststratification adjustments, examination sampling weights were incorporated into the data analysis to get bias-reduced estimates and sampling errors of estimates. Sampling weights were also used to adjust for the impact of oversampling non-Hispanic blacks, Hispanics, and individuals aged 60 years or older in the NHANES survey [18].

TABLE 1: Characteristics of participants in NHANES 1999–2010, USA.

Characteristics	Mean or percentage (95% CI)		
	Overall	NHANES 1999–2004	NHANES 2005–2010
Age (years)	54.3 (53.9, 54.6)	54.4 (54.0, 54.8)	54.2 (53.7, 54.7)
Gender			
Female, %	51.3 (50.3, 52.2)	51.2 (49.7, 52.7)	51.3 (50.1, 52.5)
Race			
Hispanic, %	10.0 (8.2, 11.8)	9.7 (6.8, 12.7)	10.2 (8.1, 12.4)
Non-Hispanic white, %	77.7 (75.5, 79.9)	78.7 (75.4, 81.9)	76.7 (73.5, 79.9)
Non-Hispanic black, %	7.8 (6.7, 8.8)	7.6 (6.1, 9.1)	7.9 (6.5, 9.4)
Other races, %	4.5 (3.9, 5.3)	4.0 (3.0, 4.9)	5.2 (4.1, 6.3)
Education			
High school or below, %	45.1 (43.3, 46.9)	46.8 (44.1, 49.4)	43.5 (40.9, 46.1)

Note: data were age-adjusted (except for age-specific estimates) by direct standardization to the 2000 projected US population.
NHANES: National Health and Nutrition Examination Survey; CI: confidence interval.

Since continuous NHANES was a national survey with a multistage clustered probability sampling design, conventional statistical analyses with underlying distributional assumptions were not appropriate for variance estimation and statistical testing [18]. Survey procedures were used to compute Taylor series standard errors, independent t-tests were used to compare means of continuous characteristics and χ^2, and the Cochran-Mantel-Haenszel tests were used for categorical survey data. We calculated age-adjusted descriptive statistics for subject characteristics using PROC SURVEYMEANS for continuous variables and PROC SURVEYREG for categorical values. The age-adjusted prevalence and 95% confidence intervals (CIs) of untreated ISH were estimated by conducting weighted simple linear models. Odds ratios (ORs) and 95% CIs of untreated ISH prevalence were calculated from weighted multiple logistic regression models to examine the impact of each demographic factor on the prevalence of untreated ISH after controlling for others. Statistical analyses were performed on PC with Microsoft Window 7 operating system, using SAS statistical software (SAS version 9.2, SAS Institute Inc., Cary, NC, USA).

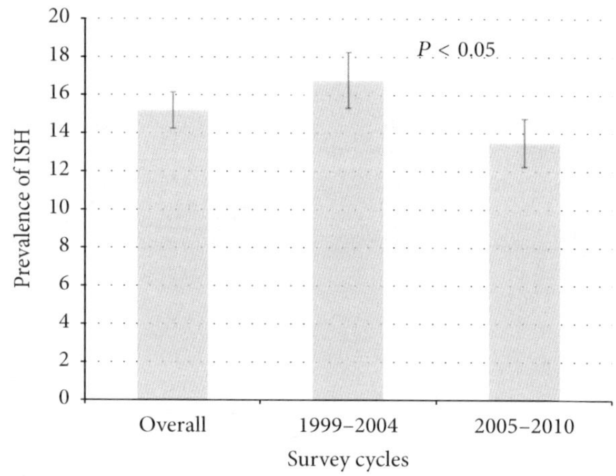

FIGURE 1: Prevalence and 95% confidence intervals of isolated systolic hypertension by survey cycles in NHANES 1999–2010, USA. (The prevalence of isolated systolic hypertension was age-adjusted by direct standardization to the 2000 projected US population. NHANES, National Health and Nutrition Examination Survey; ISH, isolated systolic hypertension. $P < 0.05$ indicates the significant difference in the prevalence of ISH between 1999–2004 and 2005–2010).

3. Results

Average age of adults in the present study was 54.3 years. 51.3% were women, 10.0% were Hispanics, 77.7% were non-Hispanic whites, and 7.8% were non-Hispanic blacks. 45.1% of adults received high school education or below. There were no significant differences in the related characteristics between NHANES 1999–2004 and NHANES 2005–2010 (Table 1).

The prevalence of untreated ISH in middle-aged and old adults is shown in Figure 1. The overall prevalence of untreated ISH during 1999–2010 is 15.2% (95% CI: 14.2–16.1%). The 6-year prevalence of untreated ISH was 16.8% in 1999–2004 and 13.5% in 2005–2010. The prevalence decreased significantly from 1999–2004 to 2005–2010 ($P < 0.05$).

Table 2 presents the prevalence and changes of untreated ISH by the 4 demographic factors in middle-aged and old adults in NHANES 1999–2010. The prevalence of untreated ISH was higher in adults aged ≥65 years than in adults aged 40–64 years. Females had higher prevalence of untreated ISH (16.9%, 95% CI: 15.8–18.1%) than males (13.3%, 95% CI: 12.1–14.4%). Non-Hispanic blacks had higher prevalence of untreated ISH (20.4%, 95% CI: 18.4–22.3%) than non-Hispanic whites (14.5%, 95% CI: 13.4–15.6%). Individuals with high school education or below had higher prevalence (17.6%, 95% CI: 16.3–18.8%) than those with college education or above (13.1%, 95% CI: 11.8–14.4%). Compared with 1999–2004, the prevalence of untreated ISH in 2005–2010 decreased significantly in old (28.0%, 95% CI: 25.1–30.9% versus 37.7%, 95% CI: 34.8–40.6%), female (14.3%, 95% CI: 12.7–15.8% versus 19.5%, 95% CI: 17.8–21.1%), and non-Hispanic white (12.7%, 95% CI: 11.3–14.2% versus 16.2%, 95% CI: 14.6–17.9%) individuals.

Prevalence estimates and changes of untreated ISH stratified by gender and race, gender and education, and education

TABLE 2: Prevalence and changes of untreated isolated systolic hypertension by age, gender, race, and education in NHANES 1999–2010, USA.

Characteristics	Prevalence (95% CI)		
	Overall, %	NHANES 1999–2004, %	NHANES 2005–2010, %
Age (years)			
40–64	15.6 (13.5, 17.7)	16.2 (13.0, 19.6)	15.1 (12.5, 17.6)
≥65	33.1 (31.1, 35.1)	37.7 (34.8, 40.6)	28.0 (25.1, 30.9)*
Gender			
Male	13.3 (12.1, 14.4)	13.8 (12.1, 15.5)	12.6 (11.1, 14.1)
Female	16.9 (15.8, 18.1)	19.5 (17.8, 21.1)	14.3 (12.7, 15.8)*
Race			
Hispanic	17.3 (14.6, 19.9)	18.3 (14.0, 22.7)	16.0 (13.4, 18.5)
Non-Hispanic white	14.5 (13.4, 15.6)	16.2 (14.6, 17.9)	12.7 (11.3, 14.2)*
Non-Hispanic black	20.4 (18.4, 22.3)	21.7 (19.2, 24.2)	18.9 (15.8, 22.0)
Other races	14.0 (9.9, 18.0)	15.7 (8.1, 23.3)	12.6 (8.2, 17.0)
Education			
High school or below	17.6 (16.3, 18.8)	18.8 (16.7, 20.9)	16.0 (14.5, 17.5)
College or above	13.1 (11.8, 14.4)	14.9 (13.2, 16.7)	11.4 (9.6, 13.3)

Note: the prevalence of isolated systolic hypertension was age-adjusted (except for age-specific estimates) by direct standardization to the 2000 projected US population.
NHANES: National Health and Nutrition Examination Survey; CI: confidence interval.
*indicates that the difference in the prevalence of untreated ISH between 1999–2004 and 2005–2010 is significant at the 0.05 level.

and race are presented in Table 3. From this table, we can see that the stratified prevalence of untreated ISH in 2005–2010 was not shown to be significantly different from that in 1999–2004 except for non-Hispanic white females (12.8%, 95% CI: 11.1–14.5% in 2005–2010 versus 18.6%, 95% CI: 16.7–20.6% in 1999–2004) and females who did not attend college (16.9%, 95% CI: 14.6–19.2% in 2005–2010 versus 21.8%, 95% CI: 19.2–24.3% in 1999–2004). Non-Hispanic black males had higher prevalence of untreated ISH than other racial males (black males: 18.0%, 95% CI: 16.0–19.9% versus white males: 13.0%, 95% CI: 11.7–14.4%; Hispanic males: 12.9%, 95% CI: 10.5–15.3%; and other males: 9.2%, 95% CI: 4.9–13.4%), and non-Hispanic black females had higher prevalence than non-Hispanic white females (22.7%, 95% CI: 19.2–26.3% versus 15.8%, 95% CI: 14.5–17.0%). Individuals with high school education or below had higher prevalence of untreated ISH than individuals with college education or above in both males (15.1%, 95% CI: 13.6–16.6% versus 11.8%, 95% CI: 10.4–13.2%) and females (19.6%, 95% CI: 17.9–21.3% versus 14.4%, 95% CI: 12.5–16.2%). Stratification analysis by education and race indicated that among individuals with high school education or below, the prevalence of untreated ISH was higher in non-Hispanic blacks (22.9%, 95% CI: 20.4–25.4%) than in non-Hispanic whites (16.9%, 95% CI: 15.3–18.4%).

Table 4 shows odds ratios and 95% confidence intervals of untreated ISH by demographic factors among middle-aged and old adults in NHANES 1999–2010. Untreated ISH was more likely to be prevalent in older adults, non-Hispanic blacks, and adults who received a high school education or below in either period of 1999–2004 or 2005–2010. Compared with males, females had higher chance to have untreated ISH in 1999–2004 but not in 2005–2010.

4. Discussion

The NHANES data have been used to study the prevalence of hypertension in the United States [19, 20], racial disparity in cardiovascular risk factors [21], and the pattern of hypertension subtypes [13, 14]. We used the NHANES 1999–2010 to estimate the prevalence and changes of untreated ISH in the population of middle-aged and old US adults by age, gender, race/ethnicity, and education. The present study demonstrated that the prevalence of untreated ISH in middle-aged and old adults decreased significantly from 16.8% in 1999–2004 to 13.5% in 2005–2010. The decrease in the prevalence of untreated ISH in old adults (37.7% versus 28.0%), females (19.5% versus 14.3%), and non-Hispanic whites (16.2% versus 12.7%) could explain this change. Females, non-Hispanic blacks, and low-educated individuals had higher prevalence of untreated ISH than males, non-Hispanic whites, and individuals with higher education, respectively. Stratified analyses showed that the decrease in the prevalence of untreated ISH in females from 1999–2004 to 2005–2010 might be contributed by the significant decrease in the prevalence in non-Hispanic white females and females with lower education and that the higher prevalence of untreated ISH in non-Hispanic blacks might be contributed by the prevalence in non-Hispanic black males higher than other racial males and the prevalence in non-Hispanic black females higher than non-Hispanic white females. Further analyses indicated that individuals with lower education had higher prevalence of untreated ISH than individuals with higher education in both males and females, and the prevalence of untreated ISH was higher in poorly educated non-Hispanic blacks.

TABLE 3: Prevalence and changes of untreated isolated systolic hypertension stratified by characteristics in NHANES 1999–2010, USA.

Characteristics	Stratified prevalence (95% CI) Overall, %	NHANES 1999–2004, %	NHANES 2005–2010, %
	Stratified by gender and race		
Male			
Hispanic	12.9 (10.5, 15.3)	12.8 (8.7, 17.0)	12.9 (10.3, 15.5)
Non-Hispanic white	13.0 (11.7, 14.4)	13.6 (11.5, 15.6)	12.4 (10.6, 14.3)
Non-Hispanic black	18.0 (16.0, 19.9)	20.6 (18.3, 23.0)	15.7 (12.7, 18.8)
Other races	9.2 (4.9, 13.4)	8.5 (1.2, 15.8)	9.5 (4.2, 14.8)
Female			
Hispanic	21.6 (17.8, 25.3)	23.4 (17.9, 28.9)	19.1 (15.0, 23.3)
Non-Hispanic white	15.8 (14.5, 17.0)	18.6 (16.7, 20.6)	12.8 (11.1, 14.5)*
Non-Hispanic black	22.7 (19.2, 26.3)	22.7 (18.5, 26.9)	22.4 (16.0, 28.7)
Other races	18.5 (12.2, 24.7)	20.8 (10.6, 31.0)	15.8 (8.3, 23.3)
	Stratified by gender and education		
Male			
High school or below	15.1 (13.6, 16.6)	15.2 (12.7, 17.7)	14.9 (13.1, 16.7)
College or above	11.8 (10.4, 13.2)	12.7 (10.8, 14.6)	10.9 (8.9, 13.0)
Female			
High school or below	19.6 (17.9, 21.3)	21.8 (19.2, 24.3)	16.9 (14.7, 19.2)*
College or above	14.4 (12.5, 16.2)	17.2 (14.4, 20.0)	11.9 (9.5, 14.3)
	Stratified by education and race		
High school or below			
Hispanic	18.6 (16.0, 21.2)	19.4 (15.2, 23.6)	17.5 (14.7, 20.3)
Non-Hispanic white	16.9 (15.3, 18.4)	18.4 (15.9, 21.0)	15.0 (13.2, 16.8)
Non-Hispanic black	22.9 (20.4, 25.4)	23.4 (20.8, 26.1)	21.8 (17.5, 26.1)
Other races	15.7 (9.6, 21.8)	15.4 (6.2, 24.6)	15.6 (8.0, 23.3)
College or above			
Hispanic	12.9 (8.2, 17.6)	15.0 (7.9, 22.1)	11.3 (5.7, 17.0)
Non-Hispanic white	12.8 (11.5, 14.2)	14.7 (12.9, 16.5)	11.1 (9.1, 13.2)
Non-Hispanic black	16.0 (12.8, 19.3)	18.1 (12.0, 24.2)	14.8 (11.0, 18.5)
Other races	12.6 (8.0, 17.2)	15.1 (5.0, 25.2)	11.2 (6.4, 15.9)

The stratified prevalence of isolated systolic hypertension was age-adjusted by direct standardization to the 2000 projected US population.
NHANES: National Health and Nutrition Examination Survey; CI: confidence interval.
*indicates that the stratified difference in the prevalence of untreated ISH between 1999–2004 and 2005–2010 is significant at the 0.05 level.

The decrease in the prevalence of untreated ISH in the overall population of adults aged ≥40 years and the population of old adults coincided with increasing trend of hypertensive patients on treatment, particularly in old people [20]. A greater percentage of hypertensive patients receiving treatment suggest that more patients with isolated systolic hypertension, particularly in old individuals, are receiving antihypertensive medications to lower high BP since ISH is a major form of hypertension subtypes in old people. Over the 12-year period from 1999 through 2010, obesity did not show the significant decrease in women and non-Hispanic whites [22]. Healthy lifestyles are an unlikely explanation for the decrease in untreated ISH prevalence in females and non-Hispanic whites from 1999–2004 to 2005–2010, because eating patterns became less "DASH-like" [23] and obesity did not decrease over time [22, 24].

Compared with non-Hispanic whites, the higher prevalence of untreated ISH in non-Hispanic blacks is consistent with the higher prevalence of hypertension from the previous study [19, 20]. Obesity has been shown to be an important determinant of untreated ISH [24]. Non-Hispanic blacks have significantly higher prevalence of obesity than in non-Hispanic whites [21, 22]. In addition, non-Hispanic blacks are poorer and receive less education than non-Hispanic whites [21]; poverty and low levels of education are associated with the increased risk of overweight or obesity [25]. The higher prevalence of untreated ISH in blacks than in whites and the higher prevalence in individuals with lower education may be attributed to the racial/ethnic differences in the prevalence of obesity.

The US population is aging and ISH is the most common hypertension subtype in middle-aged and old adults, particularly in old adults. The decreased prevalence of untreated ISH in old adults in this study may have significant clinic indications. Every 20 mm Hg increase in SBP is associated with doubling of mortality from both coronary heart disease

TABLE 4: Odds ratios and 95% confidence intervals of isolated systolic hypertension by demographic factors in NHANES 1999–2010, USA.

Factors	Odds ratios (95% CI)	
	NHANES 1999–2004	NHANES 2005–2010
Age (reference: 40–49 years)		
50–64 years	3.6 (2.7, 5.0)‡	3.3 (2.5, 4.5)‡
≥65 years	14.8 (10.5, 20.8)‡	9.90 (7.3, 13.4)‡
Gender (reference: male)		
Female	1.5 (1.3, 1.8)‡	1.1 (0.9, 1.30)
Race/ethnicity (reference: non-Hispanic white)		
Hispanic	1.0 (0.7, 1.5)	1.2 (0.9, 1.5)
Non-Hispanic black	1.6 (1.3, 2.0)†	1.8 (1.4, 2.3)‡
Other races	0.90 (0.5, 1.7)	1.1 (0.7, 1.7)
Education (reference: college or above)		
High school or below	1.4 (1.1, 1.7)†	1.5 (1.2, 1.9)†

NHANES: National Health and Nutrition Examination Survey; CI: confidence interval.
‡$P < 0.0001$ and †$P < 0.01$ for the odds ratio of isolated systolic hypertension for each factor relative to the corresponding reference category.

and stroke in people between the ages of 40 and 89 years [26]. The absolute risk of CV mortality for any given increase in SBP is much more pronounced in the older population [27]. The significant decrease in the prevalence of untreated ISH may lower the risks of coronary heart disease and stroke and extend the overall life expectancy and life expectancy free of CV disease in old adults. The reason for the lowered prevalence in recent 6 years compared with 1999–2004 may be due to the increased awareness of hypertension, greater concerns in health status, and improved lifestyles in older people [19, 28].

Non-Hispanic whites account for the majority of hypertensive population in the US [19, 20]. The significant decrease in the prevalence of untreated ISH in non-Hispanic whites may contribute to the significant decrease in the number of hypertensive patients and reduce ISH-related cardiovascular and renal outcomes in middle-aged and old population. SBP has been shown to be a stronger risk factor of myocardial infarction for women compared with men [29]. Among women aged 65–84 years, the hazard of death significantly increased with increase in SBP [30]. In this study, the decreased prevalence of untreated ISH in females, particularly in old females in 2005–2010, may reduce the risk of myocardial infarction and CV-related mortality in old women in the future. The cause of the decreased prevalence of untreated ISH in females remains unclear. The possible reasons may include the greater awareness of hypertension and the lack of increase in body mass index in females, particularly in old females [20, 23].

One of the national goals of Healthy People 2020 concerning hypertension is that the proportion of adults with hypertension should be reduced to 26.9% [30]. It seems unlikely to attain this goal because of the aging population. However, the decreased prevalence of untreated ISH in old adults, females, and non-Hispanic whites in the last few years is promising, suggesting that the target of 26.9% may be reached by 2020 with concerted efforts from health professionals and government agencies. Overall decreased trends in the prevalence of untreated ISH in the subpopulations stratified by combinations of gender, race, and education are promising although some are not statistically significant and are still in need of substantial improvement. The prevalence of untreated ISH is relatively high and does not decline from 1999–2004 to 2005–2010 in non-Hispanic females, Hispanic females, and non-Hispanic blacks with education of high school or below. To meet Healthy People 2020, the greater attention must be paid to these groups. Therefore, there is room for further improvement in the control of hypertension in the United States.

There are several limitations in our study. Hypertensive individuals who took prescribed medications for treatment were not included in the study because we could not determine what types of hypertension they had (isolated systolic hypertension, isolated diastolic hypertension, or systolic and diastolic hypertension) due to antihypertensive drug therapy. Exclusion of hypertensive adults under antihypertensive treatment may underestimate the prevalence of ISH in the general US population. The prevalence estimated in the present study is the prevalence of untreated ISH in USA. A few individuals ($n = 342$) who were diagnosed to have hypertension used nonpharmacological techniques to control hypertension. The information for hypertension subtypes in the hypertensive persons with SBP successfully controlled by physical activity, weight control, and other nonpharmacological techniques was not available. Our definition of ISH treated them as normotensive persons, and this might also underestimate the prevalence of untreated ISH in the study. The increasing rate of Type I error was another concern by using independent t-tests when multiple comparisons of the prevalence of untreated ISH occurred across the multiply stratified factors.

5. Perspectives

ISH predominates and becomes a major form of hypertension subtypes in middle-aged and old adults. Our study indicated that there were no significant changes in the prevalence of untreated ISH in middle-aged individuals and in males from 1999–2004 to 2005–2010. However, the findings that untreated ISH was more prevalent in old adults and in females and the prevalence of untreated ISH improved significantly for these two subpopulations in recent years suggest that public health measures or changes in clinical practice are in the right direction. The higher prevalence of untreated ISH in non-Hispanic blacks compared with other races and no significant improvements reveal that more attention should be paid to this racial population in the future.

Acknowledgments

Research for this study was supported by an HRSA grant. The authors would like to thank the National Center of Health Statistics for the availability of NHANES survey data.

References

[1] J. A. Chirinos, S. S. Franklin, R. R. Townsend, and L. Raij, "Body mass index and hypertension hemodynamic subtypes in the adult US population," *Archives of Internal Medicine*, vol. 169, no. 6, pp. 580–586, 2009.

[2] A. V. Chobanian, "Isolated systolic hypertension in the elderly," *The New England Journal of Medicine*, vol. 357, no. 8, pp. 789–796, 2007.

[3] E. Pinto, "Blood pressure and ageing," *Postgraduate Medical Journal*, vol. 83, no. 976, pp. 109–114, 2007.

[4] W. W. Nichols and M. F. O'Rourke, Eds., *McDonald's Blood Flow in Arteries: Theoretical, Experimental and Clinical Principles*, Hodder Headline Group, London, UK, 5th edition, 2005.

[5] C. M. McEniery, B. J. McDonnell, A. So et al., "Aortic calcification is associated with aortic stiffness and isolated systolic hypertension in healthy individuals," *Hypertension*, vol. 53, no. 3, pp. 524–531, 2009.

[6] N. M. Kaplan, "Treatment of hypertension in the elderly, particularly isolated systolic hypertension," 2012, http://www.uptodate.com/home/index.html.

[7] G. S. Stokes, "Treatment of isolated systolic hypertension," *Current Hypertension Reports*, vol. 8, no. 5, pp. 377–383, 2006.

[8] O. J. Ekundayo, R. M. Allman, P. W. Sanders et al., "Isolated systolic hypertension and incident heart failure in older adults: a propensity-matched study," *Hypertension*, vol. 53, no. 3, pp. 458–465, 2009.

[9] N. Kamath and K. A. Cappuzzo, "Review of isolated systolic hypertension in older adults," *Consultant Pharmacist*, vol. 25, no. 6, pp. 374–378, 2010.

[10] J. Huang, R. P. Wildman, D. Gu, P. Muntner, S. Su, and J. He, "Prevalence of isolated systolic and isolated diastolic hypertension subtypes in China," *The American Journal of Hypertension*, vol. 17, no. 10, pp. 955–962, 2004.

[11] J. G. Clara, M. E. de Macedo, and M. Pego, "Prevalence of isolated systolic hypertension in the population over 55 years old. Results from a national study," *Revista Portuguesa de Cardiologia*, vol. 26, no. 1, pp. 11–17, 2007.

[12] R. Antikainen, P. Jousilahti, and J. Tuomilehto, "Trends in the prevalence of isolated systolic hypertension in the middle-aged population in 1972–1992," *Journal of Human Hypertension*, vol. 13, no. 7, pp. 485–491, 1999.

[13] S. S. Franklin, M. J. Jacobs, N. D. Wong, G. J. L'Italien, and P. Lapuerta, "Predominance of isolated systolic hypertension among middle-aged and elderly US hypertensives: analysis based on National Health and Nutrition Examination Survey (NHANES) III," *Hypertension*, vol. 37, no. 3, pp. 869–874, 2001.

[14] M. R. Joffres, P. Hamet, D. R. MacLean, G. J. L'italien, and G. Fodor, "Distribution of blood pressure and hypertension in Canada and the United States," *American Journal of Hypertension*, vol. 14, no. 11 I, pp. 1099–1105, 2001.

[15] X. Liu, D. Tsilimingras, and T. K. Paul, "Prevalence and changes of isolated systolic hypertension among US Non-Hispanic black adults in 1999-2010," *Hypertension Research*, vol. 37, no. 7, pp. 685–691, 2014.

[16] National Center for Health Statistics, The National Health and Nutrition Examination Survey (NHANES) 1999–2010 Data Files, 2012, http://www.cdc.gov/nchs/nhanes/nhanes_questionnaires.htm.

[17] National Health and Nutrition Examination Survey, "Physician examination procedures manual," August 2009, http://www.cdc.gov/nchs/data/nhanes/nhanes_09_10/physician.pdf.

[18] *The National Health and Nutrition Examination Surveys: Analytic and Reporting Guidelines*, 2012, http://www.cdc.gov/nchs/data/nhanes/nhanes_03_04/nhanes_analytic_guidelines_dec_2005.pdf.

[19] K. L. Ong, B. M. Y. Cheung, Y. B. Man, C. P. Lau, and K. S. L. Lam, "Prevalence, awareness, treatment, and control of hypertension among United States adults 1999–2004," *Hypertension*, vol. 49, no. 1, pp. 69–75, 2007.

[20] B. M. Egan, Y. Zhao, and R. N. Axon, "US trends in prevalence, awareness, treatment, and control of hypertension, 1988–2008," *The Journal of the American Medical Association*, vol. 303, no. 20, pp. 2043–2050, 2010.

[21] X. F. Liu, M. Liu, D. Tsilimingras, and E. L. Schiffrin, "Racial disparities in cardiovascular risk factors among diagnosed hypertensive subjects," *Journal of the American Society of Hypertension*, vol. 5, no. 4, pp. 239–248, 2011.

[22] K. M. Flegal, M. D. Carroll, C. L. Ogden, and L. R. Curtin, "Prevalence and trends in obesity among US adults, 1999–2008," *JAMA—Journal of the American Medical Association*, vol. 303, no. 3, pp. 235–241, 2010.

[23] K. M. Flegal, D. Carroll, B. K. Kit, and C. L. Ogden, "Prevalence of obesity and trends in the distribution of body mass index among US adults, 1999–2010," *The Journal of the American Medical Association*, vol. 307, no. 5, pp. 491–497, 2012.

[24] P. B. Mellen, S. K. Gao, M. Z. Vitolins, and D. C. Goff Jr., "Deteriorating dietary habits among adults with hypertension," *Archives of Internal Medicine*, vol. 168, no. 3, pp. 308–314, 2008.

[25] M. Devaux, F. Sassi, J. Church, M. Cecchini, and F. Borgonovi, "Exploring the relationship between education and obesity," *OECD Journal: Economic Studies*, vol. 2011, no. 1, pp. 121–159, 2011.

[26] R. C. Grebla, C. J. Rodriguez, L. N. Borrell, and T. G. Pickering, "Prevalence and determinants of isolated systolic hypertension among young adults: the 1999–2004 US National Health and Nutrition Examination Survey," *Journal of Hypertension*, vol. 28, no. 1, pp. 15–23, 2010.

[27] S. Lewington, R. Clarke, N. Qizilbash, R. Peto, and R. Collins, "Age-specific relevance of usual blood pressure to vascular mortality: a meta-analysis of individual data for one million adults in 61 prospective studies," *The Lancet*, vol. 360, no. 9349, pp. 1903–1913, 2002.

[28] V. L. Roger, A. S. Go, D. M. Lloyd-Jones et al., "Heart disease and stroke statistics—2011 update: a report from the American Heart Association," *Circulation*, vol. 123, pp. e18–e209, 2011.

4

Uric Acid Levels in Normotensive Children of Hypertensive Parents

Ali Yildirim, Fatma Keles, Pelin Kosger, Gokmen Ozdemir, Birsen Ucar, and Zubeyir Kilic

Department of Pediatric Cardiology, Medical Faculty, Eskisehir Osmangazi University, 26480 Eskisehir, Turkey

Correspondence should be addressed to Ali Yildirim; yldrmaly@gmail.com

Academic Editor: Toshio Ohtsubo

This study evaluated uric acid concentrations in normotensive children of parents with hypertension. Eighty normotensive children from families with and without a history of essential hypertension were included. Concentrations of lipid parameters and uric acid were compared. Demographic and anthropometric characteristics were similar in the groups. Systolic and diastolic blood pressure were higher in the normotensive children of parents with hypertension without statistically significant difference ($P > 0.05$). Uric acid concentrations were higher in the normotensive children of parents with hypertension (4.61 versus 3.57 mg/dL, $P < 0.01$). Total cholesterol and triglyceride concentrations were similar in the two groups. Systolic and diastolic blood pressure were significantly higher in control children aged >10 years ($P < 0.01$). Uric acid levels were significantly higher in all children with more pronounced difference after age 10 of years ($P < 0.001$). Positive correlations were found between the level of serum uric acid and age, body weight, body mass index, and systolic and diastolic blood pressure in the normotensive children of parents. The higher uric acid levels in the normotensive children of hypertensive parents suggest that uric acid may be a predeterminant of hypertension. Monitoring of uric acid levels in these children may allow for prevention or earlier treatment of future hypertension.

1. Introduction

Hyperuricemia has been associated with various diseases, including gout, hypertension, atherosclerosis, cardiovascular events, the metabolic syndrome, and renal failure [1]. Studies in experimental animals have shown that increased serum levels of uric acid are related to cardiovascular risk and hypertensive cardiovascular damage [2–8]. High levels of serum uric acid in rats increased blood pressure and blood pressure decreased to normal level with treatment of hyperuricemia [9]. Moreover, hyperuricemia may lead to renal tubulopathy by decreasing the synthesis of nitric oxide [10–12]. Similarly, clinical studies have shown relationships between high levels of serum uric acid concentrations and increased blood pressure [13, 14]. For example, the incidence of hypertension was high in adolescents with high level serum uric acid, while treatment with allopurinol reduced both serum uric acid levels and blood pressure.

Several studies have investigated the relationship between hyperuricemia and hypertension in children [14–17]. Increased levels of uric acid in children were associated with increases in systolic and diastolic blood pressure, with increased uric acid being an independent risk factor for hypertension [18].

Essential hypertension is frequently observed in adults throughout the world, and its incidence is also increasing in children and adolescents [19]. Family history of essential hypertension has been shown to be a significant risk factor for essential hypertension in children [20]. Children of hypertensive parents are significantly more likely to have higher blood pressure during their adolescent years than the children of normotensive parents [19, 21]. The probability of hypertension developing in a child has been reported to be 28% if one parent has hypertension and 41% if both parents have hypertension [19].

Although several studies have assessed the relationship between essential hypertension and hyperuricemia in children, none to date has evaluated hyperuricemia in the normotensive children of hypertensive parents. This study therefore compared serum uric acid concentrations in the normotensive children of normotensive and hypertensive parents and the relationship between hyperuricemia and blood pressure in these children.

2. Materials and Methods

Of the 80 children included in the study, 36 were normotensive children from families with a history of essential hypertension, while 44 were normotensive children from families with no history of hypertension. All of these children had visited the Pediatric Cardiology Department of the Eskisehir Osmangazi University Faculty of Medicine (Eskisehir, Turkey) for murmurs, palpitations, or chest pains. The detailed medical history, background, and family history of the children were investigated. Children with a history of a chronic illness, prematurity, anemia, or use of medication for anemia, congenital heart disease, chronic renal failure, diabetes, hyperlipidemia, or obesity were excluded. Parents of the participants were provided with information on the nature and content of the study, and all provided written informed consent. The study protocol was approved by the Ethics Committee of Eskisehir Osmangazi University Medical School.

The children were divided into two groups. The study group consisted of children with a hypertensive mother and/or father ($n = 36$), while the control group consisted of children with no familial history of hypertension ($n = 44$). Parents of children in the study group had been diagnosed with essential hypertension and regularly used antihypertensive medications, with none having a history of additional illnesses causing secondary hypertension. Children of parents with a history of cardiovascular diseases, chronic renal failure, diabetes, hyperlipidemia, obesity, using the drug, and smoking were excluded from the study.

Weight and height were measured while the child was in the upright position without wearing shoes, and body mass index (BMI) was calculated as weight (kg)/height (m^2). Blood pressure was measured three times with a mercury sphygmomanometer and appropriate armband while the subject was in a sitting position after 10 minutes of rest, with the mean of the three measurements recorded. After Korotkoff sounds were heard in the brachial artery, the armband was inflated 20 mmHg above the point at which brachial pressure was not apparent and the pressure was decreased by releasing air at 2-3 mmHg/sec. Korotkoff phase 1 was considered the systolic pressure, and Korotkoff phases 4 and 5 were considered the diastolic pressure for children aged <12 and >12 years, respectively.

Venous blood samples were taken from the antecubital vein of each subject after a 12-hour fast. After clotting, the samples were centrifuged at 4000 rpm for 5 minutes; the serum samples were removed and stored at −80°C until being analyzed. Serum concentrations of total cholesterol, total triglycerides, high-density lipoprotein-cholesterol (HDL-C), low-density lipoprotein-cholesterol (LDL-C), and uric acid were measured enzymatically with a Roche modular device.

2.1. Statistical Analysis. IBM SPSS Statistics 20 software was used for all statistical analyses. The normal distribution of variables was evaluated using the Shapiro-Wilk test. Normally distributed variables were reported as mean ± standard deviation (SD) and compared using Student's *t*. The Mann-Whitney *U* test was performed for variables with nonnormal distributions, and median and percentile values (25–75%) were obtained. The numerical variables of three age groups were compared by ANOVA (one-way analysis of variance) test and pairwise comparisons were performed by post hoc test. To evaluate the relationships between the variables, a Spearman correlation analysis was performed. Statistical significance was defined as $P < 0.05$.

TABLE 1: Demographic characteristics of normotensive children of hypertensive parents (Group 1) and normotensive parents (Group 2).

	Group 1 ($n = 36$)	Group 2 ($n = 44$)	P
Age, yrs$^{\#}$	12.4 ± 3.9	12.7 ± 4.1	0.973
Female$^{\$}$ n	21	27	0.891
Male n	15	17	0.765
Weight, kg^{+}	59.2 ± 12.4	57.3 ± 13.6	0.932
Height, cm^{+}	166.5 ± 19.0	164.8 ± 17.1	0.758
BMI, kg/m^{2+}	21.2 ± 3.2	21.0 ± 2.8	0.194
SBP, mmHg$^{\#}$	113.2 ± 9.0	108 ± 8.2	0.345
DBP, mmHg$^{\#}$	69.0 ± 8.2	65.1 ± 7.0	0.621
Triglycerides, mg/dL$^{\#}$	80.7 ± 31.4	77.4 ± 30.6	0.106
HDL-cholesterol, mg/dL$^{\#}$	51.8 ± 10.4	55.7 ± 13.7	0.325
LDL-cholesterol, mg/dL$^{\#}$	86.8 ± 22.8	86.2 ± 23.4	0.156
Total cholesterol, mg/dL^{+}	148.7 ± 25.4	152.3 ± 30.1	0.765
Uric acid, mg/dL^{+}	4.31 ± 1.12	3.37 ± 0.89	0.007

BMI: body mass index; DBP: diastolic blood pressure; HDL: high-density lipoprotein; LDL: low-density lipoprotein; SBP: systolic blood pressure. All results reported as mean ± SD; $^{\#}$Student's *t*; $^{\$}$Pearson chi-square test; $^{+}$Mann-Whitney *U* test.

3. Results

The study cohort consisted of 36 normotensive children, 15 males (37.5%) and 21 females (62.5%), aged 7 to 20 years (mean age, 12.4 years), each of whom had at least one hypertensive parent (Group 1), and 44 normotensive children, 17 males (33.3%) and 27 females (66.7%), aged 6 to 20 years (mean age, 12.7 years), none of whose parents had any health problems, including hypertension (Group 2). Their anthropometric measurements, blood pressure, and laboratory values are shown in Table 1. The mean weights of the children in Groups 1 and 2 were 59.2 kg and 57.3 kg, respectively; their mean heights were 166.5 cm and 164.8 cm, respectively; and their mean BMIs were 21.2 kg/m^2 and 21.0 kg/m^2. There were no statistically significant differences ($P > 0.05$) between the study and control groups in age, gender, weight, height, or BMI. Children in Group 1 had a mean systolic blood pressure (SBP) of 113 mmHg and a mean diastolic blood pressure (DBP) of 69 mmHg, whereas children in Group 2 had a mean SBP of 108 mmHg and a

TABLE 2: Blood pressure, lipid parameters, and uric acid levels by age in normotensive children of hypertensive parents (Group 1) and normotensive parents (Group 2).

	Group 1 Age < 10 yrs	Group 2 Age < 10 yrs	Group 1 Age 10–15 yrs	Group 2 Age 10–15 yrs	Group 1 Age > 15 yrs	Group 2 Age > 15 yrs
SBP, mmHg	102 ± 6.5	99 ± 5.6	111.6 ± 8.3	108 ± 5.9	115 ± 4.9	112 ± 6.0
DBP, mmHg	60.5 ± 7.2	62.4 ± 4.6	69.0 ± 7.3	65.8 ± 5.9	71.0 ± 6.0	72.1 ± 6.4
Triglyceride, mg/dL	69.9 ± 21.6	77.0 ± 28.0	87.3 ± 30.6	83.8 ± 31.6	81.7 ± 37.3	72.0 ± 32.6
HDL-cholesterol, mg/dL	50.9 ± 10.4	57.2 ± 15.1	52.3 ± 10.7	55.5 ± 15.1	52.4 ± 10.4	55.0 ± 12.0
LDL-cholesterol, mg/dL	84.8 ± 18.6	91.4 ± 15.4	92.5 ± 28.6	86.3 ± 24.3	81.8 ± 17.0	82.6 ± 21.1
Total cholesterol, mg/dL	144.3 ± 22.8	159.1 ± 18.5	155.4 ± 31.3	153.3 ± 31.4	144.2 ± 17.1	147.0 ± 34.7
Uric acid, mg/dL	**3.68 ± 0.75**$^{\neq}$	**3.20 ± 0.56**	**4.36 ± 0.99**$^{\neq}$	**3.03 ± 0.81**	**4.61 ± 1.34**$^{\neq\neq}$	**3.57 ± 1.07**

DBP: diastolic blood pressure; HDL: high-density lipoprotein; LDL: low-density lipoprotein; SBP: systolic blood pressure. All results reported as mean ± SD; $^{\neq}P < 0.05$, $^{\neq\neq}P < 0.01$.

TABLE 3: Comparison of variables according to age groups.

Variables	Group 1				Group 2			
	P	P_{1-2}	P_{1-3}	P_{2-3}	P	P_{1-2}	P_{1-3}	P_{2-3}
SBP, mmHg	**<0.001**	**<0.001**	**<0.001**	**0.008**	**<0.001**	**<0.001**	**<0.001**	**0.002**
DBP, mmHg	**<0.001**	**<0.001**	**<0.001**	0.363	**<0.001**	**0.013**	**<0.001**	**<0.001**
Triglyceride, mg/dL	**<0.001**	**<0.001**	**<0.001**	**<0.001**	**<0.001**	**0.001**	**0.001**	**<0.001**
HDL-cholesterol, mg/dL	**0.004**	**0.003**	0.072	0.491	**0.012**	**0.022**	0.055	0.999
LDL-cholesterol, mg/dL	**<0.001**	**<0.001**	0.066	**<0.001**	**<0.001**	**<0.001**	**<0.001**	**<0.001**
Total cholesterol, mg/dL	**<0.001**	**<0.001**	0.999	**<0.001**	**<0.001**	**<0.001**	**<0.001**	**<0.001**
Uric acid, mg/dL	**<0.001**	**0.015**	**<0.001**	**0.006**	**0.036**	0.514	0.280	**0.032**

P: ANOVA test; pairwise comparisons were performed by post hoc test. DBP: diastolic blood pressure; HDL: high-density lipoprotein; LDL: low-density lipoprotein; SBP: systolic blood pressure. Comparison of groups: P_{1-2}: age < 10 yrs and age 10–15 yrs; P_{1-3}: age < 10 yrs and age > 15 yrs; P_{2-3}: age 10–15 yrs and age > 15 yrs.

mean DBP of 65 mmHg. Although both SBP and DBP were higher in Group 1 than in Group 2, these differences were not statistically significant ($P > 0.05$). Serum uric acid levels, however, were significantly higher in Group 1 than in Group 2 children (4.31 mg/dL versus 3.37 mg/dL, $P < 0.01$). Concentrations of total cholesterol, HDL-C, LDL-C, and total triglycerides, however, were similar in the two groups ($P > 0.05$ each).

In order to detect the elevation period of uric acid level and to determine whether an age-related change in variables is present, patients were divided into 3 groups according to their age. Thus, there were 9 patients < 10 years of age, 12 patients between 10 and 15 years of age, and 15 patients over 15 years of age. Control group consisted of 13 subjects under 10 years of age, 15 subjects between 10 and 15 years of age, and 16 subjects over 15 years of age. There were no significant differences regarding SBP, DBP, total cholesterol, HDL-C, LDL-C, and triglycerides between the study and control groups based on age ($P < 0.05$) (Table 2). Uric acid concentrations were significantly higher in Group 1 than in Group 2 at all ages, but this difference was especially pronounced in subjects aged >10 years ($P < 0.001$). The differences between variables according to different age groups are shown in Table 3. For all variables, a statistical difference was present according to age groups.

Correlations between uric acid and other variables are shown in Table 4. Uric acid levels showed positive correlations with age, body weight, BMI, SBP, DBP, and triglyceride concentrations in children from Group 1. Uric acid concentrations, however, did not significantly correlate with total cholesterol, HDL-C, and LDL-C concentrations in these subjects ($P > 0.05$). While there was a correlation between uric acid, DBP, and triglycerides in Group 2, no correlations with other variables were observed ($P > 0.05$).

4. Discussion

This study found no significant difference in SBP and DBP between the normotensive children of normotensive and hypertensive parents. Previous studies have shown a clear correlation between high blood pressure and a family history of hypertension [22–27], especially after adolescence [22]. Studies of prepubertal and pubertal children of normotensive and hypertensive parents showed no significant differences in blood pressure [28, 29]. For example, one study reported blood pressure was similar in the 18–22-year-old children of hypertensive and normotensive parents but aortic stiffness parameters were higher in the former group [29]. In our previous study we found that an increase in the carotid intima-media thickness in children of hypertensive parents

TABLE 4: Correlation between uric acid levels and other variables.

	Uric acid, mg/dL	Age, yrs	Height, cm	Weight, kg	BMI, kg/m^2	SBP, mmHg	DBP, mmHg	TG, mg/dL	HDL-chol., mg/dL	LDL-chol., mg/dL	Total chol., mg/dL
Group 1	r	**0.701****	**0.569****	**0.436***	**0.518***	**0.663****	**0.552****	**0.478***	0.241	−0.379	−0.062
(n = 24)	P	**<0.001**	**0.004**	**0.033**	**0.004**	**<0.001**	**0.005**	**0.007**	0.256	0.068	0.773
Group 2	r	0.094	0.060	0.048	0.204	0.100	**0.445***	**−0.408***	0.088	−0.249	−0.120
(n = 27)	P	0.640	0.767	0.810	0.307	0.621	**0.020**	**0.034**	0.662	0.210	0.551

All correlations were calculated by Spearman correlation test; DBP: diastolic blood pressure; HDL: high-density lipoprotein; LDL: low-density lipoprotein; SBP: systolic blood pressure.
$^{*}P < 0.05$, $^{**}P < 0.01$.

may indicate subclinical atherosclerosis [30]. Children of hypertensive parents may first experience hormonal and biochemical changes, followed by the development of damage to the endothelial and vascular structures and subsequent cardiac compensation, with hypertension only appearing at latter stages. Moreover, in this study the hypertensive and prehypertensive children of hypertensive parents were not included and the age range of the participants was narrow, perhaps explaining, at least in part, the similar SBP and DBP in the study and control groups.

Despite the uric acid levels of normotensive children of hypertensive parents being within normal boundaries, they were significantly higher than in normotensive children of normotensive parents. In order to detect the elevation period of uric acid level and to determine whether an age-related change in variables is present, patients were divided into 3 groups according to their age. Patients in all age groups had increased uric acid levels as compared to controls, with a more marked elevation in uric acid among those over 15 years of age. Many previous studies have reported a relationship between hyperuricemia and hypertension. For example, a study of 200 children found that 73% of those with medium and severe levels of hypertension had uric acid levels >7 mg/dL, compared with 49% of those with low levels of hypertension [15]. Hyperuricemia was observed in very young children, as well as being an early indicator of hypertension. A 13-year study of children born in Budapest, Hungary, found that the development of hypertension was associated with increased heart rate, early sexual maturity, and hyperuricemia [16]. Another study found that the development of hypertension over 10 years was associated with high levels of serum uric acid, independent of the glomerular filtration rate, alcohol consumption, smoking, and diabetes [29]. Uric acid and renin levels were found to be higher in adolescents aged 13–18 years with essential hypertension than in an age- and gender-matched normotensive control group [17]. Moreover, renin levels were normal in hypertensive individuals with normal levels of serum uric acid but higher in hypertensive individuals with high level of serum uric acid. Hyperuricemia was found to increase the synthesis of nitric oxide, increasing the release of inflammatory mediators and renin angiotensin levels and resulting in endothelial dysfunction, atherosclerosis, and hypertension [31–33]. In its early stages, hyperuricemia leads to vasoconstriction, whereas, in more advanced stages, hyperuricemia causes hypertrophy of vascular smooth muscles, increasing blood pressure. Initially, increased blood pressure responds well to treatment, but the response is reduced at more advanced stages [34]. Pharmacologic induction of hyperuricemia in mice resulted in hypertension after three weeks, whereas treatment with uricosuric agents reduced hypertension in these animals, indicating that hyperuricemia is an independent risk factor for hypertension [12]. A placebo-controlled trial in 60 pre-hypertensive and obese children found that treatment with allopurinol or probenecid reduced SBP by 10 mmHg and DBP by 9 mmHg, indicating that treatment of hyperuricemia can reduce hypertension [35]. Despite many studies of the relationship between hypertension and uric acid, none had previously investigated uric acid levels in the normotensive children of hypertensive parents. Our finding that serum uric acid levels were higher in the normotensive children of hypertensive parents than normotensive parents suggests that uric acid increases first, prior to the development of hypertension, with hypertension developing later. The higher uric acid levels in the normotensive children of hypertensive parents suggest that uric acid may be a predeterminant of hypertension. Monitoring of uric acid levels in these children may allow for prevention or earlier treatment of future hypertension. The increase in uric acid was observed at very young ages, 5–10 years, and may be followed by the development of endothelial damage and vascular stiffness and eventually the appearance of hypertension.

We observed that uric acid levels were positively correlated with SBP, DBP, BMI, age, and triglyceride concentrations. Serum uric acid levels were found to be higher in patients with essential hypertention than with secondary hypertension [14]. Serum uric acid levels were linearly correlated with SBP and DBP, with a 1 mg/mL increase in uric acid resulting in a 14 mmHg increase in SBP and a 7 mmHg increase in DBP [14]. In addition, a meta-analysis found that a 1 mg/dL increase in serum uric acid levels increased the incidence of hypertension by 13% [36]. That analysis reported a linear relationship between blood pressure and uric acid, rather than a cutoff point.

In conclusion, this study found that the levels of serum uric acid were higher at all ages in the normotensive children of hypertensive than normotensive parents. The increased levels of serum uric acid in the former may be a predeterminant of hypertension. Long term studies in large numbers of children of hypertensive parents are needed to assess the relationship between blood pressure and serum uric acid levels and the impact of diet on both levels in such children. Monitoring of uric acid may reveal early stages of hypertension in these children, allowing the implementation of measures to prevent hypertension.

References

[1] L. Billiet, S. Doaty, J. D. Katz, and M. T. Velasquez, "Review of hyperuricemia as new marker for metabolic syndrome," *ISRN Rheumatology*, vol. 2014, Article ID 852954, 7 pages, 2014.

[2] J. Sundström, L. Sullivan, R. B. D'Agostino, D. Levy, W. B. Kannel, and R. S. Vasan, "Relations of serum uric acid to longitudinal blood pressure tracking and hypertension incidence," *Hypertension*, vol. 45, no. 1, pp. 28–33, 2005.

[3] K. Yano, D. M. Reed, and D. L. McGee, "Ten-year incidence of coronary heart disease in the Honolulu Heart Program. Relationship to biologic and lifestyle characteristics," *The American Journal of Epidemiology*, vol. 119, no. 5, pp. 653–666, 1984.

[4] W. Levine, A. R. Dyer, R. B. Shekelle, J. A. Schoenberger, and J. Stamler, "Serum uric acid and 11.5-year mortality of middle-aged women: findings of the Chicago heart association detection project in industry," *Journal of Clinical Epidemiology*, vol. 42, no. 3, pp. 257–267, 1989.

[5] J. Fang and M. H. Alderman, "Serum uric acid and cardiovascular mortality: the NHANES I Epidemiologic Follow-up Study, 1971–1992," *Journal of the American Medical Association*, vol. 283, no. 18, pp. 2404–2410, 2000.

[6] M. H. Alderman, H. Cohen, S. Madhavan, and S. Kivlighn, "Serum uric acid and cardiovascular events in successfully treated hypertensive patients," *Hypertension*, vol. 34, no. 1, pp. 144–150, 1999.

[7] L. V. Franse, M. Pahor, M. D. Bari et al., "Serum uric acid, diuretic treatment and risk of cardiovascular events in the Systolic Hypertension in the Elderly Program (SHEP)," *Journal of Hypertension*, vol. 18, no. 8, pp. 1149–1154, 2000.

[8] P. Verdecchia, G. Schillaci, G. Reboldi, F. Santeusanio, C. Porcellati, and P. Brunetti, "Relation between serum uric acid and risk of cardiovascular disease in essential hypertension: the PIUMA Study," *Hypertension*, vol. 36, no. 6, pp. 1072–1078, 2000.

[9] M. Mazzali, J. Hughes, Y.-G. Kim et al., "Elevated uric acid increases blood pressure in the rat by a novel crystal-independent mechanism," *Hypertension*, vol. 38, no. 5, pp. 1101–1106, 2001.

[10] G. N. Rao, M. A. Corson, and B. C. Berk, "Uric acid stimulates vascular smooth muscle cell proliferation by increasing platelet-derived growth factor A-chain expression," *The Journal of Biological Chemistry*, vol. 266, no. 13, pp. 8604–8608, 1991.

[11] M. G. Netea, B. J. Kullberg, W. L. Blok, R. T. Netea, and J. W. M. Van der Meer, "The role of hyperuricemia in the increased cytokine production after lipopolysaccharide (LPS) challenge in neutropenic mice," *Blood*, vol. 89, no. 2, pp. 577–582, 1997.

[12] M. Mazzali, J. Kanellis, L. Han et al., "Hyperuricemia induces a primary renal arteriolopathy in rats by a blood pressure-independent mechanism," *The American Journal of Physiology—Renal Physiology*, vol. 282, no. 6, pp. F991–F997, 2002.

[13] F. N. Brand, D. L. McGee, W. B. Kannel, J. Stokes III, and W. P. Castelli, "Hyperuricemia as a risk factor of coronary heart disease: the Framingham study," *The American Journal of Epidemiology*, vol. 121, no. 1, pp. 11–18, 1985.

[14] D. I. Feig and R. J. Johnson, "Hyperuricemia in childhood primary hypertension," *Hypertension*, vol. 42, no. 3, pp. 247–252, 2003.

[15] I. Rovda, L. M. Kazakova, and E. A. Plaksina, "Parameters of uric acid metabolism in healthy children and in patients with arterial hypertension," *Pediatriya*, no. 8, pp. 19–22, 1990.

[16] E. Torok, I. Gyarfas, and M. Csukas, "Factors associated with stable high blood pressure in adolescents," *Journal of Hypertension*, vol. 3, no. 3, pp. S389–S390, 1985.

[17] A. B. Gruskin, "The adolescent with essential hypertension," *The American Journal of Kidney Diseases*, vol. 6, no. 2, pp. 86–90, 1985.

[18] D. I. Feig and R. J. Johnson, "The role of uric acid in pediatric hypertension," *Journal of Renal Nutrition*, vol. 17, no. 1, pp. 79–83, 2007.

[19] J. A. Staessen, J. Wang, G. Bianchi, and W. H. Birkenhäger, "Essential hypertension," *The Lancet*, vol. 361, no. 9369, pp. 1629–1641, 2003.

[20] B. Waeber, H. R. Brunner, and M. Burnier, "Hypertension," in *Cardiovascular Medicine*, J. T. Willerson and J. N. Cohn, Eds., pp. 1496–1511, Churchill Livingstone, Philadelphia, Pa, USA, 2nd edition, 2000.

[21] R. F. Robinson, D. L. Batisky, J. R. Hayes, M. C. Nahata, and J. D. Mahan, "Body mass index in primary and secondary pediatric hypertension," *Pediatric Nephrology*, vol. 19, no. 12, pp. 1379–1384, 2004.

[22] A. P. M. van den Elzen, M. A. J. de Ridder, D. E. Grobbee, A. Hofman, J. C. M. Witteman, and C. S. P. M. Uiterwaal, "Families and the natural history of blood pressure: a 27-year follow-up study," *American Journal of Hypertension*, vol. 17, no. 10, pp. 936–940, 2004.

[23] R. H. Myers, D. K. Kiely, L. A. Cupples, and W. B. Kannel, "Parental history is an independent risk factor for coronary artery disease: the Framingham study," *American Heart Journal*, vol. 120, no. 4, pp. 963–969, 1990.

[24] A. M. Grandi, G. Gaudio, A. Fachinetti et al., "Hyperinsulinemia, family history of hypertension, and essential hypertension," *American Journal of Hypertension*, vol. 9, no. 8, pp. 732–738, 1996.

[25] A. W. von Eiff, E. Gogolin, U. Jacobs, and H. Neus, "Ambulatory blood pressure in children followed for 3 years: influence of sex and family history of hypertension," *Clinical and Experimental Hypertension*, vol. 8, no. 4-5, pp. 577–581, 1986.

[26] R. G. Munger, R. J. Prineas, and O. Gomez-Marin, "Persistent elevation of blood pressure among children with a family history of hypertension: the Minneapolis Children's Blood Pressure Study," *Journal of Hypertension*, vol. 6, no. 8, pp. 647–653, 1988.

[27] J. Dernellis and M. Panaretou, "Aortic stiffness in children of parents with hypertension," *Journal of Human Hypertension*, vol. 20, no. 3, pp. 225–226, 2006.

[28] H. Evrengul, H. Tanriverdi, I. D. Kilic et al., "Aortic stiffness and flow-mediated dilatation in normotensive offspring of parents with hypertension," *Cardiology in the Young*, vol. 22, no. 4, pp. 451–456, 2012.

[29] A. Shankar, R. Klein, B. E. K. Klein, and F. J. Nieto, "The association between serum uric acid level and long-term incidence of hypertension: population-based cohort study," *Journal of Human Hypertension*, vol. 20, no. 12, pp. 937–945, 2006.

[30] A. Yildirim, P. Kosger, G. Ozdemir, F. M. Sahin, B. Ucar, and Z. Kilic, "Carotid intima-media thickness and elastic properties of aortas in normotensive children of hypertensive parents," *Hypertension Research*, 2015.

[31] M.-A. Yu, L. G. Sánchez-Lozada, R. J. Johnson, and D.-H. Kang, "Oxidative stress with an activation of the renin-angiotensin system in human vascular endothelial cells as a novel mechanism of uric acid-induced endothelial dysfunction," *Journal of Hypertension*, vol. 28, no. 6, pp. 1234–1242, 2010.

[32] G. Cerasola, S. Cottone, and G. Mulè, "The progressive pathway of microalbuminuria: from early marker of renal damage to strong cardiovascular risk predictor," *Journal of Hypertension*, vol. 28, no. 12, pp. 2357–2369, 2010.

[33] M. A. Gómez-Marcos, J. I. Recio-Rodríguez, M. C. Patino-Alonso et al., "Relationship between uric acid and vascular structure and function in hypertensive patients and sex-related differences," *The American Journal of Hypertension*, vol. 26, no. 5, pp. 599–607, 2013.

[34] M. Yanik and D. I. Feig, "Serum urate: a biomarker or treatment target in pediatric hypertension?" *Current Opinion in Cardiology*, vol. 28, no. 4, pp. 433–438, 2013.

[35] B. Soletsky and D. I. Feig, "Uric acid reduction rectifies prehypertension in obese adolescents," *Hypertension*, vol. 60, no. 5, pp. 1148–1156, 2012.

[36] P. C. Grayson, S. Y. Kim, M. LaValley, and H. K. Choi, "Hyperuricemia and incident hypertension: a systematic review and meta-analysis," *Arthritis Care and Research*, vol. 63, no. 1, pp. 102–110, 2011.

5

A Systematic Review of Peripheral and Central Nervous System Involvement of Rheumatoid Arthritis, Systemic Lupus Erythematosus, Primary Sjögren's Syndrome, and Associated Immunological Profiles

Anastasia Bougea, Evangelos Anagnostou, Giatas Konstantinos, Paraskevas George, Nikolaos Triantafyllou, and Evangelia Kararizou

1st Department of Neurology, University of Athens Medical School, Eginition Hospital, Athens, Greece

Correspondence should be addressed to Anastasia Bougea; annita139@yahoo.gr

Academic Editor: Gabriel J. Tobón

Both central (CNS) and peripheral nervous system (PNS) complications are frequent and varied in connective tissue diseases. A systematic review was conducted between 1989 and 2014 in the databases Medline, Scopus, and Cochrane Library using the search terms, peripheral and central nervous complications and immunological profiles, to identify studies in specific connective tissue disorders such as rheumatoid arthritis, systemic lupus erythematosus, and primary Sjögren's syndrome. A total of 675 references were identified, of which 118 were selected for detailed analysis and 22 were included in the final review with a total of 2338 participants. Our search focused only on studies upon connective tissue disorders such as rheumatoid arthritis, systemic lupus erythematosus, and primary Sjögren's syndrome associated with seroimmunological data. The reported prevalence of CNS involvement ranges from 9 to 92% across the reported studies. However, the association between CNS and PNS manifestations and seroimmunological profiles remains controversial. To date, no laboratory test has been shown as pathognomonic neither for CNS nor for PNS involvement.

1. Introduction

Connective tissue disorders are chronic inflammatory autoimmune diseases driven by an antibody or T-cell response directed against a self-antigen antibody affecting muscle, joints, and skin such as rheumatoid arthritis (RA), systemic lupus erythematosus (SLE), primary Sjögren's syndrome (pSS), and systemic sclerosis [1–3]. Both immune mediated changes in the vasculature of the vessels walls, as a hallmark of vasculitis, may be associated with central nervous system (CNS) and peripheral nervous system (PNS) symptoms. The vascular injury may be related to the presence of antibodies most commonly, but not limited to, SS or a related profile of autoantibodies including antinuclear antibody (ANA), extractable nuclear antigen antibodies (SSA/SSB), rheumatoid factor (RF), anticardiolipin antibodies (ACA), cryoglobulins, and anti-double-stranded DNA antibody (A-ds DNA) [4] (Table 1). Anti-ribosomal P antibodies have been associated with CNS SLE disease [5].

To our knowledge this is the first systematic review focused in both most common CNS and PNS complications of RA, SLE, and pSS emphasizing the associated immunological features of these specific connective tissue.

2. Methods

2.1. Eligibility Criteria and Source Selection. This is a systematic review of literature, based on the PRISMA guidelines. We search for relevant studies in English in the following databases, from the emergence of the condition to October 2014: Medline (from 1989 to 2014), Scopus (from 1983 to 2012), and Cochrane Library (from 1993 to

Table 1: Most frequent autoantibodies in nervous system involvement in connective tissue diseases SLE, SS, and RA.

Connective tissue diseases	Autoantibodies (% of positive patients, clinical association)
SLE	ANA Anti-dsDNA (nephritis, disease activity) Anti-ribosomal P (disease activity, NPSLE) Anti-Sm (highly specific for SLE) Anti-Ro (DD Sjögren's syndrome) Anti-La (DD Sjögren's syndrome) Antiphospholipid (thrombosis) AQP-4 (overlap NMO spectrum)
SS	ANA Anti-Ro (DD SLE) Anti-La (DD SLE) RF (lymphoma) Cryoglobulins (vasculitis, lymphoma) AQP-4 (overlap NMO spectrum)
RA	ANA

SLE: systemic lupus erythematosus, NP: neuropsychiatric, SS: Sjögren's syndrome, RA: rheumatoid arthritis, ANA: antinuclear antibodies, Anti-Sm: anti-Smith, Anti-Ro: Ro antigen, Anti-La: lupus anticoagulant, anti-dsDNA: anti-double-stranded DNA, RF: rheumatoid factor, DD: differential diagnosis, AQP-4: Aquaporin, and NMO: Neuromyelitis optica.

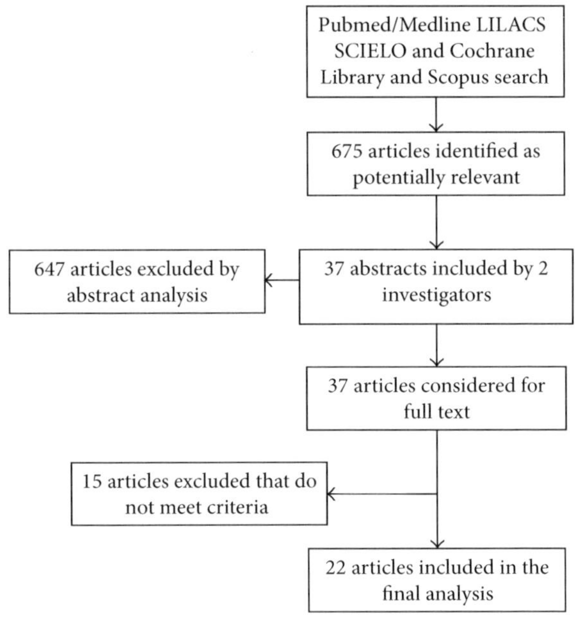

Figure 1: Research process flowchart.

2014). The keywords used for the study were the following: "peripheral nervous and central nervous manifestations," "myositis," "cranial neuropathy," "mononeuropathy," "polyneuropathy," "myelopathy," "myelitis," "multiple sclerosis," "Neuromyelitis optica spectrum (NMO)," "headaches," "seizures," "psychosis," "depression," "connective tissue disorders," "rheumatoid arthritis, systemic lupus erythematosus, primary Sjögren's syndrome," "Immunological profiles," "ANA," "anti-ribosomal P antibodies," "Antiphospholipid antibodies," "SSA/SSB," "RF," "ACA," "cryoglobulins," "A-ds DNA," and "AQ4 antibody".

2.2. Inclusion and Exclusion Criteria. Articles not published in English, letters, summaries, dissertations, theses, and case reports were excluded, as well as studies that used children or animal models and studies that were not related to central and peripheral nervous complications of RA, SLE, and pSS. Studies were included only if diagnosis of neurological complications was made by expert neurologists. Only studies with neurological complications primary or secondary to RA, SLE, and PSS with associated immunological features were included. Immunological tests (i.e., gamma globulins, ANA, anti-ribosomal P antibodies, anti-Ro/SSA and anti-La/SSB antibodies, RF, AQ4 antibody, and cryoglobulins) were included if they were performed at the time of diagnosis and at least yearly during follow-up.

3. Results

The described search identified six hundred seventy-five relevant studies (Figure 1), 107 of which were excluded based on abstract analysis. The remaining 37 studies were reviewed on its full text and 22 were included in this systematic review that addressed the inclusion criteria (a total of 2338 patients). The majority of them were cohort studies (18); 1 was case-control and 1 was randomized controlled trial. Of these, 12 studies focused on SLE and 9 on SS. Only one study was found regarding patients with RA. Classification of each connective tissue disorders was assessed according to established criteria for SLE [6], SS [7], and RA [8].

We performed qualitative data synthesis, organizing the results by connective tissue type. We did not attempt to perform meta-analysis because of the heterogeneity of the study designs, populations, and results. Using our critical appraisal of individual studies and the body of evidence for each study design, we identified strengths and weaknesses of each study in the discussion. We did not assess publication bias. Table 2 summarizes the main methodologic characteristics and results of the included studies.

In 1989, Mellgren et al. [29] reviewed 33 cases of primary SS and peripheral neuropathy evaluated at the Mayo Clinic from 1976 to 1988 and studied sural nerve biopsy specimens in 11 of them. Based on analytical clinical and electrophysiological (electromyography and sensory and motor conduction study) nerve features, 23 patients had PNS features such as distal sensorimotor neuropathy, 10 had a sensory neuropathy, five had trigeminal neuropathy, and two had carpal tunnel syndrome. The authors did not report any correlation between neuropathy and laboratory findings such as anti-SS-A/Ro antibodies, cryoglobulins, and RF in patients with SS.

In Andonopoulos et al.'s study [30], 10 of the 14 patients with evidence of PNS disease had a mild peripheral neuropathy of the glove and stocking distribution; six of them were mixed and four were sensory only. Two of those, plus one more, had trigeminal neuropathy. Two patients had abnormal terminal latencies of the peroneal nerves, indicative of motor neuropathy. Six of our primary SS subjects

Table 2: Characteristics of the selected clinical trials focusing on PNS and CNS complications of SLE, pSS, and RA.

Authors/year	Type of study	Sample characteristics (sex, years in median or mean ± SD)	Type of CNS involvement % (n) of patients	Type of PNS involvement	Clinical associations with immunological profiles
			SLE patients*		
Schneebaum et al., 1991 [9]	Cohort	269 patients with SLE	Depression 88% ($n = 8$), 45% psychosis ($n = 29$)	NM	The serum level of anti-P antibodies correlates with the activity of psychiatric disease
Isshi and Hirohata, 1998 [10]	Cohort	87 SLE patients	Psychosis 39% ($n = 34$), nonpsychotic CNS lupus 29,9% ($n = 26$)	NM	Serum anti-P levels were significantly elevated in patients with lupus psychosis compared with those with non-CNS SLE or those with nonpsychotic CNS lupus
Tzioufas et al., 2000 [11]	Cohort	28 patients with NPSLE	Psychiatric disorders 25% ($n = 7$), grand mal seizures 14,2% ($n = 4$), focal signs 46,4% ($n = 13$)	NM	Overall prevalence of anti-P antibodies in active CNS disease patients was statistically and significantly higher, as compared to unselected SLE patients
Kasitanon et al., 2002 [12]	Cohort	91 patients with NPSLE (90 F, 1 M, 30,7 ± 10,9)	Seizures 58,3% ($n = 53$), psychosis 14,3% ($n = 13$), acute confusion state 12% ($n = 11$), cerebral infraction 2,2% ($n = 2$), abnormal consciousness 6,6% ($n = 6$), transverse myelitis 6,6% ($n = 6$), aseptic meningitis 2,2% ($n = 2$)	MM 3,3% ($n = 3$), polyneuropathy 2,2% ($n = 2$)	Patients with NPSLE had significantly more cutaneous vasculitis and less arthritis than those without NPSLE
Sanna et al., 2003 [13]	Cohort	185 patients with NPSLE	Headache 24% ($n = 78$), CD 14.5% ($n = 47$), mood disorders 16.7% ($n = 54$), cognitive disorders 10.8% ($n = 35$), seizures 8.3% ($n = 27$), psychosis 7.7% ($n = 25$), anxiety 3.7% ($n = 24$), acute confusional state 3.7% ($n = 12$)	NM	The presence of aPL was associated with NP manifestations
Chiewthanakul et al., 2012 [14]	Cohort	97 patients with NPSLE (84 F, 13 M, 35.1 ± 11.7)	Seizures 33% ($n = 32$), CD 23,7% ($n = 23$), psychoses 24% ($n = 23$), myelopathy 6,2% ($n = 6$), headaches 2% ($n = 2$), mood disorders 1% ($n = 1$)	13 patients with polyneuropathy 77% ($n = 10$), GB 7,7% ($n = 1$), mononeuropathy 7,7% ($n = 1$), cranial neuropathy 7,7% ($n = 1$)	ANA and antibodies to dsDNA did not correlate with NP manifestations
Závada et al., 2013 [15]	Cohort	50 patients with NPSLE (5 M, 45 F 43 years (±16))	Cognitive disorder 50% ($n = 25$), mood disorder 28% ($n = 14$), CD 26% ($n = 13$), headache 26% ($n = 13$), seizure 22% ($n = 11$), psychosis 16% ($n = 8$), aseptic meningitis 4% ($n = 2$)	Polyneuropathy 8% ($n = 4$), cranial neuropathy 6% ($n = 3$), mononeuropathy 4% ($n = 2$), transverse myelitis 2% ($n = 1$)	NMO-IgG/AQP4-Ab in NPSLE were present only in a patient with TM and were not detectable in NPSLE patients with other neurological manifestations

Table 2: Continued.

Authors/year	Type of study	Sample characteristics (sex, years in median or mean ± SD)	Type of CNS involvement % (n) of patients	Type of PNS involvement	Clinical associations with immunological profiles
Hanly et al., 2004 [16]	Cohort	111 patients with SLE (96 F, 15 M, 44.7 ± 1.2 years)	Headaches 9% ($n = 10$), CD 3,6% ($n = 4$), mood disorders 3,6% ($n = 4$), cognitive dysfunction 2,7% ($n = 3$), acute confusional state 2,7% ($n = 3$), psychoses 2,7% ($n = 3$), seizures 0,9% ($n = 1$), anxiety 0,9% ($n = 1$), aseptic meningitis 0,9% ($n = 1$)	Cranial neuropathy 1,8% ($n = 2$), polyneuropathy 1,8% ($n = 2$)	No correlations were found
Kluz et al., 2007 [17]	Cohort	15 F mean age: 38.33 ± 11.02 years with SLE	Organic brain syndrome 13,3% ($n = 2$), cranial nerve disorder 6,6% ($n = 1$), headache 6,6% ($n = 1$), seizures 6,6% ($n = 1$)	NM	CNS complications were associated with aPL antibodies in patients with severe disease activity and microangiopathic complications compared with those with less active disease
Briani et al. 2009 [18]	Cohort	85 SLE patients (NM sex and mean age)	Headache 41,2% ($n = 35$), CD 12,3% ($n = 11$), epilepsy 11,8% ($n = 10$), psychiatric disorders 3% ($n = 6$), myelopathy 2,4% ($n = 2$)	Symmetric polyneuropathy 20% ($n = 17$), mononeuropathy 15,3% ($n = 13$), median nerve 3,6% ($n = 3$) sciatic nerve 3,6% ($n = 3$) involvement, MM 2,4% ($n = 2$)	Abs to ribosomal P proteins are associated with psychosis and MM
Florica et al., 2011 [19]	Case-control (retrospective)	207 SLE patients, F 86.3% (125 SLE-related PN 35.2 ± 14.4 years and 82 non-SLE-related PN 38.6 ± 15.4)	NM	PM 11,1% ($n = 23$), cranial neuropathy 12,5% ($n = 26$), MM 9,2% ($n = 19$), CIDP 0,9% ($n = 2$)	There was no significant difference in lupus serology such as antinuclear antibody, anti-double-stranded DNA antibody, and antibodies to the extractable nuclear antigens between the two groups
Hirohata et al., 2014 [20]	Cohort	72 patients with NPSLE (49 with diffuse NPSLE 38.3 ± 14.4, 23 with neurological syndromes or peripheral neuropathy 42.0 ± 15.2) 32 M, 50 F	Diffuse NPSLE: acute confusional state 38,7% ($n = 19$), anxiety 6,1% ($n = 3$), cognitive disorder 6,1% ($n = 3$), psychosis 14,2% ($n = 7$); focal NPSLE: headache 8,7% ($n = 2$), movement disorder 8,7% ($n = 2$), seizure 8,7% ($n = 7$), aseptic meningitis 4,3% ($n = 1$), demyelinating syndrome 4,3% ($n = 1$)	Polyneuropathy 4,3% ($n = 1$)	Anti-Sm and anti-RNP in CSF and sera were elevated in NPSLE compared with non-SLE control
			SS patients		
Spezialetti et al., 1993 [21]	Cohort	77 patients with pSS	Severe depression 13% ($n = 10$), psychosis 8% ($n = 6$), cognitive dysfunction 69% ($n = 54$)	NM	No correlation between CNS diseases, including the presence of anti-ribosomal P antibodies

Table 2: Continued.

Authors/year	Type of study	Sample characteristics (sex, years in median or mean ± SD)	Type of CNS involvement % (n) of patients	Type of PNS involvement	Clinical associations with immunological profiles
Alexander et al., 1994 [22]	Cohort	Group 1: 52 SS patients Group 2: 49 patients	Group 1: focal CNS disease 60% ($n = 26/43$), nonfocal CNS disease 22% ($n = 2/9$) Group 2: focal CNS disease 63% ($n = 19/30$), nonfocal CNS disease 37% ($n = 7/19$)	Not available	Anti-Ro antibodies were positive in 48% of patients with CNS compared to only 24% of all patients with pSS
Delalande et al., 2004 [23]	Cohort	82 patients (65 F, 17 M 48,6 years)	Seizures 8,5% ($n = 7$), cognitive dysfunction 11% ($n = 9$), encephalopathy 2,4% ($n = 2$), optic neuropathy 15% ($n = 13$), MS 28% ($n = 23$)	SMN 34,1% ($n = 28$), cranial neuropathy 19,5% ($n = 16$), MN 8,5% ($n = 7$), myositis 2,4% ($n = 2$), polyradiculoneuropathy 1,2% ($n = 1$)	Anti-Ro/SSA or anti-La/SSB antibodies were more frequently observed in patients with PNS involvement than in those with CNS involvement
Pittock et al., 2008 [24]	Cohort	14 patients with SS/SLE with neurological manifestations	NM	NM	SSA, SSA, ANA, and dsDNA antibodies were found in these patients but not NMO-IgG
Sène et al., 2011 [25]	Cohort	120 patients with pSS (106 F, 14 M 50.4 ± 14.0)	NM	SMN 23% ($n = 7$), ASN 10% ($n = 3$), NSN 67% ($n = 20$)	Patients with NSN with lower prevalence of ANA (60% versus 90%; $P = 0.003$), anti-SSA (Ro) (40% versus 72%; $P = 0.009$), anti-SSB (La) (15% versus 41%; $P = 0.039$), RF (37% versus 67%; $P = 0.02$), and hypergammaglobulinemia (35% versus 64%; $P = 0.023$)
Jamilloux et al., 2014 [26]	Cohort	420 patients with pSS (377 F, 43 M, 53.6 ± 14.8)	Acute ischemic stroke-like symptoms 1,4% ($n = 6$), dysarthria 0,2% ($n = 1$), seizures 0,2% ($n = 1$), cerebellar ataxia 0,4% ($n = 2$) central neuronitis 0,4% ($n = 2$), acute encephalopathy 2,1% ($n = 9$), cognitive impairment 0,4% ($n = 2$), aseptic meningitis 0,2% ($n = 1$), transverse myelitis ($n = 12$), optic neuritis 1,2% ($n = 5$), MS-like syndrome 1,2% ($n = 5$), cerebral venous thrombosis 0,2% ($n = 1$)	SMN 0,6% ($n = 25$), MM 0,7% ($n = 3$), SN 4,5% ($N = 19$), SGN 2,1% ($n = 9$), DPN 0,2% ($n = 1$), cranial neuropathy 1,9% ($n = 8$)	Patient with SN had more frequent cryoglobulinemia and lymphopenia ($P < 0.05$) but lower prevalence of anti-Ro/SSA antibodies and hypergammaglobulinemia ($P < 0.05$)
Morreale et al. 2014 [27]	Cohort	120 patients (12 M, 108 F; 58.3 ± 14.2 years)	Headache 46.9% ($n = 30$), cognitive disorder 44.4% ($n = 28$), mood disorders 38.3% ($n = 6$)	NM	Headache, cognitive disorders, and psychiatric symptoms were significantly associated with anti-SSA

TABLE 2: Continued.

Authors/year	Type of study	Sample characteristics (sex, years in median or mean ± SD)	Type of CNS involvement % (n) of patients	Type of PNS involvement	Clinical associations with immunological profiles
			RA		
Sivri and Güler-Uysal, 1999 [28]	Cohort	33 RA patients (28 F, 5 M; 46.7 ± 13.7 years)	NM	6% (n = 2) carpal tunnel syndrome, 18% (n = 6) MM	No correlation between neuropathy and RF

n: number of patients, F: female, M: male, SD: standard deviation, pSS: primary Sjögren syndrome, RA: rheumatoid arthritis, RF: rheumatoid factor, NMO: Neuromyelitis optica, PN: peripheral neuropathy, SMN: sensorimotor neuropathy, ASN: ataxic sensory neuropathy, NSN: nonataxic sensory neuropathy, SFN: small fiber neuropathy, PN: peripheral mononeuropathy, MM: mononeuritis multiplex, SN: sensory neuropathy, SGN: sensory ganglionopathy, DPN: demyelinating polyradiculoneuropathy, ANS: autonomous nervous symptoms, PNS: peripheral nervous system, CNS: central nervous system, CD: cerebrovascular disease, MS: multiple sclerosis, NP: neuropsychiatric disease, SLE: systemic lupus erythematosus, aPL: antiphospholipid antibodies, CIDP: chronic inflammatory demyelinating polyradiculoneuropathy, AIDP: acute inflammatory demyelinating polyradiculoneuropathy, focal CNS disease: one or more fixed focal clinical deficits of brain or spinal cord with or without psychiatric or cognitive dysfunction, nonfocal CNS disease: psychiatric or cognitive dysfunction or both without focal neurologic deficit, and NM: not mentioned; *according to the 1999 ACR definition of NPSLE.

had skin vasculitis, all anti-SS-A/Ro positive. Two of those, with cryoglobulinemia and low C, had PNS disease (one with mononeuritis multiplex). Only one patient with severe primary SS, manifested by cryoglobulinemia, vasculitis, and glomerulonephritis, presented with mononeuritis multiplex that partially responded to intravenous cyclophosphamide and high-dose steroids. Of interest is the absence of any statistically significant correlation between the observed PNS pathology and any other clinical or immunologic feature.

Among 33 RA patients, Sivri and Güler-Uysal [28] found 2 (6%) patients to have carpal tunnel syndrome, while 6 (18%) patients had mononeuritis multiplex. Impaired nerve conduction velocities were detected in 6 (18%) of 33 RA patients suggesting CNS involvement with intact PNS (however, there is no information about CNS involvement). Of note, there was not any clear correlation between neuropathy and clinical or laboratory data (RF).

Kasitanon et al. [12] studied 91 patients (90 females, 1 male) fulfilling standardized criteria of ACR nomenclature for neuropsychiatric SLE (NPSLE) [31]. CNS manifestations included seizures in 53 patients (54.1%), psychosis in 13 (13.3%), acute confusion state in 11 (11.2%), abnormal consciousness in 6 (6.1%), transverse myelitis in 6 (6.1%), cerebral infarction in 2 (2.0%), and aseptic meningitis in 2 (2.0%). PNS manifestations such as peripheral neuropathy were reported in 5 (5.1%) patients. However, patients with NPSLE had significantly more cutaneous vasculitis than those without associations between NPSLE and immunoserological data.

In Schneebaum et al. study [9], 19% of 269 patients with SLE demonstrated elevated levels of IgG or IgM anti-P antibodies, including 14% of 187 patients without and 29% of 82 patients with neuropsychiatric manifestations. The frequency in patients with severe depression ($n = 8$) and psychosis ($n = 29$) was 88% and 45%, respectively, compared with only 9% in patients with nonpsychiatric neurologic disease ($n = 45$). For the entire SLE group, the odds ratio for the association of anti-P antibodies and severe psychiatric manifestations was 7.63 with a 95% confidence interval of 3.61 to 16.14.

Isshi and Hirohata [10] also analyzed sera from 87 SLE patients (27 with non-CNS SLE, 34 with lupus psychosis, and 26 with nonpsychotic CNS lupus) and from 20 control patients with neurologic manifestations without SLE and cerebrospinal fluid (CSF) from 41 patients with CNS lupus and from the 20 control patients for IgG anti-P. Serum anti-P levels were significantly elevated in patients with lupus psychosis compared with those with non-CNS SLE or those with nonpsychotic CNS lupus, indicating that anti-P in the systemic circulation are involved in the development of lupus psychosis.

In Tzioufas et al. study [11], serum was obtained from 28 SLE patients during active CNS involvement. Eleven patients had diffuse CNS involvement (seven had psychiatric disorders and four had grand mal seizures), 13 patients had focal CNS involvement, seven of whom were associated with antibodies to cardiolipin, and four patients had a mixed form of CNS disease. The overall prevalence of anti-P antibodies in active CNS disease patients was statistically and significantly higher, as compared to unselected SLE patients ($\chi^2 = 6.04$, $P < 0.05$). These antibodies are associated with active SLE and CNS involvement particularly in patients without anticardiolipin antibodies.

In Sanna et al. study [13], 185 SLE patients (57.3%) had NP manifestations at any time during follow-up. Headache was the most frequent manifestation, present in 78 patients (24%). Cerebrovascular disease (CD) was diagnosed in 47/323 patients (14.5%), with a total of 57 events. Mood disorders were found in 54 (16.7%), cognitive disorders in 35 (10.8%), and seizures in 27 patients (8.3%). Psychosis was diagnosed in 25 (7.7%), anxiety disorder in 24 (3.7%), and acute confusional state in 12 patients (3.7%). NP manifestations are significantly associated with aPL. CD, headache, and seizures were independently associated with these antibodies.

In Hirohata et al. study [20], 23 patients showed that CNS manifestations other than diffuse NPSLE, including neurologic syndromes and PNS involvements (focal NPSLE), according to the ACR nomenclature for NPSLE anti-Sm levels in CSF and sera were measured using enzyme-linked immunosorbent assay (ELISA) kits. Anti-Sm in CSF were significantly elevated in NPSLE compared with non-SLE control. Among subsets of NPSLE, CSF anti-Sm was significantly elevated in acute confusional state compared with nonacute confusional state diffuse NPSLE ($P = 0.0028$) or with focal NPSLE ($P = 0.0008$).

In Závada et al. study [15], sera of 76 patients with SLE and neurological symptoms, 50 of whom met the ACR nomenclature for NPSLE, were tested for AQP4-Ab in an indirect immunofluorescence assay employing HEK293 cells transfected with recombinant human AQP4. Only one of the examined sera was positive for NMO-IgG/AQP4-Ab. None of the 75 NPSLE without was found to be seropositive for NMO-IgG/AQP4-Ab. NMO-IgG/AQP4-Ab in NPSLE were present only in a patient with transverse myelitis and were not detectable in NPSLE patients with other neurological manifestations.

Hanly et al. [16] identified 41 NPSLE patients. CNS manifestations accounted for 92% of the events compared to involvement of the PNS in 8%. In patients with NP, the occurrence of renal disease was significantly associated with use of prednisone and immunosuppressive drugs. However, associations between positive antinuclear antibodies (97%) and elevated anti-dsDNA antibodies were not examined.

According to 1997 American College of Rheumatology diagnostic criteria [6], 15 women were enrolled in the study of Kluz et al. [17] with severe disease activity (a modified SLE Disease Activity Index (SLEDAI) of >12 points) and inflammatory microangiopathy-related complications such as systemic CNS affection and/or vasculitis and/or nephritis. In 6 of them, CNS complications were seizure ($n = 1$), organic brain syndrome ($n = 2$), cranial nerve disorder ($n = 1$), and headache ($n = 2$). Significantly higher levels of both fractions of ACA and IgM ACA and of both fractions of ACA and IgM ACA and antiphospholipid antibodies (repeatedly positive test for serum ACA and/or lupus anticoagulant) were determined in patients with severe disease activity and microangiopathic complications compared with those with less active disease.

Briani et al. [18] presented 85 SLE patients (39%) with neurological manifestations. Both central (53 patients) and peripheral (23 patients) nervous systems were involved (Table 2). In 9 patients CNS and PNS manifestations concurred. The most common CNS manifestation was headache (35 cases, 58%) followed by cerebrovascular diseases (11 cases, 17%), epilepsy (10 cases, 16%), psychiatric disorders (6 cases, 10%), and myelopathy (2 cases, 3%). PNS manifestations included symmetric polyneuropathy (17 cases, 20%), mononeuropathy (13 cases, 10 with median nerve and 3 with sciatic nerve involvement, 35%), and mononeuropathy multiplex (2 cases, 5%). One patient with mononeuropathy multiplex underwent sural nerve biopsy, which showed vasculitic axonal injury. Of the 7 sera and CSF samples with Abs to ribosomal P proteins, these autoantibodies are associated with CNS manifestations such as psychosis ($P = 0.017$) and PNS mononeuropathy multiplex ($P = 0.040$).

Gono et al. [32] enrolled 20 patients with pSS. PNS involvement regarded seven patients with cranial neuropathy, nine patients with polyneuropathy, and three patients with mononeuritis multiplex (Table 2). Seven patients with cranial neuropathy included three with optic neuritis, two with trigeminal neuralgia, one with facial nerve palsy, and one with glossopharyngeal and vagus nerve palsy. Eight of the nine patients with polyneuropathy revealed pure sensory neuropathy. Two of the three patients with mono neuritis multiplex revealed motor sensory neuropathy. CNS involvement included three patients with encephalopathy and two patients with aseptic meningitis. One patient with optic neuritis had spinal cord lesions and cerebral focal symptoms, such as right hemiparesis, which are similar findings in multiple sclerosis. Moreover, AQ4 antibody was detected in the other one of the three patients with optic neuritis. This patient was diagnosed with Neuromyelitis optica (NMO) associated with pSS.

Among 207 SLE patients Florica et al. [19] showed that 125 had SLE-related PN involvement and 82 had non-SLE-related PN. The most frequent etiologies of non-SLE-related PN were compressive neuropathy (nerve or root compression) in 35 (42.6%), followed by medication toxicity in 23 (28%), hypothyroidism in 19 (23.1%), and diabetes mellitus in 14 (17%). Other causes of non-SLE-related PN included ethanol abuse, paraproteinemia, uremia, and viral hepatitis in a limited number of patients.

Patients with PNS were more likely to have also CNS involvement (14.2%) compared with patients without PN (CNS involvement: 6.6%, $P = 0.02$). The most common PN observed was peripheral polyneuropathy, with a predominance of the sensory form, present in 76 (36.7%) patients and the sensory-motor variant in 39 (18.8%) patients. Twenty-three (11.1%) patients had a peripheral mononeuropathy and 26 (12.5%) had a cranial neuropathy. Nineteen (9.2%) patients suffered from mononeuritis multiplex and only 11 (5.3%) were diagnosed with chronic inflammatory demyelinating polyradiculoneuropathy (CIDP). There was no difference between PNS features and SLE immune markers (presence of antiphospholipid antibodies).

In study of Chiewthanakul et al. [14], CNS manifestations accounted for 87% (84/97 patients), while involvement of the PNS was 13% (13/97 patients). The three most frequent CNS manifestations included seizures (33%), psychoses (22.7%), and cerebrovascular disease (22.3%), composed of 82.6% cerebral infarction, 8.7% transient ischemic attack, and 8.7% venous sinus thrombosis. ANA and antibodies to dsDNA did not correlate with NP manifestations.

In 2014 study by Jamilloux et al. [26], 420 patients fulfilled the 2002 American-European pSS criteria [7]. Within 93 (22%) patients with neurological manifestations, PN and CNS were involved in 66% and 44%, respectively. The number of extraglandular manifestations was increased in patients with sensorimotor neuropathies (3.3 ± 1.9 versus 2 ± 1.5, $P < 0.05$). This subgroup had more frequent cryoglobulinemia and lymphopenia ($P < 0.05$) but lower prevalence of anti-Ro/SSA antibodies and hypergammaglobulinemia ($P < 0.05$). Authors also confirmed cryoglobulinemia as unique predictive factor of PNS disease.

In Spezialetti et al. study [21], from 77 patients with pSS and CNS involvement, psychiatric or cognitive impairment, usually mild or moderate, occurred in over 80% (63 of 77) of this highly selected population of SS patients, and more than 60% of patients (48 of 77) had both. Anti-ribosomal P antibodies occurred in six (4.6%) patients with SS and related disorders. None of the patients with primary SS had anti-ribosomal P antibodies. There was no correlation between nonfocal CNS disease, including psychosis or severe depression, and the presence of anti-ribosomal P antibodies. Paired serum CSF samples from 34 SS patients with active CNS disease, including 6 with psychosis and 5 with severe depression, did not contain anti-ribosomal P.

In Sène et al. study [25], patients with pSS and PNS involvement and nonataxic sensory neuropathy were characterized by a higher age (57.5 ± 10.7 versus 48.7 ± 14.3 years; $P = 0.007$), more frequent CNS involvement (15% versus 2%; $P = 0.04$), and lower prevalence of ANA (60% versus 90%; $P = 0.003$), anti-SSA (Ro) (40% versus 72%; $P = 0.009$), anti-SSB (La) (15% versus 41%; $P = 0.039$), RF (37% versus 67%; $P = 0.02$), and hypergammaglobulinemia (35% versus 64%; $P = 0.023$). In multivariate analysis, nonataxic sensory neuropathy was associated with the presence of CNS involvement (OR, 17.0; $P = 0.025$) and ANA (OR, 0.07; $P < 0.001$).

In Delalande et al. study [23], fifty-six patients with pSS had CNS disorders, which were mostly focal or multifocal. Twenty-nine patients had spinal cord involvement (acute myelopathy ($n = 12$), chronic myelopathy ($n = 16$), or motor neuron disease ($n = 1$)). The disease mimicked relapsing-remitting multiple sclerosis (MS) in 10 patients and primary progressive MS in 13 patients. CNS symptoms included seizures ($n = 7$), cognitive dysfunction ($n = 9$), and encephalopathy ($n = 2$). Fifty-one patients had PNS involvement: symmetric axonal sensorimotor polyneuropathy with a predominance of sensory symptoms or pure sensory neuropathy occurred most frequently ($n = 28$), followed by cranial nerve involvement affecting trigeminal, facial, or cochlear nerves ($n = 16$). Multiple mononeuropathy ($n = 7$), myositis ($n = 2$), and polyradiculoneuropathy ($n = 1$) were also observed. Anti-Ro/SSA or anti-La/SSB antibodies were detected in 21% of patients at the diagnosis of SS, more frequently observed in patients with PNS involvement than in those with CNS involvement ($P < 0.01$).

Alexander et al. [22] examined 49 SS patients (group I) for the potential relationship between anti-Ro(SS-A) antibodies and active CNS disease by double immunodiffusion. In group 2 with 52 SS patients and active CNS disease, the anti-SSA antibodies were detected by ELISA. This study showed that anti-Ro antibodies were positive in 48% of patients with CNS manifestations and serious complications compared to only 24% of all patients with pSS.

Pittock et al. [24] detected NMO-IgG in 5 of 14 patients (35.7%) with NMOSDs and SS/SLE and in 2 of 4 patients (50.0%) with NMO without SS/SLE ($P = 0.59$). SSA, SSA, ANA, and dsDNA antibodies were found in these patients but not NMO-IgG.

4. Discussion

In this first systematic review of both CNS and PNS involvement in *RA*, *SLE*, and *pSS*, our results indicate that CNS complications (9–92%) are much more frequent than those of PNS (8–66%) across the various studies (total of 2338 patients). These findings are compatible with previous results in the literature. In this review, the majority of reported studies attributable in SLE CNS manifestations range from 13 to 92% of the events compared to PNS in 8–56%. The most frequent NP syndromes were headache, mood disorders, and seizures which are consistent with previous meta-analysis [33]. Ours finding are also consistent with previous studies where SLE CNS manifestations range from 33% to 75% [34, 35]. In SS studies, CNS manifestations range between 9 and 44% and PNS ranged between 24 and 68%, which agree with previous studies [36]. In this review, the frequency of PNS (mononeuritis) in RA patients is 18% lower as compared to other study, while for entrapment neuropathy (6% in our patients) it varies from 4% to 54.6% [37, 38].

Overall prevalence is seen to vary widely among the studies and is mainly attributed to a number of factors including bias in selection of patients for study, disease duration, and lack of uniformity in diagnostic criteria. With this in mind, we sought to expand the probability of specific manifestations by using established criteria and double-reading (by a certified neurologist), and excluding uncertain cases.

Among the most interesting points of this review is the correlation between CNS/PNS manifestations and immune activation markers (i.e., antinuclear antibodies ANA, anti-Ro/SSA, anti-La/SSB, RF, and hypergammaglobulinemia). Anti-Ro and anti-La seem to be less frequent in pSS patients with neurological involvement (40%) compared to patients without neurological manifestations (60% of positivity), so, it is necessary for more markers are necessary in pSS to better classify subpopulations of patients with neurological involvement [39]. Jamilloux et al. [26] claimed that the implication that the immunological profile (as potential serological markers) may only be a signature related to distinct neurological rather than a reflection of the pathogenic mechanism could not be dismissed. Nonetheless, given the apparent association with Raynaud's phenomenon, cutaneous vasculitis, and renal involvement, they proposed that sensorimotor neuropathy or mononeuritis multiplex originates from immunovascular injury. Contrary to other studies, Jamilloux et al. showed that sensory ganglionopathy is associated with lymphocytic infiltration and not cryoglobulinemia. In the same manner, Mellgren et al. showed that sensory ganglionopathy in pSS was related to lymphocyte infiltration of the dorsal root ganglia. In addition, Gono et al. reported optic neuropathy in one patient with SS and NMO (Aquaporin Ab positive) and MS, suggesting the implication of more mechanisms associated with the pathogenesis of neurological involvement in SS rather than the previously described vasculopathy. In the same context, Pittock et al. concluded that NMO disorders with seropositive findings for NMO-IgG occurring with SS/SLE or non-organ-specific autoantibodies is an indication of coexisting NMO rather than a vasculopathic or other complication of SS/SLE. Florica et al. observed that the group of SLE-related PN patients had more frequent CNS involvement and a higher score of disease activity, indicating that the immune response shows a preference toward neurological tissue. This is the first large study solely focused on peripheral neuropathy in SLE which suggests an autoimmune etiology for PN manifestations in SLE. It remains undetermined whether any of these clinical characteristics could predict the onset of PNS or/and CNS in either SS or SLE or other connective tissue disorders.

Several specific autoantibodies are associated with NPSLE (antiphospholipid, serum anti-ribosomal P antibodies, ANA, and antibodies to dsDNA). The presence of antiphospholipid antibodies is significantly associated with cerebrovascular disease and cognitive dysfunction, whereas serum anti-ribosomal P antibodies are strongly associated with psychosis and depression in SLE as discussed in this review [9, 10, 13, 20]. These findings are consistent with one multicenter study [40]. Moreover, the presence of cutaneous vasculitic lesions was significantly associated with NPSLE in the study by Kasitanon et al., rather than thrombocytopenia, as suggested by other studies [41]. According to Chiewthanakul et al., cutaneous vasculitis was only marginally related to active CNS involvement. Notably, in this study, neither ANA and antibodies to dsDNA nor anti-ribosomal P antibodies correlated with NP manifestations. In the same line is Spezialetti et al. study [21]. It seems that the independent associations of such manifestations with NPSLE have been difficult to study so far. This is partly explained by the difficulty to conduct studies with an adequate sample size.

However, Andonopoulos et al. failed to find a statistically significant correlation between the observed PNS pathology and any other clinical or immuno/serologic data. In the absence of any obvious reason, it is tempting to ascribe PNS symptoms to vasculitis of the vasa nervorum, but the data provided cannot fully support this hypothesis. The classical severe picture of a patient presenting with mononeuritis multiplex, associated with vasculitis in other organs, as already mentioned, leaves little doubt as to the pathogenesis of the neurologic syndrome. However, no patient has been reported to exhibit additional features of CNS disease that could be clinically detected.

Similarly, Sivri and Güler-Uysal found no correlation between mononeuritis and the immunological data in the serum of RA patients (i.e., RF), which is in contrast with the finding by other study [42]. This could be explained by the implication of a number of multiple factors in determining the clinical signs of disease (i.e., nonsteroidal anti-inflammatory drugs, NSAIDs). The single center, tertiary referral center-based patient population and small number of subjects might also explain the result.

Several limitations which compromised their external validity were identified in the specific studies, mainly by their authors. In terms of reporting complications, methods varied considerably. In this review, incidence was determined from studies of varying sample sizes across multiple age groups. Data collection was retrospective [14, 19, 29, 32]. Hence, patient assessment might have been incomplete, rendering it difficult to analyze details of NPSLE syndromes [13] or missing PN initial events [20]; secondly, other CNS manifestations, such as headaches, anxiety, cognitive dysfunction, and autonomic disorders, may have been missed; thus, their prevalence has been underestimated [19, 30]. Finally, the cause of death by autopsy was not always performed; thus, authors could not conclude whether death was related to SLE-mediated organ dysfunction or other diseases [15]. Perhaps due to methodological limitations it was not possible to determine if the associations between medication use with the occurrence of NP events and renal disease were independent of each other [9].

Notwithstanding, this review is not without its limitations. There are a small number of studies available for analysis. One limitation of this review is that a limited number of databases were searched. Consequently, there is always the possibility that we overlooked studies in other databases published before 1980. In addition, there is always the possibility of publication bias due to underreported negative results and grey literature. However, the use of fewer search limits increases the sensitivity of the search method.

5. Conclusions

Despite the abovementioned limitations, this systematic review provides foundation for further research on the pathophysiology of immune system among the vasculature of the CNS and PNS. It is still a matter of debate whether the CNS and PNS manifestations of RA, SLE, and pSS are direct effect of these diseases or secondary such as side effects of corticosteroids and other immunosuppressive therapies or multiple systemic organ dysfunction (i.e., drug or SLE-mediated multiorgan induced psychosis). To date, no laboratory test, that is, autoantibodies, has been shown as pathognomonic neither for CNS nor for PNS involvement in these connective tissue disorders. Prospective multicenter studies are warrant for further confirmations.

References

[1] J. E. Riggs, "Neurological consequences of systemic disease," in *Neurology in Clinical Practice*, W. Bradley, R. Daroff, G. Fenichel, and D. Marsden, Eds., pp. 841–860, Butterworth-Heinemann, Boston, Mass, USA, 1991.

[2] C. Chalk, J. Dyck, and D. Conn, "Vasculitic neuropathy," in *Peripheral Neuropathy*, P. K. Thomas and P. J. Dyck, Eds., pp. 1424–1430, Saunders, Philadelphia, Pa, USA, 1993.

[3] G. Midroni and J. Bilbao, "Vasculitic neuropathy," in *Biopsy Diagnosis of Peripheral Neuropathy*, G. Midroni and J. Bilbao, Eds., pp. 241–262, Butterworth-Heinemann, Boston, Mass, USA, 1995.

[4] E. V. Voss and M. Stangel, "Nervous system involvement of connective tissue disease: mechanisms and diagnostic approach," *Current Opinion in Neurology*, vol. 25, no. 3, pp. 306–315, 2012.

[5] S. Sciascia, M. L. Bertolaccini, D. Roccatello, M. A. Khamashta, and G. Sanna, "Autoantibodies involved in neuropsychiatric manifestations associated with systemic lupus erythematosus: a systematic review," *Journal of Neurology*, vol. 261, no. 9, pp. 1706–1714, 2014.

[6] M. C. Hochberg, "Updating the American College of Rheumatology revised criteria for the classification of systemic lupus erythematosus [letter]," *Arthritis & Rheumatism*, vol. 40, no. 9, p. 1725, 1997.

[7] C. Vitali, S. Bombardieri, R. Jonsson et al., "Classification criteria for Sjögren's syndrome: a revised version of the European criteria proposed by the American-European Consensus Group," *Annals of the Rheumatic Diseases*, vol. 61, no. 6, pp. 554–558, 2002.

[8] D. Aletaha, T. Neogi, A. J. Silman et al., "2010 rheumatoid arthritis classification criteria: an American College of Rheumatology/European League Against Rheumatism collaborative initiative," *Annals of the Rheumatic Diseases*, vol. 69, no. 9, pp. 1580–1588, 2010.

[9] A. B. Schneebaum, J. D. Singleton, S. G. West et al., "Association of psychiatric manifestations with antibodies to ribosomal p proteins in systemic lupus erythematosus," *The American Journal of Medicine*, vol. 90, no. 1, pp. 54–62, 1991.

[10] K. Isshi and S. Hirohata, "Differential roles of the anti-ribosomal P antibody and antineuronal antibody in the pathogenesis of central nervous system involvement in systemic lupus erythematosus," *Arthritis and Rheumatism*, vol. 41, no. 10, pp. 1819–1827, 1998.

[11] A. G. Tzioufas, N. G. Tzortzakis, E. Panou-Pomonis et al., "The clinical relevance of antibodies to ribosomal-P common epitope in two targeted systemic lupus erythematosus populations: a large cohort of consecutive patients and patients with active central nervous system disease," *Annals of the Rheumatic Diseases*, vol. 59, no. 2, pp. 99–104, 2000.

[12] N. Kasitanon, W. Louthrenoo, S. Piyasirisilp, W. Sukitawut, and R. Wichainun, "Neuropsychiatric manifestations in Thai patients with systemic lupus erythematosus," *Asian Pacific Journal of Allergy and Immunology*, vol. 20, no. 3, pp. 179–185, 2002.

[13] G. Sanna, M. L. Bertolaccini, M. J. Cuadrado et al., "Neuropsychiatric manifestations in systemic lupus erythematosus: prevalence and association with antiphospholipid antibodies," *Journal of Rheumatology*, vol. 30, no. 5, pp. 985–992, 2003.

[14] P. Chiewthanakul, K. Sawanyawisuth, C. Foocharoen, and S. Tiamkao, "Clinical features and predictive factors in neuropsychiatric lupus," *Asian Pacific Journal of Allergy and Immunology*, vol. 30, no. 1, pp. 55–60, 2012.

[15] J. Závada, P. Nytrová, K. P. Wandinger et al., "Seroprevalence and specificity of NMO-IgG (anti-aquaporin 4 antibodies) in patients with neuropsychiatric systemic lupus erythematosus," *Rheumatology International*, vol. 33, no. 1, pp. 259–263, 2013.

[16] J. G. Hanly, G. McCurdy, L. Fougere, J.-A. Douglas, and K. Thompson, "Neuropsychiatric events in systemic lupus erythematosus: attribution and clinical significance," *The Journal of Rheumatology*, vol. 31, no. 11, pp. 2156–2162, 2004.

[17] J. Kluz, W. Kopeć, U. Jakobsche, I. Prajs, and R. Adamiec, "Vasculitis in systemic lupus erythematosus (SLE)—assessment of peripheral blood mononuclear cell activation and the degree of endothelial dysfunction: initial report," *Postpy Higieny I Medycyny Doświadczalnej*, vol. 61, pp. 725–735, 2007.

[18] C. Briani, M. Lucchetta, A. Ghirardello et al., "Neurolupus is associated with anti-ribosomal P protein antibodies: an inception cohort study," *Journal of Autoimmunity*, vol. 32, no. 2, pp. 79–84, 2009.

[19] B. Florica, E. Aghdassi, J. Su, D. D. Gladman, M. B. Urowitz, and P. R. Fortin, "Peripheral neuropathy in patients with systemic lupus erythematosus," *Seminars in Arthritis and Rheumatism*, vol. 41, no. 2, pp. 203–211, 2011.

[20] S. Hirohata, Y. Sakuma, T. Yanagida, and T. Yoshio, "Association of cerebrospinal fluid anti-Sm antibodies with acute confusional state in systemic lupus erythematosus," *Arthritis Research & Therapy*, vol. 16, no. 5, article 450, 2014.

[21] R. Spezialetti, H. G. Bluestein, J. B. Peter, and E. Alexander, "Neuropsychiatric disease in Sjögren's syndrome: anti-ribosomal P and anti-neuronal antibodies," *American Journal of Medicine*, vol. 95, no. 2, pp. 153–160, 1993.

[22] E. L. Alexander, M. R. Ranzenbach, A. J. Kumar et al., "Anti–Ro(SS–A) autoantibodies in central nervous system disease associated with Sjögren's syndrome (CNS–SS)," *Neurology*, vol. 44, no. 5, pp. 899–908, 1994.

[23] S. Delalande, J. de Seze, A.-L. Fauchais et al., "Neurologic manifestations in primary Sjögren syndrome: a study of 82 patients," *Medicine*, vol. 83, no. 5, pp. 280–291, 2004.

[24] S. J. Pittock, V. A. Lennon, J. de Seze et al., "Neuromyelitis optica and non-organ-specific autoimmunity," *Archives of Neurology*, vol. 65, no. 1, pp. 78–83, 2008.

[25] D. Sène, M. Jallouli, J.-P. Lefaucheur et al., "Peripheral neuropathies associated with primary sjögren syndrome: immunologic profiles of nonataxic sensory neuropathy and sensorimotor neuropathy," *Medicine*, vol. 90, no. 2, pp. 133–138, 2011.

[26] Y. Jamilloux, L. Magy, J.-F. Hurtevent et al., "Immunological profiles determine neurological involvement in Sjögren's syndrome," *European Journal of Internal Medicine*, vol. 25, no. 2, pp. 177–181, 2014.

[27] M. Morreale, P. Marchione, P. Ciacomini et al., "Neurological involvement in primary Sjögren syndrome: a focus on central nervous system," *PLoS ONE*, vol. 9, no. 1, Article ID e84605, 2014.

[28] A. Sivri and F. Güler-Uysal, "The electroneurophysiological findings in rheumatoid arthritis patients," *Electromyography and Clinical Neurophysiology*, vol. 39, no. 7, pp. 387–391, 1999.

[29] S. I. Mellgren, D. L. Conn, J. C. Stevens, and P. J. Dyck, "Peripheral neuropathy in primary Sjogren's syndrome," *Neurology*, vol. 39, no. 3, pp. 390–394, 1989.

[30] A. P. Andonopoulos, G. Lagos, A. A. Drosos, and H. M. Moutsopoulos, "Neurologic involvement in primary Sjögren's syndrome: a preliminary report," *Journal of Autoimmunity*, vol. 2, no. 4, pp. 485–488, 1989.

[31] "The American College of Rheumatology nomenclature and case definitions for neuropsychiatric lupus syndromes," *Arthritis & Rheumatism*, vol. 42, no. 4, pp. 599–608, 1999.

[32] T. Gono, Y. Kawaguchi, Y. Katsumata et al., "Clinical manifestations of neurological involvement in primary Sjögren's syndrome," *Clinical Rheumatology*, vol. 30, no. 4, pp. 485–490, 2011.

[33] A. Unterman, J. E. S. Nolte, M. Boaz, M. Abady, Y. Shoenfeld, and G. Zandman-Goddard, "Neuropsychiatric syndromes in systemic lupus erythematosus: a meta-analysis," *Seminars in Arthritis and Rheumatism*, vol. 41, no. 1, pp. 1–11, 2011.

[34] G. A. W. Bruyn, "Controversies in lupus: nervous system involvement," *Annals of the Rheumatic Diseases*, vol. 54, no. 3, pp. 159–167, 1995.

[35] R. L. Brey, S. L. Holliday, A. R. Saklad et al., "Neuropsychiatric syndromes in lupus: prevalence using standardized definitions," *Neurology*, vol. 58, no. 8, pp. 1214–1220, 2002.

[36] J. Font, M. Ramos-Casals, G. De la Red et al., "Pure sensory neuropathy in primary Sjögren's syndrome. Longterm prospective followup and review of the literature," *Journal of Rheumatology*, vol. 30, no. 7, pp. 1552–1557, 2003.

[37] V. Agarwal, R. Singh, Wiclaf et al., "A clinical, electrophysiological, and pathological study of neuropathy in rheumatoid arthritis," *Clinical Rheumatology*, vol. 27, no. 7, pp. 841–844, 2008.

[38] S. A. Hamed, E. A. Hamed, A. M. Elattar, M. S. A. Rahman, and N. F. Amine, "Cranial and peripheral neuropathy in rheumatoid arthritis with special emphasis to II, V, VII and XI cranial nerves," *APLAR Journal of Rheumatology*, vol. 9, no. 3, pp. 216–226, 2006.

[39] G. J. Tobn, J.-O. Pers, V. Devauchelle-Pensec, and P. Youinou, "Neurological disorders in primary Sjögren's syndrome," *Autoimmune Diseases*, vol. 2012, Article ID 645967, 11 pages, 2012.

[40] M. Mahler, K. Kessenbrock, M. Szmyrka et al., "International multi-center evaluation of autoantibodies to ribosomal P proteins," *Clinical and Vaccine Immunology*, vol. 13, no. 1, pp. 77–83, 2006.

[41] F. B. Karassa, J. P. A. Ioannidis, G. Touloumi, K. A. Boki, and H. M. Moutsopoulos, "Risk factors for central nervous system involvement in systemic lupus erythematosus," *QJM*, vol. 93, no. 3, pp. 169–174, 2000.

[42] M. Biswas, A. Chatterjee, S. K. Ghosh, S. Dasgupta, K. Ghosh, and P. K. Ganguly, "Prevalence, types, clinical associations, and determinants of peripheral neuropathy in rheumatoid patients," *Annals of Indian Academy of Neurology*, vol. 14, no. 3, pp. 194–197, 2011.

Relationship between *Helicobacter pylori* Infections in Diabetic Patients and Inflammations, Metabolic Syndrome, and Complications

Yusuf Kayar,[1] Özgül Pamukçu,[2] Hatice Eroğlu,[2] Kübra Kalkan Erol,[2] Aysegul Ilhan,[3] and Orhan Kocaman[1]

[1]*Division of Gastroenterology, Internal Medicine Department, Bezmialem Vakif University, Turkey*
[2]*Internal Medicine Department, Şişli Etfal Training and Research Hospital, Turkey*
[3]*Sisli Etfal Hamidiye Education and Research Hospital, Clinics of Internal Medicine, Turkey*

Correspondence should be addressed to Özgül Pamukçu; pamgul@hotmail.com

Academic Editor: Kathleen Gillespie

Helicobacter pylori infection and diabetes mellitus are two independent common diseases. It is showed that the worsening glycemic and metabolic control increases the rates of *Helicobacter pylori* infections and *Helicobacter pylori* is shown as one of the common problems in diabetic patients with complaints of gastrointestinal diseases. In this study, we aimed to investigate the prevalence and eradication rates of *Helicobacter pylori* in diabetic patients and the relationship of *Helicobacter pylori* with the risk factors and diabetic complications. In our study, in which we have included 133 patients, we have shown a significant relationship between *Helicobacter pylori* infections and metabolic syndrome, insulin resistance, inflammations, and diabetic complications.

1. Introduction

Helicobacter pylori (HP) infections are very common worldwide, affecting approximately 50% of the world's population, and are more common especially in developing countries [1]. Although the findings of various studies are inconsistent, the presence of *H. pylori* is found to be higher in diabetic patients compared to nondiabetic patients [2–4]. *H. pylori* colonizes in the gastric antrum in all patients, particularly in diabetic patients with impaired metabolic control [2–5]. Beside the well-defined gastric effects of *H. pylori* infection, some studies are also published pointing the extragastric effects of *H. pylori* infection which plays an additional role for the vascular damage in course of atherosclerosis [5, 6].

The presence of *H. pylori* and diabetes mellitus (DM) is one of the main causes of gastrointestinal diseases [2, 7]. Additionally, the presence of *H. pylori* in DM cases plays an important role in the development of gastrointestinal diseases [7]. In particular, the worsening of glycemic and metabolic control increases the incidence of *H. pylori* infections and complaints of dyspepsia [2, 7]. A significant relationship between dyslipidemia and *H. pylori* has been reported. In prospective studies, it has been shown that *H. pylori* eradication improves dyslipidemia and insulin resistance and decreases inflammation [6]. Although the relationship between *H. pylori* infection and DM and the complications secondary to diabetes is not clear, it is known that neuropathy and hyperglycemia play an important role in *H. pylori* colonization in the gastric epithelium [8]. Although the findings of various studies are inconsistent, it has been shown that there is a significant relationship between microvascular complications (nephropathy, neuropathy, and retinopathy) and *H. pylori* [6, 9, 10].

Although there is no clear-cut consensus in the literature, it has been reported that HPeradication is noticeably lower in diabetic patients. There are a limited number of studies on the factors that play a role in HPeradication. We investigated the HP prevalence, HP eradication rates, and confounding factors affecting HP eradication in diabetic patients.

TABLE 1: The relationship between *H. pylori* positivity and inflammatory parameters.

Variables	Total	*H. pylori* (+) subjects	*H. pylori* (−) subjects	*P* value
CRP*	4.8 ± 3.4	5.5 ± 3.9	3.9 ± 2.3	<0.05
Leukocytes	7.0 ± 1.8	7.1 ± 1.6	6.9 ± .9	NS
Thrombocytes	250 ± 65	252 ± 69	248 ± 61	NS
Sedimentation*	9.4 ± 8.2	11.3 ± 8.9	7.3 ± 6.8	<0.05
Ferritin*	86.5 ± 91.7	122 ± 105	45.6 ± 47	<0.05
Fibrinogen*	321 ± 77	336 ± 82	303 ± 67	<0.05

*Significant variables.

2. Materials and Methods

133 dyspeptic patients aged 18 to 65 and recruited from the internal medicine outpatient clinic were included into the study. All patients provided written informed consent to participate. 62 out of 133 patients had Type 2 DM. Exclusion criteria were (1) patients over 65 years; (2) patients having diabetes for more than 5 years; (3) patients with apparent proteinuria, creatinine values of >1.2 mg/dL, triglyceride levels of >400 mg/dL, and HbA1C of >8% with positive urine culture; (4) patients who received ulcer treatment within the last three months; (5) patients currently using proton pump inhibitor or H2 receptor blockers; (6) patients with a history of *H. pylori* eradication treatment; and (7) patients with vascular and inflammatory diseases.

Demographics (age, gender, and duration of disease) of the patients were documented. Height, weight, and waist circumference were measured and BMI was calculated as weight/height^2 (kg/m^2). Systolic and diastolic blood pressure measurements using standard sphygmomanometry were performed. Biochemical investigation including hemoglobin A1C (HbA1C), cholesterol, triglyceride, HDL, LDL, fasting blood glucose, leukocyte count, thrombocyte count, erythrocyte sedimentation rate, C reactive protein, and fibrinogen levels was performed in all patients. Approval of the local ethics committee was obtained for the study.

Peripheral vascular disease was assessed based on the presence of intermittent claudication clinically and the absence of pulse in physical examinations. Retinopathy was determined with standard fundus examination. The presence of neuropathy was determined as per abnormal sensorimotor findings in examinations. Patients with a protein amount of 30 to 300 mg in 24-hour urine were considered cases with microalbuminuria, and those with ≥300 mg were considered cases with apparent proteinuria. In order to determine HP infection, the HPantigen stool test was used as it is a useful method for detection of active and repetitive HP infections [11]. The success rate of eradication was checked four weeks after the end of all treatments.

In all patients with dyspeptic complaints, the presence of *H. pylori* was investigated by the *H. pylori* antigen stool test, and the patients were compared by dividing them into two groups (Type 2 DM patients and nondiabetic patients). The relationship between *H. pylori* positivity and demographic clinical anthropometric and inflammatory parameters was investigated in all patients. The relationship between *H. pylori* positivity and retinopathy, nephropathy, neuropathy, and HbA1C was investigated in diabetic patients.

Eradication treatment (clarithromycin, amoxicillin, and omeprazole) was given to *H. pylori* positive patients for two weeks. Additional omeprazole treatment without antibiotics was continued for 4 weeks. Two weeks after cessation of all treatments, eradication rates were determined by stool antigen test and a comparison was made.

2.1. Statistical Analysis. SPSS 17.0 package program was used for statistical analysis of data. The data were summarized in percentage, mean ± SD, and median values. The presence of *H. pylori* and eradication of *H. pylori*, as well as the relationship with demographic clinical anthropometric and inflammatory parameters, were analyzed using chi-square test, Fischer's exact test, and independent T-sample test. The relationship between the presence of *H. pylori* and eradication of *H. pylori* in diabetic patients was analyzed using chi-square test and Fischer's exact test. The results were assessed with hazard ratio and in a 95% confidence interval. A $P < 0.05$ value was considered statistically meaningful in the analyses.

3. Results

H. pylori positivity was detected in 64.5% of the diabetic patients and in 43.6% of the control group. *H. pylori* positivity was detected in 53.4% of all patients. The relationship between *H. pylori* positivity and inflammatory, demographic, clinical, and anthropometric parameters was shown in Tables 1 and 2.

When the relationship between the complications in diabetic patients and *H. pylori* positivity was evaluated, *H. pylori* positivity was significantly associated with the presence of nephropathy and neuropathy. Although retinopathy was more common in patients with *H. pylori* positivity, no statistical significance was found between groups. Additionally, a significant relationship between glycemic control and the presence of *H. pylori* was detected. While 48.5% of the patients with HbA1C ≤7 were *H. pylori* positive, 82.8% of the patients with HbA1C >7 were found to be *H. pylori* positive (Table 3).

The rate of *H. pylori* eradication in diabetic and control groups was 62.5% and 93.5%, respectively. The factors affecting the rate of *H. pylori* eradication were shown in Table 4.

When the relationship between the complications in diabetic patients and *H. pylori* eradication was evaluated, a significant relationship between nephropathy and neuropathy with successful eradication of *H. pylori* was detected. Although retinopathy is more common in patients without *H. pylori* eradication, no statistical significance was detected.

TABLE 2: The relationship between *H. pylori* positivity and demographic, clinical, and anthropometric parameters.

Variables	Total	*H. pylori* (+) subjects	*H. pylori* (−) subjects	*P* value
Gender				
Female	70	34 (48.5%)	36 (51.5%)	NS
Male	63	37 (58.7%)	26 (41.3%)	NS
Age	47 ± 12	48.7 ± 12.1	46.9 ± 13.1	NS
Body mass index				NS
Normal	30	12 (40%)	18 (60%)	NS
Overweight	53	31 (58.4%)	22 (41.6%)	NS
Obese	50	28 (56%)	22 (44%)	NS
Waistline*	94 ± 11	95.7 ± 10	91.9 ± 11.8	<0.05
Hypertension				
Yes*	49	34 (69.3%)	15 (30.7%)	<0.05
No	84	37 (44%)	47 (56%)	NS
Cholesterol				NS
≥200	67	38 (56.7%)	29 (43.3%)	NS
<200	66	33 (50%)	33 (50%)	NS
Triglyceride				
≥150*	42	30 (71.4%)	12 (28.6%)	<0.05
<150	91	41 (45%)	50 (55%)	NS
Low density lipoprotein				
≥100	87	51 (58.6%)	36 (41.4%)	NS
<100	46	20 (43.4%)	26 (56.6%)	NS
High density lipoprotein				
Male ≥40, female ≥50	98	47 (%47.9)	51 (52.1%)	NS
Male <40, female <50*	35	24 (68.5%)	11 (31.5%)	<0.05
Glucose*	106 ± 35	117 ± 41	93 ± 21	<0.05
Creatinine	0.8 ± 0.2	0.84 ± 0.23	0.78 ± 0.19	NS
Patient groups				
DM*	62	40 (64.5%)	20 (35.5%)	<0.05
Non-DM	71	31 (43.6%)	40 (56.7%)	NS

*Significant variables.

TABLE 3: The relationship between the complications in diabetic patients and *H. pylori* positivity.

Variables	Total DM	*H. pylori* (+) subjects	*H. pylori* (−) subjects	*P* value
Nephropathy				
Yes*	23	21 (91.3%)	2 (8.7%)	<0.05
No	39	19 (48.7%)	20 (51.3%)	
Neuropathy				
Yes*	29	24 (82.8%)	5 (18.2%)	<0.05
No	33	16 (48.4%)	17 (51.6%)	
Retinopathy				
Yes	20	14 (70%)	6 (30%)	NS
No	42	24 (57.1%)	18 (42.9%)	
HbA1C				
6-7*	33	16 (48.5%)	17 (51.5%)	<0.05
7-8	29	24 (82.8%)	5 (17.2%)	

*Significant variables.

Additionally, a significant relationship between glycemic control and the presence of *H. pylori* eradication was detected. While *H. pylori* were successfully eradicated in 81.2% of the patients with HbA1C ≤7, *H. pylori* could be eradicated in 50% of the patients with HbA1C (Table 5).

4. Discussion

DM patients are usually prone to chronic infections. While the findings of studies on the prevalence of *H. pylori* in DM patients are contradictory, in our study, *H. pylori* positivity was detected in 64.5% of the DM patients and in 43.6% of the control group ($P < 0.05$). While Gentile et al. found that the prevalence of *H. pylori* infection was 74.4% in DM patients and 50% in the control group ($P < 0.01$), Gentile et al. found that the prevalence of *H. pylori* was significantly higher in the DM group compared to the control group [12, 13]. However, some studies did not find any significant difference in the DM group and the control group with regard to *H. pylori* infections [9, 14]. It is well known that diabetic patients are prone to chronic infections because of cellular and humoral immune deficiency. As a result of delayed gastric emptying due to gastroparesis diabeticorum, bacterial overgrowth occurs and this poses a risk for *H. pylori* infections. Achlorhydria and reduced acid secretion are a negative factor for *H. pylori* infections. Additionally, leukocyte dysfunction and hyperglycemia are a predisposing factor for infections

Table 4: The factors affecting the rate of *H. pylori* eradication.

Variables	Total	Those eradicated	Those not eradicated	*P* value
Gender				
Female	34	25 (73.5%)	9 (26.5%)	NS
Male	37	29 (78.3%)	8 (21.7%)	
Age	48.7 ± 12.1	48.1 ± 13.3	50.8 ± 7.2	NS
Body mass index				
Normal	12	12 (100%)	0 (0%)	
Overweight	31	28 (90.3%)	3 (9.7%)	
Obese*	28	14 (50%)	14 (50%)	<0.05
Waistline*	95.7 ± 10	94.3 ± 9.8	100 ± 9.4	<0.05
Hypertension				
Yes*	34	22 (64.7%)	12 (35.3%)	<0.05
No	37	32 (86.4%)	5 (13.6%)	
Cholesterol				
≥200*	38	24 (63.1%)	14 (36.9%)	<0.05
<200	33	30 (90.9%)	3 (9.1%)	
Triglyceride				
≥150*	30	19 (63.3%)	11 (36.7%)	<0.05
<150	41	35 (85.3%)	6 (14.7%)	
Low density lipoprotein				NS
≥100	51	37 (72.5%)	14 (27.5%)	
<100	20	17 (85%)	3 (15%)	
High density lipoprotein				NS
Male ≥40, female ≥50	47	38 (80.8%)	9 (19.2%)	
Male <40, female <50	24	16 (66.6%)	8 (33.4%)	
Glucose*	117 ± 42	110 ± 39	140 ± 41	<0.05
Patient groups				
DM*	40	25 (62.5%)	15 (37.5%)	<0.05
Non-DM	31	29 (93.5%)	2 (6.5%)	

*Significant variables.

Table 5: The relationship between the complications in diabetic patients and *H. pylori* eradication.

Variables	Total DM	Those eradicated	Those not eradicated	*P* value
Nephropathy				
Yes*	22	10 (45.4%)	12 (54.6%)	<0.05
No	18	15 (83.8%)	3 (16.7%)	
Neuropathy				
Yes*	24	11 (45.8%)	13 (54.2%)	<0.05
No	16	14 (87.5%)	2 (22.5%)	
Retinopathy				
Yes	16	9 (56%)	7 (44%)	NS
No	24	16 (66.6%)	8 (33.4%)	
HbA1C				
6-7*	16	13 (81.2%)	3 (18.8%)	<0.05
7-8	24	12 (50%)	12 (50%)	

*Significant variables.

and facilitate secondary *H. pylori* colonization to antibiotics taken. Based on all these factors, it can be said that the prevalence of *H. pylori* is increased in diabetics [9].

Studies report that HP infections cause microvascular damage and trigger premature development of atherosclerosis in patients [5, 6]. Although the underlying mechanism is not fully known, there are many findings which support this [5]. First of all, it has been shown that HP plays a role in the thickening of the intima media, atherosclerotic plaque destabilization, and atherosclerotic plaque development after vessel wall invasion [5, 15]. Due to vessel wall invasion of the bacteria, an increase in maturation and activation of monocytes and an increase in the proliferation of smooth muscle or endothelial cells occur, and, as a result, thrombosis and ischemia develop. It is thought that the endotoxins produced by the bacteria play a role in the maturation of monocytes. Activation of monocytes leads to the production of inflammatory cytokines, after which it triggers platelet aggregation and procoagulant activity [16]. Secondly, atherosclerotic plaques due to HP trigger high amounts of IL-6 and TNF-α. An increase in these cytokines causes endothelial dysfunction and insulin resistance. While IL-6 increases the production of hepatic gluconeogenesis and triglycerides, TNF-α modifies the lipid levels by inhibiting the lipoprotein lipase activity and activating hepatic lipogenesis [17]. Thirdly, the inflammation secondary to the plaque which forms due to HP triggers the peroxidation of membrane lipids, oxidation of LDL cholesterol, antioxidant loss, an increase in production of various superoxidases, and activation of macrophages, T-lymphocytes, and lipoprotein-a [18]. Additionally, chronic HP infection causes atrophic gastritis, and, as a result of this, it reduces absorption of folate and B12. B12 and folate are required for conversion of homocysteine to methionine. However, the homocysteine level increases due to the deficiency of B12 and folate in HP infections. Homocysteine plays a role in vascular endothelial damage and increases atherogenesis and thrombogenesis. It also increases platelet functions, coagulation, and LDL oxidation [19]. Similar to our study, many other studies have shown that, in the presence of HP infection, inflammatory indicators increase significantly [5, 20]. It has been reported that, as a result of an increase in inflammation due to HP infection and the triggering of arthrosclerosis, insulin resistance and metabolic syndrome increase, and the complications also increase in diabetic patients. A study on the Japanese population has shown that metabolic syndrome increases in HP infection [21]. Gunji et al. have shown in their study that HP infection significantly increases insulin resistance in asymptomatic patients [22]. Similar to the said studies, our study has also shown that metabolic syndrome significantly increases in patients with HP infection. Hamed et al. have shown in their study that, in HP-positive diabetic patients, the prevalence of macrovascular (cardiovascular and cerebrovascular diseases) and microvascular (nephropathy, neuropathy, and retinopathy) complications is significantly higher [5]. Furthermore, there are studies which report that microalbuminuria is significantly higher in HP-positive patients, regardless of the development of diabetes [6]. Demir et al. have reported that there is a significant relationship between HP-positivity and neuropathy, but there is no significant relationship between HP-positivity and retinopathy and neuropathy [9]. Similar to the said studies, our study has found a significant relationship between HP-positivity and neuropathy but has not found a significant relationship between HP-positivity and retinopathy.

HP eradication is more difficult in diabetic patients. Sargýn et al. attained 50% HP eradication in DM patients and 85% HP eradication in non-DM patients [7]. Zojaji et al. attained successful eradication in 62% of DM patients, and a significant relationship was found between eradication and HbA1C [23]. In a study by Tseng, it was reported that comorbid conditions such as obesity, dyslipidemia, retinopathy, and neuropathy were significantly associated with HP eradication [10]. Our study has also shown that HP eradication is significantly lower in diabetic patients with retinopathy and neuropathy and with impaired glycemic and metabolic control. The fact that the HP eradication percentage is low in diabetic patients can be explained by the immunosuppressive condition in DM patients. Additionally, frequent bacterial and mycotic infections and the development of resistance due to drug use also play an important role [24].

As a result, we have shown in our study that there is a significant relationship between HP infections and metabolic syndrome, insulin resistance, inflammations, and diabetic complications. We have also shown that similar parameters are effective in HP eradication. In the light of the studies, we think that patients with impaired metabolic and glycemic control should be treated in case of HP infection.

References

[1] R. E. Pounder and D. Ng, "The prevalence of *Helicobacter pylori* infection in different countries," *Alimentary Pharmacology & Therapeutics*, vol. 9, supplement 2, pp. 33–39, 1995.

[2] B. R. Devrajani, S. Z. A. Shah, A. A. Soomro, and T. Devrajani, "Type 2 diabetes mellitus: a risk factor for *Helicobacter pylori* infection: a hospital based case-control study," *International Journal of Diabetes in Developing Countries*, vol. 30, no. 1, pp. 22–26, 2010.

[3] J. Vafaeimanesh, M. Parham, M. Seyyedmajidi, and M. Bagherzadeh, "*Helicobacter pylori* infection and insulin resistance in diabetic and nondiabetic population," *Scientific World Journal*, vol. 2014, Article ID 391250, 5 pages, 2014.

[4] M. Talebi-Taher, M. Mashayekhi, M. H. Hashemi, and V. Bahrani, "*Helicobacter pylori* in diabetic and non-diabetic patients with dyspepsia," *Acta Medica Iranica*, vol. 50, no. 5, pp. 315–318, 2012.

[5] S. A. Hamed, N. F. Amine, G. M. Galal et al., "Vascular risks and complications in diabetes mellitus: the role of *Helicobacter pylori* infection," *Journal of Stroke and Cerebrovascular Diseases*, vol. 17, no. 2, pp. 86–94, 2008.

[6] G. E. Chung, N. J. Heo, M. J. Park, S. J. Chung, H. Y. Kang, and S. J. Kang, "*Helicobacter pylori* seropositivity in diabetic patients is associated with microalbuminuria," *World Journal of Gastroenterology*, vol. 19, no. 1, pp. 97–102, 2013.

[7] M. Sargin, O. Uygur-Bayramiçli, H. Sargýn, E. Orbay, D. Yavuzer, and A. Yayla, "Type 2 diabetes mellitus affects eradication rate of *Helicobacter pylori*," *World Journal of Gastroenterology*, vol. 9, no. 5, pp. 1126–1128, 2003.

[8] N. J. Talley, L. Young, P. Bytzer et al., "Impact of chronic gastrointestinal symptoms in diabetes mellitus on health-related quality of life," *The American Journal of Gastroenterology*, vol. 96, no. 1, pp. 71–76, 2001.

[9] M. Demir, H. S. Gokturk, N. A. Ozturk, M. Kulaksizoglu, E. Serin, and U. Yilmaz, "*Helicobacter pylori* prevalence in diabetes mellitus patients with dyspeptic symptoms and its relationship to glycemic control and late complications," *Digestive Diseases and Sciences*, vol. 53, no. 10, pp. 2646–2649, 2008.

[10] C.-H. Tseng, "Diabetes, insulin use and *Helicobacter pylori* eradication: a retrospective cohort study," *BMC Gastroenterology*, vol. 12, article 46, 2012.

[11] Y.-H. Ni, J.-T. Lin, S.-F. Huang, J.-C. Yang, and M.-H. Chang, "Accurate diagnosis of *Helicobacter pylori* infection by stool antigen test and 6 other currently available tests in children," *Journal of Pediatrics*, vol. 136, no. 6, pp. 823–827, 2000.

[12] S. Gentile, S. Turco, B. Oliviero, and R. Torella, "The role of autonomic neuropathy as a risk factor of *Helicobacter pylori* infection in dyspeptic patients with type 2 diabetes mellitus," *Diabetes Research and Clinical Practice*, vol. 42, no. 1, pp. 41–48, 1998.

[13] M. Marrollo, G. Latella, D. Melideo et al., "Increased prevalence of *Helicobacter pylori* in patients with diabetes mellitus," *Digestive and Liver Disease*, vol. 33, no. 1, pp. 21–29, 2001.

[14] R. Anastasios, C. Goritsas, C. Papamihail, R. Trigidou, P. Garzonis, and A. Ferti, "*Helicobacter pylori* infection in diabetic patients: prevalence and endoscopic findings," *European Journal of Internal Medicine*, vol. 13, no. 6, pp. 376–379, 2002.

[15] F. Franceschi, A. R. Sepulveda, A. Gasbarrini et al., "Cross-reactivity of anti-CagA antibodies with vascular wall antigens: possible pathogenic link between *Helicobacter pylori* infection and atherosclerosis," *Circulation*, vol. 106, no. 4, pp. 430–434, 2002.

[16] C. M. Bliss Jr., D. T. Golenbock, S. Keates, J. K. Linevsky, and C. P. Kelly, "*Helicobacter pylori* lipopolysaccharide binds to CD14 and stimulates release of interleukin-8, epithelial neutrophil-activating peptide 78, and monocyte chemotactic protein 1 by human monocytes," *Infection and Immunity*, vol. 66, no. 11, pp. 5357–5363, 1998.

[17] J. E. Crabtree, T. M. Shallcross, R. V. Heatley, and J. I. Wyatt, "Mucosal tumour necrosis factor α and interleukin-6 in patients with *Helicobacter pyloris* associated gastritis," *Gut*, vol. 32, no. 12, pp. 1473–1477, 1991.

[18] A. E. Kratnov and O. N. Pavlov, "*Helicobacter pylori* infection and state of antioxidant protection in patients with the unstable course of ischemic disease," *Eksperimental'naia i Klinicheskaia Gastroenterologiia*, vol. 145, no. 5, pp. 4–9, 2004.

[19] L. A. Harker, R. Ross, S. J. Slichter et al., "Homocystine induced arteriosclerosis. The role of endothelial cell injury and platelet response in its genesis," *The Journal of Clinical Investigation*, vol. 58, no. 3, pp. 731–741, 1976.

[20] J. Majka, T. Róg, P. C. Konturek et al., "Influence of chronic *Helicobacter pylori* infection on ischemic cerebral stroke risk factors," *Medical Science Monitor*, vol. 8, no. 10, pp. 675–684, 2002.

[21] T. Gunji, N. Matsuhashi, H. Sato et al., "*Helicobacter pylori* infection is significantly associated with metabolic syndrome in the Japanese population," *American Journal of Gastroenterology*, vol. 103, no. 12, pp. 3005–3010, 2008.

[22] T. Gunji, N. Matsuhashi, H. Sato et al., "*Helicobacter pylori* infection significantly increases insulin resistance in the asymptomatic Japanese population," *Helicobacter*, vol. 14, no. 5, pp. 144–150, 2009.

[23] H. Zojaji, E. Ataei, S. J. Sherafat, M. Ghobakhlou, and S. R. Fatemi, "The effect of the treatment of *Helicobacter pylori* infection on the glycemic control in type 2 diabetes mellitus," *Gastroenterology and Hepatology from Bed to Bench*, vol. 6, no. 1, pp. 36–40, 2013.

[24] V. Zweet and F. Megraud, "Diagnosis," *Current Opinion in Gastroenterology*, vol. 14, supplement 1, pp. S27–S33, 1998.

7

Effect of Aerobic Exercise Training on Blood Pressure in Indians

Sonu Punia,[1] Sivachidambaram Kulandaivelan,[1] Varun Singh,[1] and Vandana Punia[2]

[1]*Department of Physiotherapy, GJUST, Hisar 125001, India*
[2]*Human Resource Development Center, GJUST, Hisar 125001, India*

Correspondence should be addressed to Sivachidambaram Kulandaivelan; tryhard2024@yahoo.co.in

Academic Editor: Tadeusz Robak

Introduction. High blood pressure (BP) is one of the most important modifiable risk factors for cardiovascular diseases, which accounts for one in every eight deaths worldwide. It has been predicted that, by 2020, there would be 111% increase in cardiovascular deaths in India. Aerobic exercise in the form of brisk walking, jogging, running, and cycling would result in reduction in BP. Many meta-analytical studies from western world confirm this. However, there is no such review from Indian subcontinent. *Objective*. Our objective is to systematically review and report the articles from India in aerobic exercise on blood pressure. *Methodology*. Study was done in March 2016 in Google Scholar using search terms "Aerobic exercise" AND "Training" AND "Blood pressure" AND "India." This search produced 3210 titles. *Results*. 24 articles were identified for this review based on inclusion and exclusion criteria. Total of 1107 subjects participated with median of 25 subjects. Studies vary in duration from +3 weeks to 12 months with each session lasting 15–60 minutes and frequency varies from 3 to 8 times/week. The results suggest that there was mean reduction of −05.00 mmHg in SBP and −03.09 mmHg in DBP after aerobic training. *Conclusion*. Aerobic training reduces the blood pressure in Indians.

1. Introduction

Elevated blood pressure, also known as hypertension, is one of the most important modifiable risk factors for cardiovascular disease and is accounting for 10% of overall deaths in India [1]. In a meta-analysis of 142 studies from rural and urban populations of India, it was concluded that hypertension is emerging as a major health problem in India [2] and is more in urban than in rural subjects [3] and is associated with a higher risk of developing coronary heart disease (CHD), congestive heart failure, and stroke [4, 5].

Aerobic exercises are advised for health promotion and prophylaxis for many cardiovascular diseases. They refer to all exercises that involve major muscle groups and improve oxygen consumption by the body. Many methods of aerobic exercise are available like walking, jogging, running, cycling, and others. Recent meta-analytical study from western world confirms that aerobic exercise would result in clinically significant reduction in blood pressure [6]. Aerobic exercise such as walking not only improves fitness but also improves overall quality of life and decreases all-cause mortality [7, 8].

Even though it is confirmed from western world that exercises are helpful, there is little available evidence from India. Many of Indian literatures are grey in nature, that is, short studies done for postdoctoral dissertation or doctoral thesis which are not available in standard electronic database, namely, Pubmed, CINHAL, and EMBASE. However, recent rise in electronic journals with or without print copy encourages young researchers from India to publish their research in them. But these journals are not indexed in major databases and hence are not noticed and reported by other authors. Thus the objective of this paper is to collect the available literature from India using secondary search engine "Google Scholar" and derive the conclusion whether aerobic exercise is reducing blood pressure in normal and pathological conditions or not in Indians.

2. Methodology

Computerized literature search was performed using "Google Scholar" search engine during March 2016. Keywords or search protocol used for this review is "Aerobic Exercise" AND "Training" AND "Blood Pressure" AND "India." Inclusion criteria for this review were as follows: (i) experimental study with post-premeasurement of BP, (ii) aerobic exercise as the exercise intervention with minimal duration of 3 weeks, (iii) full-text articles in English published in journals with ISSN number, (iv) study done in any part of India without any time limitation, and (v) subjects being either normal or with following clinical conditions: obesity, hypertension, and diabetes. A main exclusion criterion was other clinical conditions (2 articles were excluded based on this criterion). Search protocol resulted in 3210 articles. Authors Sonu Punia and Sivachidambaram Kulandaivelan reviewed 3210 titles individually and selected articles based on inclusion and exclusion criteria. Sonu Punia selected 19 articles and Sivachidambaram Kulandaivelan selected 24 articles. Authors Vandana Punia and Varun Singh studied 43 articles and selected 25 articles (18 were duplicates). Results were prepared by Varun Singh. During this, we found two articles which used the same results in their papers [9, 10]. Recent one was excluded from the review [9].

Mean difference with 95% CI (confidence interval) for individual studies was calculated using mean, standard deviation (SD), and sample size (this was not possible in [11–15] due to nonavailability of SD). If there are 2 or more groups in an article [12, 15–17], standard mean of all groups BP values was used as single measure. Subtotal and overall reduction in SBP and DBP were calculated by adding individual BP values divided by number of studies ([18] was excluded from analysis due to this criterion). Mean difference with 95% CI was calculated using standard formula as described earlier.

3. Results

We selected 24 articles [10–33] with 1107 subjects (mean: 46; median: 25) for this review. Even though we did not use any time limits, all articles included in this reviews were from 2009 to 2015. Out of 24 articles, 13 articles [10–13, 16, 19–26] used healthy subjects and 11 articles [14, 15, 17, 18, 27–33] used clinical condition subjects with hypertension [14, 18, 27, 28] and diabetes [15, 17, 29–33]. Aerobic exercise was performed for the mean period of 40 minutes (median: 30) with a frequency of 4.8 days·week^{-1} (median: 5) and total duration of 12.5 weeks (median: 12) (Table 1).

A total of 5 articles [11, 16, 19–21] were included in young healthy adults population with total of 165 participants (mean: 33; median: 15; males/females: 73/92). The number of sessions in a week ranged from 3 to 8 sessions (mean: 5; median: 4). Total duration of program ranged from 4 to 16 weeks (mean: 11.2; median: 12.0). A total of 6 articles [12, 13, 22–25] were included in healthy middle and old age population with total of 541 participants (mean: 90; median: 25). Four articles mentioned the duration of session which ranged from 15 minutes to 45 minutes (mean: 35; median: 30). The number of sessions in a week ranged from 3 to 6 sessions (mean: 4.7; median: 5). Total duration of program ranged from 3 to 16 weeks (mean: 9; median: 11). A total of 2 articles [10, 26] were included in obese adults population with total of 40 participants (mean: 20; male/female: 30/10) (Table 1).

A total of 4 articles [14, 18, 27, 28] were included in aerobic exercise in hypertensive patients population with total of 122 participants (mean: 30.5; median: 28.5). Duration of exercise in single session ranged from 30 minutes to 60 minutes (mean: 40; median: 40). Frequency of exercise per week ranged from 3 to 5 days (mean: 4; median: 4). Total duration of exercise program ranged from 6 to 8 weeks (mean: 6.5; median: 6). A total of 7 articles [15, 17, 29–33] were included in aerobic exercise in diabetic patients population with total of 239 participants (mean: 34; median: 24). Duration of single session ranged from 15 minutes to 45 minutes (mean: 34; median: 30). Frequency of exercise per week ranged from 3 days to 7 days (mean: 5.3; median: 6). Total duration of the program ranged from 7 weeks to 52 weeks (mean: 21; median: 16) (Table 1).

Table 2 shows the effect of aerobic training of 3 weeks or more on blood pressure in individual studies basis. The results are classified into healthy adults and other clinical conditions, that is, hypertension and diabetes.

Figure 1 shows summary of aerobic training on SBP in Indians. There is a mean reduction of 3.71 mmHg (95% CI: −2.74 to −4.68) in healthy Indians, 5.38 mmHg (95% CI: −2.99 to −7.77) in hypertensive Indians, and 7.24 mmHg (95% CI: −5.89 to −8.59) in diabetic Indians. Overall, aerobic training with mean duration of 12.5 weeks reduced SBP to 05.00 mmHg (95% CI: −4.18 to −5.82) in Indians.

Figure 2 shows summary of aerobic training on DBP in Indians. There is a mean reduction of 2.79 mmHg (95% CI: −2.12 to −3.46) in healthy Indians, 3.66 mmHg (95% CI: −2.02 to −5.30) in hypertensive Indians, and 3.41 (95% CI: −2.61 to −4.21) in diabetic Indians. Overall, aerobic training with mean single session duration of 40 minutes reduced DBP to 3.09 mmHg (95% CI: −2.57 to −3.61) in Indians.

Out of 24 included articles (23 for meta-analysis), 10 studies used control group (5 healthy subjects and 5 subjects with clinical condition) [10, 12, 14, 17, 23, 24, 26, 30, 32, 33]. Subgroup analysis of control versus experimental group in healthy Indian subjects showed mean reduction of 2.92 mmHg in SBP and 2.25 mmHg in DBP in favor of experimental group. The same analysis in clinical condition showed mean reduction of 5.4 mmHg in SBP and 2.6 mmHg in DBP in favor of experimental group.

4. Discussion

Primary objective of this review is to collect and present the literature from India of aerobic exercise on blood pressure. We found 24 articles from different parts of India (north, 5, south, 10, east, 3, and west, 6). Results show 5.00 mmHg reduction in SBP and 3.09 mmHg reduction in DBP. This result is supported by several meta-analyses from western population [6, 34–36]. Cornelissen and Smart [6] studied the effect of aerobic exercise on blood pressure in 105 study groups (93 RCTs) with 3500 subjects. Their results showed

TABLE 1: Basic characteristics of included studies.

Author et al., year	Population (male/female)	Intensity	Session duration	Frequency	Total duration
Healthy young adults (n = 165)					
Dureja and Bardhan, 2014 [19]	05 (05/00)	7–10 Km/hr	15–25 minutes	6 days/week	4 weeks
Munieskhar et al., 2014 [20]	50 (00/50)	NA	30 minutes	7 days/week	12 weeks
Golda and Margaret, 2013 [11]	10 (10/00)	65–80% HRR	90 minutes	3 days/week	12 weeks
Harsoda and Purohit, 2013 [21]	15 (15/00)	10 Km/hr	30 minutes	5 days/week	12 weeks
Hulke et al., 2012 [16]	85 (43/42)	RPE	60 minutes	8 sessions/week	16 weeks
Middle and old age (n = 541)					
Karadkhedkar and Somwanshi, 2015 [22]	30 (00/30)	60–75% HR_{max}	30 minutes	5 days/week	16 weeks
Selvakumar and Raja, 2015 [12]	20	NA	NA	5 days/week	12 weeks
Singh et al., 2015 [23]	17 (06/11)	50–75% APMHR	30 minutes	5 days/week	3 weeks
Raja, 2014 [24]	15	NA	NA	6 days/week	13 weeks
Subitha et al., 2012 [25]	38 (18/20)	NA	15 minutes	3 days/week	10 weeks
Lakshminarayanan et al., 2012 [13]	421	Brisk	30 minutes	4 days/week	10 weeks
Obese adults (n = 40)					
Chaudhary et al., 2010 [10]	10 (00/10)	60–70% MHR	Till exhaustion	3 days/week	6 weeks
Raju, 2014 [26]	30 (30/00)	Varying	60 minutes	6 days/week	12 weeks
Hypertensive adults (n = 122)					
Jaiswal et al., 2015 [27]	15	50–80% HRR	30 minutes	5 days/week	6 weeks
Patel and Desai, 2014 [18]	30 (21/09)	NA	30 minutes	NA	6 weeks
Bose and Dhanalakshmi, 2012 [28]	50	60–75% HR_{max}	50 minutes	3 days/week	6 weeks
Saptharishi et al., 2009 [14]	27 (19/08)	Brisk	50–60 minutes	4 days/week	8 weeks
Diabetic adults (n = 239)					
Sadhesh and Kumar, 2014 [15]	15	NA	45 minutes	7 days/week	7 weeks
Ghosh and Roy, 2013 [29]	24 (00/24)	65–75% run/walk	15 minutes	6 days/week	25 weeks
Sanghani et al., 2013 [30]	74	Varying	45 minutes	6 days/week	26 weeks
Tiwari et al., 2012 [17]	51 (28/23)	NA	30 minutes	NA	12 weeks
Sridhar et al., 2010 [31]	55 (30/25)	NA	45 minutes	7 days/week	52 weeks
Arora et al., 2009 [32]	10 (06/04)	NA	30 minutes	3 days/week	8 weeks
Shenoy et al., 2009 [33]	10 (06/04)	NA	30 minutes	3 days/week	16 weeks

APHRM, age predicted heart rate maximum; HR_{max}, heart rate maximum; HRR, heart rate reserve; MHR, maximal heart rate; NA, not available; RPE, ratings of perceived exertion.

mean difference (MD) of −3.5 mmHg in SBP and −2.5 mmHg in DBP. Whelton et al. [35] studied effect of aerobic exercise on blood pressure in 53 RCTs (2419 subjects). They found MD of −3.84 mmHg in SBP (−4.97 to −2.72) and −2.58 mmHg in DBP (−3.35 to −1.81). Halbert et al. [36] analyzed 26 RCTs of at least 4-week aerobic training on blood pressure. Their results are similar to our findings (SBP, −04.70 mmHg, and DBP, −03.10 mmHg). All the three meta-analyses included here used either normotensive or hypertensive subjects only; diabetes was not reported in these meta-analyses. So we did another subanalysis for healthy and hypertensive studies which showed mean reduction of 4.03 mmHg (95% CI: −3.05 to −5.01) in SBP and of 2.96 mmHg (95% CI: −2.29 to −3.63) in DBP.

As compared to control group, aerobic training reduced 4.16 mmHg in SBP and 2.43 mmHg in DBP in experimental group of Indians which is lower end of 95% CI in post-premean MD of present study. This is in agreement with western meta-analysis [6, 35, 36]. We compared individual studies' SBP MD (95% CI) with overall meta-analysis' SBP mean (Figure 1) and results showed that 16 of 23 studies are in agreement with meta-analysis' SBP mean. Three articles (2 healthy subjects [16, 22] and 1 diabetic subject [31]) only deviated from meta-analysis' SBP mean. 17 of 23 studies' DBP MD (95% CI) are in agreement with meta-analysis' DBP mean (Figure 2). Two articles (both of diabetic population [29, 31]) only deviated from meta-analysis' DBP mean. This suggests that all articles' results are reliable to each other. The mean reduction of BP in all the three western meta-analyses [6, 35, 36] is within 95% CI of present meta-analysis; hence, we could predict that future studies from India will reproduce the same reduction after aerobic training.

TABLE 2: Effect of aerobic exercise training on blood pressure in Indians.

Author et al., year	Before SBP	After SBP	Before DBP	After DBP	Mean difference (MD)
Healthy young adults (n = 165)					
Dureja and Bardhan, 2014 [19]	116.00 ± 5.47	110.00 ± 6.07	79.00 ± 8.94	69.00 ± 7.41	SBP −06.00 DBP −10.00
Munieskhar et al., 2014 [20]	99.6 ± 8.38	95.1 ± 6.9	66.2 ± 5.67	62.15 ± 3.43	SBP −04.50 DBP −04.05
Golda and Margaret, 2013 [11]	128.5	121.7	80.52	78.27	SBP −06.80 DBP −02.25
Harsoda and Purohit, 2013 [21]	120.2 ± 7.55	112.2 ± 6.88	78.4 ± 8.01	75.6 ± 6.73	SBP −08.00 DBP −02.80
Hulke et al., 2012 [16]	113.74 ± 8.36	112.36 ± 6.16	73.72 ± 8.4	72.29 ± 6.56	SBP −01.38 DBP −01.43
Middle and old age (n = 541)					
Karadkhedkar and Somwanshi, 2015 [22]	126.46 ± 6.30	124.39 ± 1.86	86.03 ± 7.12	83.60 ± 7.57	SBP 02.07 DBP 02.43
Selvakumar and Raja, 2015 [12]	Control 134.34	131.48	Control 90.18	86.96	SBP −02.86 DBP −03.22
Singh et al., 2015 [23]	120.3 ± 6.6	118.1 ± 6.0	82.7 ± 6.3	81.5 ± 3.6	SBP −02.20 DBP −01.20
Raja, 2014 [24]	129.87 ± 7.96	128.60 ± 7.92	85.60 ± 5.65	84.33 ± 5.51	SBP −01.27 DBP −01.27
Subitha et al., 2012 [25]	126.89 ± 16.9	122.71 ± 14.4	77.84 ± 10.5	75.82 ± 9.46	SBP −04.18 DBP −02.02
Lakshminarayanan et al., 2012 [13]	122.40	120.84	76.81	76.07	SBP −01.56 DBP −00.74
Obese Adults (n = 40)					
Chaudhary et al., 2010 [10]	128.10 ± 4.95	124.20 ± 2.82	85.00 ± 3.27	81.80 ± 3.12	SBP −03.90 DBP −03.20
Raju, 2014 [26]	131.03 ± 4.642	127.93 ± 4.89	84.00 ± 4.02	82.33 ± 3.88	SBP −03.10 DBP −01.67
Hypertensive adults (n = 122)					
Jaiswal et al., 2015 [27]	129.46 ± 2.87	124.6 ± 1.95	81.37 ± 2.37	79.86 ± 2.56	SBP −04.86 DBP −01.51
Patel and Desai, 2014 [18]					SBP −03.35 DBP −02.00
Bose and Dhanalakshmi, 2012 [28]	145.87 ± 5.73	139.87 ± 5.92	94.80 ± 2.86	91.33 ± 2.59	SBP −06.00 DBP −03.47
Saptharishi et al., 2009 [14]	128.6	123.3	87.4	81.4	SBP −05.30 DBP −06.00
Diabetic adults (n = 239)					
Sadhesh and Kumar, 2014 [15]	119.69	112.89	74.45	74.45	SBP −06.80 DBP 00.00
Ghosh and Roy, 2013 [29]	139.66 ± 14.38	127.83 ± 13.9	80.00 ± 5.57	72.25 ± 5.46	SBP −11.80 DBP −07.75
Sanghani et al., 2013 [30]	133.47 ± 13.23	131.20 ± 10.36	84.29 ± 9.38	83.24 ± 9.02	SBP −02.27 DBP −01.05
Tiwari et al., 2012 [17]	131.92 ± 18.25	121.84 ± 15.03	84.76 ± 12.12	79.50 ± 7.48	SBP −10.08 DBP −05.26
Sridhar et al., 2010 [31]	144.24 ± 2.87	135.53 ± 3.54	88.59 ± 3.92	82.82 ± 1.07	SBP −08.71 DBP −05.77
Arora et al., 2009 [32]	132 ± 8.5	124 ± 11.6	84 ± 5.3	81 ± 8.2	SBP −08.00 DBP −03.00
Shenoy et al., 2009 [33]	132 ± 8.5	129 ± 11.6	84 ± 5.3	83 ± 7.4	SBP −03.00 DBP −01.00

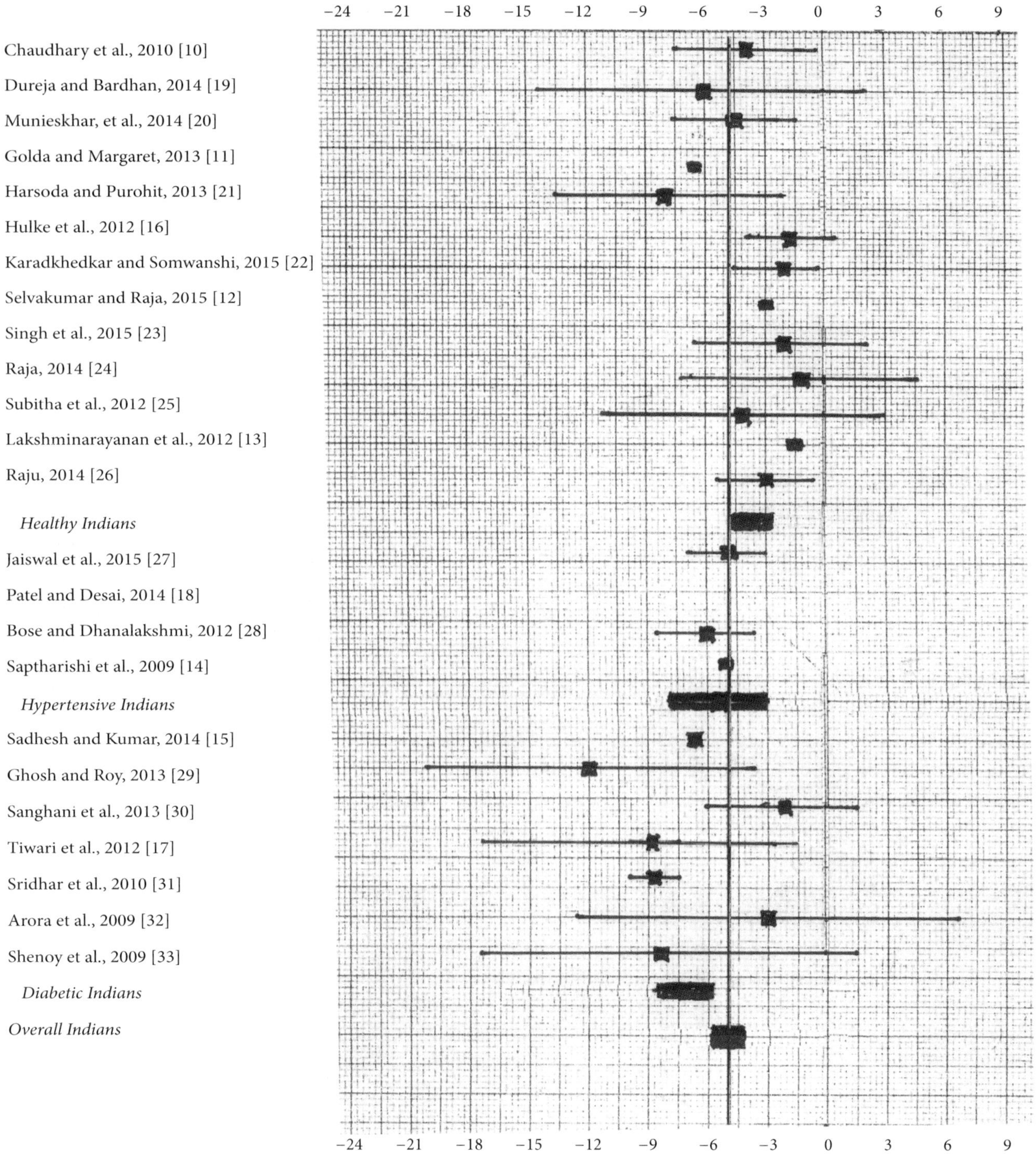

FIGURE 1: Summary of aerobic training on SBP (mean difference with 95% CI) in Indians. Bold vertical line is meta-analysis mean ($n = 23$).

Hypertension is a growing problem in India with every third to fifth Indian as hypertensive [2, 37, 38]. Approximately 10% of death in India was attributable to high blood pressure [39]. It is the third leading risk factor for disease burden in both developed and developing nations worldwide [40]. According to SEEK study, ischemic heart disease, stroke, and peripheral vascular diseases are significantly higher in hypertensive Indian population than in control [41]. In a recent meta-analysis of 18 prospective cohorts, compared to normotension, prehypertension elevated the risk of cardiovascular disease (CVD) by 1.55 (relative risk, RR), coronary heart disease (CHD) by 1.50, and stroke by 1.71 [4]. It is one of the most common modifiable risk factors in CVD. Mean reduction of 3.0 mmHg in SBP could reduce mortality from CHD by 6% and from stroke by 9% [42]. Another study found that rise of SBP by 3.0 mmHg and DBP by 2.3 mmHg

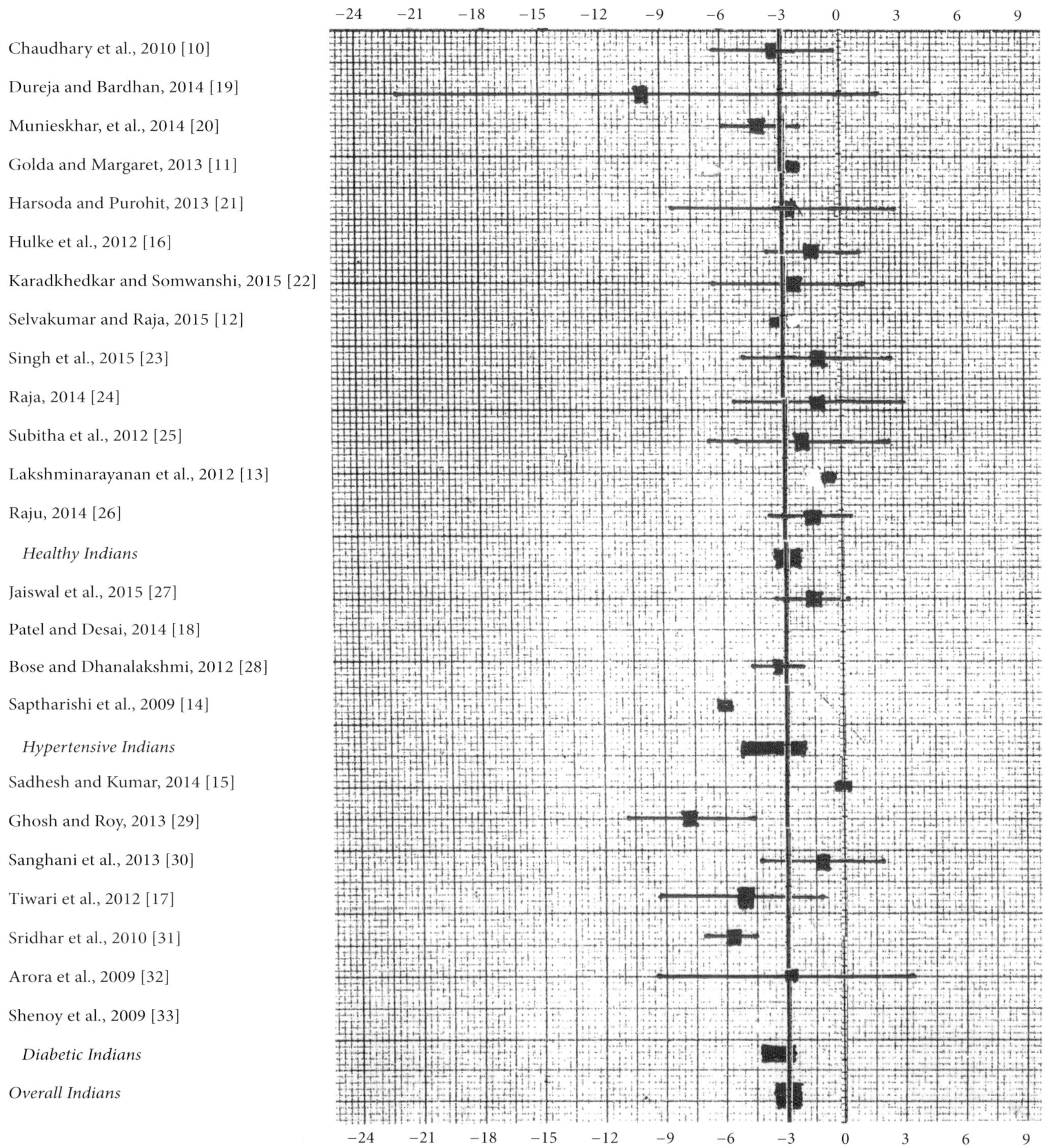

FIGURE 2: Summary of aerobic training on DBP (mean difference with 95% CI) in Indians. Bold vertical line is meta-analysis mean ($n = 23$).

would result in estimated 12% increased risk for CHD and 24% increased risk for stroke [43].

There are some limitations observed in this review. We used improvement in BP using after minus before values, except one study [12], and one study used MD instead of blood pressure values [18]. Sample size, training duration, session duration, and frequency of training are varied between studies which may underestimate or overestimate our interpretations in results and we do not use any statistical tests to see their association with BP lowering effect.

5. Conclusion

Aerobic training of 4-week duration would reduce BP to a clinically significant level in Indian population. This reduction is more pronounced in clinical conditions like hypertension and diabetes. So this type of training should be used as primary prevention in high risk population and as secondary prevention in hypertension, diabetes, and so forth.

Competing Interests

The authors declare that there are no competing interests regarding the publication of this paper.

References

[1] V. Patel, S. Chatterji, D. Chisholm et al., "Chronic diseases and injuries in India," *The Lancet*, vol. 377, no. 9763, pp. 413–428, 2011.

[2] R. Anchala, N. K. Kannuri, H. Pant et al., "Hypertension in India: a systematic review and meta-analysis of prevalence, awareness, and control of hypertension," *Journal of Hypertension*, vol. 32, no. 6, pp. 1170–1177, 2014.

[3] R. Gupta, "Convergence in urban-rural prevalence of hypertension in India," *Journal of Human Hypertension*, vol. 30, no. 2, pp. 79–82, 2016.

[4] Y. Huang, S. Wang, X. Cai et al., "Prehypertension and incidence of cardiovascular disease: a meta-analysis," *BMC Medicine*, vol. 11, no. 1, article 177, pp. 1–9, 2013.

[5] J. Hsia, K. L. Margolis, C. B. Eaton et al., "Prehypertension and cardiovascular disease risk in the women's health initiative," *Circulation*, vol. 115, no. 7, pp. 855–860, 2007.

[6] V. A. Cornelissen and N. A. Smart, "Exercise training for blood pressure: a systematic review and meta-analysis," *Journal of the American Heart Association*, vol. 2, no. 1, Article ID e004473, 2013.

[7] K. Ueshima, K. Ishikawa-Takata, T. Yorifuji et al., "Physical activity and mortality risk in the Japanese elderly. A cohort study," *American Journal of Preventive Medicine*, vol. 38, no. 4, pp. 410–418, 2010.

[8] M. Reiner, C. Niermann, D. Jekauc, and A. Woll, "Long-term health benefits of physical activity—a systematic review of longitudinal studies," *BMC Public Health*, vol. 13, no. 1, article 813, pp. 1–9, 2013.

[9] P. K. Changela, "A study to compare the effect of aerobic and resistance training on cardiovascular fitness in young obese sedentary females," *International Journal of Scientific and Research Publications*, vol. 3, no. 2, 9 pages, 2013.

[10] S. Chaudhary, M. K. Kang, and J. S. Sandhu, "The effects of aerobic versus resistance training on cardiovascular fitness in obese sedentary females," *Asian Journal of Sports Medicine*, vol. 1, no. 4, pp. 177–184, 2010.

[11] J. Golda and J. G. D. Margaret, "Impact of cardio-respiratory endurance training resistance training and core strength training on selected physiological variables among college athletes," *Journal of Academic Sports Scholar*, vol. 2, no. 12, 5 pages, 2013.

[12] S. Selvakumar and S. C. Raja, "Effects of aerobic exercise programme on different terrains on blood pressure and assertiveness," *International Journal of Recent Research and Applied Studies*, vol. 2, no. 13, pp. 55–58, 2015.

[13] S. Lakshminarayanan, S. M. Bala, M. Ramanujam, and G. Kannan, "Effectiveness of physical activity promotion in blood pressure and blood sugar reduction: a community-based intervention study in rural south India," *Journal of Family and Community Medicine*, vol. 19, no. 2, pp. 81–87, 2012.

[14] L. G. Saptharishi, M. B. Soudarssanane, D. Thiruselvakumar et al., "Community-based randomized controlled trial of non-pharmacological interventions in prevention and control of hypertension among young adults," *Indian Journal of Community Medicine*, vol. 34, no. 4, pp. 329–334, 2009.

[15] A. Sadhesh and G. V. Kumar, "Influence of low to moderate intense training between type 1 and type 2 diabetic," *International Journal of Health, Physical Education & Computer Science in Sports*, vol. 16, pp. 68–72, 2014.

[16] S. M. Hulke, Y. P. Vaidya, and A. R. Ratta, "Effects of sixteen weeks exercise training on left ventricular dimensions and function in young athletes," *National Journal of Physiology, Pharmacy & Pharmacology*, vol. 2, no. 2, pp. 152–158, 2012.

[17] S. Tiwari, S. Gehlot, S. K. Tiwari, and G. Singh, "Effect of walking (aerobic isotonic exercise) on physiological variants with special reference to *Prameha* (diabetes mellitus) as per *Prakriti*," *AYU*, vol. 33, no. 1, pp. 44–49, 2012.

[18] H. Patel and D. Desai, "A study to evaluate the changes in blood pressure values of hypertensive patients post aerobic and progressive resistance exercise (PRE)," *International Journal of Health Sciences and Research*, vol. 3, no. 2, pp. 183–189, 2014.

[19] G. Dureja and S. Bardhan, "Effect of treadmill training on blood pressure among young adult boys," *Education Practice and Innovation*, vol. 1, no. 1, pp. 1–5, 2014.

[20] K. Munieskhar, M. V. Muralidhar, M. Venkatachalam, and D. Hemalatha, "Comparision of heart rate and blood pressure changes during walking and running before and after training in healthy adult women," *International Journal of Physiotherapy and Research*, vol. 2, no. 3, pp. 537–541, 2014.

[21] J. M. Harsoda and G. Purohit, "Effect of different modes of aerobic exercise on cardiorespiratory efficiency and exercise performance in sedentary males," *International Journal of Basic and Applied Physiology*, vol. 2, no. 1, p. 72, 2013.

[22] S. Karadkhedkar and N. D. Somwanshi, "Effect of aerobic training on VO_2 max and other physiological parameters in working women," *Indian Journal of Clinical Anatomy and Physiology*, vol. 2, no. 2, pp. 105–107, 2015.

[23] V. Singh, P. Thakur, and B. Khandelwal, "Effectiveness of short-term aerobic exercise program on cardiovascular risk profile in moderate risk adults: a randomized controlled pilot study," *CHRISMED Journal of Health and Research*, vol. 2, no. 1, pp. 38–45, 2015.

[24] S. C. Raja, "Effect of yogic practices and physical exercises on strength endurance self-concept and blood pressure," *International Journal of Physical Education Sports Management and Yogic Sciences*, vol. 4, no. 3, pp. 7–11, 2014.

[25] L. Subitha, S. M. Bala, and M. Ramanujam, "Community based physical exercise program for the elderly in South India," *National Journal of Community Medicine*, vol. 3, no. 4, pp. 675–680, 2012.

[26] P. S. Raju, "Twelve weeks of aerobic dance impact on cardiovascular parameters of male obese adults," *International Journal of Physical Education, Fitness & Sports*, vol. 3, no. 1, pp. 51–55, 2014.

[27] A. V. Jaiswal, A. H. Kazi, S. B. Gunjal, P. M. Tawde, A. A. Mahajan, and S. M. Khatri, "Effectiveness of interval training versus circuit training exercises on blood pressure, heart rate

and rate of perceived exertion in individual with prehypertension," *International Journal of Health Sciences and Research*, vol. 5, no. 10, pp. 149–156, 2015.

[28] M. Bose and V. Dhanalakshmi, "Effect of short duration aerobic exercises on resting blood pressure and heart rate in prehypertensive and stage 1 hypertensive subjects," *International Journal of Physiotherapy and Occupational Therapy*, vol. 6, no. 4, pp. 191–195, 2012.

[29] S. S. Ghosh and G. S. Roy, "Effects of six month aerobic training on selected physiological variables of moderately active female NIDDM," *International Journal of Movement Education and Social Science*, vol. 2, no. 2, pp. 4–8, 2013.

[30] N. B. Sanghani, D. N. Parchwani, K. M. Palandurkar, A. M. Shah, and J. V. Dhanani, "Impact of lifestyle modification on glycemic control in patients with type 2 diabetes mellitus," *Indian Journal of Endocrinology and Metabolism*, vol. 17, no. 6, pp. 1030–1039, 2013.

[31] B. Sridhar, N. Haleagrahara, R. Bhat, A. B. Kulur, S. Avabratha, and P. Adhikary, "Increase in the heart rate variability with deep breathing in diabetic patients after 12-month exercise training," *Tohoku Journal of Experimental Medicine*, vol. 220, no. 2, pp. 107–113, 2010.

[32] E. Arora, S. Shenoy, and J. S. Sandhu, "Effects of resistance training on metabolic profile of adults with type 2 diabetes," *Indian Journal of Medical Research*, vol. 129, no. 5, pp. 515–519, 2009.

[33] S. Shenoy, E. Arora, and J. Sandhu, "Effects of progressive resistance training and aerobic exercise on type 2 diabetics in Indian population," *International Journal of Diabetes & Metabolism*, vol. 17, pp. 27–30, 2009.

[34] V. A. Cornelissen and R. H. Fagard, "Effects of endurance training on blood pressure, blood pressure-regulating mechanisms, and cardiovascular risk factors," *Hypertension*, vol. 46, no. 4, pp. 667–675, 2005.

[35] S. P. Whelton, A. Chin, X. Xin, and J. He, "Effect of aerobic exercise on blood pressure: a meta-analysis of randomized, controlled trials," *Annals of Internal Medicine*, vol. 136, no. 7, pp. 493–503, 2002.

[36] J. A. Halbert, C. A. Silagy, P. Finucane, R. T. Withers, P. A. Hamdorf, and G. R. Andrews, "The effectiveness of exercise training in lowering blood pressure: a meta-analysis of randomised controlled trials of 4 weeks or longer," *Journal of Human Hypertension*, vol. 11, no. 10, pp. 641–649, 1997.

[37] T. Midha, B. Nath, R. Kumari, Y. K. Rao, and U. Pandey, "Prevalence of hypertension in India: a meta-analysis," *World Journal of Meta-Analysis*, vol. 1, no. 2, pp. 83–89, 2013.

[38] P. Devi, M. Rao, A. Sigamani et al., "Prevalence, risk factors and awareness of hypertension in India: a systematic review," *Journal of Human Hypertension*, vol. 27, no. 5, pp. 281–287, 2013.

[39] V. Patel, S. Chatterji, D. Chisholm et al., "Chronic diseases and injuries in India," *The Lancet*, vol. 377, no. 9763, pp. 413–428, 2011.

[40] M. Ezzati, A. D. Lopez, A. Rodgers, S. Vander Hoorn, and C. J. L. Murray, "Selected major risk factors and global and regional burden of disease. Comparative risk assessment collaborating Group," *The Lancet*, vol. 360, no. 9343, pp. 1347–1360, 2002.

[41] Y. M. K. Farag, B. V. Mittal, S. R. Keithi-Reddy et al., "Burden and predictors of hypertension in India: results of SEEK (Screening and Early Evaluation of Kidney Disease) study," *BMC Nephrology*, vol. 15, article 42, 2014.

[42] J. Stamler, G. Rose, R. Stamler, P. Elliott, A. Dyer, and M. Marmot, "INTERSALT study findings. Public health and medical care implications," *Hypertension*, vol. 14, no. 5, pp. 570–577, 1989.

[43] P. Poirier, T. D. Giles, G. A. Bray et al., "Obesity and cardiovascular disease: pathophysiology, evaluation, and effect of weight loss: an update of the 1997 American Heart Association Scientific Statement on Obesity and Heart Disease from the Obesity Committee of the Council on Nutrition, Physical Activity, and Metabolism," *Circulation*, vol. 113, no. 6, pp. 898–918, 2006.

Exploring the Unmet Needs of the Patients in the Outpatient Respiratory Medical Clinic: Patients versus Clinicians Perspectives

Lone Birgitte Skov Jensen,[1,2] Ulf Brinkjær,[1] Kristian Larsen,[3] and Hanne Konradsen[4]

[1] *Department of Education, University of Aarhus, 2400 Copenhagen, Denmark*
[2] *Respiratory Department, Gentofte University Hospital, 2900 Gentofte, Denmark*
[3] *Department of Education, Learning and Philosophy, University of Aalborg, 2450 Copenhagen, Denmark*
[4] *Gentofte University Hospital, 2900 Gentofte, Denmark*

Correspondence should be addressed to Lone Birgitte Skov Jensen; lonebirgitteskovjensen@gmail.com

Academic Editor: Karen Hirschman

Aim. Developing a theoretical framework explaining patients' behaviour and actions related to unmet needs during interactions with health care professionals in hospital-based outpatient respiratory medical clinics. *Background*. The outpatient respiratory medical clinic plays a prominent role in many patients' lives regarding treatment and counselling increasing the need for a better understanding of patients' perspective to the counselling of the health care professionals. *Design*. The study is exploratory and based on Charmaz's interpretation of grounded theory. *Methods*. The study included 65 field observations with a sample of 43 patients, 11 doctors, and 11 nurses, as well as 30 interviews with patients, conducted through theoretical sampling from three outpatient respiratory medical clinics in Denmark. *Findings*. The patients' efforts to share their significant stories triggered predominantly an adaptation or resistance behaviour, conceptualized as "fitting in" and "fighting back" behaviour, explaining the patients' counterreactions to unrecognized needs during the medical encounter. *Conclusion*. Firstly this study allows for a better understanding of patients' counterreactions in the time-pressured and, simultaneously, tight structured guidance program in the outpatient clinic. Secondly the study offers practical and ethical implications as to how health care professionals' attitudes towards patients can increase their ability to support emotional suffering and increase patient participation and responsiveness to guidance in the lifestyle changes.

1. Introduction

The burden of chronic respiratory diseases (CRDs) is increasing worldwide, and knowledge about the physical, mental, and social consequences of these diseases is extensive [1–4]. Generally, hospital outpatient clinics play a prominent role in the Nordic countries' health care systems. In Denmark, the number of outpatient visits to somatic hospital departments increased by 34% from 4,917,000 in 2002 to 6,612,000 in 2009 [5]. The outpatient respiratory medical clinic (ORMC) receives referrals after the patients' discharge from medical wards or by their general practitioner for the purpose of processing diagnosis, rehabilitation, and counselling or drug treatment. Many patients with CRD suffering from severe or very severe CRD are followed up regularly in the ORMC, according to the "chronic care model" guidelines and recommendations [6]. Patients who suffer from CRD may be vulnerable in many ways: CRD is associated with increased risk of anxiety, insomnia, fatigue, anorexia, loneliness, guilt, isolation, and depression [7–13]. As CRD progresses, it is characterized by severe daily symptoms such as shortness of breath, cough, and increased mucus production [1]. Thus, these diseases have not only physical but also existential implications in terms of their existence-threatening progressive and, over time, terminal character [14–16]. At the same time, it is well documented that many patients suffering from

CRD may have limited economic and educational resources and, over time, a reduced and limited network [17–19]. In light of the fact that CRDs are characterized by their chronic, progressive, and lethal nature, there is a growing awareness of the need for more palliative-directed treatment and care for these patients [20, 21]. As suggested in other studies, the outpatient clinics are subject to many temporal, structural, and substantial requirements that may impact what may be talked about and how long the conversation can last [22–24]. These factors may limit opportunities to recognize and listen to patients' experiences during interactions [25]. Several studies suggest that patients' stories may offer important knowledge of how patients overcome, adapt to, and understand life with CRD [10, 26].

Furthermore, these stories may reveal strong emotions and existential suffering in patients [27–29]. The aspects of limited time and the many demands on the content of the consultation seem to influence what the health care professional (HCP) can hope to accomplish during counselling [22]. Several studies point to external factors affecting the lack of patient involvement and HCPs' responsiveness to patients' existential and emotional suffering [30], including aspects such as increasing work pressure, numerous changes in the structure of tasks, implementation of new or changed administrative tasks, and increasing demands for documentation [25, 31]. Furthermore, the demands of patients regarding empathy and the recognition of their suffering may exhaust HCPs and cause burnout [25, 31]. At the same time, many studies suggest that HCPs have a large potential to be instrumental in facilitating patients' coping and self-care management and optimizing their quality of life or, conversely, damaging these processes [8, 21, 32, 33].

Over the last several decades, the former authoritative approach of the HCP has been replaced by an ideological, institutional, and also vocational desire to include chronically ill patients in their own care and treatment [34–36]. Today, being patient-oriented is immensely popular with health authorities in many Western countries, as it reflects a moral philosophical approach in which the patient is regarded as unique and the multidimensionality of the human experience of illness is recognized through a relation that builds on multiple understandings of the patient's situation [37, 38]. Studies show that this paradigm change is not always implemented and present during the patient-HCP interaction [19, 39]. The studies emphasized here, based primarily on hospitalized CRD patients, suggest that the interaction with patients may be difficult for multiple reasons. The assumption was, consistent with other studies in related areas [22], that several specific characteristics affect the outpatient interaction. These characteristics arise from the typically short-term and very structured content and time frame for each consultation, which is of relevance to the extent and the content of the interaction since the demarcated time for counselling and treatment may create limitations for the interaction and HCPs' ability to meet the needs of patients. Whether this is the case in the ORMC has not been addressed in other studies exploring how the short time sessions affect the interaction in similar or particular ways. There seems to be a lack of studies exploring the clinical encounter in the ORMC [23, 24, 40] and none exploring the processes of interaction between patients and HCPs. Targeted attention to the patient's perspectives, reactions to actions, and behaviour could contribute to increased insight into patient's concerns and expectations. This study aims to contribute with knowledge in this area concerning the needs and behaviour of the patients and patients' reactions to the actions of the HCP's during the short-term counselling in the ORMC.

2. The study

2.1. Aim. The aim of the study was to develop a theoretical framework explaining patients' behaviour and actions related to unmet needs during interactions with health care professionals in hospital-based outpatient respiratory medical clinics.

2.2. Participants. This study includes 65 field observations and 30 individual interviews with patients with a sample of 43 patients, 11 doctors, and 11 nurses, in total 22 HCPs, from three ORMCs in Denmark during a period of 18 months in 2012-2013. The patients all suffered from CRD and were aged 45 to 91 years. The patients' experiences with the ORMC varied and spanned from initial contact to four years' association with several annually recurring consultations. The first 13 patients, 7 women and 6 men, were included exclusively for purposeful sampling conducting the initial field observations during patient-HCP interactions in clinic 3. Nine patients suffered from COPD and 2 from fibrosis, and 3 did not have a definitive diagnosis at the inclusion time. The purpose of the initial field observations was to explore possible central interactional themes. Out of the subsequent 30 included patients, 17 had COPD exclusively, 4 had COPD and asthma, 3 had emphysema, 2 had fibrosis, and 3 had other interstitial lung diseases. Demographic data of the participating patients are shown in Table 1.

A total of 22 HCPs, 11 doctors and 11 nurses, were included from the same 3 ORMCs as the patients in the field observations. The number and the distribution of field observations on patient/health care professional interactions are shown in Table 2. The HCPs were included to the extent that they were communicating with participating patients during the field observations, as illustrated in Table 2.

2.3. The Outpatient Respiratory Medical Clinic. The nurses and doctors worked in separate premises and with different tasks related to the patients. Doctor-patient conversation lasted 15–20 minutes and typically referred to the status of the disease, the effect of medicine, and possible revision, referring to rehabilitation in the municipality or hospital for further investigation and assessment. Nurse-patient conversation lasted 15–45 minutes and covered disease status, lung function tests, MRC breathlessness scale, and body mass index, as well as guidance in lifestyle changes and advice and recommendations related to these subjects. All included clinics used a primary nurse and doctor system for all CRD patients, and nurses and doctors held separate individual consultations in the included clinics.

TABLE 1: Demographic data, included patients.

Participant patients	Age	Clinic	Education	Employment	Lung disease	Stage	Chronic diseases
01–013 (7 female, 6 male)	—	3	—	—	6 COPD; 3 lung fibrosis; 3 without diagnosis	—	—
1 Female	68	1	White collar	Pensioner	Sarcoidosis	Mild	4
2 Male	52	1	Blue collar	Working	Alpha-1 antitrypsin deficiency	Severe	2
3 Male	59	1	Blue collar	Working		Moderate	2
4 Female	52	1	White collar	Working	Asthma; COPD	Moderate	2
5 Male	79	1	Blue collar	Pensioner	Emphysema	Mild	4
6 Female	45	1	Blue collar	Early retirement	COPD	Moderate	6
7 Male	49	1	Blue collar	Early retirement	Alpha-1 antitrypsin deficiency	Severe	1
8 Female	58	3	Academician	Working	COPD, asthma	Severe	2
9 Male	82	3	White collar	Pensioner	Emphysema	Moderate	2
10 Female	74	3	Employer	Pensioner	COPD	Moderate	2
11 Female	82	3	White collar	Pensioner	COPD	Moderate	3
12 Female	53	2	Blue collar	Working	COPD	Mild	2
13 Female	55	2	Blue collar	Sickness benefit	Asthma; COPD	Severe	2
14 Female	78	2	White collar	Pensioner	COPD	Moderate	2
15 Female	82	2	White collar	Pensioner	COPD	Moderate	2
16 Male	85	2	Blue collar	Pensioner	COPD	Moderate	1
17 Male	72	2	White collar	Pensioner	COPD	Severe	1
18 Female	91	2	White collar	Pensioner	COPD	Mild	2
19 Female	75	2	Academician	Pensioner	COPD	Moderate	1
20 Female	62	2	Academician	Early retirement	Emphysema	Severe	3
21 Female	66	3	Blue collar	Early retirement	COPD	Moderate	6
22 Male	52	3	White collar	Sickness benefit	COPD	Severe	3
23 Male	71	3	Blue collar	Pensioner	Pulmonary fibrosis	Severe	2
24 Male	59	2	Academician	Pensioner	COPD	Mild	2
25 Male	73	3	Blue collar	Pensioner	COPD	Moderate	2
26 Male	71	3	Blue collar	Pensioner	COPD	Moderate	1
27 Male	67	3	Blue collar	Pensioner	Pulmonary fibrosis	Severe	2
28 Male	62	3	Blue collar	Early retirement	COPD	Moderate	1
29 Female	82	3	White collar	Pensioner	COPD	Moderate	1
30 Female	58	2	Academician	Early retirement	Asthma; COPD	Severe	2

Stage: Spirometry measures airflow. Classification of patients' lung function is highlighted by the HCP during HCP-patient interaction and written down by researcher during the field observations.

2.4. Data Collection. The patients were included and observed at different stages of the outpatient clinic course, including initial consultations, subsequent visits, diagnosis meetings, and conclusive meetings. The patients were included upon arrival to the outpatient clinic and invited to participate, thus giving the researcher permission to observe the interaction during the visit. The patients were followed during the waiting time before and in between the conversations, which often included conversations with a nurse and then a doctor and occasionally a follow-up conversation with the nurse concerning medication intake or a new appointment in the ORMC. The field observations lasted between 20 minutes and 2.5 hours. All patients were followed during their entire stay in the clinic. Before the patient left, a home visit or a phone interview was scheduled. The researcher's field observations were nonparticipatory in the ORMC during the counselling and interactions between the patients and HCPs. Between examinations and interviews, the researcher participated in conversations with the patients, brought coffee, and listened to stories about, for example, everyday life, individual coping with illness and disease, and the patient's individual experiences of interactions with HCPs. While listening and talking, the interviewer wrote down important points, ideas, and statements as memos [41]. These relaxed and unrecorded conversations gave important information about the patients'

TABLE 2: Field observations during patient-HCP interaction in ORMC.

HCP-nr.	Sex	Clinic	Profession	HCP counselling PT nr.
HCP 1	Female	3	RN	22; 29
HCP 2	Female	3	RN	26; 27
HCP 3	Female	3	RN	23; 28
HCP 4	Female	3	RN	2; 10
HCP 5	Female	3	RN	8; 9; 11; 24
HCP 6	Male	3	MD	9; 10; 23
HCP 7	Male	3	MD	24; 26; 27
HCP 8	Male	3	MD	01–013; 11; 22
HCP 9	Female	1	RN	2; 4
HCP 10	Female	1	RN	1; 3; 6
HCP 11	Female	1	MD	7
HCP 12	Male	1	MD	1; 3
HCP 13	Male	1	MD	5; 4; 6
HCP 14	Female	2	RN	16; 15; 17
HCP 15	Female	2	RN	20; 21; 30
HCP 16	Female	2	RN	13; 19
HCP 17	Female	2	RN	12; 14; 18
HCP 18	Male	2	MD	12; 13
HCP 19	Female	2	MD	21; 14
HCP 20	Female	2	MD	19; 25
HCP 21	Female	2	MD	15; 20
HCP 22	Male	2	MD	13; 14
Field observations in total:				**65**

HCP: healthcare professionals; RN: registered nurse; MD: medical doctor.

experiences regarding the ORMC, everyday life at home, and relations with close relatives. Insofar as it was possible for the patient, the follow-up interview was performed within a week of the visit to strengthen both the patient's and the researcher's ability to remember important topics for conversation or other areas that the researchers wanted to cover. Out of the 30 interviews, 19 took place in the patients' own homes and 11 interviews were performed by phone, in accordance with the patient's needs and preferences. The interviews lasted between 25 minutes and 3 hours. All interviews were tape-recorded and transcribed verbatim afterwards. The interview guide was initially loosely structured, exploring issues concerning the patient's perspectives, expectations, experiences and outcome of the interaction, view on health and illness, and the personal and unique challenges and joys of everyday life. The focus of data collection of the included HCPs was to understand and explain how the HCP actions during the interaction triggered counterreactions and actions in patients.

The included field observations of the HCPs had the purpose of exploring the actions of the HCPs to increase the understanding of what patients reacted to and how patients reacted and identifying the meaning and significance attributed to the interaction when the needs of the patients were predominantly unmeet.

2.5. Ethical Considerations. All interviews and field observations have been carried out with respect to the HCPs' and patients' experiences and actions. It has been a balancing act to be loyal to the participants' understanding of their actions and interpretations while being able to say something more and something different than the respondents could say. The project was carried out in accordance with ICN's code of ethics for nursing research [42] and approved by the Danish Data Protection Agency (j.nr. 2011-41-6670). Oral and written information about the study was given to the participants, including information on anonymity, informed consent, confidentiality, and the right to end participation at any time without stating any reason. All personal identifiers have been removed or disguised, and the participants are not identifiable and cannot be identified through the details of the stories.

2.6. Design and Data Analysis. The study is exploratory and based on Charmaz's social constructionist interpretation of grounded theory [43–45]. An important source of inspiration from symbolic interactionism is an approach to the research field in which social processes are regarded as not only structural but also situational and changeable over time [46]. In line with this way of thinking, this study's focus is on researching the meaning and action in specific situations as close to an inner perspective as possible, acknowledging that it is not possible to duplicate the participants' experiences [45]. The coding process led to identifying what was happening in the data, explaining the elements of the emergent theory generating categories that were made more and more abstract as data were gathered to refine the theory. During *initial coding*, fragments of data—words, lines, segments, and incidents—were closely studied for their analytic import. During *focused coding*, the most fruitful initial codes were selected and tested against extensive data to determine their analytical importance to categories in accordance with the constant comparative method in grounded theory studies. The process of data collection and initial and focused coding ended when the categories were saturated and when gathering fresh data no longer revealed new theoretical insights or new properties of the categories. During the data coding and analysis, the focus was directed towards the fact that many patients apparently felt a lack of HCPs' responsiveness to their problems and perspectives during interactions and was given limited possibilities to influence what the conversation could include, which was found to be a prominent frustration for patients in the follow-up interview.

2.7. Rigour. The criteria for validating the findings followed Charmaz's credibility, originality, resonance, and usefulness [45, 47]. A clear and rigorous working process, as described in the data analysis, assured credibility. *Originality* can be met by the fact that this study offers new knowledge regarding patients' responses to unmet needs during interactions in an underexposed area where knowledge is limited. To achieve *resonance*, the study must be relevant to the participants. Several of the participating patients pointed out the importance of developing better understanding and visibility of their needs in the ORMC. At the same time, the participating HCPs showed great interest in the study and recognized, among other things, the need of the patients to express feelings during their stories in the time-pressed ORMC, and they confirmed and recognized the experience of not having the time to examine patients' perspectives of life experiences with illness. *Usefulness* may be difficult to assess at this stage. Subsequent studies should examine, adjust, and adapt the findings to further shape the theory and identify possible practical implications for HCPs' practice.

3. Findings: Striving to Share the Significant Story

During the coding and analysis process, it became clear that the unmet needs of the patient triggered counterreactions initially conceptualized as resistance and adaptation behaviour.

Based on the data, a decision was made to pursue the findings of the unmet needs of patients based on patients' perspective. This does not mean that no positive and stimulating interactions were identified. But a research decision based on the data led us to unfold the patients' behaviour and experiences related to interactions in which they did not feel seen, heard, and recognized focusing on partially as well as predominantly failed interactions on the basis of the patients' comprehension. To investigate and compare processes related to patients' need to be seen and heard, subsequent patients were sampled to ensure a variation in patient experiences to unmet needs. Further investigation during data collection verified or modified this first impression and led to the sample included in this study as listed in Table 1.

The analysis generated a substantive theory explaining how a main concern of many patients was "striving to share the significant story" comprising the significant individual issues related to their coping of illness or existential aspects of their everyday life. Regardless of the patients' behaviour, they rarely had the opportunity to tell their stories during the interactions. Patients' efforts to share their story and their reactions when this demand was unmet by the HCP triggered an adaptation or resistance behaviour, conceptualized as a "fitting in" or "fighting back" behaviour, explaining the patients' counterreactions when they were not seen, heard, and recognized during the medical encounter. The lack of shared understanding to the content of the interaction is illustrated in Figure 1.

When the patients responded through "fitting in" behaviour, the HCP apparently assumed as if the patients were responsive and adaptive to the organized agenda. When patients responded through a "fighting back" behaviour, the HCP reacted with resignation, discomfort, frustration, or resentment. The "fitting in" and "fighting back" behaviour could overlap, balance, and shift during the interaction, and both behaviours could appear in the same interaction with varying strength at various times. Sometimes they would emerge during the interaction, and, in other situations, the patient had already chosen behaviour to the expected responses from the HCP. Neither of these two reactions created a basis for mutual understanding of the interaction, whether the patient adapted to a "fitting in" or "fighting back" behaviour. The counterreactions of the patients to HCPs' responses were affected by individual negotiation and adaptation in interactions regarding patients' efforts to play an active role during the interaction, their wanting of the HCP to respond to emotional statements, and their opportunities to modify their own expectations of content and counselling during the interaction. These recurring structural modes of patients were conceptualized as *role negotiation*, *emotional resonance*, and *perspective modification* modes and determinations of the meaning and significance attributed to the interactions when the needs of the patients were predominantly unmet. The process attributed to the interactions when the needs of the patients were predominantly unmet is explained in Figure 2.

The outcome of role negotiation, perspective modification, and emotional resonance in patients determined the behaviour of either "fitting in" or "fighting back" and whether the patient adapted to or resisted the HCP-planned guidance for procedures and issues during counselling.

The HCPs displayed several actions to modify, maintain, and control the content of the conversation. This includes HCPs' resignation to "let the patients talk" when they finished practical tasks. In other cases, the HCP could elude the patient's story by interruption, distraction, or an appeal to the fixed programme of the counselling session in order to win back control of the conversation. In other cases, the time for each session was used as an argument to prevent the patient from telling his or her story:

> *We have to move on to... (HCP 14), if we are to finish all of this in time, we need to... (HCP 20), Let's stick with the lungs, shall we? (HCP 8)*

The various modification mechanisms used to minimize or exclude patients' stories included lack of reply, interruptions, listening in silence, lack of eye contact or physical contact, or referral to limited time. In some cases, the actions of the HCP resulted in the patient continuously insisting on telling the story, but mostly they closed down the patient's stories.

3.1. "Fitting In" Behaviour. "Fitting in" behaviour conceptualized a passive patient role, which maintained a mutually recognizable and, on the surface, smooth, evolving, and developing framework for interactions. "Fitting in" consisted of resignation, adjustment, and surrender behaviour during interactions by handing over control and the power to distinguish between important and less important topics of conversation. Patients gave up telling their significant story and adjusted to the HCP's objectives for conversation related to treatment or illness subjects concerning CRD recommendations, hospital standards, and guidelines. The HCP could reward "fitting in" behaviour with recognition of and attention to the patient's cooperation. "Fitting in" behaviour created a harmonic and consensual interaction concerning the content of the case and a mutual confirmation of the good atmosphere.

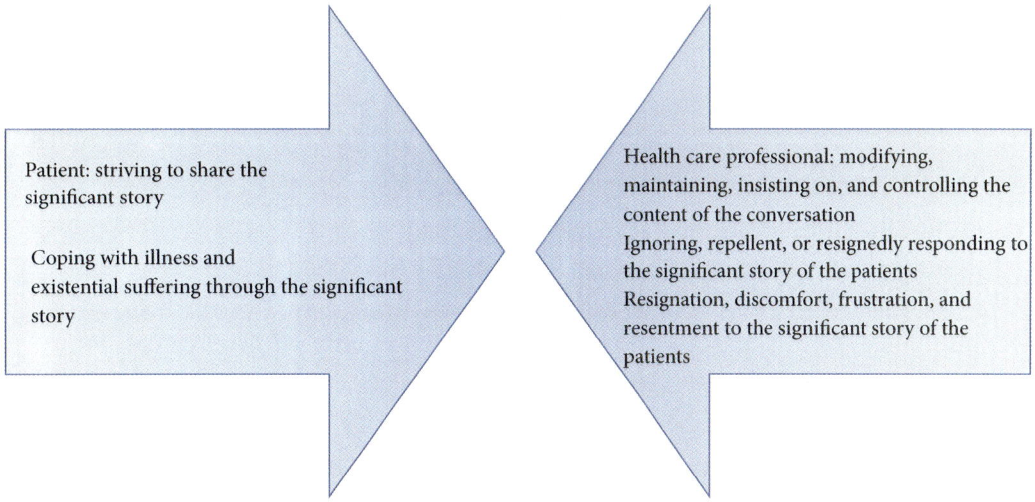

FIGURE 1: Lack of shared understanding to the content of the interaction in the outpatient respiratory medical clinic.

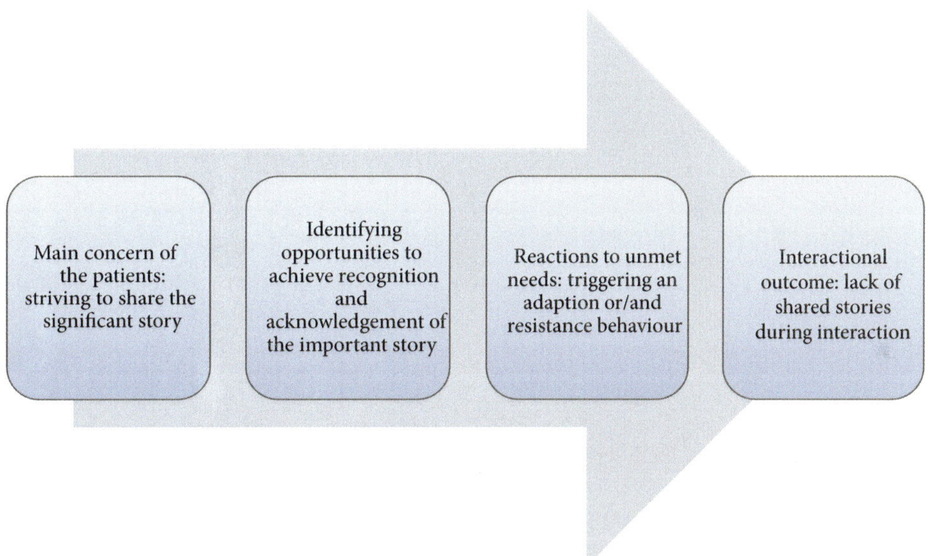

FIGURE 2: Core processes to unmet needs of the patients triggering counterreactions.

3.1.1. Pretending Shared Understanding. Despite the fact that "fitting in" behaviour could be met with recognition and attention, this did not necessarily mean that patients were satisfied with the conversation or considered the interaction meaningful or relevant. On the other hand, "fitting in" behaviour often caused the HCP to assume the patient understood and recognized the importance and relevance of the counselling and treatment. The "fitting in" mode did not necessarily result in patients' receptiveness to counselling and information, as many patients silently resisted guidance while appearing responsive during the interaction. Below is an example showing a patient's "fitting in" behaviour and at the same time a resistance to counselling in the patient. During a field observation, the patient silently nods and does not argue with the HCP, who strongly disapproves of the patient's continued use of cough medicine. The patient explains in a subsequent interview:

> *And I was thinking... "Don't talk to me that way,"... but then I thought, "No! Just finish your speech... I'm not listening anyway." (Laughing out loud) (pt. 15)*

The "fitting in" behaviour resulted in patients rarely expressing their concerns, strategies, and emotions to the HCP. Several patients were preoccupied with symptoms of their other chronic diseases, which they found to be even more disabling, or troubled by a lack of understanding from relatives or feelings of loneliness or anxiety, which the interaction often rendered impossible to discuss. By contrast, the patient's questions could be context-related and in accordance with the HCP's predefined subjects, resulting in patient-directed and problem-based counselling.

3.2. "Fighting Back" Behaviour. "Fighting back" behaviour demonstrated resistance, retention, and frustration to the unmet needs of the patient. The role of the patient and of the HCP could be challenged or disturbed by the story. A patient's fighting back to create opportunities for the story without obtaining the HCP's responsiveness could furthermore create emotions such as anxiety, anger, despair, or resignation in the patient, as exemplified below:

> *X (HCP), who we went to see, was very nice... and I think that she was very careful taking notes... So I got angry when we went to see Y (HCP)... Who does she think she is... talking about my back instead of talking about my lungs... I know how to treat my back... So that was not at all what I needed... And this commanding tone in her voice... "Do this and do that...." (pt. 15)*

Resignation could cause that patients gave up "fighting back" and reverted to "fitting in" behaviour, which was less energy demanding and made the interaction more predictable and less exhausting for them. The "fighting back" behaviour could relate to greater or lesser part of the interaction and consist of more or less important elements of patient's stories. "Fighting back" behaviour was often visible throughout the interaction. It was particularly evident in the many interactions where patients wanted to bring up other topics than planned or where patients considered the counselling dull, time-consuming, offensive, or invading.

> *Well,... I had absolutely no impression that there was any contact between him and me. It was at the end, as he was becoming kind of offended and sulky. And my annoyance was particularly with the fact that I felt he started to become a little rude. However, it is non sequitur. You do not get any answers. In principle, I do not care whether it is negative or positive, but you must have some answers as to what the hell is wrong, has it become better or worse, what do we do and why not. And I do not think I got any answers at all. And as I said earlier... it's my big problem, or my big concern. It's my concern for people who cannot answer for themselves. So to me, the counselling, it's quite a waste of time. (pt. 24)*

In other cases, patients' "fighting back" behaviour seemed more veiled and expressed through a return to issues that the HCP had attempted to finish or through insistence on sharing a narrative or expressing their views on alternative treatment or the way they tackled common problems related to the illness. Many patients considered the bodily learned knowledge as important and tried to share these stories, even though the HCP rarely called for or responded to their experiences.

In Figure 3 the overall grounded theory is presented. This explains how "striving to share the significant story"

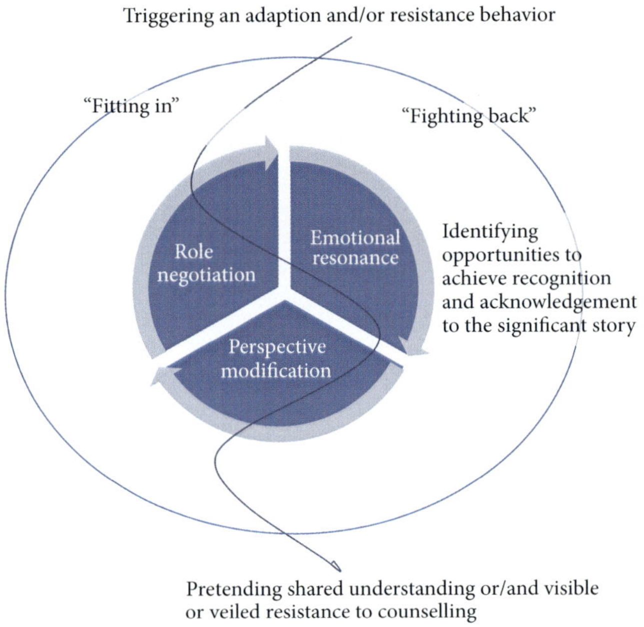

Figure 3: Striving to share the significant story. Triggering an adaption and/or resistance behaviour.

triggered a "fitting in" or "fighting back" behaviour based on a process of *role negotiation*, *emotional resonance*, and *perspective modification* leading to the meaning and significance in patients attributed to the interactions when the needs of the patients were predominantly unmet. The wavy arrow-line down the centre of the figure illustrates how a "fitting in" as well as a "fighting back" behaviour in patients undergoes the same process of identifying perceived opportunity to achieve recognition through the process of role negotiation, emotional resonance, and perspective modification. The text below the figure explains how these processes in patients are leading to either a pretended shared understanding or a visible or veiled resistance to counselling (Figure 3).

3.3. Role Negotiation. Role negotiation describes the struggle for allocation of roles during the interaction and conceptualizes how the patient, silently or vocally, negotiates the patient role, including the right to define the content, the subject, and the framework for the interaction.

Patients could basically resist or adapt to the expected passive patient role the HCP expected them to undertake during interactions. At the same time, the HCP strived to uphold the dominant expert role and the right to define the content of the interaction, reacting with irritation, resignation, or frustration when challenged in the distribution of roles during the interaction. HCPs displayed several actions to accommodate this, including disregard, interruption, or breakdown of the story. Therefore, the patient could either fulfill or challenge the passive patient role. Role negotiation can be explained as patient-driven breakdowns, surrender, or attempt to control the content of the interaction in the ORMC.

3.3.1. Breakdowns. When the interaction caused breakdowns, it was often clear to both parties. Many of the HCPs experienced these situations as unpleasant and tried to prevent or alleviate the disharmony caused by it. Breakdown situations clarified the patient's anger or frustration when the HCP's abortive assessment of the patient's emotional state became visible to both sides.

In one of the field observations, a dialogue between a patient and a nurse takes place illustrating the breakdown of the counselling. The patient suffers from posttraumatic stress syndrome, which, according to the patient, is a much greater challenge in his everyday life than his COPD. Early in the observed conversation, the HCP asks about the patient's daily number of cigarettes. The following dialogue takes place:

> *(pt. 22): 15 cigarettes... Since August... only 15... I actually enjoy smoking.*
>
> *HCP.1: How about electronic cigarettes?*
>
> *(pt. 22): It's simply overrated... It's just bullshit... To quit smoking when you have PTSS (shakes his head).*
>
> *HCP.1: How about nicotine patches?*
>
> *(pt. 22): Yes, but I can't light them up, can I! (laughs) (field observation, pt. 22)*

The patient explained that he did not have the power to continue trying to make the HCP understand what his self-perceived biggest problems were: anxiety and water retention. In the follow-up interview, he pointed out that cigarettes were his only consolation and relief, the only thing that could alleviate his anxiety and ease his suffering. Even though patients mostly were aware that the HCP was not receptive to their story, it did not necessarily mean a change of behaviour. Patients' fighting back against the expected patient role rarely created opportunities for their story but instead complicated and disturbed the maintenance of the planned content at the ORMC. On the other hand, breaking or challenging the patient role created an opportunity to prevent the HCP from communicating information or recommendations to the patients they did not want to receive. This happened through irony, anger, humour, laughter, or bodily nonverbal rejection of the counselling. There was a connection between breaking or challenging the traditional patient role and the patient's experience of anger directed at the HCP and, at the same time, an experience of the ORMC as a place where the patient's problems were neither met nor recognized.

3.3.2. Surrender. Patients could mitigate any previous challenge of the patient role by surrender through recognizing the HCP's advice or showing gratitude for the HCP's efforts to help them. When accepting the passive role, the patients surrendered and gave up expressing their wishes for the conversation and their needs to share and explore hope, emotions, and strategies. Instead, the patients followed the HCP's agenda during interaction and counselling. During the follow-up interview, the patients often expressed feelings of disappointment and dwindling expectations for the ORMC and the HCP.

3.3.3. Control. Breakdowns often allowed the patient to take control of the interaction for a limited period of time. It rarely meant that the patient achieved breakthroughs in sharing perspectives and experiences. Regardless of the outcome of the "role distribution," the patients' need and effort to share their significant story transformed their hope of creating opportunities during the interaction to a state of resignation, anger, or disappointment.

3.4. Perspective Modification. The patients' self-perception was often challenged and negotiated during interactions with the HCP in which patients tested their own attitudes and actions. Through this, patients were able to adjust to the situation and modify their own reactions to the actions of the HCP.

3.4.1. Adjusting and Modifying. The HCP's violation, indifference, or recognition was thereby turned into something meaningful or meaningless by the patient. Through the story, patients modified and tested their own stances towards everyday life and the disease, strategies, self-perception, and the things perceived as important/not important for living with CRD. A consensus emerged between the HCP and the patient that it was the HCP's prerogative to comment on and reprimand the patient on issues such as weight, alcohol consumption, smoking, social network, moods, and strategies. The story of coping with CRD was important to many patients. These stories involved compromises on lifestyle changes that the HCP encouraged the patients to follow. The HCPs displayed inertia in their response to these compromises and a lack of involvement in the patients' own experiences of and tricks for coping with CRD. A pattern emerged in which the HCP often displayed an inflexible approach to counselling on lifestyle changes, regardless of the prerequisites, interest, or motivation of the patient. The HCP rarely responded to patients' own suggestions of strategies for living with breathlessness, which sometimes decreased patients' adjustment to the HCP counselling.

> *Yes, I often see sulky attitudes at that outpatient clinic, actually... I mean, I don't think that they are very... enthusiastic... encouraging... making people want to pitch in... I think that they are a bunch of grumpy ladies... and I think that I wasted my time... by driving up here... I'd much rather go see XX, because he's sympathetic and seems enthusiastic about the things that you tell him... and what you accomplish on your own, right? (pt. 4)*

Some patients pointed to individual HCPs whom they considered to be particularly skilled and motivating in their effort to create lifestyle changes by adjusting and finding new ways and strategies. These HCPs displayed a recognizing approach to the patients' own actions in relation to lifestyle changes and reacted to the patients' emotional condition with advice, comfort, or encouragement.

3.5. Emotional Resonance. The presence or absence of emotional resonance was the key determinant of patients' self-perceived satisfaction or dissatisfaction to interactions and was characterized by patients' need to achieve emotional response and recognition during the interaction.

3.5.1. Unrecognized Emotions. When the patients experienced a lack of emotional response to their story's emotional content, it resulted in additional suffering and discouragement in the patients. Many patients were striving to share some kind of hope expressed by the story and, at the same time, a need to have the emotions related to hope in the story recognized.

The HCP's rejection, ignoring, or lack of recognition of the emotional part of the story contributed to extinguishing the hope of less suffering, distress, and worries of everyday life. Many patients expressed the importance of emotional responsiveness during the interviews:

> *I told her that I would like to quit the medicine... and she told me to forget about it, ... but I told her that I had hoped, ... but she wouldn't listen... And at that point in time, I just really needed the hope... I mean... that they understood that it was a hope of mine... or a milestone to me, right ? (pt. 4)*

The lack of emotional resonance negatively affected the patients' self-perceived motivation and courage to create everyday lifestyle changes. Furthermore, the HCPs' lack of emotional reflection on patients' challenges tended to increase the patients' "fighting back" mode to recommended lifestyle changes. The patients often reflected upon their own health and disease related choices and actions. Patients were aware that emotions such as triumph, pride, and satisfaction from reducing cigarettes or reducing medicine would not give rise to recognition by the HCP. Even if they wanted to share their enthusiasm for their own lifestyle changes, these stories were rarely considered good stories from the HCP's point of view. Apparently, there was a discrepancy between patients' and HCPs' experience of what a good patient story might imply. In some cases, the patients reacted to the discrepancy with anger, frustration, or fighting back towards the HCP. Other patients regarded the interaction as violating and did not feel encouraged to enter into a dialogue about lifestyle habits.

> *No one bloody told me... "Damn, you managed to go from 30 cigarettes per day to 5, well done." Nooo [sic]... "You need to quit smoking." That's the way it is. (pt. 7)*

When the emotions in the story remained unrecognized, counselling sometimes became more anxiety provoking, incomprehensible, or less relevant, resulting in increased disappointment, despair, or hopelessness in patients.

3.5.2. Emotional Recognition. When the HCP recognized and reflected the story about anxiety, despair, joy, victory, insecurity, resignation, or annoyance, it had a tremendous effect on patients. It was consistent across the data that patients responded positively and often with gratitude and appreciation when the HCP recognized and positively indicated an understanding of their difficult everyday life. It motivated them when the HCP recognized and really listened to the story and had great importance when they felt emotionally understood, when they were awarded a significant role, and when their effort to find strategies and perspectives was recognized. Some of the HCPs had the ability to reflect the patients' emotions by acting interested and engaged in their life. Comments like "It's not easy for you" and "I understand your plight" or leave-takings like "Keep up your spirit till we meet again" had great value for patients, who mentioned these HCPs as particularly talented, caring, and encouraging. The patients' stories of hope could be expressed by and converted into, for example, striving for more good days with less breathlessness, reducing the number of cigarettes, or using less medicine. It was consistent across data that, to the extent the patients were emotionally reflected, they found counselling to be more relevant and were more willing to explore the perspectives regarding the HCPs' attitudes to an optimal life with CRD.

4. Discussions

The original intention of this study was to explain interpretations and counterreactions to unmet needs in the patients during counselling with HCPs in hospital-based outpatient respiratory medical clinics. Patients' efforts to share their story and the subsequent rejection or ignoring of this pursuit triggered predominantly an adaptation or resistance behaviour, conceptualized as "fitting in" and "fighting back," explaining the patients' counterreactions to unrecognized needs during the medical encounter, which turned out to be an exhausting but necessary behaviour to maintain perspectives and stories during the interactions. In addition, the patients' counterreactions were based on whether it was possible to play an active role during the interaction, the extent to which HCPs responded to the emotional intentions, and how the patients were able to change their own expectations of content during the interaction. These recurring structural patterns of interpretations of the patients, which were conceptualized as role negotiation, emotional resonance, and perspective modification conditions, turned out to be decisive of the meaning and significance patients attributed to the interaction and thus whether the patient adapted to a "fitting in" or "fighting back" behaviour. In accordance with the findings in this study, the patients' capability of being open to guidance was related to the extent to which they felt recognized and experienced the opportunity to share their concerns, suffering, and hopes with the HCP. The findings do not provide any answers to what seems to be a significantly greater degree of willingness to adhere to disease related issues and, to a lesser extent, an attachment to the emotional needs of patients. In addition, other studies have suggested that CRD patients lack knowledge of the disease and its long-term effects [48, 49] and that patients experience limited access to specialized nurses and doctors within the field of lung diseases [48, 50]. At the same time, it has been shown that lifestyle-related counselling and medicinal treatment at outpatient clinics can prevent readmittance, increase the level of patient satisfaction, and increase patients' ability to cope with illness and optimize drug compliance [15, 24, 51, 52]. However, before discussing the implication of these patterns of behaviour for clinical practice, it is essential to emphasize that although a general pattern of lacking commitment and responsiveness to patients' suffering in the ORMC was found, it may have complex causes and contexts, as suggested in other studies [25, 30]. Since this study maintains a patient-oriented perspective on the interaction, it is central to outline the limits and possibilities that affect the HCPs' actions in and attitudes to the interaction in the ORMC. Several studies suggest possible explanations for the lack of commitment to patients' emotional needs. Studies have shown that it is a difficult and complex task to maintain individual patient-oriented and emotionally responsive counselling, pointing to a high risk level of burnout and emotional exhaustion in many HCPs caused by the emotional needs, expectations, and demands of responsiveness from patients [25, 30, 31]. In terms of emotional burnout, lack of reciprocity, and attached concern, many studies suggest that the lack of responsiveness to patients' needs may be a way to resist emotional strain and stress [53, 54]. It may be a difficult task to listen to patients' stories of suffering, not knowing how to help [55]. Patients are often severely ill, treatment options poor, and healing possibilities nonexistent, and the existential suffering may be overwhelming to patients [1, 34]. At the same time, demands to navigate a time-constrained and topic-bounded guidance session involving many compulsory subjects to be documented may leave limited time for individual and patient defined selection of topics for conversation [22]. Additionally, HCPs are portrayed in a highly critical light in several studies, expressed particularly through the postmodern critique emerging from concepts like discipline, power, and individual control as problematic in the health care system [56–58]. The criticism that this study to some extent supports can give a misleading picture of the knowledge that HCPs possess and the practices associated with it. It needs to be taken into account that the HCPs included in this study had extensive knowledge and experience with CRD. Mostly they played a central role for patients in treatment and disease control, and they expressed a desire to support and help patients who suffered from CRD in the best possible way within the framework they had and the possibility they could recognize. At the same time, it is important to stress that the participating HCPs had extensive practical and theoretical knowledge regarding the consequences of the lifestyle choices made by patients suffering from CRD that they wish to introduce to patients, including knowledge on topics such as the benefit of exercise, smoking cessation, body weight, and medicine intake that may lead to extended life span and higher quality of everyday life in CRD patients [1, 34]. This means that there are many and often medically rational explanations to the HCPs' focus on control, monitoring, and treatment as found in this study. The vulnerability of patients suffering from CRD, which is prominent in our study and confirmed in other studies, stresses the importance of a supporting, empathic, and encouraging approach in HCP counselling [19, 39]. Although several other studies examine patient behaviour and actions [28, 39, 59], no other studies provide knowledge about the processes that constitute CRD patients' behaviour of fitting in or fighting back to counselling during interactions with HCPs in the ORMC. This study underlines the possibility of improving the experiences of being recognized in the ORMC through susceptibility of HCPs to listen to the stories of illness and suffering of the patients. The findings in this study suggest that an increasingly empathetic and extensive understanding of patients' concerns may possibly lead to a lesser degree of patients' resistance to advice and counselling during interactions. The findings suggest that patients rarely expected solutions to problems and concerns but rather anticipated an empathetic approach and willingness to listen to and understand their stories of suffering, hope, and ways of overcoming illness. This study offers new knowledge in an underexposed research field where the interaction is characterized by short meetings subject to a well-defined agenda during the clinical encounter. In accordance with other studies, our findings point to the importance of supplementing the disease-oriented perspective with a perspective increasingly inclusive of an empathetic and extensive understanding of patients' concerns and an appreciative view of patients [56, 60]. Further research is required to explore patients' counterreactions to unmet needs and further disclose the content and importance to patients with CRD in the ORMC.

5. Limitations

This study explores the patient's behaviour and actions related to interactions with HCPs in the ORMC. This study is limited by the fact that the voice of the HCPs is not explored in this study. Further exploration of the HCP's perspectives may provide further understanding of the knowledge of the ORMC interaction, which this study cannot provide. Future research should explore the HCP's reactions to the patient's actions and behaviour in the ORMC to provide an overall picture of reactions and counterreactions of both patients and HCPs.

6. Conclusion

The findings of this study allow for a better understanding of patients' counterreactions in the time-pressured and, simultaneously, tight structured guidance program in the ORMC. Firstly, the findings show that patients' efforts to share their story triggered predominantly an adaptation or resistance behaviour, conceptualized as "fitting in" and "fighting back," explaining the patients' counterreactions to unrecognized needs during the medical encounter. Secondly, counterreactions of the patients were based on whether it was possible to play an active role during the interaction, the extent to which HCPs responded to the emotional intentions, and how the patients were able to change their own expectations of content during the interaction. The patients' capacity to receive help and guidance was related to the extent to which they felt recognized and experienced the opportunity to share their concerns, suffering, and hopes with the HCP. The study offers new knowledge in an underexposed research field where the interaction is characterized by short meetings subject to a well-defined agenda during the clinical encounter. The findings point to the importance of supplementing the disease-oriented perspective with a perspective increasingly inclusive of an empathetic and extensive understanding of patients' concerns and an appreciative view of patients. An increasingly empathetic understanding of patients' concerns may lead to less resistance in patients to HCP advice and counselling during interactions. Further research is required to explore patients' counterreactions to unmet needs and further disclose the content and importance to patients during counselling in the CRD.

7. Implications for Practice

The findings of patients' counterreactions to unmet needs provide new knowledge to HCP practice regarding the interactional possibilities and limitations in the ORMC. The findings offer practical and ethical implications as to how HCPs' attitudes towards patients can increase their ability to support emotional suffering and increase patient participation and guidance in the lifestyle changes that many HCPs hope to achieve during counselling.

Throughout this paper, how the lack of emotional responsiveness and recognition triggered a fitting in or fighting back behaviour has been outlined and analysed, explaining the patients' counterreactions to unmet needs during the interaction in the ORMC. This paper emphasizes a lack of shared expectations between the patient and HCP as being a central problem in the interaction, proposing that HCP may involve utilising the already available time frame to conduct an open dialogue with patients and prioritising the tasks and issues that are most important for the patient quality of life and health at the time. The need to develop specific models or guidelines, while focusing on the time-dependent ORMC interaction, is crucial in order to develop and strengthen an ORMC based on empathy, ethics, and emotional responsiveness to patients' needs and suffering during interaction in the ORMC. Future studies would benefit from examining how a narrative medicine could be implemented. A concrete proposal could be, for example, that future ORMC visits included an initial exploration of patients' experiences with the disease, hopes, ambitions, and expectations for the ORMC interaction. Furthermore, not only may a narrative approach be used in academic writing, but at the same time, it should be implemented as a way to forward the development of the ORMC. Actively using patient's stories is a way of understanding how the patient experiences can be understood and what is perceived as meaningful to patients regarding support, treatment, and guidance. Through this, the ORMC could gain development of the ORMC practice. Narrative methods seem to embrace the possibility of a more individual and patient-directed guidance, focusing on patient experienced problems rather than on the prospects based on the problems that HCPs perceive as typical, general, and specific to patient groups in the ORMC [39]. This approach would consequently be a shift in perspective and complement the HCP's understanding of the ORMC aims, tasks, and possibilities.

References

[1] A. Cruz, E. Mantzouranis, P. Matricardi et al., *Global Surveillance, Prevention and Control of Chronic Respiratory Disease*, edited by: T. Bousquet, N. Khaltaev, WHO, Geneva, Switzerland, 2007.

[2] M. Giacomini, D. DeJean, D. Simeonov, and A. Smith, "Experiences of living and dying with COPD: a systematic review and synthesis of the qualitative empirical literature," *The Ontario Health Technology Assessment Series*, vol. 12, no. 13, pp. 1–47, 2012.

[3] GOLD, *Global Strategy for the Diagnosis, Management, and Prevention of Chronic Obstructive Pulmonary Disease*, Global Initiative for Chronic Obstructive Lung Disease (GOLD), 2014.

[4] M. B. Parshall, R. M. Schwartzstein, L. Adams et al., "An official American thoracic society statement: update on the mechanisms, assessment, and management of dyspnea," *American Journal of Respiratory and Critical Care Medicine*, vol. 185, no. 4, pp. 435–452, 2012.

[5] H. O. Birk, R. Gut, and L. O. Henriksen, "Patients' experience of choosing an outpatient clinic in one county in Denmark: results of a patient survey," *BMC Health Services Research*, vol. 11, article 262, 2011.

[6] J. Blands and L. Bælum, *KOL—KRONISK OBSTRUKTIV LUNGESYGDOM Anbefalinger for Tidlig Opsporing, Opfølgning, Behandling og Rehabilitering/COPD—Chronic OBSTRUCTIVE PULMONARY DISEASE Recommendations for Early Detection, Monitoring, Treatment and Rehabilitation the 2007*, Sundhedsstyrelsen/National Board of Health, Copenhagen, Denmark, 2007.

[7] C. R. Borge, A. K. Wahl, and T. Moum, "Association of breathlessness with multiple symptoms in chronic obstructive pulmonary disease," *Journal of Advanced Nursing*, vol. 66, no. 12, pp. 2688–2700, 2010.

[8] M. Gysels and I. J. Higginson, "The experince of breathlessness: the social course of chronic obstructive pulmonary disease," *Journal of Pain and Symptom Management*, vol. 39, no. 3, pp. 555–563, 2010.

[9] G. Lindquist and L. Hallberg, "'Feelings of guilt due to Self-inflicted Disease' a grounded theory of suffering from Chronic Obstructive Pulmonary Disease (COPD)," *Journal of Health Psychology*, vol. 15, no. 3, pp. 456–467, 2010.

[10] K. Ek, E. Sahlberg-Blom, B. Andershed, and B.-M. Ternestedt, "Struggling to retain living space: patients' stories about living with advanced chronic obstructive pulmonary disease," *Journal of Advanced Nursing*, vol. 67, no. 7, pp. 1480–1490, 2011.

[11] P. Karakurt and A. Ünsal, "Fatigue, anxiety and depression levels, activities of daily living of patients with chronic obstructive pulmonary disease," *International Journal of Nursing Practice*, vol. 19, no. 2, pp. 221–231, 2013.

[12] M. Kvangarsnes, H. Torheim, T. Hole, and L. S. Öhlund, "Narratives of breathlessness in chronic obstructive pulmonary disease," *Journal of Clinical Nursing*, vol. 22, no. 21-22, pp. 3062–3070, 2013.

[13] C. Giot, M. Maronati, I. Becattelli, and G. Schoenheit, "Idiopathic pulmonary fibrosis: an EU patient perspective survey," *Current Respiratory Medicine Reviews*, vol. 9, no. 2, pp. 112–119, 2013.

[14] K.-H. Chen, M.-L. Chen, S. Lee, H.-Y. Cho, and L.-C. Weng, "Self-management behaviours for patients with chronic obstructive pulmonary disease," *Journal of Advanced Nursing*, vol. 64, no. 6, pp. 595–604, 2008.

[15] J. Bourbeau, D. Nault, and T. Dang-Tan, "Self-management and behaviour modification in COPD," *Patient Education and Counseling*, vol. 52, no. 3, pp. 271–277, 2004.

[16] L. Cicutto, D. Brooks, and K. Henderson, "Self-care issues from the perspective of individuals with chronic obstructive pulmonary disease," *Patient Education and Counseling*, vol. 55, no. 2, pp. 168–176, 2004.

[17] K. O. Juel, M. Døssing, and Udgiver, *KOL i Danmark. Sygdommen der Hver dag Koster 10 Danskere Livet*, Statens Institut for Folkesundhed, 2003.

[18] J. Gullick and M. C. Stainton, "Living with chronic obstructive pulmonary disease: developing conscious body management in a shrinking life-world," *Journal of Advanced Nursing*, vol. 64, no. 6, pp. 605–614, 2008.

[19] R. T. Disler, A. Green, T. Luckett et al., "Experience of advanced chronic obstructive pulmonary disease: metasynthesis of qualitative research," *Journal of Pain and Symptom Management*, vol. 48, no. 6, pp. 1182–1199, 2014.

[20] S. Bajwah, I. J. Higginson, J. R. Ross et al., "The palliative care needs for fibrotic interstitial lung disease: a qualitative study of patients, informal caregivers and health professionals," *Palliative Medicine*, vol. 27, no. 9, pp. 869–876, 2013.

[21] C. Gardiner, M. Gott, N. Small et al., "Living with advanced chronic obstructive pulmonary disease: patients concerns regarding death and dying," *Palliative Medicine*, vol. 23, no. 8, pp. 691–697, 2009.

[22] K. Fiscella and R. M. Epstein, "So much to do, so little time: care for the socially disadvantaged and the 15-minute visit," *Archives of Internal Medicine*, vol. 168, no. 17, pp. 1843–1852, 2008.

[23] B. Kayahan, H. Karapolat, E. Atýntoprak, A. Atasever, and Ö. Öztürk, "Psychological outcomes of an outpatient pulmonary rehabilitation program in patients with chronic obstructive pulmonary disease," *Respiratory Medicine*, vol. 100, no. 6, pp. 1050–1057, 2006.

[24] P. Lange, K. K. Andersen, E. Munch et al., "Quality of COPD care in hospital outpatient clinics in Denmark: the KOLIBRI study," *Respiratory Medicine*, vol. 103, no. 11, pp. 1657–1662, 2009.

[25] A. B. Bakker, W. B. Schaufeli, H. J. Sixma, W. Bosveld, and D. Van Dierendonck, "Patients demands, lack of reciprocity, and burnout: a five-year longitudinal study among general practitioners," *Journal of Organizational Behavior*, vol. 21, no. 4, pp. 425–441, 2000.

[26] P. H. Bailey, "The dyspnea-anxiety-dyspnea cycle—COPD patients' stories of breathlessness: 'it's scary /when you can't breathe'," *Qualitative Health Research*, vol. 14, no. 6, pp. 760–778, 2004.

[27] W. G. Anderson, S. Kools, and A. Lyndon, "Dancing around death: hospitalist-patient communication about serious illness," *Qualitative Health Research*, vol. 23, no. 1, pp. 3–13, 2013.

[28] G. Lucius-Hoene, U. Thiele, M. Breuning, and S. Haug, "Doctors' voices in patients' narratives: coping with emotions in storytelling," *Chronic Illness*, vol. 8, no. 3, pp. 163–175, 2012.

[29] A. W. Frank, "'How can they act like that?' Clinicians and patients as characters in each other's stories," *The Hastings Center report*, vol. 32, no. 6, pp. 14–22, 2002.

[30] J. J. Michaelsen, "Emotional distance to so-called difficult patients," *Scandinavian Journal of Caring Sciences*, vol. 26, no. 1, pp. 90–97, 2012.

[31] B. A. Potter, "Job burnout and the helping professional," *Clinical Gerontologist*, vol. 2, no. 2, pp. 63–65, 1983.

[32] S. Thorne, "Patient-provider communication in chronic illness: a health promotion window of opportunity," *Family & Community Health*, vol. 29, supplement 1, no. 1, pp. 4s–18s, 2006.

[33] S. Lawn, T. Delany, L. Sweet, M. Battersby, and T. C. Skinner, "Control in chronic condition self-care management: how it occurs in the health worker-client relationship and implications for client empowerment," *Journal of Advanced Nursing*, vol. 70, no. 2, pp. 383–394, 2014.

[34] K. F. Rabe, S. Hurd, A. Anzueto et al., "Global strategy for the diagnosis, management, and prevention of chronic obstructive pulmonary disease: GOLD executive summary," *American Journal of Respiratory and Critical Care Medicine*, vol. 176, no. 6, pp. 532–555, 2007.

[35] K. Larsen, M. P. Cutchin, and I. Harsløf, "Health capital: new health and personal investment in the body in the context of changing Nordic welfare states," in *Changing Social Risks and Social Policy Responses in the Nordic Welfare States*, I. Harsløf and R. Ulmestig, Eds., Palgrave Macmillan, New York, NY, USA, 2013.

[36] J. K. Shim, "Cultural health capital: a theoretical approach to understanding health care interactions and the dynamics of unequal treatment," *Journal of Health and Social Behavior*, vol. 51, no. 1, pp. 1–15, 2010.

[37] L. A. Dubbin, J. S. Chang, and J. K. Shim, "Cultural health capital and the interactional dynamics of patient-centered care," *Social Science and Medicine*, vol. 93, pp. 113–120, 2013.

[38] R. M. Epstein, K. Fiscella, C. S. Lesser, and K. C. Stange, "Why the nation needs a policy push on patient-centered health care," *Health Affairs*, vol. 29, no. 8, pp. 1489–1495, 2010.

[39] S. S. L. Wong, N. Abdullah, A. Abdullah et al., "Unmet needs of patients with chronic obstructive pulmonary disease (COPD): a qualitative study on patients and doctors," *BMC Family Practice*, vol. 15, article 67, 2014.

[40] J. M. Seymour, L. Moore, C. J. Jolley et al., "Outpatient pulmonary rehabilitation following acute exacerbations of COPD," *Thorax*, vol. 65, no. 5, pp. 423–428, 2010.

[41] P. Montgomery and P. H. Bailey, "Field notes and theoretical memos in grounded theory," *Western Journal of Nursing Research*, vol. 29, no. 1, pp. 65–79, 2007.

[42] ICN, *The ICN Code of Ethics for Nurses*, International Council of Nurses (ICN), Geneva, Switzerland, 2012.

[43] K. Charmaz, "'Discovering' chronic illness: using grounded theory," *Social Science and Medicine*, vol. 30, no. 11, pp. 1161–1172, 1990.

[44] K. Charmaz, "Premises, principles, and practices in qualitative research: revisiting the foundations," *Qualitative Health Research*, vol. 14, no. 7, pp. 976–993, 2004.

[45] C. Charmaz, *Constructing Grounded Theory. A Practical Guide through Qualitative Analysis*, Sage Publications, London, UK, 2006.

[46] H. Blumer, *Symbolic Interactionism: Perspective and Method*, University of California Press, Berkeley, Calif, USA, 1969.

[47] C. Charmaz, "Grounded theory methods in social justice research," in *The Sage Handbook of Qualitative Research*, N. L. Y. Denzin, Ed., pp. 359–380, SAGE, Thousand Oaks, Calif, USA, 2011.

[48] C. Shipman, S. White, M. Gysels, and P. White, "Access to care in advanced COPD: factors that influence contact with general practice services," *Primary Care Respiratory Journal*, vol. 18, no. 4, pp. 273–280, 2009.

[49] J. S. Wilson, J. S. Elborn, and D. Fitzsimons, "'It's not worth stopping now': why do smokers with chronic obstructive pulmonary disease continue to smoke? A qualitative study," *Journal of Clinical Nursing*, vol. 20, no. 5-6, pp. 819–827, 2011.

[50] J. M. Habraken, J. Pols, P. J. E. Bindels, and D. L. Willems, "The silence of patients with end-stage COPD: a qualitative study," *The British Journal of General Practice*, vol. 58, no. 557, pp. 844–849, 2008.

[51] E. Ö. Efraimsson, B. Fossum, A. Ehrenberg, K. Larsson, and B. Klang, "Use of motivational interviewing in smoking cessation at nurse-led chronic obstructive pulmonary disease clinics," *Journal of Advanced Nursing*, vol. 68, no. 4, pp. 767–782, 2012.

[52] P. Almagro and A. Castro, "Helping COPD patients change health behavior in order to improve their quality of life," *International Journal of COPD*, vol. 8, pp. 335–345, 2013.

[53] U. Rout, C. L. Cooper, and J. K. Rout, "Job stress among British general practitioners: predictors of job dissatisfaction and mental ill-health," *Stress Medicine*, vol. 12, no. 3, pp. 155–166, 1996.

[54] P. Conway, "Characteristics or traits of patients which may result in their being considered as 'difficult' by nurses," in *Proceedings of the Qualitative Evidence-Based Practice Conference*, Coventry University, Coventry, UK, May 2000.

[55] A. W. Frank, *The Wounded Storyteller. Body Illness, and Ethics*, The University of Chicago Press, Chicago, Ill, USA, 1995.

[56] A. W. Frank, M. Corman, J. Gish, and P. Lawton, "Healer-patient interaction: new mediations in clinical relationships," in *Qualitative Methods in Health Research*, I. Bourgeault, R. Dingwall, and R. Vries, Eds., pp. 34–52, SAGE Publications, London, UK, 2010.

[57] L. M. L. Ong, J. C. J. M. de Haes, A. M. Hoos, and F. B. Lammes, "Doctor-patient communication: a review of the literature," *Social Science and Medicine*, vol. 40, no. 7, pp. 903–918, 1995.

[58] W. R. Arney and B. J. Bergen, "The anomaly, the chronic patient and the play of medical power," *Sociology of Health and Illness*, vol. 5, no. 1, pp. 1–24, 1983.

[59] V. Zoffmann and M. Kirkevold, "Relationships and their potential for change developed in difficult type 1 diabetes," *Qualitative Health Research*, vol. 17, no. 5, pp. 625–638, 2007.

[60] R. Charon, *Narrative Medicine: Honoring the Stories of Illness*, Oxford University Press, New York, NY, USA, 2006.

9

Antihypertensive Medications and Change in Stages of Chronic Kidney Disease

Marina Komaroff,[1] Fasika Tedla,[2] Elizabeth Helzner,[1] and Michael A. Joseph[1]

[1] *School of Public Health, Department of Epidemiology and Biostatistics, State University of New York Downstate Medical Center, Brooklyn, NY, USA*
[2] *College of Medicine, Department of Medicine, State University of New York Downstate Medical Center, Brooklyn, NY, USA*

Correspondence should be addressed to Marina Komaroff; genmar2k@gmail.com

Academic Editor: Katarzyna Zorena

Objectives. The goal of this study is to estimate the change in the relationships between use of five classes of antihypertensive medications and stages of Chronic Kidney Disease (CKD) in American adults treated for hypertension. *Methods.* The US National Health and Nutrition Examination Survey (NHANES) data sets 1999–2012 were used with the final analytical sample of 3,045 participants. Population prevalence estimates were calculated using the NHANES survey design weights. Inferential analyses were done with binomial logistic regression models. *Results.* The odds of advanced (3, 4, and 5 combined) versus early CKD stages (1 and 2 combined) were significantly higher among patients treated with Angiotensin Receptor Blockers (ARB) versus those not treated with ARB in 2009–2012 (adjusted odds ratio (95% confidence interval) = 2.52 (1.32–4.80)). From 1999 to 2012, the increase in this relationship was significant ($p = 0.0023$) for users of ARB polytherapy and in users of ARB in patients with albuminuria ($p = 0.0031$). *Conclusion.* Aggressive pharmacological management of hypertension with ARB as add-on therapy may have accelerated kidney damage in American adults. However, prospective longitudinal studies are needed to establish proper temporal sequence in this relationship.

1. Introduction

Hypertension (HTN) is the second leading cause of kidney failure [1–7]. Thus, effective treatment of hypertension for American adults with CKD to slow the progression of the disease is important. In the Seventh Report of the Joint National Committee on Prevention, Detection, Evaluation, and Treatment of High Blood Pressure (JNC 7, 2003), Angiotensin Converting Enzyme (ACE) Inhibitors or Angiotensin II Receptor Blockers (ARBs) were recommended as initial or add-on pharmacological therapy particularly for patients with CKD [5, 7]. There has been a considerable increase in treatment and control of hypertension with antihypertensive medications in patients with CKD since release of JNC 7, 2003 [8–14]. Recent studies suggest a potential relationship between use of antihypertensive medications and deterioration in kidney function [15, 16]. The major point was that antihypertensive agents to control blood pressure may also impact kidney function independently of their effect on blood pressure [6].

This study examines the relationships between use of antihypertension medications and CKD stages among American adults (18 years or older) treated for hypertension and determines whether these relationships have changed from 1999 to 2012 (stacked cross-sectional design). There was public health campaign during this time period to aggressively treat and lower blood pressure particularly by use of ACE I and ARBs in patients with CKD. We hypothesized that if the recommended treatment of hypertension in patients with CKD worked as intended then the associations with stages of CKD should be moving towards a decrease in the prevalence of advanced stages or at least stay stable; otherwise, the recommended therapy might appear to be more harmful than beneficial and should perhaps be revised.

2. Material and Methods

2.1. Database Overview. The US National Health and Nutrition Examination Survey (NHANES) is a representative sample of noninstitutionalized US civilian residents that are currently conducted every 2 years. NHANES data are obtained using a complex, multistage, cluster, and probability sampling design that incorporates differential probabilities of selecting participants. The data collection, reporting, and analyses followed consistent definitions that can be found on the websites [17].

2.2. Study Design. Three time points (NHANES cycles 1999–2004, 2005–2008, and 2009–2012) were utilized to determine if these relationships have changed over time (stacked cross-sectional design).

2.3. Study Population. Inclusion criteria were participants 18 years of age or older, who completed questionnaire and underwent a physical examination, reported demographic information (age, gender, and race), provided self-reported information on hypertension including treatment, had blood pressure measured, had estimated glomerular filtration rate (eGFR) and urine albumin/creatinine ratio (ACR), and were not pregnant if female. Population of interest was participants with hypertensive CKD, who satisfied inclusion criteria, and were treated for hypertension.

2.4. Definitions. CKD was defined by the level of glomerular filtration rate (GFR) and the urine albumin-to-creatinine ratio (ACR) [6, 18]. The stages of CKD and albumin to creatinine ratio (ACR) were classified following the National Kidney Foundation (NKF) Kidney Disease Outcomes Quality Initiative (KDOQI) [6, 18].

Hypertension for participants with CKD was present if systolic blood pressure is greater than or equal to 130 mm Hg or diastolic blood pressure greater than or equal to 80 mm Hg, or subject currently was taking medication to lower high blood pressure [7, 19].

Treatment of high blood pressure was defined by an affirmative response to the question "Have you ever been told by a doctor or health professional that you had hypertension, also called high blood pressure?" and to the following questions: "Because of your high blood pressure/hypertension, have you ever been told to take prescribed medicine?" and "Are you now following this advice to take prescribed medicine?" [7, 19].

Diabetes was present if glycohemoglobin (HbA1c) was equal to or greater than 6.5% [20].

The five antihypertensive classes of medications were (1) ACE I (Angiotensin Converting Enzyme Inhibitors); (2) ARB (Angiotensin Receptor Blockers); (3) BB (β-blockers); (4) CCB (Calcium Channel Blockers); and (5) Diuretics [5, 7]. Monotherapy was defined when participates reported use of only one antihypertensive drug, and polytherapy which is the same as combination therapy was defined when participants reported use of more than one antihypertensive agent. When single pill of antihypertensive combination was reported, it was classified as polytherapy.

Data from seven NHANES surveys 1999–2012 included 71,916 records. The analytical sample of hypertensive participants with CKD who were treated for HTN and satisfied inclusion criteria was 3,045; see consort flow diagram, Figure 1.

2.5. Statistical Analyses. The prevalence of CKD by classes of antihypertensive medications was age-standardized to the 2000 US standard population using 4 age groups [19, 21]. Variance estimation was performed utilizing Taylor series method. Relative standard errors (RSE) were calculated, and those greater than 30% were considered potentially statistically unreliable per NHANES Analytic Guidance and marked with the asterisk ($*$) in the tables [21]. Because of small sample size of severe advanced stages (4 or 5), the main analyses were focused on CKD early stages 1 and 2 combined and advanced stages 3, 4, and 5 combined.

2.5.1. Model Description. Binomial logistic regression models were used to test the hypotheses of the study. In the models for three time points (NHANES cycles 1999–2004, 2005–2008, and 2009–2012), the ordinal coded dichotomous variable for stages of CKD was the dependent variable (outcome), time was independent variable, and class of antihypertensive medication was the independent variable (effect modifier). Interaction terms (time $\times$ class of medication) or (time $\times$ mono- or polytherapy) were used to test the null hypothesis of no difference in change in the odds ratios for patients treated versus untreated with particular class of medication over 14-year time period. The models included the following covariates: age, gender, race/ethnicity, body mass index (BMI), smoking status, diabetes, and albuminuria to adjust for potential confounding. The models accommodated the complex multistage sample survey design following NHANES Analytic and Reporting guidance [21]. To preserve Type I error in multiple subgroup analyses, the Bonferroni correction α/k was used where k is the number of analyses.

2.5.2. Trend Analyses. Trend was determined with the statistically significant interaction between class of medication and time (ordinal variable) indicating that their relationships had changed over time. In the models, the outcome variable was modeled as Logits that contrasted advanced (3, 4, and 5 combined) with the earlier (1 and 2 combined) stages of CKD. The odds ratios (95% Confidence Interval) were reported for each of five classes of medications: ACEI, ARB, BB, CCB, DIU, and poly- or monotherapy.

Exploratory Analyses. Subgroup analyses were performed with the same model and covariates for the following groups: diabetes (absent/present); albuminuria/ACR >30 mg/g (absent/present); microalbuminuria/ACR 30–<300 mg/g (absent/present); macroalbuminuria/ACR >300 mg/g (absent/present); diabetes with albuminuria; diabetes with microalbuminuria; diabetes with macroalbuminuria; diabetes without albuminuria; diabetes without microalbuminuria; diabetes without macroalbuminuria; no diabetes and albuminuria; no diabetes and microalbumin-uria; no diabetes and macroalbuminuria.

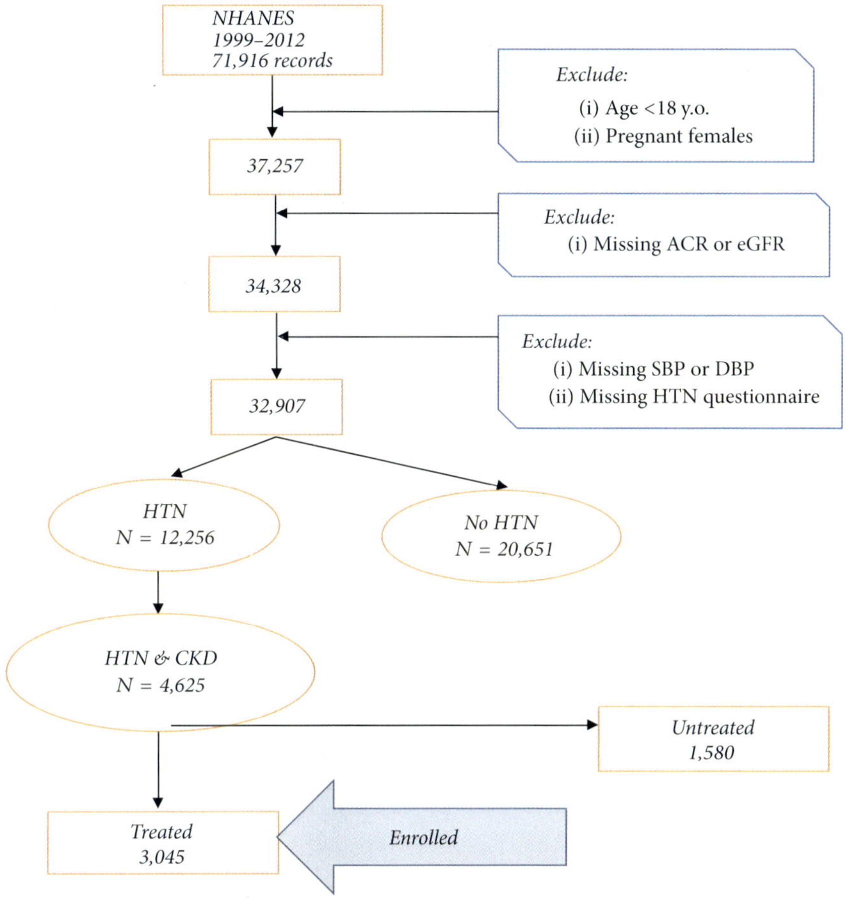

FIGURE 1: Consort flow diagram.

Statistical analyses were conducted using the SAS® System for Windows (release 9.3; SAS® Institute Inc., Cary, NC) and utilized the SURVEY procedures that account for NHANES survey multistage complex design [21].

3. Results

The use of medications other than the five major classes decreased from about 6.5% in 1999–2004 to 4.6% in 2005–2008 and 3.9% in 2009–2012. Those "other" included miscellaneous cardiovascular agents, vasodilators, vasopressors, agents for pulmonary hypertension, aldosterone receptor antagonists, and renin inhibitors; and they were not considered in this study. The use of alpha-1 blockers increased from 4.27% in 1999–2004 to 5.44% in 2005–2008 and 6% in 2009–2012. Similarly, the use of central alpha-2 antagonists and other centrally acting antiadrenergic agents increased from 3.58% in 1999–2004 to 3.81% in 2005–2008 and 5.28% in 2009–2012. This study did not examine alpha-blockers, but focused only on the use of five major classes of antihypertensive medications recommended by JNC-7 to treat hypertension in patients with CKD [7].

3.1. Prevalence of Use of Antihypertensive Medications. From 1999 to 2012, the prevalence % (SE) of adults with CKD and HTN who were treated for HTN increased from 55.58% (1.81) to 64.76% (1.91). Among five classes of medications, the use of ARB polytherapy increased the most: from 12.26% (1.44) to 21.56% (2.22); and the use of DIU polytherapy decreased the most: from 49% (2.55) to 42.05% (2.35); from 1999–2004 to 2009–2012. Two out of three patients with CKD and HTN received combination of classes (Table 1).

The prevalence of users of more than one class decreased from 65.76% (2.24) to 62.21% (3.31); however, the distributions by CKD stages for these users demonstrated increase in advanced stages, from 55.45% (2.28) to 56.20% (3.59) in stage 3 and from 7.33% (1.62) to 8.97% (1.85) in stages 4 and 5 combined, and decrease in early stages (1 and 2) from 37.21% to 34.82% (Table 1). The prevalence of patients was consistently greater in advanced (3) versus any early stages (1 or 2) among uses of each class. However, the increase in advanced stages was observed for ARB polytherapy and Diuretics monotherapy. The most increase in advanced stages was observed for ARB polytherapy: from 49.97% (5.61) to 70.72% (5.06) for stage 3 and from 5.7% (1.96) to 7.42% (1.94) for stages 4 and 5; while the early stages decreased from 29.58% (6.57) to 15.87% (4.38) for stage 2 and from 14.74% (5.72) to 5.98% (2.48) for stage 2.

3.2. Antihypertensive Medications and CKD Stages: Trend Analyses. The significant increase in the odds of advanced

Table 1: Age-standardized[$] prevalence of American adults (18 years of age or older) with hypertensive CKD treated for hypertension by five classes of medications and CKD stages: NHANES 1999–2012.

Population	CKD	1999–2004 % (SE)	2005–2008 % (SE)	2009–2012 % (SE)
CKD & HTN treated	Total	*N* = 1122 55.58 (1.81)	*N* = 916 62.13 (1.87)	*N* = 1007 64.76 (1.91)
	Stage 1	17.80 (2.15)	17.18 (1.83)	16.65 (2.01)
	Stage 2	24.81 (2.43)	26.64 (2.36)	25.06 (2.68)
	Stage 3	51.38 (2.68)	52.08 (3.40)	52.10 (3.19)
	Stages 4 & 5	6.00 (1.34)	4.09 (0.78)	6.17 (1.02)
Poly- or monotherapy		*N* = 1049	*N* = 874	*N* = 968
Angiotensin Converting Enzyme Inhibitors (ACE I)	Total	462 42.48 (1.93)	395 47.68 (1.68)	424 40.40 (2.08)
	Stage 1	13.91 (2.98)	17.38 (2.58)	20.49 (3.22)
	Stage 2	28.61 (4.46)	31.59 (3.58)	28.40 (3.38)
	Stage 3	51.40 (3.89)	48.42 (3.89)	46.14 (4.03)
	Stages 4 & 5	6.08* (1.89)	2.60 (0.70)	4.96* (1.79)
Angiotensin Receptor Blockers (ARB)	Total	176 15.93 (1.78)	218 22.30 (2.30)	282 26.10 (2.37)
	Stage 1	18.28 (4.76)	12.13* (4.04)	5.83* (2.24)
	Stage 2	24.88 (5.42)	22.72 (5.47)	19.56 (5.32)
	Stage 3	52.17 (5.07)	59.24 (6.43)	66.56 (5.16)
	Stages 4 & 5	4.65* (1.50)	5.89* (2.08)	8.03 (1.89)
β-blockers (BB)	Total	365 38.14 (2.35)	434 43.62 (2.70)	465 41.64 (3.16)
	Stage 1	13.07 (3.13)	14.41 (3.76)	9.29 (2.27)
	Stage 2	23.04 (3.02)	24.95 (3.51)	26.90 (3.84)
	Stage 3	55.20 (3.58)	53.36 (4.96)	54.38 (4.00)
	Stages 4 & 5	8.69 (2.12)	7.27 (1.58)	9.41 (2.16)
Calcium Channel Blockers (CCB)	Total	427 32.39 (1.92)	332 32.84 (2.17)	339 30.34 (3.21)
	Stage 1	14.69 (3.18)	16.46 (3.64)	20.29 (4.08)
	Stage 2	26.76 (4.21)	25.41 (4.15)	21.51 (3.89)
	Stage 3	47.83 (3.82)	53.15 (5.71)	48.53 (4.69)
	Stages 4 & 5	10.71 (2.89)	4.98 (1.47)	9.66 (2.14)
Diuretics (DIU)	Total	549 51.95 (2.68)	495 51.06 (2.50)	494 47.77 (2.35)
	Stage 1	15.21 (2.53)	13.86 (2.87)	15.34 (2.90)
	Stage 2	22.19 (3.10)	26.82 (3.53)	18.80 (2.73)
	Stage 3	58.07 (3.27)	54.33 (4.04)	58.62 (3.94)
	Stages 4 & 5	4.51 (1.10)	4.98 (1.26)	7.23 (1.60)
Polytherapy				
Angiotensin Converting Enzyme Inhibitors (ACE I)	Total	345 31.10 (1.62)	317 34.68 (2.19)	324 28.81 (2.42)
	Stage 1	11.49 (2.45)	14.85 (2.42)	18.46 (3.73)
	Stage 2	23.99 (4.32)	30.01 (3.47)	27.24 (4.25)
	Stage 3	55.36 (4.21)	51.72 (4.40)	48.53 (3.86)
	Stages 4 & 5	9.16* (3.07)	3.41 (1.01)	5.76* (2.03)

Table 1: Continued.

Population	CKD	1999–2004 % (SE)	2005–2008 % (SE)	2009–2012 % (SE)
Angiotensin Receptor Blockers (ARB)	Total	144	189	227
		12.26 (1.44)	18.17 (2.21)	21.56 (2.22)
	Stage 1	14.74* (5.72)	14.58* (4.86)	5.98* (2.48)
	Stage 2	29.58 (6.57)	24.02 (6.03)	15.87 (4.38)
	Stage 3	49.97 (5.61)	55.15 (6.53)	70.72 (5.06)
	Stages 4 & 5	5.70* (1.96)	6.24* (1.87)	7.42 (1.94)
β-blockers (BB)	Total	315	370	404
		32.45 (2.06)	36.08 (2.39)	34.33 (2.71)
	Stage 1	10.92 (2.93)	12.26* (3.91)	11.50 (2.94)
	Stage 2	23.47 (3.37)	25.75 (3.65)	20.72 (3.90)
	Stage 3	56.55 (3.65)	54.99 (5.21)	54.89 (4.35)
	Stages 4 & 5	9.06 (2.17)	6.99 (1.78)	12.87 (3.28)
Calcium Channel Blockers (CCB)	Total	309	298	285
		24.72 (1.91)	29.81 (2.22)	24.64 (3.10)
	Stage 1	9.88 (2.55)	14.00 (3.41)	18.49 (4.37)
	Stage 2	26.28 (4.79)	25.47 (4.38)	19.55 (4.24)
	Stage 3	50.59 (4.29)	55.01 (6.18)	50.64 (4.80)
	Stages 4 & 5	13.24 (3.46)	5.51 (1.60)	11.31 (2.61)
Diuretics (DIU)	Total	511	470	460
		49.36 (2.55)	46.98 (2.34)	42.05 (2.35)
	Stage 1	14.76 (2.57)	15.68 (3.51)	12.04 (3.20)
	Stage 2	22.09 (3.19)	26.32 (3.98)	19.00 (3.14)
	Stage 3	58.61 (3.31)	52.71 (4.21)	59.86 (4.48)
	Stages 4 & 5	4.53 (1.16)	5.28 (1.34)	9.09 (2.43)
Monotherapy				
Angiotensin Converting Enzyme Inhibitors (ACE I)	Total	117	78	100
		11.38 (1.59)	13.00 (2.18)	11.59 (1.78)
	Stage 1	16.63* (5.53)	21.82 (4.47)	24.97 (5.16)
	Stage 2	36.24 (6.89)	33.29 (5.41)	32.19 (6.85)
	Stage 3	45.40 (5.76)	44.49 (5.70)	41.60 (6.72)
	Stages 4 & 5	1.72* (1.19)	0.39* (0.41)	1.24* (0.65)
Angiotensin Receptor Blockers (ARB)	Total	32	29	55
		3.67 (0.99)	4.13 (1.08)	4.54 (0.74)
	Stage 1	27.57* (9.96)		4.85* (3.12)
	Stage 2	9.41* (4.24)		37.07* (12.63)
	Stage 3	62.22 (10.37)		47.57 (8.88)
	Stages 4 & 5	0.79* (0.81)		10.50* (5.34)
β-blockers (BB)	Total	50	64	61
		5.69 (1.36)	7.55 (1.42)	7.31 (1.75)
	Stage 1		25.90 (6.64)	1.43* (1.18)
	Stage 2		22.04* (7.71)	43.74 (10.40)
	Stage 3		44.35 (9.61)	54.53 (10.46)
	Stages 4 & 5		7.69* (4.15)	0.29* (0.29)

Table 1: Continued.

Population	CKD	1999–2004 % (SE)	2005–2008 % (SE)	2009–2012 % (SE)
Calcium Channel Blockers (CCB)	Total	118	34	54
		7.67 (1.21)	3.03 (0.71)	5.70 (1.29)
	Stage 1	28.52 (5.62)		27.20 (7.21)
	Stage 2	28.85 (6.87)		30.38 (7.91)
	Stage 3	39.36 (5.46)		39.04 (10.77)
	Stages 4 & 5	3.26* (1.28)		3.38* (2.04)
Diuretics (DIU)	Total	38	25	34
		2.59 (0.62)	4.08* (1.34)	5.73 (1.65)
	Stage 1	20.99* (8.61)	6.71* (4.92)	29.59 (6.83)
	Stage 2	29.29* (11.04)	19.98* (8.86)	11.98* (5.43)
	Stage 3	45.03 (11.72)	73.31 (8.34)	58.41 (7.14)
	Stages 4 & 5	4.69* (3.15)	0	0
Monotherapy Number of class meds = 1	Total	382	241	312
		31.69 (2.18)	32.51 (2.68)	35.24 (2.94)
	Stage 1	22.71 (3.83)	20.64 (2.06)	19.11 (3.37)
	Stage 2	28.15 (4.43)	26.10 (4.31)	32.31 (3.75)
	Stage 3	46.37 (3.59)	50.82 (4.68)	46.21 (4.63)
	Stages 4 & 5	2.76 (0.83)	2.43* (0.97)	2.35* (0.81)
Polytherapy Number of class meds > 1	Total	667	633	656
		65.76 (2.24)	66.32 (2.71)	62.21 (3.31)
	Stage 1	13.93 (2.49)	14.35 (2.43)	14.65 (2.94)
	Stage 2	23.28 (2.86)	26.65 (2.80)	20.17 (2.86)
	Stage 3	55.45 (2.82)	53.97 (4.13)	56.20 (3.59)
	Stages 4 & 5	7.33 (1.62)	5.03 (1.10)	8.97 (1.85)

*Potentially statistically unreliable estimates with relative standard errors > 30%. $Age-standardized to the 2000 US standard population using 4 age groups.

versus early stages was observed for ARB users ($p = 0.0069$), users of ARB polytherapy ($p = 0.0023$), and for users of poly- versus monotherapy ($p = 0.0063$); see Table 2 and Figure 2. Table 3 summarizes the prevalence of combinations of five antihypertensive classes of medication. The least prevalent was combination of ARB with ACEI therapy. Moreover, combinations of ARB with ACEI demonstrated decreased prevalence from 2005 through 2012: from 0.33% (SE = 0.18) to 0.04% (SE = 0.03) for ARB + ACEI; 0.57% (SE = 0.51) to 0.14% (SE = 0.11) for ARB + ACEI + BB; 0.22% (SE = 0.20) to 0.06% (SE = 0.04) for ARB + ACEI + CCB; 0.21% (SE = 0.12) to 0.03% (SE = 0.03) for ARB + ACEI + DIU; 0.33% (SE = 0.21) to 0.03% (SE = 0.03) for ARB + ACEI + BB + CCB; and 0.21% (SE = 0.15) to 0.17% (SE = 0.11) for ARB + ACEI + BB + DIU. Increased prevalence of medication combinations was observed only for ARB + ACEI + CCB + DIU from 0.08% (SE = 0.06) to 0.14% (SE = 0.08) and for ARB + ACEI + CCB + DIU + BB from 0.17% (SE = 0.10) to 0.49% (0.24) from 2005 through 2012. The most prevalent combinations with ARB were ARB + DIU and ARB + DIU + BB with the prevalence above 4% from 2005 through 2012. During the same period of time, the use of combinations with ARB increased more than 2% for ARB + BB + CCB: from 0.40% (SE = 0.14) to 2.29% (SE = 0.88). The other combination with ARB was above 1% and increased from 1.11% (SE = 0.21) to 1.92% (SE=0.76) for ARB + BB, from 1.81% (SE = 0.61) to 2.88% (SE = 0.81) for ARB + CCB + DIU, and from 1.67% (SE = 0.61) to 1.88% (SE = 0.52) for ARB + BB + CCB + DIU and slightly decreased from 1.88% (SE=0.64) to 1.82% (SE = 1.12) for ARB + CCB. None of the combinations of classes of medications with ARB demonstrated significant change in the relationships between advanced versus earlier stages of CKD from 1999 through 2012, except ARB + CCB ($p = 0.0065$). However, complete analysis cannot be performed, particularly for ARB combinations with ACEI due to small sample sizes.

The exploratory analyses were conducted with level of significance $\alpha/15 = 0.0033$ (Bonferroni correction for $\alpha = 0.05$) where 15 is the number of analyses. The same models stratified by subgroups demonstrated significant increase in odds of advanced versus early stages of CKD for: (1) ARB users among patients with albuminuria ($p = 0.0031$) and (2) users of more than one class of medications with albuminuria ($p = 0.002$); table is not present.

TABLE 2: Adjusted[##] odds ratios (95% CI) for advanced (3, 4, and 5) versus early (1 and 2) stages of CKD by use of each class of medication.

Model: class med[$]	1999–2004 odds ratio (95% CI)	2005–2008 odds ratio (95% CI)	2009–2012 odds ratio (95% CI)	$p^{\#}$
ACE I				
Overall	1.08 (0.69–1.70)	0.85 (0.63–1.14)	0.67 (0.43–1.04)	0.1574
Polytherapy	0.93 (0.57–1.52)	0.83 (0.60–1.15)	0.74 (0.46–1.20)	0.5417
Monotherapy	1.59 (0.91–2.80)	1.06 (0.65–1.73)	0.70 (0.33–1.48)	0.0713
ARB				
Overall	0.67 (0.36–1.23)	1.30 (0.87–1.94)	2.52 (1.32–4.80)	**0.0069**
Polytherapy	0.55 (0.29–1.03)	1.20 (0.80–1.80)	2.63 (1.37–5.07)	**0.0023**
Monotherapy	1.97 (0.63–6.18)	1.66 (0.83–3.31)	1.39 (0.56–3.46)	0.6575
BB				
Overall	1.05 (0.71–1.57)	1.19 (0.87–1.61)	1.34 (0.82–2.17)	0.4637
Polytherapy	1.05 (0.67–1.65)	1.23 (0.89–1.69)	1.43 (0.91–2.27)	0.3490
Monotherapy	0.98 (0.43–2.28)	0.88 (0.47–1.64)	0.78 (0.29–2.13)	0.7414
CCB				
Overall	1.28 (0.85–1.93)	1.17 (0.86–1.59)	1.08 (0.67–1.72)	0.5953
Polytherapy	1.14 (0.73–1.78)	1.22 (0.88–1.70)	1.31 (0.77–2.22)	0.7036
Monotherapy	1.24 (0.63–2.46)	0.78 (0.45–1.36)	0.49 (0.24–1.02)	**0.0359**
DIU				
Overall	1.27 (0.81–2.00)	1.49 (1.13–1.98)	1.76 (1.16–2.67)	0.3344
Polytherapy	1.37 (0.88–2.13)	1.65 (1.24–2.20)	1.99 (1.29–3.06)	0.2665
Monotherapy	0.31 (0.11–0.91)	0.30 (0.12–0.73)	0.29 (0.06–1.29)	0.9288
Number of Classes med >1 (polytherapy) versus = 1 (monotherapy)				
Combination	1.12 (0.74–1.70)	1.73 (1.30–2.30)	2.67 (1.74–4.09)	**0.0063**

[$]ACEI = Angiotensin Converting Enzyme Inhibitors; ARB = Angiotensin Receptor Blockers; BB = β-blockers; CCB = Calcium Channel Blockers; DIU = Diuretics; [#]PROC SURVEYLOGISTIC was used to test the trend; [##]Adjusted for: age, gender, race, body mass index, smoking status diabetes, and albuminuria; *NOTE.* Significant associations and p-values with level of significance $\alpha = 0.05$ are presented *in bold.*

4. Discussion

The major finding is that there was significant increase in this relationship for the users of ARB polytherapy ($p = 0.0023$) from 1999 through 2012. The trend can be explained by the increase in prevalence of advanced stages CKD and decrease or stable prevalence in early stages among users of ARB polytherapy. Such increase in advanced CKD stages may have been explained by use of ARB combinations with ACEI that was particularly warned by JNC-7, but those combinations were least prevalent and decreased during the investigated time period. Possibly, change in the relationship was driven by ARB combinations with other classes, particularly with CCB where odds of advanced stages significantly increased compared to the odds of earlier stages, from 1999 through 2012. A significant increase in advanced stages was observed for ARB users among people with albuminuria. The results suggest that increase in ARB polytherapy may have increased advanced stages of CKD among American adults, particularly among people with albuminuria.

In this study for American adults 18 years or older with CKD, the changes in age-standardized prevalence were from 55.58% to 64.76%, from 1999–2004 to 2009–2012 (Table 1). Gu et al. reported similar significant ($p = 0.03$) increase in unadjusted prevalence of users of multiple antihypertensive drugs in this population of adults with CKD from 54.2% (3.5) to 65.6% (3.0), from 2001-2002 to 2009-2010 [22]. But the prevalence by five classes of medications reported by Gu et al. was smaller to that reported in this study that can be explained by having population of adults with CKD as comorbid condition in this study. For example, in the Gu et al. study the change in prevalence of ARB users went from 10.5% (1.1) to 22.2% (1.6) for poly- or monotherapy, from 7.6% (0.9) to 16.1% (1.1) for polytherapy, and from 3.0% (0.4) to 4.9% (0.7) for monotherapy: NHANES from 2001-2002 to 2009-2010 [22]. In the present study, the increase in ARB users among hypertensive adults with CKD went from 15.93% (1.78) to 26.1% (2.37) for poly- or monotherapy, from 12.26% (1.44) to 21.56% (2.22) for polytherapy, and from 3.67% (0.99) to 4.54% (0.74) for monotherapy: NHANES from 1999–2004 to 2009–2012. The prevalence of advanced stages for the users of ARBs polytherapy increased from about 49.97% (5.61) to 70.72% (5.06) in stage 3 and from 5.70% (1.96) to 7.42% (1.94) in stages 4 and 5 combined, while the early stages decreased about half as much. The strength of the association suggests that the aggressive treatment of patients with CKD by ARB

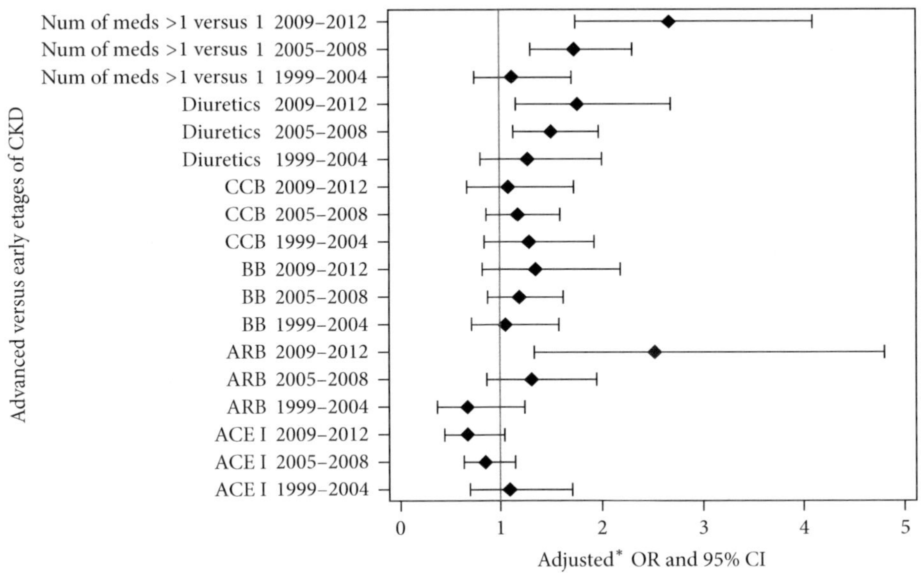

*Adjusted for age, gender, race/ethnicity, body mass index, smoking status, diabetes, albuminuria, and use of other classes

FIGURE 2: Forest-plots of adjusted* odds ratios (95% CI) for advanced (3, 4, and 5) versus early (1 and 2) stages of CKD by use of five classes of medication. *Note.* ACEI = Angiotensin Converting Enzyme Inhibitors; ARB = Angiotensin Receptor Blockers; BB = β-blockers; CCB = Calcium Channel Blockers; DIU = Diuretics.

could be responsible for kidney damage and the increase in advanced stages of CKD. A first population-based ecological study in the United Kingdom demonstrated an association between the increase in hospital admission rates for acute kidney injury (AKI) and the increase in prescriptions of antihypertensive medications (ACE inhibitors/ARA) in medical practices over a 4-year time period [15]. The authors concluded that 15% of the increase in AKI admission was potentially attributable to increased prescriptions of ACE I and ARBs [15].

The current study is the first study to the authors' knowledge that estimated changes in relationships between use of antihypertensive medications and stages of CKD for American hypertensive adults with CKD. The results are consistent with the population-based ecological study in the United Kingdom and suggest that significant increase in advanced stages of CKD can be potentially attributable to the treatment with ARB polytherapy, perhaps, damaging the kidney and increasing albuminuria. However, the temporal relationship between ARB therapy and increase in advanced stages of CKD cannot be established because of the cross-sectional nature of this study. It is possible that increase in ARB therapy resulted from the increase in advanced stages of CKD. Prospective longitudinal studies are needed to establish proper temporal sequence of this relationship.

4.1. Limitations and Strengths. The major limitation is that cross-sectional NHANES data does not allow assessing the relationship between CKD and treatment of hypertension longitudinally within patients. Another limitation is that blood pressure was measured on a single day versus on more than two separate days as was recommended by JNC 7 guidance [7]. However, three measurements were taken that might have minimized this misclassification. Similarly, CKD was defined based on single laboratory measurements versus multiple measurements during more than three months defined by KDOQI guidance [18]. However, the bias is minimal for the estimates that were the goal of this study. NHANES is a representative sample of the noninstitutionalized US population; yet, older people or people with severe cases, such as stage 3 or 4 of CKD, might have been underreported because usually weaker populations were less likely to attend MEC examination. Combining the advanced versus early stages in the statistical analyses minimized the population selection bias. Small sample size per each stage of CKD did not allow separate analysis by each stage. The combinations of classes of antihypertensive medications cannot be fully examined due to small sample sizes. Lastly, although the relationships between antihypertension medications and CKD stages are intriguing, NHANES data does not permit analysis of prescribing practices of physicians. The strength of the study is the use of NHANES data with a large sample size, good quality control, and comprehensive data collection. The long period of consistent data collected gives change to investigate the trend in the relationships between CKD stages and treatment of HTN before and after publishing JNC-7 guidelines. The presence of major risk factors for CKD and HTN was also consistently collected that gives us confidence in the results.

5. Conclusions

The link between ARBs and acute kidney injures was recognized recently by KDIOGO and UK National Institute for

Table 3: Age-standardized prevalence of American adults (18 years of age or older) with hypertensive CKD treated For hypertension by combination of five classes of medications: NHANES 1999–2012.

Combination of classes	1999–2004 % (SE)	2005–2008 % (SE)	2009–2012 % (SE)
ACE I + ARB	0.12* (0.09)	0.33* (0.18)	0.04* (0.03)
ACE I + BB	3.41 (0.89)	4.06 (1.02)	4.24 (0.73)
ACE I + CCB	4.59 (0.86)	4.39 (0.88)	3.24* (1.22)
ACE I + DIU	10.82 (1.54)	6.84 (1.17)	7.36 (1.33)
ARB + BB	0.52* (0.19)	1.11 (0.21)	1.92* (0.76)
ARB + CCB$	0.44* (0.16)	1.88* (0.64)	1.82* (1.12)
ARB + DIU	4.22 (0.91)	4.31 (1.05)	4.64 (0.85)
BB + CCB	2.12 (0.51)	2.88 (0.64)	1.44 (0.41)
BB + DIUX	12.11 (1.72)	5.48 (0.92)	5.21 (1.37)
CCB + DIUX	3.85 (0.69)	3.28 (0.96)	1.91* (0.82)
ACE I + ARB + BB	0.00 (0.00)	0.57* (0.51)	0.14* (0.11)
ACE I + ARB + CCB	0.22* (0.16)	0.22* (0.20)	0.06* (0.04)
ACE I + ARB + DIU	0.17* (0.14)	0.21* (0.12)	0.03* (0.03)
ACE I + BB + CCB	2.45* (0.91)	2.40* (0.96)	2.00 (0.48)
ACE I + BB + DIU	2.23 (0.50)	6.79 (1.22)	5.74 (1.13)
ACE I + CCB + DIU	3.09 (0.70)	5.02 (1.30)	2.39* (0.82)
ARB + BB + CCB	0.34* (0.26)	0.40* (0.14)	2.49* (0.88)
ARB + BB + DIU	3.08 (0.69)	4.70 (0.81)	4.66 (1.27)
ARB + CCB + DIU	1.57* (0.50)	1.81* (0.61)	2.88 (0.81)
BB + CCB + DIU	2.13 (0.55)	2.25 (0.52)	1.11* (0.35)
ACE I + ARB + BB + CCB	0.04* (0.04)	0.33* (0.21)	0.03* (0.03)
ACE I + ARB + BB + DIU	0.35* (0.19)	0.21* (0.15)	0.17* (0.11)
ACE I + ARB + CCB + DIU	0.48* (0.48)	0.08* (0.06)	0.14* (0.08)
ARB + BB + CCB + DIU	0.31* (0.12)	1.67* (0.61)	1.88 (0.52)
ACEI + ARB + BB + CCB + DIU	0.20* (0.16)	0.17* (0.10)	0.49* (0.24)

ACEI = Angiotensin Converting Enzyme Inhibitors; ARB = Angiotensin Receptor Blockers; BB = β-blockers; CCB = Calcium Channel Blockers; DIU = Diuretics. *Potentially statistically unreliable estimates with relative standard errors > 30%. $The use of this combination demonstrated significant increase in odds of advanced stages of CKD compared to odd of early stages, 1999 through 2012 ($p = 0.0065$).

Health and Clinical Excellence (NICE) [23, 24]. The results from this study suggest that increase in treatment with ARB possibly increased the prevalence of advanced CKD stages among American adults by damaging the kidneys. However, the temporal relationship cannot be claimed from this cross-sectional study. Prospective studies will be necessary to establish proper temporal sequence.

References

[1] "U.S. Department of Health and Human Services, Office of Disease Prevention and Health Promotion. Healthy People 2020. Washington, DC," http://www.healthypeople.gov/2020/default.aspx.

[2] Kidney Disease Outcomes Quality Initiative (K/DOQI), "K/DOQI clinical practice guidelines on hypertension and antihypertensive agents in chronic kidney disease," *Kidney Disease Outcomes Quality Initiative (K/DOQI)*, vol. 43, pp. S1–S290, 2004.

[3] The National Kidney and Urologic Diseases Information Clearinghouse (NKUDIC)/ National Institute of Diabetes and Digestive and Kidney Diseases (NIDDK). NIH Publication No. 14-4572 February 2014.

[4] Annals of Internal Medicine-In the Clinic® Chronic Kidney Disease American College of Physicians 2015.

[5] A. V. Chobanian, G. L. Bakris, H. R. Black et al., "The seventh report of the joint national committee on prevention, detection, evaluation, and treatment of high blood pressure: the JNC 7 report," *The Journal of the American Medical Association*, vol. 289, no. 19, pp. 2560–2572, 2003.

[6] Kidney Disease: Improving Global Outcomes (KDIGO) CKD Work Group, "KDIGO 2012 clinical practice guideline for the evaluation and management of chronic kidney disease," *Kidney International Supplements*, vol. 3, pp. 1–150, 2013.

[7] The Seventh Report of the Joint National Committee on Prevention, Detection, Evaluation, and Treatment of High Blood Pressure; U.S. DEPARTMENT OF HEALTH AND HUMAN SERVICES; National Institutes of Health National Heart, Lung, and Blood Institute National High Blood Pressure Education Program NIH Publication No. 04-5230; August 2004.

[8] T. H. Hostetter and M. Lising, "National kidney disease education program," *Journal of the American Society of Nephrology*, vol. 94, 8, pp. 114S–116S, 2002.

[9] T. F. Parker III, R. Blantz, T. Hostetter et al., "The Chronic Kidney Disease Initiative," *Journal of the American Society of Nephrology*, vol. 15, no. 3, pp. 708–716, 2004.

[10] S. S. Yoon, V. Burt, T. Louis, and M. D. Carroll, *Hypertension among adults in the United States, 2009–2010. NCHS data brief, no 107*, MD: National Center for Health Statistics, Hyattsville, Md, USA, 2012, http://www.cdc.gov/nchs/data/databriefs/db107.pdf.

[11] B. M. Egan, Y. Zhao, and R. N. Axon, "US trends in prevalence, awareness, treatment, and control of hypertension, 1988–2008," *The Journal of the American Medical Association*, vol. 303, no. 20, pp. 2043–2050, 2010.

[12] T. Nwankwo, S. S. S. Yoon, R. N. Vicki Burt, and Gu. Qiuping, *Hypertension Among Adults in the United States: National Health and Nutrition Examination Survey*, US Department of Health and Human Services, CDC/NCHS No.133, October 2013.

[13] K. L. Ong, A. W. K. Tso, K. S. L. Lam, and B. M. Y. Cheung, "Gender difference in blood pressure control and cardiovascular risk factors in Americans with diagnosed hypertension," *Hypertension*, vol. 51, no. 4, pp. 1142–1148, 2008.

[14] USRDS Annual Data Report; Volume1-Chronic Kidney Disease ;Volume2-End-Stage Renal Disease; 2014.

[15] L. A. Tomlinson, G. A. Abel, A. N. Chaudhry et al., "ACE inhibitor and angiotensin receptor-II antagonist prescribing and hospital admissions with acute kidney injury: A longitudinal ecological study," *PLoS ONE*, vol. 8, no. 11, Article ID e78465, 2013.

[16] The SPRINT Research Group, "A randomized trial of intensive versus standard blood-pressure control," *The New England Journal of Medicine*, vol. 373, no. 22, pp. 2103–2116, 2015, ClinicalTrials.gov number, NCT01206062.

[17] National Center for Health Statistics, *National Health and Nutrition Examination Survey (NHANES) manuals (1999-2000, 2001-2002, 2003-2004, 2005-2006, 2007-2008, 2009–2010, 2011–2012, and 2013-2014)*, 2013, http://www.cdc.gov/nchs/nhanes/nhanes.

[18] National Kidney Foundation, "K/DOQI clinical practice guidelines for chronic kidney disease: evaluation, classification, and stratification," *American Journal of Kidney Diseases*, vol. 39, 1, pp. S1–S266, Feb 2002.

[19] M. T. Crim, S. S. Yoon, E. Ortiz et al., "National surveillance definitions for hypertension prevalence and control among adults," *Circulation: Cardiovascular Quality and Outcomes*, vol. 5, no. 3, pp. 343–351, 2012.

[20] American Diabetes Association, "Standards of medical care in diabetes—2010," *Diabetes Care*, vol. 33, supplement 1, pp. S11–S61, 2010.

[21] Centers for Disease Control and Prevention, *National Center for Health Statistics Division of Health and Nutrition Examination Surveys: National Health and Nutrition Examination Survey: Analytic Guidelines*, 2013, http://www.cdc.gov/nchs /nhanes/.

[22] Q. Gu, V. L. Burt, C. F. Dillon, and S. Yoon, "Trends in antihypertensive medication use and blood pressure control among United States adults with hypertension: the national health and nutrition examination survey, 2001 to 2010," *Circulation*, vol. 126, no. 17, pp. 2105–2114, 2012.

[23] D. C. Wheeler and G. J. Becker, "Summary of KDIGO guideline. What do we really know about management of blood pressure in patients with chronic kidney disease?" *Kidney International*, vol. 83, no. 3, pp. 377–383, 2013.

[24] National Institute for Health and Clinical Excellence, NICE clinical guidance. Chronic kidney disease: early identification and management of chronic kidney disease in adults in primary and secondary care. 2008.

10

Does Intensive Glucose Control Prevent Cognitive Decline in Diabetes?

Carlos Peñaherrera-Oviedo,[1] Daniel Moreno-Zambrano,[1] Michael Palacios,[1] María Carolina Duarte-Martinez,[1] Carlos Cevallos,[1] Ximena Gamboa,[1] María Beatriz Jurado,[1] Leonardo Tamariz,[2] Ana Palacio,[2] and Rocío Santibañez[1]

[1]*Universidad Catolica de Santiago de Guayaquil, 090112 Guayas, Ecuador*
[2]*Miller School of Medicine, University of Miami, Miami, FL 33136, USA*

Correspondence should be addressed to Carlos Peñaherrera-Oviedo; ca_penaherrera@hotmail.com

Academic Editor: Katarzyna Zorena

Diabetes mellitus is associated with cognitive decline and impaired performance in cognitive function tests among type 1 and type 2 diabetics. Even though the use of tight glucose control has been limited by a reported higher mortality, few reports have assessed the impact of treatment intensity on cognitive function. We conducted a meta-analysis to evaluate if an intensive glucose control in diabetes improves cognitive function, in comparison to standard therapy. We included 7 studies that included type 1 or type 2 diabetics and used standardized tests to evaluate various cognitive function domains. Standardized mean differences (SMDs) were calculated for each domain. We found that type 1 diabetics get no cognitive benefit from a tight glucose control, whereas type 2 diabetics get some benefit on processing speed and executive domains but had worse performances in the memory and attention domains, along with a higher incidence of mortality when using intensive glucose control regimes.

1. Introduction

Diabetes mellitus (DM) is a chronic metabolic condition that affects 8.3% of the world population and causes significant morbidity and mortality. The number of people suffering from diabetes is expected to increase beyond 592 million people over the next 25 years [1, 2]. Endothelial damage in diabetes leads to damage of multiple organs and an increased risk of myocardial infarction, stroke, and peripheral vascular disease, along with other chronic complications such as kidney disease or retinopathy [1]. Diabetes also increases the risk of cognitive dysfunction and both vascular dementia and Alzheimer's disease [3–5]. This association is more prominent in elderly diabetics, although mild cognitive impairment may be present also in relatively younger diabetics [6–8]. The impact of diabetes in cognitive function may become more apparent as the life expectancy has significantly increased over the past years [2].

A recent meta-analysis determined that type 2 diabetics had worse performance in neuropsychological tests when compared to normal subjects [9]. As for type 1 diabetes, which is less common and has an onset in childhood, information relating to cognitive function is relatively scarce [1]. There is, however, evidence of an overall decrease in pediatric cognitive performance for diabetic children except in the memory and language domains [10]. A more recent study showed a nonstatistically significant reduction of intellectual function for type 1 diabetics when compared to normal children [11].

Although recent data has found that intensive glucose control could be associated with increased mortality among diabetics, the impact on cognitive function is less understood [12]. We conducted a meta-analysis to determine if intensive glucose control can actually prevent or delay the onset of cognitive decline both in type 1 and in type 2 diabetics. As we move to achieve patient centered care, having information for patients regarding the balance between quantity and quality of life will be useful.

2. Materials and Methods

2.1. Search Strategy. PubMed (MEDLINE) database was searched for randomized controlled trials published from January 1, 1980, to June 1, 2014, using MeSH terms and keywords. Search terms used included "type 1 diabetes mellitus," "type 2 diabetes mellitus," "drug therapy," and "cognitive function." The full search including MeSH terms was (((diabetes mellitus, type 1/drug therapy [MeSH Terms] OR diabetes mellitus, type 2/drug therapy [MeSH Terms]) OR diabetes mellitus, type 1/therapy [MeSH Terms]) OR diabetes mellitus, type 2/therapy [MeSH Terms]) AND (cognitive [All Fields] AND ("physiology" [Subheading] OR "physiology" [All Fields] OR "function" [All Fields] OR "physiology" [MeSH Terms] OR "function" [All Fields])) AND ((Clinical Trial [ptyp] OR Randomized Controlled Trial [ptyp]) AND ("1980/01/01" [PDAT]: "2014/12/31" [PDAT])). We also reviewed the reference list of the identified articles looking for additional studies that might be included in this meta-analysis.

2.2. Inclusion Criteria. We included randomized controlled trials (RCT), which analyzed patients with either type 1 or type 2 diabetes, had at least one group of patients receiving intensive glucose control and another receiving conventional antidiabetic treatment, and provided information regarding assessment of cognitive function after a follow-up period using a standardized method.

2.3. Exclusion Criteria. The exclusion criteria we used were as follows: studies which included patients already diagnosed with cognitive dysfunction or established dementia, studies that used only the Minimental Score Examination (MMSE) as an assessment of cognitive function, and studies that utilized a cognitive testing method which was not comparable to those used in any of the other articles included.

2.4. Definition of the Exposure. We defined interventions as "intensive" if they tailored care to reach a glycated hemoglobin (HbA1c) goal of less than 7% or a fasting glucose level of less than 130 mg/dL. The format and content of the interventions could vary. Conventional treatment was defined simply as the continuation of the regular treatment the patient was already receiving.

The definition of intensive glucose control varied among the included studies. Four of them intended to achieve levels of HbA1c below 6%, while another one targeted HbA1c levels below 7% [14–16, 18, 19]. Two more studies did not report a goal level of glycated hemoglobin, one of them targeted preprandial glucose levels below 130 mg/dL instead, and the last one adjusted goals of glycaemia and HbA1c individually with each patient [13, 17]. Treatment goals are summarized in Table 1. The methods used to achieve these goals ranged from multifactorial behavioral interventions to adjusted doses of oral antidiabetics to 3 or more insulin injections per day or continuous insulin infusion with an external pump.

TABLE 1: Treatment goals for the definition of intensive glucose control.

Study	HbA1c (%)	Preprandial glucose level (mg/dL)
Reichard et al. [13]	Individual adjustment	Individual adjustment
DCCT [14]	<6.05	70–120
EDIC [15]	<6	70–120
Musen et al. [16]	<6.05	70–120
Naor et al. [17]	N/A	<130
Launer et al. [18]	<6	N/A
Koekkoek et al. [19]	<7	N/A

2.5. Outcome. The main outcome was cognitive dysfunction classified into the following domains based on standard domain definitions: information processing speed, executive function, attention/concentration, verbal memory, and motor function.

The domains were evaluated using validated neuropsychological tests. Information processing speed was assessed through the Digit-Symbol Substitution Subtest (DSST) of the Wechsler Assessment of Intelligence Scale (WAIS), in which the participant is initially shown a key containing symbol-digit pairs and must later copy the corresponding symbol under a series of numbers with empty boxes below [20]. Total score is given by the number of correct pairings within a 90-second limit. As measures of executive functioning, participants were assessed using the Trail Making Test part B (TMT-B) and the Similarities subtest of the WAIS. The TMT-B measures the time a subject needs to draw lines connecting 25 encircled letters and numbers distributed over a sheet of paper in alternating order [21]. For the Similarities subtest, subjects are asked in what way two words are alike (i.e., poem and statue). The scores for the Similarities task are presented in age-adjusted scaled scores.

Memory function was evaluated using the Rey Auditory Verbal Learning Test (RAVLT), a verbal learning task where the participant is given a list of 15 unrelated words repeated over 5 trials [22]. A delayed-recall trial is administered 30 minutes after the initial learning phase and the number of freely recalled words is recorded. Reaction time to auditory and visual stimuli was measured through computerized tasks where participants had to press a key immediately after presentation of visual (light) or auditory (tone) stimuli. The Finger Tapping Test was administered as a measure of motor function. In this test, participants place their hand on a board with a lever and tap their index finger on the lever as quickly as possible, using their dominant and nondominant hands, within a 10-second time interval. Scores are calculated by averaging the number of taps over five consecutive trials within a 5-point range with each hand [23]. The Stroop test is a measure of selective attention, cognitive flexibility, and cognitive inhibition [24]. It consists of three parts. In the first part subjects read a list of color names printed in black ink. In the second part they must name the color of a list of X's or color patches, depending on the version used. In the third

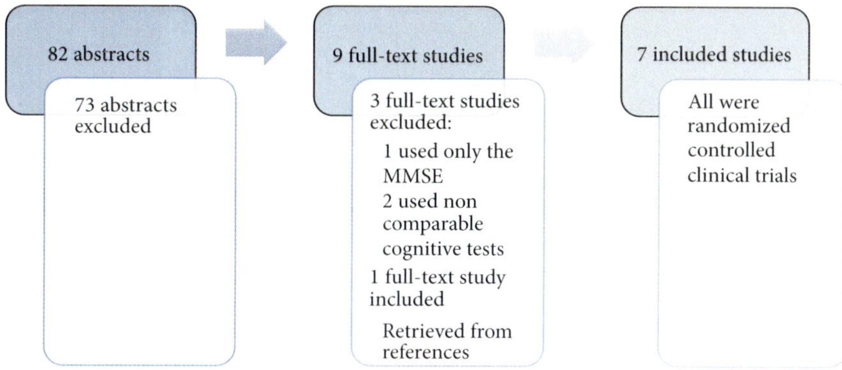

Figure 1: Summary of database search conducted on PubMed and details of study selection.

part of the task the subject must name the color of a color word written in nonmatching ink color (e.g., the word green printed in red). A Stroop interference effect occurs when color-naming speed is significantly reduced as the subject must inhibit an automatic reading response to produce a more effortful color-naming response [25].

2.6. Statistical Analysis. We reported relevant baseline characteristics for each study as mean and percentage as reported. To aggregate unweighted results for all studies we report the median and interquartile range for continuous variables and for HbA1c we report the mean values before and after the intervention per randomized group. To assess for heterogeneity across studies we used the Cochran Q chi-square (significance level <0.10) and the I-squared statistic (>50%).

For the mathematical pooling we stratified the analysis by type of diabetes and calculated the standardized mean difference (SMD) with the corresponding 95% confidence interval and p value. The SMD represents the difference between the mean and standard deviation of the cognitive test in the intensive control group minus that of the conventional group for each study. The SMD was weighted by the sample size of each individual study per randomized group. We used Comprehensive Meta-Analysis software (Biostat Inc., Englewood, NJ) for the quantitative analysis.

3. Results

Our search strategy yielded 82 articles, from which we excluded 73 abstracts because they were not RCT or did not meet inclusion criteria. From the remaining 9 studies from the original search, we removed 3 more articles after exclusion criteria were applied. One additional study was retrieved from the references of the articles reviewed and was included for analysis as it did not meet exclusion criteria [16]. A total of 7 articles were finally included in the meta-analysis, of which 4 analyzed type 1 diabetics and 3 studied type 2 diabetics (Figure 1).

The combined sample size was 6056 patients (3011 under intensive glucose control and 3045 under conventional treatment). The median age was 27 years for type 1 diabetics and 62.4 years for type 2 diabetics. The median follow-up time was for type 1 and type 2. Only two studies had more than 50% female patients. Median baseline levels of HbA1c were 9.24% for the intensive treatment group and 9.07% for the conventional treatment patients, while HbA1c levels after treatment follow-up were 7.43% for the intensive group and 8.17% for the conventional treatment patients. Study characteristics are presented in Table 2.

Table 3 describes the results of each test per arm. The most commonly reported tests where the DSST, trail making, finger tap, and RAVLT. The univariate results show that on each test there is a difference between the intensive treatment group and the control group. Table 4 shows the weighted SMDs of each test stratified by type of diabetes. All tests for type 1 diabetes were nonsignificant. For type 2 diabetes the DSST SMD had a positive direction (0.71), while the Trail Making Test, Stroop test, and RAVLT had a negative direction. However, a negative direction on the SMD for Trail Making Test also favors intensive glucose control due to the nature of the test. These results are summarized in Figure 2, where results for TMT have been mirrored to a positive sense for a better presentation.

4. Discussion

Our meta-analysis demonstrates that tight glucose control is not superior to conventional care at preventing cognitive decline among type 1 diabetics and has a positive impact only on the information processing speed and executive functions among type 2 diabetics.

The lack of effect seen for type 1 diabetics could be related to the nonsignificant differences described to date in cognitive function between diabetics and healthy control groups [11]. Among young diabetic patients who are free of multiple comorbidities, the effect of hyperglycemia may not be severe enough to cause a significant cognitive impairment, and thus the glucose lowering regime used to treat diabetes becomes unimportant regarding prevention of cognitive function loss. An alternative explanation is that the small cognitive decline reported among type 1 diabetics is related to the effect of repeated hypoglycemic events which may cause white matter damage but would not be reduced by tight glucose control [10, 26].

In contrast, the effect of tight glucose control varied across cognitive domains among type 2 diabetics. The intensive

Table 2: Characteristics of included studies.

Study*	Country	DM type	(*n*)	Intensive treatment (*n*)	Conventional treatment (*n*)	Mean (SD) age (years)		Follow-up time (months)	Female patients (%)	
						Intensive	Conventional		Intensive	Conventional
Reichard et al. [13]	Sweden	1	96	44	52	29.5 ± 1.1	31.6 ± 1	50	50	48
DCCT [14]	USA/Canada	1	1441	711	730	27.1 ± 7.1	26.5 ± 7.1	60	48.5	45.9
EDIC [15]	USA/Canada	1	1144	588	556	27 ± 7	27 ± 7	144	49	45
Musen et al. [16]	USA/Canada	1	175	82	93	16 ± 2	16 ± 2	144	50	62
Naor et al. [17]	Germany	2	40	20	20	63.6 ± 5.3	63.8 ± 5.5	2	60	65
Launer et al. [18]	USA/Canada	2	2977	1469	1508	62.3 ± 5.7	62.7 ± 5.9	40	48	49
Koekkoek et al. [19]	Netherlands	2	183	97	86	59.3 ± 5.6	59.5 ± 5.3	120	42.3	35.7

* All included studies were randomized controlled clinical trials (RCCT).
DCCT: Diabetes Control and Complications Trial; EDIC: Epidemiology of Diabetes Interventions and Complications Study.

TABLE 3: Mean (SD) results from each cognitive function test utilized in the studies included.

Study	DM type	DSST (number of correct pairings in 50 seconds)		Trail Making Test (seconds)		Similarities subtest of WAIS (age-adjusted score 0–19)		Visual reaction time (milliseconds)		Auditory reaction time (milliseconds)		RAVLT (number of freely recalled words)		Stroop test (number of correct items in 45 seconds)		Finger tap for dominant hand (taps in 10 seconds)		Finger tap for nondominant hand (taps in 10 seconds)	
		I	C	I	C	I	C	I	C	I	C	I	C	I	C	I	C	I	C
Reichard et al. [13]*	1	—	—	39.9	45.6	—	—	241	241	209	207	—	—	—	—	6.8	6.5	6.2	6.1
DCCT [14]	1	64.7 (11.3)	64.8 (11.2)	52.9 (16.7)	53.5 (19.6)	12.5 (2.4)	12.6 (2.3)	—	—	—	—	15.4 (1.7)	15.3 (1.9)	—	—	4.9 (0.7)	4.9 (0.7)	4.4 (0.6)	4.5 (0.6)
EDIC [15]	1	62.3 (11.4)	61.9 (11.4)	54.4 (20)	55 (18.8)	14 (2.2)	13.9 (2.3)	—	—	—	—	14.7 (2.2)	15 (2)	—	—	5.1 (0.7)	5.1 (0.8)	4.5 (0.7)	4.5 (0.7)
Musen et al. [16]	1	67.8 (10.5)	66.3 (9.1)	45.6 (12.8)	48.9 (15.1)	13.8 (2.2)	13.1 (2.4)	—	—	—	—	15.5 (1.4)	15.3 (1.7)	—	—	5.2 (0.7)	5.1 (0.7)	4.7 (0.6)	4.5 (0.7)
Naor et al. [17]	2	—	—	93.8 (17.1)	140 (35.6)	—	—	284.7 (22.8)	309.1 (54.7)	211.4 (42.8)	218.1 (38.1)	—	—	—	—	—	—	—	—
Launer et al. [18]	2	50.93 (0.43)	50.61 (0.42)	—	—	—	—	—	—	—	—	7.98 (0.1)	7.99 (0.09)	31.45 (0.36)	32.06 (0.36)	—	—	—	—
Koekkoek et al. [19]	2	55.6 (17.4)	57 (15.5)	93.5 (39.4)	96.5 (50.2)	—	—	8.3 (3.5)	8.1 (3)	—	—	8.3 (3.5)	8.1 (3)	50.2 (8.4)	50.1 (11.6)	—	—	—	—

*Standard deviation (SD) not reported.
I: intensive glucose control group.
C: conventional therapy group.
"—" denotes that such test was not carried out in the corresponding study.

Weighted SMD for type 1 diabetes

Study	SMD	Lower CI	Upper CI	p
(1) DSST				
DCCT (1996)	−0,009	−0,112	0,094	0,866
EDIC (2007)	0,035	−0,081	0,151	0,553
Musen et al. (2008)	0,153	−0,144	0,451	0,312
Overall	0,020	−0,055	0,094	0,607
(2) TMT (results inverted for presentation)				
Reichard et al. (1991)	1,000	0,574	1,426	<0,01
DCCT (1996)	0,033	−0,070	0,136	0,532
EDIC (2007)	0,031	−0,085	0,147	0,602
Musen et al. (2008)	0,235	−0,063	0,532	0,123
Overall	0,073	−0,000	0,147	0,051
(3) Similarities subtest of WAIS				
DCCT (1996)	−0,043	−0,146	0,061	0,419
EDIC (2007)	0,044	−0,071	0,160	0,452
Musen et al. (2008)	0,303	0,005	0,602	0,047
Overall	0,015	−0,060	0,090	0,691
(4) RAVLT				
DCCT (1996)	0,055	−0,048	0,159	0,293
EDIC (2007)	−0,143	−0,259	−0,026	0,016
Musen et al. (2008)	0,128	−0,170	0,425	0,400
Overall	−0,022	−0,097	0,053	0,565
(5) Finger tap for dominant hand				
Reichard et al. (1991)	0,750	0,335	1,165	<0,01
DCCT (1996)	0,000	−0,103	0,103	1,000
EDIC (2007)	0,000	−0,116	0,116	1,000
Musen et al. (2008)	0,143	−0,154	0,440	0,346
Overall	0,032	−0,041	0,106	0,390
(6) Finger tap for nondominant hand				
Reichard et al. (1991)	0,500	0,092	0,908	0,016
DCCT (1996)	−0,167	−0,270	−0,063	0,002
EDIC (2007)	0,000	−0,116	0,116	1,000
Musen et al. (2008)	0,305	0,007	0,604	0,045
Overall	−0,049	−0,123	0,024	0,188

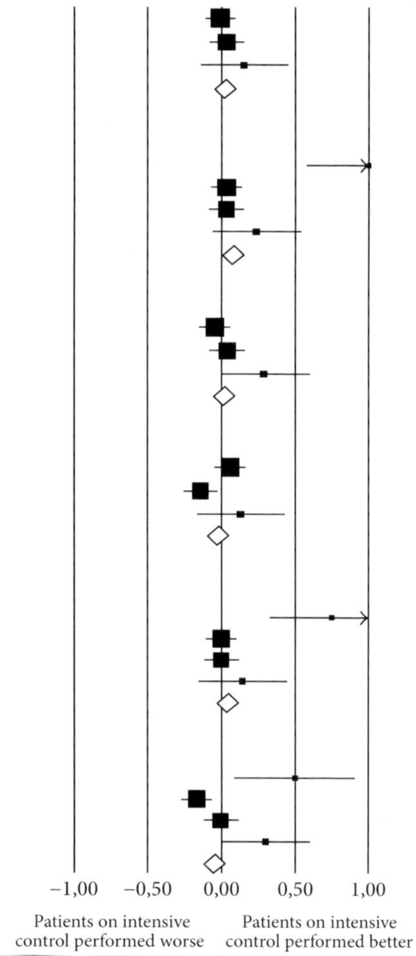

Weighted SMD for type 2 diabetes

Study	SMD	Lower CI	Upper CI	p
(1) DSST				
Launer et al. (2011)	0,753	0,679	0,827	<0,01
Koekkoek et al. (2012)	−0,085	−0,375	0,206	0,568
Overall	0,701	0,629	0,774	<0,01
(2) TMT (results inverted for presentation)				
Naor et al. (1997)	1,654	0,936	2,372	<0,01
Koekkoek et al. (2012)	0,067	−0,223	0,357	0,651
Overall	0,290	0,021	0,559	0,035
(3) RAVLT				
Launer et al. (2011)	−0,200	−0,272	−0,128	<0,01
Koekkoek et al. (2012)	0,061	−0,229	0,351	0,680
Overall	−0,185	−0,255	−0,115	<0,01
(4) Stroop test				
Launer et al. (2011)	−0,847	−0,922	−0,772	<0,01
Koekkoek et al. (2012)	0,010	−0,280	0,300	0,946
Overall	−0,794	−0,866	−0,721	<0,01

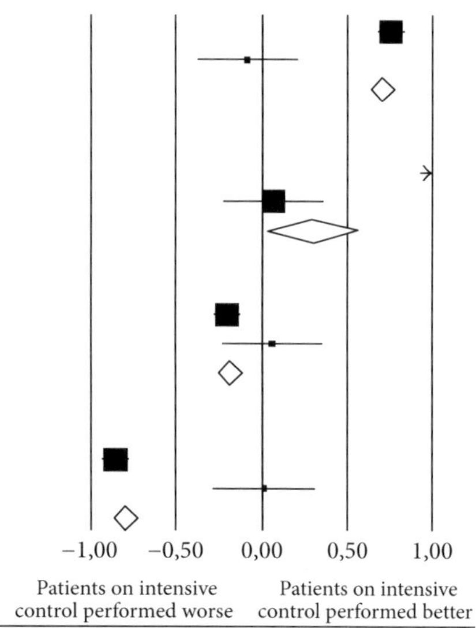

FIGURE 2: Summary of standardized mean differences for each cognitive test, divided by type of diabetes. Results for TMT have been mirrored for a more uniform presentation.

Table 4: Results of weighted SMDs for each cognitive test.

Cognitive test	Number of studies	Weighted SMD (95% CI)	I-squared	p
		Type 1 diabetes		
DSST	3	0.02 (−0.05 to 0.09)	0%	0.60
Trail Making Test	4	−0.07 (−0.14 to 0.00)	85%	0.05
Similarities subtest of WAIS	3	0.015 (−0.06 to 0.09)	60%	0.69
RAVLT	3	−0.022 (−0.09 to 0.05)	72%	0.56
Finger tap from the dominant hand	4	0.032 (−0.04 to 0.106)	76%	0.39
Finger tap from nondominant hand	4	−0.045 (−0.123 to 0.024)	83%	0.19
		Type 2 diabetes		
DSST	2	0.71 (0.64 to 0.78)	97%	<0.01
Trail Making Test	2	−0.29 (−0.55 to −0.02)	94%	0.04
RAVLT	2	−0.185 (−0.26 to −0.16)	66%	<0.01
Stroop test	2	−0.79 (−0.87 to −0.72)	97%	<0.01

control group performed significantly better on the DSST and TMT but did worse than the conventional treatment group on the Stroop test and the RAVLT. From these results we can conclude that tight glucose control favors the domains of information processing speed and executive function, but at the cost of negatively affecting attention and memory functions. The presence of comorbidities at the age of onset of diabetes, which is much later than that for type 1 diabetics, may help explain these results. Also, it has been described that insulin is one of the molecules that regulate tau protein phosphorylation in neurons, and thus insulin resistance may disrupt this process, causing tau to bind to microtubules, giving rise to the pathogenesis of Alzheimer's disease and dementia [27]. Educational level is also an important confounding factor in this population, as it has been observed that cognitive performance correlates directly with the amount of years of completed study [28]. However, there are no enough data to test the impact of these confounders in the current meta-analysis.

In regard to the higher risk of mortality previously reported for tight glucose control regimes, only two of the studies included reported a mortality outcome [15, 18]. Thus, evaluating the relationship between cognitive decline, mortality, and tight glucose control was not possible. To date, age, the increased risk of hypoglycemia, and the presence of important comorbidities are factors that favor the increased incidence of deaths in type 2 population, while in type 1 diabetics, though there was an increased risk of hypoglycemic events, the great majority were nonfatal [12, 15]. Further studies are needed to understand the relationship between cognitive decline and mortality.

Our study has several limitations. First, while there is significant evidence on the relationship of diabetes and cognitive decline, very few trials have addressed the impact of different glucose control regimes on cognitive function. More so, many studies evaluating this question could not be included because they either used noncomparable tests or reported cognitive decline using only the MMSE [26, 28–30]. The MMSE does not offer enough information to rigorously evaluate cognitive function. Also, the large variation in sample size among type 2 diabetes studies caused one of the studies to carry more significant weight than the others.

In conclusion, we observed that there is no benefit from intensive glucose lowering regarding cognitive function for the young type 1 diabetics, while the older type 2 diabetics benefit from this therapy in the domains of information processing speed and executive function but find their attention and memory hindered. These findings provide insight into the pathophysiology of different types of cognitive impairment and possible therapeutic avenues in the future. Some studies have shown an increased risk of cardiovascular mortality and hypoglycemia when using intensive glucose control regimes. Thus, each case should be evaluated individually to assess the benefits of a tight glycemic control against the observed risks. Since these complications are more common in older diabetic patients, intensive control of the glucose levels might be safer and more recommendable in type 1 diabetics, most of which are children or young adolescents, regarding noncognitive benefits.

References

[1] American Diabetes Association, "Standards of medical care in diabetes—2014," *Diabetes Care*, vol. 37, supplement 1, pp. S14–S80, 2014.

[2] International Diabetes Federation, *IDF Diabetes Atlas*, International Diabetes Federation, Brussels, Belgium, 6th edition, 2013.

[3] S. C. M. Croxson and C. Jagger, "Diabetes and cognitive impairment: a community-based study of elderly subjects," *Age and Ageing*, vol. 24, no. 5, pp. 421–424, 1995.

[4] T. Ohara, Y. Doi, T. Ninomiya et al., "Glucose tolerance status and risk of dementia in the community: the Hisayama study," *Neurology*, vol. 77, no. 12, pp. 1126–1134, 2011.

[5] A. Ott, R. P. Stolk, A. Hofman, F. van Harskamp, D. E. Grobbee, and M. M. B. Breteler, "Association of diabetes mellitus and

dementia: the Rotterdam Study," *Diabetologia*, vol. 39, no. 11, pp. 1392–1397, 1996.

[6] S. Kalmijn, E. J. M. Feskens, L. J. Launer, T. Stijnen, and D. Kromhout, "Glucose intolerance, hyperinsulinaemia and cognitive function in a general population of elderly men," *Diabetologia*, vol. 38, no. 9, pp. 1096–1102, 1995.

[7] J. Dey, A. Misra, N. G. Desai, A. K. Mahapatra, and M. V. Padma, "Cognitive function in younger type II diabetes," *Diabetes Care*, vol. 20, no. 1, pp. 32–35, 1997.

[8] C. M. Ryan and M. O. Geckle, "Circumscribed cognitive dysfunction in middle-aged adults with type 2 diabetes," *Diabetes Care*, vol. 23, no. 10, pp. 1486–1493, 2000.

[9] P. Palta, A. L. C. Schneider, G. J. Biessels, P. Touradji, and F. Hill-Briggs, "Magnitude of cognitive dysfunction in adults with type 2 diabetes: a meta-analysis of six cognitive domains and the most frequently reported neuropsychological tests within domains," *Journal of the International Neuropsychological Society*, vol. 20, no. 3, pp. 278–291, 2014.

[10] P. A. Gaudieri, R. Chen, T. F. Greer, and C. S. Holmes, "Cognitive function in children with type 1 diabetes: a meta-analysis," *Diabetes Care*, vol. 31, no. 9, pp. 1892–1897, 2008.

[11] M. A. Cato, N. Mauras, J. Ambrosino et al., "Cognitive functioning in young children with type 1 diabetes," *Journal of the International Neuropsychological Society*, vol. 20, no. 2, pp. 238–247, 2014.

[12] The Action to Control Cardiovascular Risk in Diabetes Study Group, "Effects of intensive glucose lowering in type 2 diabetes," *The New England Journal of Medicine*, vol. 358, no. 24, pp. 2545–2459, 2008.

[13] P. Reichard, A. Britz, and U. Rosenqvist, "Intensified conventional insulin treatment and neuropsychological impairment," *British Medical Journal*, vol. 303, no. 6815, pp. 1439–1442, 1991.

[14] The Diabetes Control and Complications Trial Research Group, "Effects of intensive diabetes therapy on neuropsychological function in adults in the diabetes control and complications trial," *Annals of Internal Medicine*, vol. 124, no. 4, pp. 379–388, 1996.

[15] Diabetes Control and Complications Trial/Epidemiology of Diabetes Interventions and Complications Study Research Group, "Long-term effect of diabetes and its treatment on cognitive function," *The New England Journal of Medicine*, vol. 356, no. 18, pp. 1842–1852, 2007.

[16] G. Musen, A. M. Jacobson, C. M. Ryan et al., "Impact of diabetes and its treatment on cognitive function among adolescents who participated in the diabetes control and complications trial," *Diabetes Care*, vol. 31, no. 10, pp. 1933–1938, 2008.

[17] M. Naor, H. J. Steingrüber, K. Westhoff, Y. Schottenfeld-Naor, and A. F. Gries, "Cognitive function in elderly non-insulin-dependent diabetic patients before and after inpatient treatment for metabolic control," *Journal of Diabetes and Its Complications*, vol. 11, no. 1, pp. 40–46, 1997.

[18] L. J. Launer, M. E. Miller, J. D. Williamson et al., "Effects of intensive glucose lowering on brain structure and function in people with type 2 diabetes (ACCORD MIND): a randomised open-label substudy," *The Lancet Neurology*, vol. 10, no. 11, pp. 969–977, 2011.

[19] P. S. Koekkoek, C. Ruis, M. van den Donk et al., "Intensive multifactorial treatment and cognitive functioning in screen-detected type 2 diabetes—the ADDITION-Netherlands study: a cluster-randomized trial," *Journal of the Neurological Sciences*, vol. 314, no. 1-2, pp. 71–77, 2012.

[20] D. Wechsler, *Wechsler Adult Intelligence Scale*, The Psychological Corporation, Harcourt Brace, San Antonio, Tex, USA, 3rd edition, 1997.

[21] War Department Adjutant General's Office, *Army Individual Test Battery: Manual of Directions and Scoring*, War Department Adjutant General's Office, Washington, DC, USA, 1944.

[22] M. Schmidt, *Rey Auditory and Verbal Learning Test: A Handbook*, Western Psychological Services, Los Angeles, Calif, USA, 1996.

[23] R. M. Reitan, *The Halstead-Reitan Neuropsychological Test Battery: Theory and Clinical Interpretation*, Neuropsychology Press, S. Tucson, Ariz, USA, 2nd edition, 1993.

[24] J. R. Stroop, "Studies of interference in serial verbal reactions," *Journal of Experimental Psychology*, vol. 18, no. 6, pp. 643–662, 1935.

[25] E. Strauss, E. M. S. Sherman, and O. Spreen, *A Compendium of Neuropsychological Tests: Administration, Norms, and Commentary*, Oxford University Press, New York, NY, USA, 3rd edition, 2006.

[26] T. Hershey, N. Bhargava, M. Sadler, N. H. White, and S. Craft, "Conventional versus intensive diabetes therapy in children with type 1 diabetes: effects on memory and motor speed," *Diabetes Care*, vol. 22, no. 8, pp. 1318–1324, 1999.

[27] M. Hong and V. M.-Y. Lee, "Insulin and insulin-like growth factor-1 regulate tau phosphorylation in cultured human neurons," *The Journal of Biological Chemistry*, vol. 272, no. 31, pp. 19547–19553, 1997.

[28] R. D. Lindeman, L. J. Romero, A. Larue et al., "A biethnic community survey of cognition in participants with type 2 diabetes, impaired glucose tolerance, and normal glucose tolerance—the New Mexico elder health survey," *Diabetes Care*, vol. 24, no. 9, pp. 1567–1572, 2001.

[29] J. Hung, L. Menth, M. J. Thompson, B. Saner, K. V. Rao, and J. Barbosa, "The Minnesota diabetes complications clinical trial cognitive functions under long term maximized and standard metabolic controls," *Diabète et Métabolisme*, vol. 10, no. 1, pp. 48–51, 1984.

[30] A. Araki, S. Iimuro, T. Sakurai et al., "Long-term multiple risk factor interventions in Japanese elderly diabetic patients: the Japanese Elderly Diabetes Intervention Trial—study design, baseline characteristics and effects of intervention," *Geriatrics and Gerontology International*, vol. 12, supplement 1, pp. 7–17, 2012.

11

Burden of Self-Reported Noncommunicable Diseases in 26 Villages of Anand District of Gujarat, India

Dinesh Kumar,[1] Shyamsundar J. Raithatha,[1] Shanti Gupta,[2] Ravi Raj,[2] and Nikhil Kharod[1]

[1]*Pramukhswami Medical College, Karamsad, Gujarat 388325, India*
[2]*Extension Programmes Department, HM Patel Center for Medical Care and Education, Karamsad, Gujarat 388325, India*

Correspondence should be addressed to Dinesh Kumar; drdineshkl@charutarhealth.org

Academic Editor: Jose Tellez-Zenteno

Introduction. Noncommunicable diseases (NCDs) account for 53% of deaths and 44% of disability adjusted life years lost in India. A survey was undertaken to measure the prevalence of tobacco and alcohol use and self-reported NCDs in a rural community in western part of India. *Methodology.* Trained Village Health Workers did the survey in the years 2012-13 under supervision. The data was collected for five NCDs, namely, hypertension, diabetes mellitus, cancer, heart disease, and mental illnesses. *Results.* 18,269 households with a population of 89755 were covered. Prevalence of any form of tobacco use in the age group of >20 years was 34.5 and 52.7% and 15.2% in males and females, respectively. Prevalence of any NCD was 5.3% with a slightly higher prevalence in females (5.4%) than males (5.2%) in the age group of 20–69 years. Prevalence of NCD multimorbidity (≥2 NCDs) was 0.7% in the age group of 20–69 years. 80.7% of hypertensives and 94.9% of diabetics were taking treatment. More females than males were taking antihypertensive treatment. *Conclusion.* Tobacco use was high. Prevalence of NCDs was less than that reported in other studies. Data generated from this study can be useful in planning a community based NCD programme.

1. Introduction

Noncommunicable diseases (NCDs) comprising heart diseases, diabetes, cancer, respiratory diseases, and others contributed to 63% of the 57 million global deaths in 2008 [1]. Eighty percent (80%) of all of these deaths occurred in low- and middle-income countries [1, 2]. These deaths are projected to rise by 15% globally between 2010 and 2020 and with the greatest increases expected to be in low- and middle-income regions [1]. India is undergoing an epidemiological transition with changing patterns of diseases. According to a report, NCDs accounted for a 53% of all deaths and 44% of the disability adjusted life years (DALYs) lost in the year 2005 [3]. The age standardized mortality rate for the NCDs for males and females has been reported to be 757.7 and 537.9 deaths per 100000, respectively [4]. Cardiovascular diseases are the most common diseases contributing to 29% of all the deaths followed by cancer, chronic respiratory diseases, and diabetes which contribute to 7%, 7%, and 2% of the deaths, respectively. As the population of India ages, total number of deaths will increase and the proportion of the deaths due to the chronic diseases will increase as well. The high NCD burden poses a significant challenge to the health care system by accounting for 35% of all outpatient and 40% of inpatient hospitalization bed-days in 2004 [5]. NCDs have a significant effect on the financial condition of households considering the fact that 86.4% of the total expenditure on health care is borne out of pocket in India [6]. According to a World Bank report, the annual income losses to households associated with NCDs account to roughly INR 280 billion (USD 6222 million). It has also been found that 25% of families with a member with CVD experience catastrophic expenditure (health expenditure that is more than 40% of the total nonfood consumption expenditure) [7]. The situation is much worse with cancer, where almost 50% of households with a member with cancer experience catastrophic spending and 25% are driven to poverty by health care expenses [5]. In such a scenario, significant steps are required to be taken at the community level for prevention and control of these diseases. There are very few community based models available in India to address this problem. In order to develop such a model, one of the prerequisites is availability of baseline data on the burden of diseases. It will help in better planning of the resources required for the project. This study reports the findings of a survey related to the burden of self-reported NCDs and tobacco and alcohol use in the community.

2. Materials and Methods

Our institute is involved in testing and developing a three-tier health care delivery model with a major focus on noncommunicable diseases. It works in 90 villages and has a network of 5 extension centers (health centers) in the community. A household survey was undertaken in 26 of these villages in the years 2012-13 to identify the catchment population for the programme, estimate the population size for screening of the three cancers, and estimate the burden of tobacco and alcohol use in the population. Moreover data was also collected on prevalence, duration, and treatment status of five self-reported NCDs (hypertension, diabetes mellitus, cancer, heart disease, and mental illnesses). The operational definition for the presence of an NCD was "Whether the doctor has told you that you are suffering from this disease and/or advised treatment for the same?" The survey is repeated annually for updating of the database. The findings of the first survey are presented in this study. The information about all the members of the household was obtained from one of the adult members of the household. If any chronic disease other than these 5 NCDs was present, it was reported as well. The data was collected by Village Health Workers (VHWs) belonging to each of the villages through a one-page questionnaire in local language (Gujarati). The VHWs were females belonging to the village in which they conducted the survey. Their mean age and mean years of schooling were 44.65 years and 9 years, respectively. A one-day training programme comprising didactic sessions and hands on exercises was organised for the VHWs for the data collection process. The training was extended on field as well where the VHWs did the data collection under supervision in the initial phase. The process of data collection lasted from September 2012 to December 2013. The data collection process was supervised by 3 Field Supervisors (FS) and 3 Programme Executives (PEs). The FS checked all the forms for completeness and 10% for quality of data collection by cross verification through home visits. The PEs verified 5% of the forms for completeness and 5% of the forms for quality of data collection by cross verification through home visits. The data was entered in a data entry software designed specifically for this project, by five data entry operators. The PEs checked 5% of the entered forms for accuracy and 5% for completeness during the data entry process. A daily backup and online storage process through Dropbox was established to prevent loss of data. Moreover postentry data quality checks were run through Statistical Package for Social Science (SPSS) 16 wherein a descriptive analysis was done to identify outliers which were cross-checked with the hard copies of the forms. Ethical clearance was obtained from the institutional Human Research Ethics Committee (HREC) for publishing the findings of the survey.

Table 1: Age and sex distribution and education status of the study population.

Variable	Frequency	Percent
Total population	89755	100%
Age groups		
Children (0–9 years)	16067	17.9%
Adolescents (10–19 years)	15098	16.8%
Adults (≥20 years)	58590	65.2%
Elderly (>60 years)	8288	9.2%
Sex		
Male	46903	52.3%
Female	42852	47.7%
Education status in adults (aged 20–69 years)		
Illiterate	10372	18.7%
≤8 years of schooling	21547	38.9%
8–12 years of schooling	29852	35.8%
>12 years of schooling	3680	6.6%

Analysis. Age-sex pyramid was created. Proportions were calculated for self-reported prevalence of five NCDs. Crude as well as age adjusted prevalence was calculated. The prevalence was adjusted by direct standardization method using the standard WHO population [8]. Chi-square test was applied for testing statistical significance of difference in the prevalence of NCDs between different groups.

3. Results

There were 18,269 households contributing to a population of 89755 with an average family size of 4.91. 70.2% of the population comprised adults >20 years of age (Table 1). The overall gender ratio and the gender ratio in the 0–6 years' age group were 914 and 894 females per 1000 males, respectively. Agriculture (46.8%) was the major occupation for heads of the households followed by labour work in nonagricultural jobs (22%). 34.7% of the population (age group 20–69 years) reported at least some form of tobacco (oral tobacco, beedi, and cigarettes) or alcohol use. Similarly 2.5% of the population in the age group of 5–19 years (children) reported at least some form of tobacco or alcohol use. The prevalence of tobacco and alcohol use among males was significantly higher than that among females (Table 2). The prevalence of any NCD in the population was 5.3% and it was slightly higher in females 5.4% as compared to males 5.2% (Table 3). 80.7% of hypertensives and 94.9% of the diabetics were taking treatment. The proportion of hypertensive females (82.5%) taking treatment was significantly higher than that for males (78.3%) with a p value of 0.003. In case of diabetes, this difference was not significant. The prevalence of NCDs increased with the age ($p < 0.001$, chi-square for trend) except for mental illnesses. Increasing educational status also showed association with prevalence of hypertension and diabetes mellitus ($p < 0.001$, chi-square for trend). Substance use did not show any statistical association with self-reported NCD prevalence. The details for association of age, education, and substance use categories are provided in Table 4.

TABLE 2: Prevalence of substance abuse in the total population and genderwise (in adults aged 20–69 years).

Substance abuse	Total prevalence (%)	Prevalence in females (%)	Prevalence in males (%)	p value* (chi-square test)
Any	34.7	15.2	53.1	<0.001
Any tobacco	34.5	15.2	52.7	<0.001
Oral tobacco	27.7	14.8	39.8	<0.001
Beedi	9.3	0.5	17.6	<0.001
Cigarette	0.4	0	0.7	<0.001
Alcohol	2.1	0.2	3.9	<0.001
Tobacco + alcohol	0.6	0.000	1.1	<0.001

* p value is for difference between genders and is based on chi-square test.

TABLE 3: Prevalence of self-reported noncommunicable diseases (NCDs) in the adult population (aged 20–69 years).

NCD	Age adjusted prevalence*	Crude prevalence	Prevalence in males	Prevalence in females	p value# (Chi-square test)
Hypertension	4.2%	3.7%	3.7%	4.4%	<0.001
Diabetes mellitus	1.5%	1.3%	1.5%	1.2%	0.003
Cancer	0.1%	0.1%	0.1%	0.1%	0.090
Heart disease	0.44	0.39%	0.5%	0.3%	<0.001
Mental illnesses	0.3%	0.3%	0.3%	0.3%	0.264
Any disease	5.9%	5.3%	5.2%	5.4%	0.690

* Adjusted with WHO standard population [8].
# For crude prevalence between males and females.

TABLE 4: Prevalence of self-reported noncommunicable diseases in adults (20–69 years) compared with respect to various sociodemographic variables.

Variable	Any NCD	Hypertension	Diabetes mellitus	Heart disease	Cancer	Mental illness
Age groups						
20–40 years	389 (1.3%)	209 (0.7%)	53 (0.2%)	22 (0.1%)	12 (0.1%)	77 (0.3%)
40–60 years	1571 (7.9%)	1135 (5.7%)	428 (2.1%)	127 (0.6%)	27 (0.1%)	66 (0.3%)
60–69 years	993 (19.5%)	748 (14.7%)	264 (5.2%)	71 (1.4%)	20 (0.4%)	20 (0.4%)
Education						
Illiterate	571 (5.5%)	390 (3.8%)	72 (0.7%)	35 (0.3%)	5 (0.0%)	57 (0.5%)
≤8 years of schooling	1057 (4.9%)	760 (3.5%)	231 (1.1%)	88 (0.4%)	31 (0.1%)	54 (0.3%)
8–12 years of schooling	1083 (5.5%)	778 (3.9%)	364 (1.8%)	81 (0.4%)	19 (0.1%)	45 (0.2%)
>12 years of schooling	242 (6.6%)	164 (4.5%)	78 (2.1%)	16 (0.4%)	4 (0.1%)	7 (0.2%)
Substance use						
Oral tobacco	629 (4.1%)	464 (3%)	144 (0.9%)	56 (0.4%)	16 (0.1%)	41 (0.3%)
Smoking	442 (8.4%)	263 (5%)	84 (1.6%)	48 (0.9%)	12 (0.2%)	17 (0.3%)
Oral tobacco and smoking	982 (5.1%)	670 (3.5%)	213 (1.1%)	94 (0.5%)	24 (0.1%)	51 (0.3%)
Alcohol	56 (4.8%)	33 (2.8%)	9 (0.8%)	9 (0.8%)	1 (0.1%)	4 (0.3%)
Any addiction	987 (5.1%)	672 (3.5%)	214 (1.1%)	96 (0.5%)	24 (0.1%)	53 (0.3%)
All three	12 (3.7%)	8 (2.5%)	1 (0.3%)	2 (0.6%)	0 (0%)	0 (0%)

The prevalence of any NCD and NCD multimorbidity (≥2 NCDs [9]) in the population of >20 years of age was 4.5% and 0.7%, respectively (Table 5). The mean age at diagnosis of hypertension and diabetes mellitus in our study was 49.9 (SD-9.0) and 49.2 (SD-9.6) years, respectively (Table 6). It was significantly higher in those who were illiterate as compared to those who had more than 8 years of schooling (primary education).

4. Discussion

This survey conducted by trained Village Health Workers reports prevalence of self-reported NCDs and substance use patterns (tobacco and alcohol) in a rural population of the Gujarat state located in the western part of India. The adult gender ratio and the child gender ratio (0–6 years) reported in the study were 914 and 894 females per 1000 males,

TABLE 5: Association between number of NCDs with other variables (age group 20–69 years).

Variable	Number of NCDs 0	1	≥2
Overall (for adults >20 years)	52576 (94.8%)	2152 (4.5%)	363 (0.7%)
Age groups			
20–39 years	30043 (98.9%)	333 (1.1%)	13 (0.0%)
40–59 years	18388 (92.1%)	1401 (7.0%)	184 (1.0%)
60–69 years	4145 (81.5%)	778 (15.3%)	166 (3.3%)
Gender (for adults >20 years)			
Male	27134 (95.1%)	1214 (4.3%)	189 (0.7%)
Female	25442 (94.5%)	1298 (4.8%)	174 (0.6%)
Education (for adults >20 years)			
Illiterate	9851 (95%)	486 (4.7%)	35 (0.3%)
≤8 years of schooling	20517 (95.2%)	915 (4.2%)	115 (0.5%)
8–12 years of schooling	18760 (94.5%)	914 (4.6%)	178 (0.9%)
>12 years of schooling	3448 (93.7%)	197 (5.4%)	35 (1%)
Substance use			
Oral tobacco	14726 (96%)	538 (3.5%)	83 (0.5%)
Smoking	4894 (93%)	323 (6.1%)	45 (0.9%)
Oral tobacco and smoking	18197 (95.2%)	797 (4.2%)	116 (0.6%)
Alcohol	1111 (95.8%)	42 (3.6%)	7 (0.6%)
Any substance	18337 (95.2%)	804 (4.2%)	116 (0.6%)
All three	315 (96.6%)	11 (3.4%)	0

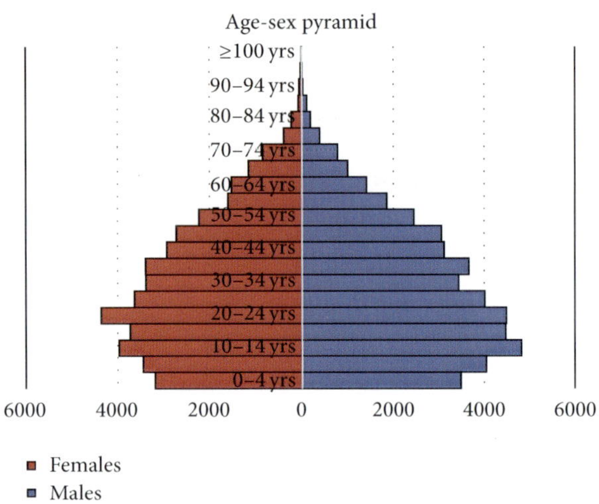

FIGURE 1: Population pyramid for the study population.

respectively. Similar figures for Anand District, Gujarat, and India were 925 and 884, 919 and 890, and 943 and 919, respectively [10]. The age-gender pyramid (Figure 1) shows bulge in the 10–25 years' group compared to the wide base in under 5 years' age group seen in the developing countries. This probably indicates the demographic transition through which the community is passing.

The prevalence of tobacco use in the age group of 20–69 years was found to be 34.5% (52.7% and 15.2% in males and females, resp.). The prevalence of oral tobacco use was 27.7% (39.8% and 14.8% in males and females, resp.). As per the National Family Health Survey 3 (NFHS 3), the prevalence of any form of tobacco use in the age group of 15–49 years was found to be 60.2% in rural Gujarat with prevalence of 63.4% and 11.3% for males and females, respectively. The prevalence of oral tobacco consumption was found to be 45.2% and 6% among males and females, respectively. However, the data was based on the responses of 737 male participants and 2114 female participants only. Also NFHS 3 had preceded our survey by about 6 years during which the prevalence might have changed [9].

The prevalence of any NCD was 5.3% in the age group of 20–69 years (5.4% in males and 5.2% in females). In a multisite study conducted in 5 Asian countries in 2005, 22.7% of men and 31.6% of women in the age group of 25–64 years reported having at least 1 of the chronic health conditions of interest. 5.1% of men and 9.2% of women reported having 2 or more chronic conditions. Women had more NCDs than men, the prevalence of NCDs increased with age, and people with the least education were more likely to have chronic conditions [11]. In the WHO-SAGE study conducted on nationally representative data in India, 28.5% of the sample population had at least one NCD and 8.9% had NCD multimorbidity. The prevalence of multimorbidity increased from 1.3% in 18–29-year-olds to 30.6% in those aged 70 years and above [12]. The reasons for low prevalence reported in our study could be multiple such as information collected from a representative of the household, rural population having lower burden of the disease, or greater portion of the disease being undiagnosed. The prevalence of any NCDs and that of hypertension, diabetes mellitus, and heart disease increased with the increasing age as observed in other studies in India and outside as well [11–13]. The difference in the prevalence

TABLE 6: Self-reported age at diagnosis of hypertension and diabetes mellitus in adults (20–69 years) with respect to various sociodemographic variables.

Variable	Mean age at diagnosis of hypertension in years (SD)	Mean age at diagnosis of diabetes mellitus in years (SD)
Overall	49.9 (9.0)	49.2 (9.6)
Age groups		
20–39 years	31.0 (5.8)	30.3 (4.7)
40–59 years	46.4 (6.1)	46.2 (6.0)
60–69 years	57.0 (5.5)	58.5 (4.9)
Gender		
Male	50.3 (9.0)	48.8 (9.1)
Female	49.7 (10.0)	49.7 (9.2)
Education		
Illiterate	51.9 (9.5)	52.4 (9.6)
≤8 years of schooling	50.3 (9.8)	49.3 (10.0)
8–12 years of schooling	48.9 (11.0)	48.4 (10.9)
>12 years of schooling	48.7 (9.9)	50.0 (7.4)
Substance abuse		
Oral tobacco	50.3 (10.0)	49.8 (9.0)
Smoking	51.5 (10.0)	49.3 (9.6)
Alcohol	52.9 (6.7)	49.4 (13.4)
Oral tobacco and smoking	50.9 (9.5)	49.7 (9.3)
Any	52.8 (7.8)	49.7 (9.3)
All three	50.8 (9.5)	49.2 (9.3)
Number of NCDs		
1	49.7 (9.8)	47.9 (9.4)
2	51.2 (8.5)	51.5 (7.9)
≥3	50.1 (9.2)	49.4 (10.2)

of any NCDs in males and females was not significant in our study. The prevalence for any NCD and hypertension was higher in the illiterate groups than that in the group having education of ≤8 years of schooling. Thereafter it increased progressively with increasing education. Such a phenomenon was not observed for other NCDs.

The prevalence of hypertension reported in our study was 4.2% with 3.7% and 4.4% prevalence reported in males and females, respectively (Table 3). It has been reported to be in the range between 20–40% in urban adults and 12–17% among rural adults [14]. In the multicountry study conducted in the year 2005, it was reported to be 7.4% across all the sites and 3.2% in the Indian site which is comparable with our finding [12]. 80.7% of all the hypertensive patients in our study were receiving treatment for their disease status. In a systematic review, the pooled estimate for the percentage of hypertensive patients being treated was found to be 24.9% (16.7–33.0) [15] which was quite low as compared to that reported in our study. This could be due to the fact that majority of those who reported to be suffering from hypertension in our study reported so because they were taking treatment while there might be a significant portion who might be suffering from hypertension but not taking regular treatment or taking irregular treatment and might not have reported the same.

The prevalence of diabetes in the adult population (>20 years) in our study was 1.5%. As per the 6th Edition (2013) of the International Diabetes Federation Atlas, it is estimated that around 50% of the diabetics are not aware of their condition; that is, they are not diagnosed [16]. Considering this fact, the actual prevalence of diabetes in our population can be estimated to be around 3.5%. The multicountry study reported prevalence of 2.2% across all the sites and 1.7% in India [11]. The ICMR India Diabetes (ICMR-INDIAB) study reported prevalence of 2.3–5.2% for diabetes in rural parts of 4 states of India by conducting diagnostic tests on the population, which is comparable with our estimates [17]. However, in the WHO-ICMR Indian NCD risk factor surveillance study, the prevalence of self-reported diabetes mellitus was found to be 3.1% in a sample of 13,524 individuals (age group: 15–64 years) from different geographical locations in the country [18]. The mean age at diagnosis for diabetes mellitus in our study was 49.2 (SD-9.6) years. In a nationwide survey conducted in 2011 for 6168 patients taking treatment at 330 centers comprising general hospitals, diabetes clinics, and referral clinics in India, the mean age at diagnosis was reported to be 45.4 (±10.9) [19]. However it was a predominantly urban population, reflecting a greater awareness and a greater access to health care services as compared to our study population which was in a rural setting. The higher mean age at diagnosis for hypertension and diabetes mellitus in our study for those who were illiterate as compared to those with more than 8 years of schooling reflects the effect of education on awareness about the need for screening and early diagnosis and access to health care services.

The prevalence of heart disease in the study population was found to be 0.6%. The estimated prevalence of coronary heart disease is around 3-4% in rural areas and 8–10% in urban areas among adults older than 20 years [20].

The self-reported prevalence of chronic conditions is subject to recall bias and may not reflect the true prevalence. Reporting also can be affected by respondents' knowledge, manifestations of the illness in everyday life, their willingness to report the condition, and frequency of contact with a physician [21], although it has been found in studies conducted in Western countries that self-reports of chronic conditions are quite accurate when compared with physician diagnoses [22–24]. Due to different sociodemographic characteristics of our population and the study design followed in our population, the self-reported prevalence might be reported to be lower as compared to other studies [11, 15, 17].

5. Conclusions

Prevalence of NCDs in our study was found to be less than that reported in other studies. The prevalence increased with age and there was no significant difference in the prevalence in males and females. Effect of education on the age of diagnosis of hypertension and diabetes mellitus could be documented in the study. The percentage of hypertensives and diabetics taking treatment was significantly high with more females taking treatment for hypertension as compared to males. Data generated from this study can be useful in planning a community based NCD programme. It provides the much needed population denominator which can be utilised to calculate various incidence, prevalence, and mortality rates which can serve as impact indicators for various community based programmes. Moreover it provides information on the number of patients of NCDs which are in need of treatment. It is useful information for calculating the need of resources and better planning of the programme related activities. Further studies may be undertaken to identify the actual burden of these diseases through more objective assessments and investigation by trained paramedical personnel. High prevalence of tobacco use calls for developing community based tobacco control and cessation activities.

References

[1] World Health Organization, *Global Status Report on Noncommunicable Diseases*, World Health Organization (WHO), Geneva, Switzerland, 2011, http://www.who.int/chp/ncd_global_status_report/en/.

[2] World Health Organization, "Global burden of disease: 2004 update," WHO, 2008, http://www.who.int/healthinfo/global_burden_disease/2004_report_update/en/.

[3] K. Srinath Reddy, B. Shah, C. Varghese, and A. Ramadoss, "Responding to the threat of chronic diseases in India," *The Lancet*, vol. 366, no. 9498, pp. 1744–1749, 2005.

[4] WHO, *Noncommunicable Diseases Coutnry Profiles*, 2011, http://whqlibdoc.who.int/publications/2011/9789241502283_eng.pdf?ua=1.

[5] A. Mahal, A. Karan, and M. Engelgau, *The Economic Implications of Non-Communicable Diseases for India*, World Bank, 2010, http://siteresources.worldbank.org/HEALTHNUTRITIONANDPOPULATION/Resources/281627-1095698140167/EconomicImplicationsofNCDforIndia.pdf.

[6] National Health Accounts Cell and Ministry of Health and Family Welfare-India, "National health accounts India 2004-05," MOHFW, New Delhi, India, September 2009, http://planningcommission.nic.in/reports/genrep/health/National_Health_Account_04_05.pdf.

[7] World Health Organization, *Health Systems: Improving Performance*, WHO, Geneva, Switzerland, 2000.

[8] O. R. Ahmad, C. Boschi-Pinto, A. D. Lopez, C. J. Murray, R. Lozano, and M. Inoue, *Age Standardization of Rates: A New WHO Standard*, World Health Organization, Geneva, Switzerland, 2001, http://www.who.int/healthinfo/paper31.pdf?ua=1.

[9] National Family Health Survey 3 Gujarat state report, 2015, http://www.rchiips.org/nfhs/NFHS-3%20Data/gujarat_state_report_for_website.pdf.

[10] Anand District Population Census 2011, Gujarat literacy sex ratio and density, 2015, http://www.census2011.co.in/census/district/196-anand.html.

[11] H. Van Minh, N. Ng, S. Juvekar et al., "Self-reported prevalence of chronic diseases and their relation to selected sociodemographic variables: a study in INDEPTH Asian sites, 2005," *Preventing Chronic Disease*, vol. 5, no. 3, article A86, 2008.

[12] S. Basu and A. C. King, "Disability and chronic disease among older adults in India: detecting vulnerable populations through the WHO SAGE Study," *American Journal of Epidemiology*, vol. 178, no. 11, pp. 1620–1628, 2013.

[13] S. Pati, S. Agrawal, S. Swain et al., "Non communicable disease multimorbidity and associated health care utilization and expenditures in India: cross-sectional study," *BMC Health Services Research*, vol. 14, article 451, 2014.

[14] R. Gupta, "Trends in hypertension epidemiology in India," *Journal of Human Hypertension*, vol. 18, no. 2, pp. 73–78, 2004.

[15] R. Anchala, N. K. Kannuri, H. Pant et al., "Hypertension in India: a systematic review and meta-analysis of prevalence, awareness, and control of hypertension," *Journal of Hypertension*, vol. 32, no. 6, pp. 1170–1177, 2014.

[16] International Diabetes Federation, *IDF Diabetes Atlas*, International Diabetes Federation, Brussels, Belgium, 6th edition, 2013, http://www.idf.org/diabetesatlas.

[17] R. M. Anjana, R. Pradeepa, M. Deepa et al., "Prevalence of diabetes and prediabetes (impaired fasting glucose and/or impaired glucose tolerance) in urban and rural India: phase i results of the Indian Council of Medical Research-INdia DIABetes (ICMR-INDIAB) study," *Diabetologia*, vol. 54, no. 12, pp. 3022–3027, 2011.

[18] V. Mohan, P. Mathur, R. Deepa et al., "Urban rural differences in prevalence of self-reported diabetes in India—the WHO-ICMR Indian NCD risk factor surveillance," *Diabetes Research and Clinical Practice*, vol. 80, no. 1, pp. 159–168, 2008.

[19] V. Mohan, S. N. Shah, S. R. Joshi et al., "Current status of management, control, complications and psychosocial aspects of patients with diabetes in India: results from the DiabCare India 2011 Study," *Indian Journal of Endocrinology and Metabolism*, vol. 18, no. 3, pp. 370–378, 2014.

[20] A. Ghaffar, K. S. Reddy, and M. Singhi, "Burden of non-communicable diseases in South Asia," *British Medical Journal*, vol. 328, no. 7443, pp. 807–810, 2004.

[21] J. A. A. Dalstra, A. E. Kunst, C. Borell et al., "Socioeconomic differences in the prevalence of common chronic diseases: an overview of eight European countries," *International Journal of Epidemiology*, vol. 34, no. 2, pp. 316–326, 2005.

[22] D. M. W. Kriegsman, B. W. J. H. Penninx, J. T. M. Van Eijk, A. J. P. Boeke, and D. J. H. Deeg, "Self-reports and general practitioner information on the presence of chronic diseases in community dwelling elderly. A study on the accuracy of patients' self-reports and on determinants of inaccuracy," *Journal of Clinical Epidemiology*, vol. 49, no. 12, pp. 1407–1417, 1996.

[23] N. Goldman, I.-F. Lin, M. Weinstein, and Y.-H. Lin, "Evaluating the quality of self-reports of hypertension and diabetes," *Journal of Clinical Epidemiology*, vol. 56, no. 2, pp. 148–154, 2003.

[24] R. Kehoe, S.-Y. Wu, M. C. Leske, and L. T. Chylack Jr., "Comparing self-reported and physician-reported medical history," *American Journal of Epidemiology*, vol. 139, no. 8, pp. 813–818, 1994.

12

Cervical Cancer Awareness among Women in Tanzania: An Analysis of Data from the 2011-12 Tanzania HIV and Malaria Indicators Survey

Fabiola V. Moshi, Elisa B. Vandervort, and Stephen M. Kibusi

College of Health Sciences, School of Nursing and Public Health, University of Dodoma, Dodoma, Tanzania

Correspondence should be addressed to Fabiola V. Moshi; fabiola.moshi@gmail.com

Academic Editor: Sally Guttmacher

Background. Awareness about cervical cancer is a first step in the process of screening and early treatment. The purpose of this study was to provide better understanding of basic knowledge about cervical cancer among women of reproductive age in Tanzania. *Method.* Data were analyzed from the 2011-2012 Tanzania HIV and Malaria Indicators Survey (THMIS) and a sample of 5542 sexually active women from 15 to 49 years of age were included in the analysis. *Results.* Overall knowledge about cervical cancer was high among interviewed women. Only 30.9% of women had never heard about cervical cancer. The predictors of awareness were having secondary or more level of education (AOR = 3.257, 95% CI 2.328–4.557, $p < 0.001$), residing in urban (AOR = 1.365, 95% CI 1.093–1.705, $p < 0.01$), being affluent (AOR = 2.685, 95% CI 2.009–3.587, $p < 0.001$), having one to four children (AOR = 1.36, 95% CI 1.032–1.793), and age of 30–34 years (AOR = 3.15, 95% CI 2.353–4.220, $p < 0.001$), 35–39 years (AOR = 2.46, 95% CI 1.831–3.308, $p < 0.001$), and 40–44 years (AOR = 3.46, 95% CI 2.497–4.784, $p < 0.001$). *Conclusion.* While the cervical cancer landscape in Tanzania has evolved since this survey, coverage has not yet been achieved and access to cervical cancer prevention services for rural women and girls remains a concern. Women who were least likely to be aware of cervical cancer were rural women, less affluent women, those with limited education, and those with limited access to the formal economy. Arguably, these are the women who are most at risk for cervical cancer. To close this gap, Tanzania's ongoing efforts to increase access to high-quality cervical cancer prevention services for all women at risk are commendable.

1. Introduction

Cervical cancer is caused by the human papilloma virus (HPV), the most common viral infection of the reproductive tract. Almost all sexually active individuals will become infected with HPV at some point in their lives, and some may repeatedly be infected. The peak time for infection is shortly after becoming sexually active, and most individuals with healthy immune systems will clear the virus within a few years [1]. Prolonged infection with high-risk oncogenic types of HPV puts women at risk for development of cervical cancer. To mitigate this risk, primary and secondary prevention strategies have been implemented in the global north, dramatically reducing the rate of cervical cancer diagnosis and death [1, 2].

In the global south, cervical cancer remains the second most common cancer (after breast cancer) among women of reproductive age. Worldwide, it is the third most common carcinoma after breast cancer and colorectal cancer [1, 3]. Unlike other cancers, cervical cancer is almost 100% preventable by ensuring that women receive quality screening and treatment of precancerous lesions. The impact of secondary prevention efforts for cervical cancer prevention in high resource settings is impressive [3]. Despite this, the World Health Organization (WHO) estimates of global cervical cancer rates remain sobering, with more than 500,000 new cases diagnosed each year. Of those cases, more than 85% of women hail from developing countries where access to primary and secondary prevention is far from universal [3, 4]. In these settings, most women diagnosed with cervical cancer in developing countries present at late stages when curative treatments are often no longer possible [1].

East Africa has the highest rate of cervical cancer in the world. In this region, the age-standardized incidence rate (ASR) is estimated at 42.7 new cases per 100,000 women [3]. ASR rates range from Malawi at 75.9/100,000 to Kenya at 40.1/100.000 [3]. Tanzania ranks second in the region with an ASR of 54.9/100,000 women [3]. Similar to other East African countries, cervical cancer is the leading cause of cancer and cancer-related death among Tanzanian women. Each year more than 7,300 Tanzanian women are diagnosed with cervical cancer [3]. More than half of these women die as they are diagnosed at a late stage of the disease [3].

The variation in cervical cancer rates by region mirrors access to primary and secondary cervical cancer prevention. Given the tremendous burden in Sub-Saharan Africa, the impact of HIV cannot be overlooked. It is well known that women with HIV are at unique risk for persistent HPV infection and cervical dysplasia. As such, women with HIV in Sub-Saharan Africa may have access to effective treatments for HIV but lack access to life-saving screening and treatment for precancer of the cervix [1, 5].

Effective screening and treatment for precancer of the cervix are a secondary prevention strategy that has been implemented globally to prevent cervical cancer. Commonly used screening tests include cytology (Pap), HPV testing, and visual inspection with acetic acid (VIA). Myriad studies have examined and reexamined the risks and benefits of each screening approach [1, 6, 7]. Regardless, highly effective modalities for screening and treatment of cervical precancer are widely available in the global north to prevent cervical cancer. For most women in the global south, universal access to high-quality cost-effective screening and treatment remains a distant goal and access to HPV vaccines for primary prevention also remains unequal [1].

Similar to women in other developing countries, most Tanzanian women with cervical cancer are diagnosed at late stages when curative treatments are no longer possible. Since 2002, the Tanzanian Ministry of Health and Social Welfare (MoHSW) has collaborated with the WHO, the International Agency for Research on Cancer (IARC), the international nonprofit Jhpiego, and numerous other local and international NGO partners to scale up cervical cancer prevention efforts for Tanzanian women [8, 9]. In accordance with the MoHSW's Service Delivery Guidelines for Cervical Cancer Prevention Services, the use of visual inspection with acetic acid (VIA) and cryotherapy is the secondary prevention approach that has been widely implemented in Tanzania [8]. This secondary prevention strategy is well supported by the research as a cost-effective strategy for cervical cancer prevention [1, 7] and is a recommended strategy by the WHO for cervical cancer prevention in low resource settings [1].

At a fundamental level, cervical cancer prevention programming focuses on two main areas: (1) the supply of prevention services on the part of health systems and (2) generating demand for services at the community level. Knowledge about an illness does not necessarily translate into a demand for services, but it is a first step in the process [1]. To better understand baseline community knowledge about cervical cancer in Tanzania at the time when the MoHSW was scaling prevention efforts, we reviewed data from the 2011-2012 Tanzania HIV and Malaria Indicators Survey.

2. Materials and Methods

2.1. The Study Area and Period. The study was conducted among women of reproductive age, aged 15–49 years living in Tanzania sampled from a population of 10,905,117 women accounting for 47.3% of women in Tanzania [10].

2.2. Design. A nationally based cross-sectional survey of a representative sample of individuals aged 15–49 years living in Tanzania was conducted in the period between December 2011 and May 2012.

2.3. Data Sources. The source of data was the 2011-2012 Tanzania HIV and Malaria Indicators Survey (THMIS). The survey was conducted by the National Bureau of Statistics (NBS) in collaboration with the Tanzania Commission for AIDS (TACAIDS) and the Zanzibar AIDS Commission (ZAC), the Ministry of Health and Social Welfare (MoHSW), and the USAID-funded Measure DHS project from December 16, 2011, to May 24, 2012.

2.4. Sampling Technique and Sample Size. The 2002 Population and Housing Census (PHC) which covered all of the 30 regions of Tanzania was used as a sampling frame. The first stage involved selecting sample points (clusters) consisting of enumeration areas (EAs) delineated for the 2002 PHC. A total of 583 clusters were selected. On Tanzania's mainland, 30 sample points were selected in Dar es Salaam. Additional 20 data points were selected in each one of the other 24 regions. In Zanzibar, 15 sample points were selected in each of Zanzibar's five regions. The second stage of selection involved systemic sampling of households. Prior to fieldwork, a household listing operation was undertaken in all the selected areas. From these lists, households to be included in the survey were then selected. A total sample size of 10,496 households was identified through the following process: approximately 18 households were selected from each sample point thereby determining the total. Weighting factors were utilized to obtain results proportional at the national level. Eligible respondents included all women and men aged 15–49 who either permanently live in the selected household or were visitors who stayed in the home on the night prior to the survey. In total, 10,067 women completed interviews, with a response rate of 96%. The main reason for nonresponse among eligible women was the failure to find them at home despite repeated visits to the households.

The question regarding cervical cancer awareness was given to women of reproductive age of 15–49 years. Of the 10,967 women who completed interviews, 9693 responded to the question regarding cervical cancer awareness. From this sample, 8365 participants were further selected for being sexually active. Participants with missing data on important covariates particularly regarding assertive safe sexual behavior were excluded, remaining with a final sample of 5542 women included in this analysis

2.5. Data Collection Tools. The 2011-12 THMIS utilized two questionnaires: a Household Questionnaire and an Individual Questionnaire. These questionnaires were based on the Measure DHS standard AIDS Indicator Survey and Malaria Indicator Survey questionnaires. The questionnaires were adapted to reflect Tanzanian population and relevant health issues of Tanzania. Following adaption, the questionnaires were translated into Kiswahili, Tanzania's national language. The data presented in this study is based on the individual questionnaire.

2.6. Variables. Guided by literature review, key variables were identified from the 2011-12 THMIS individual questionnaires. A conceptual framework was developed comprising a list of primary independent variables (such as socioeconomic and demographic variables), intermediate independent variables (such as number and timing of antenatal visits), and the outcome variable, cervical cancer awareness.

2.7. Outcome Measures. The outcome was an awareness about cervical cancer (which was a dichotomous variable) whereby a participant was or was not aware of cervical cancer.

2.8. Independent Variables. The socioeconomic and demographic variables that have been theoretically and empirically reported to influence women's awareness of health issues were included in this study. Demographic characteristics included variables such as age grouping by 5-year intervals, the location of residence (rural or urban), education level, a woman's marital status, and occupation status. Other sociodemographic characteristics included parity, Tanzanian zone of residence, and wealth index categorized as poorest, poorer, middle income, richer, and richest. The survey also included intermediate factors potentially related to cervical cancer awareness. These included a woman's assertiveness regarding safe sexual behavior, access to reproductive health services, and indicators for sexually transmitted infections.

2.9. Statistical Analyses. Descriptive statistics for sample's sociodemographic characteristics and cervical cancer awareness were calculated. Sociodemographic differences in cervical cancer awareness were assessed by chi-square testing. For all the analyses, the level of significance was set at $p < 0.05$ (2-tailed). To generate crude (OR) and adjusted odds ratios (AOR) both bivariate and multiple logistic regression were employed. Odds ratios were estimated to determine the strength of the associations. Confidence intervals (CIs) of 95% were used for significance testing. Covariates were simultaneously entered into the multiple regression models. Analyses were performed using SPSS version 16. To allow for adjustments for the cluster sampling design and sampling probabilities across clusters and strata, sample weighting was applied.

2.10. Ethical Considerations. The procedures for the THMIS data collection and the survey content and protocol were approved by Tanzania's National Institute for Medical Research (NIMR), the Zanzibar Medical Ethics and Research Committee (ZAMREC), the Institutional Review Board of ICF International, and the Centers for Disease Control and Prevention in Atlanta, USA. After being read a document emphasizing the voluntary nature of the survey, participants provided verbal informed consent. The household interviews took place under the most private conditions afforded by the environments encountered. If privacy could not be insured, the interviewers were instructed to skip the module.

3. Results and Discussion

3.1. Results. Table 1 shows the sociodemographic characteristics of participants and their awareness about cervical cancer. Most of the participants had completed at least primary education. There was a significant relationship ($p < 0.001$) between education level and awareness about cervical cancer. Among women without education, 44.3% had never heard of cervical cancer. Young respondents (ages 15 to 19 years) had the highest percentage of women (50.2%) who had never heard about cervical cancer ($p < 0.001$). There was also a statistically significant relationship ($p < 0.001$) between the women's occupation and awareness about cervical cancer. Among self-employed women, 32.9% were not aware of cervical cancer.

Table 2 shows the distribution of participants by potential factors which may affect awareness about cervical cancer. When analyzed by income, the most affluent group had the highest awareness about cervical cancer (87.1%). This was contrasted by a much lower awareness among less affluent women. Among those women, only 57.4% had ever heard about cervical cancer ($p < 0.001$). When comparing different zones of Tanzania, women from Eastern Tanzania had the highest percentage (85%) of women who had heard about cervical cancer, while women from the South Western Highlands had the lowest percentage (59.9%) of women who had ever heard about cervical cancer ($p < 0.001$). Awareness about cervical cancer was also compared to parity (reported number of children delivered). Respondents with no children had the lowest percentage (58.6%) of awareness about cervical cancer and women who had one to four children had the highest awareness (71.4%) about cervical cancer ($p < 0.001$). When considering the place of residence, women from urban areas had the highest percentage (84.6%) of knowledge about cervical cancer while among women, only 65% had ever heard about cervical cancer ($p < 0.001$).

The results of the logistic regression analysis are presented in Table 3. This analysis demonstrated that a woman was aware of cervical cancer if she had the following characteristics: aged between 30 and 49 years, more affluent, having had completed at least secondary school, living in an urban area, and self-employed. Interestingly, employed women were less (4%) likely to have had heard about cervical cancer compared to unemployed women.

4. Discussion

Through this review of the data, a profile emerges of a Tanzanian woman most likely to know about cervical cancer in 2011-2012. She was more likely to live in an urban setting, be older than 30 years of age, have completed secondary

TABLE 1: The distribution by sociodemographic characteristics and awareness about cervical cancer.

Variables	Awareness about cervical cancer				p value
	Not aware		Aware		
	n	%	n	%	
Education:					
No education	528	44.3	663	55.7	
Primary incomplete	250	35.8	448	64.2	***
Primary completed	867	27.3	2307	72.7	
Secondary or more	67	14	413	86	
Age groups:					
15–19	218	50.2	216	49.8	
0–24	334	35	619	65	
25–29	374	32	794	68	***
30–34	224	23.5	731	76.5	
35–39	287	30.7	647	69.3	
40–44	155	24.6	475	75.4	
45–49	119	25.4	350	74.6	
Occupation:					
Unemployed	162	27.3	432	72.7	
Self-employed	1494	32.9	3050	67.9	***
Employed	56	13.8	349	86.2	

Here *** indicates $p < 0.001$. $N = 5543$; 2 participants were missing some information on independent variables: 2 on occupation.

TABLE 2: Distribution of participants by awareness about cervical cancer and the potential factors affecting awareness (chi-square).

Variables	Awareness about cervical cancer				p value
	Not aware		Aware		
	n	%	n	%	
Wealth index:					
Poorest	441	42.6	595	57.4	
Poorer	433	37.8	712	62.2	***
Middle	378	34.6	713	65.4	
Richer	318	27.3	847	72.7	
Richest	142	12.9	962	87.1	
Zones:					
Eastern	90	15	510	85	
Western	138	31.6	299	68.4	
Southern	112	36.1	198	63.9	***
Southern Highlands	244	38.7	386	61.3	
SW Highlands	240	40.1	359	59.9	
Central	129	20.1	513	79.9	
Northern	188	30.2	434	69.8	
Lake	507	33.1	1025	66.9	
Zanzibar	64	37.4	107	62.6	
Parity:					
0	146	41.4	207	58.6	
1–4	933	28.6	2332	71.4	***
>4	633	32.9	1292	67.1	
Place of Residence:					
Urban	180	15.5	989	84.6	***
Rural	1532	35	2843	65	

Here *** indicates $p < 0.001$.

TABLE 3: Adjusted odds ratios (AOR) for factors associated with awareness about cervical cancer among women of reproductive age (15–49 yrs) in Tanzania 2011-2012 ($N = 5543$).

Variable	AOR	95% CI	p value
Age groups:			
15–19	1		
20–24	1.58	1.212–2.054	***
25–29	1.80	1.377–2.348	***
30–34	3.15	2.353–4.220	***
35–39	2.46	1.831–3.308	***
40–44	3.46	2.497–4.784	***
45–49	1.35	2.370–4.733	***
Zones:			
Eastern	1		
Western	0.75	0.543–1.044	
Southern	0.49	0.345–0.691	***
Southern Highlands	0.40	0.297–0.543	***
SW Highlands	0.47	0.343–0.629	***
Central	1.43	1.036–1.971	*
Northern	0.61	0.452–0.830	**
Lake	0.69	0.527–0.909	**
Zanzibar	0.21	0.133–0.318	***
Parity:			
No child	1		
One to four children	1.36	1.032–1.793	*
More than four children	0.95	0.694–1.301	
Employment status:			
Unemployed	1		
Employed	0.96	0.758–1.205	
Self-employed	1.51	1.091–2.085	*
Wealth:			
Poorest	1		
Poorer	1.237	1.032–1.482	*
Middle	1.383	1.147–1.668	**
Richer	1.706	1.396–2.084	***
Richest	2.685	2.009–3.587	***
Level of education:			
No education	1		
Primary incomplete	1.434	1.17–1.758	**
Primary completed	1.704	1.463–1.985	***
Secondary or more	3.257	2.328–4.557	***
Area of residence:			
Rural	1		
Urban	1.365	1.093–1.705	**

Here *, **, and *** indicate $p < 0.05$, $p < 0.01$, and $p < 0.001$, respectively.

education, be self-employed, and be affluent. In contrast, those most at risk for lack of awareness about cervical cancer were rural Tanzanian women with limited education and limited access to the formal economy and women of young reproductive age. Despite the scaling up of secondary cervical cancer prevention efforts with VIA and cryotherapy in Tanzania since 2011-2012, the availability of high-quality cervical cancer prevention services for rural populations is uncertain. Even today, one wonders about the availability of screening and treatment for cervical precancer for rural women who know about the service availability and somehow manage to surmount the many barriers to accessing services [11, 12]. Despite impressive local efforts to scale up effective cervical cancer prevention services since 2011-2012, it is likely that not all Tanzanian women know about their risk for cervical cancer or where to access screening services. As such not all women in Tanzania have equal access to services [11, 12].

This analysis found that the vast majority of study participants (69%) had heard about cervical cancer as of 2011-2012. A similar study performed in Kilimanjaro Region among rural and urban women reported that the majority of women were knowledgeable about cervical cancer [11]. Given the high rates of cervical cancer in Tanzania, this knowledge is not surprising. Rural and urban Tanzanians have significant experience caring for family and community members with end-stage cervical cancer. It is possible that cervical cancer awareness was underreported in this 2011-2012 survey as less educated and less affluent Tanzanians may not have been familiar with the medical terminology used by the interviewers.

Rural women who are more apt to be poor and less educated were less knowledgeable about cervical cancer (65%), but overall knowledge was quite high in this survey. Knowledge among urban women (84.6%) mirrors findings from a Kenyan study where 87% of urban women were aware of cervical cancer [13]. This current analysis also found that the level of education of the respondents influenced their awareness of cervical cancer. With increasing education, a woman was more likely to be aware. This finding is consistent with other studies demonstrating cervical cancer knowledge correlating with higher education [14].

Our analysis of the 2011-2012 THMIS data found that the vast majority of women knew something about cervical cancer and that basic knowledge also increased as women aged. This has been demonstrated in other settings [15]. Unfortunately, this knowledge may be more linked with personal experience rather than effective community health education and personal experience with cervical cancer screening services. As the leading cause of cancer and cancer death among women ages 15 to 44 years of age in Tanzania, it is common for Tanzanian men and women to have a personal connection with someone who has had cervical cancer.

As such, in this setting there is a relatively robust awareness of the existence of cervical cancer among women of reproductive age. They know that this illness exists but commonly lack knowledge about the availability of screening and treatment services [11]. To increase screening and treatment coverage for cervical precancer, we must devise strategies to deepen knowledge at the community level and drive a demand for effective primary and secondary prevention services. By increasing core knowledge about cervical cancer risk and available prevention services, it may be possible to cultivate a demand for screening services for all women at risk.

Some programs have focused on increasing community awareness about signs and symptoms of cancer to strengthen a person's ability to detect early signs and symptoms of cancer.

Studies have reported that knowledge and understanding of cancer risk factors and outcomes of cancer treatments influenced individual's intentions and participation in cancer prevention programs [16, 17]. In the case of cervical cancer, the early stages of cervical cancer are commonly silent, without symptoms. As such, women presenting with symptoms of cervical cancer usually have late-stage disease, and curative treatments are unlikely [1].

Luckily, cervical cancer tends to have a relatively long precancer stage, providing a convenient window for preventive screening and treatment for precancer. To prevent progression to cancer, women require access to early detection and treatment of precancerous lesions [1]. In Tanzania, women and men know that cervical cancer exists. But further intensive outreach and education are needed at the community level to deepen knowledge about prevention of cervical cancer and meaningfully connect women and girls with primary and secondary prevention services. A crucial layer of this process is for an individual to possess knowledge and understanding about woman's risk for cervical cancer and the local options available for prevention. If such information is not widely available and community structures are not engaged to assist with reproductive health education and mobilization, it understandably increases the risk that women will not receive quality screening and treatment, even if such is available.

The reasons for the high cervical cancer mortality burden in East Africa and Tanzania are complex. Regardless, it is evident that to reduce cervical cancer incidence in Tanzania and beyond, creative strategies must continue to be implemented to increase coverage of preventive services for cervical cancer. There are complex factors that contribute to Tanzania's continued high rates of death from cervical cancer. Simply put, if at least 80% of women had access to quality screening and treatment for precancer at least once in their life (when most at risk), cervical cancer rates in Tanzania could plunge rapidly [7]. With more than 5 million Tanzanian women between 30 and 50 years of age [18], there is a vast population to reach with cervical cancer screening services. Given the current health policy and funding climate, it is likely unwise for women of Tanzania to patiently wait for the health system and NGO partners to provide optimal screening and treatment services, especially for rural populations. It may be that cultivating a grassroots demand for services becomes a more effective way to influence the supply of primary and secondary cervical cancer prevention services. By driving demand at a local level, the health system may be encouraged to strengthen and respond.

To that end, continued engagement at the community level should engender creative and sustainable ways to increase knowledge and awareness about cervical cancer to drive a demand for effective primary and secondary prevention services. As demonstrated by the 2011-2012 THMIS data and numerous other studies in Tanzania [11, 12], women know about cervical cancer but often do not realize that there are effective preventive services available. To close this gap, we need creative multisectoral collaborations that will prioritize investments in effective reproductive health services for all women at risk in the global south, including a focus on primary and secondary cervical cancer prevention.

This study has some limitations, as it utilized data that is now relatively old. Knowledge today is likely increased given MoHSW and NGO partners' secondary prevention achievements, especially in communities where screening access and uptake have been high. Regardless, it is interesting to such a high baseline level of awareness at a time when MoHSW had really just begun to scale up cervical cancer prevention efforts.

5. Conclusion

This analysis looked at the 2011-2012 THMIS data to better understand cervical cancer knowledge among Tanzanian women at a time when the MoHSW was scaling up cervical cancer prevention efforts. While the cervical cancer landscape in Tanzania has evolved since this survey, coverage has not yet been achieved, and access to cervical cancer prevention services especially for rural women and girls remains a concern. Overall knowledge about cervical cancer was quite high among surveyed women, most likely due to personal experiences caring for someone with cervical cancer. Women who were least likely to be aware of cervical cancer were rural women, less affluent women, those with limited education, and those with limited access to the formal economy. Arguably, these are the women who are most at risk for cervical cancer. Since this survey, impressive gains have been made in the access to screening and treatment for precancer in Tanzania through the efforts of the MoHSW and NGO partners. Meanwhile, the vast majority of women at risk have not yet been screened, such women may not know of available screening services, and most Tanzanian girls have not yet received the HPV vaccine. To close this gap, Tanzania's efforts to increase access to high-quality cervical cancer prevention services for all women at risk are commendable. These efforts deserve continued local and international support to reduce unnecessary deaths from cervical cancer. Increasing demand at the community level for such services will continue to be a crucial component of the equation, especially among rural populations.

Abbreviations

ASR:	Age-standardized incidence rate
HIV:	Human immunodeficiency virus
HPV:	Human papilloma virus
MoHSW:	Ministry of Health and Social Welfare
NBS:	National Bureau of Statistics
NGO:	Non-Governmental Organization
TACAIDS:	Tanzania Commission for AIDS
THMIS:	Tanzania HIV and Malaria Indicators Survey
VIA:	Visual inspection with acetic acid
WHO:	World Health Organization
ZAC:	Zanzibar AIDS Commission.

Ethical Approval

The procedures for THMIS data collection were approved by the following organizations: Tanzania's National Institute for Medical Research (NIMR), the Zanzibar Medical Ethics and Research Committee (ZAMREC), the Institutional Review

Board of ICF International, and the Centers for Disease Control and Prevention in Atlanta, USA.

Authors' Contributions

Fabiola V. Moshi drafted the manuscript and led the process of critical revision of the manuscript. Stephen M. Kibusi developed the study framework and study design, performed the statistical analysis, drafted the methods section of the paper, and participated in critical revision of the manuscript. Elisa B. Vandervort contributed to the cervical cancer prevention literature review, discussion, critical review, and editing of the manuscript. All authors have read and approved this manuscript to be processed for publication.

Acknowledgments

The authors are grateful to MEASURE DHS for providing them with the data set.

References

[1] World Health Organisation, *Comprehensive Cervical Cancer Control. A Guide to Essential Practice*, WHO Library Cataloguing-in-Publication Data, 2014, http://www.who.int/reproductivehealth/publications/cancers/cervical-cancer-guide/en/.

[2] UNAIDS, *HPV, HIV And Cervical Cancer Leveraging Synergies to save Women's Lives*, 2016, http://www.unaids.org/sites/default/files/media_asset/JC2851_HPV-HIV-cervicalcancer_en.pdf.

[3] F. Bray, J.-S. Ren, E. Masuyer, and J. Ferlay, "Global estimates of cancer prevalence for 27 sites in the adult population in 2008," *International Journal of Cancer*, vol. 132, no. 5, pp. 1133–1145, 2013.

[4] L. A. Torre, F. Bray, R. L. Siegel, J. Ferlay, and J. Lortet-Tieulent, "Global cancer statistics, 2012," *CA: A Cancer Journal for Clinicians*, vol. 65, no. 2, pp. 87–108, 2015.

[5] A. Ntekim, "Cervical Cancer in Sub Sahara Africa," in *Topics on Cervical Cancer With an Advocacy for Prevention*, 75, p. 51, InTech, 2012.

[6] N. G. Campos, P. E. Castle, T. C. Wright, and J. J. Kim, "Cervical cancer screening in low-resource settings: A cost-effectiveness framework for valuing tradeoffs between test performance and program coverage," *International Journal of Cancer*, vol. 137, no. 9, pp. 2208–2219, 2015.

[7] S. J. Goldie, L. Gaffikin, J. D. Goldhaber-Fiebert et al., "Cost-effectiveness of cervical-cancer screening in five developing countries," *The New England Journal of Medicine*, vol. 353, no. 20, pp. 2158–2168, 2005.

[8] R. McCree, M. R. Giattas, V. V. Sahasrabuddhe et al., "Expanding cervical cancer screening and treatment in Tanzania: stakeholders' perceptions of structural influences on scale-Up," *The Oncologist*, vol. 20, no. 6, pp. 621–626, 2015.

[9] WHO, *Prevention of Cervical Cancer through Screening Using Visual Inspection with Acetic Acid (VIA) And Treatment with Cryotherapy*, African Population and Health Research Center, 2012, http://www.who.int/reproductivehealth/publications/cancers/9789241503860/en/.

[10] National Bureau of Statistics (NBS), *Office of Chief Government Statistician (OCGS). Population Distribution by Age and Sex: The United Republic of Tanzania*, 2013, http://ihi.eprints.org/2169/1/Age_Sex_Distribution.pdf.

[11] M. S. Cunningham, E. Skrastins, R. Fitzpatrick et al., "Cervical cancer screening and HPV vaccine acceptability among rural and urban women in Kilimanjaro Region, Tanzania," *BMJ Open*, vol. 5, no. 3, Article ID e005828, 2015.

[12] C. Kahesa, S. Kjaer, J. Mwaiselage et al., "Determinants of acceptance of cervical cancer screening in Dar es Salaam, Tanzania," *BMC Public Health*, vol. 12, article 1093, 2012.

[13] O. Elizabeth, M. Anne, and W. Peter, "Awareness of cervical cancer risk factors and practice of Pap smear testing among female primary school teachers in Kasarani division, Nairobi Kenya," *African Journal of Health Sciences*, vol. 21, no. 2, pp. 121–132, 2012.

[14] O. A. Akinlaja and R. Anorlu, "Knowledge of cervical cancer, awareness and attitude to screening among patients at a cytology clinic," *Austin Journal of Obstetrics and Gynecology*, vol. 1, no. 1, pp. 1–4, 2014.

[15] M. R. Balogun, O. O. Odukoya, M. A. Oyediran, and P. I. Ujomu, "Cervical cancer awareness and preventive practices: a challenge for female urban slum dwellers in Lagos, Nigeria," *African Journal of Reproductive Health*, vol. 16, no. 1, pp. 75–82, 2012.

[16] A. E. Simon, J. Waller, K. Robb, and J. Wardle, "Patient delay in presentation of possible cancer symptoms: the contribution of knowledge and attitudes in a population sample from the United Kingdom," *Cancer Epidemiology, Biomarkers & Prevention*, vol. 19, no. 9, 2010.

[17] A. D. Mwaka, C. G. Orach, E. M. Were, G. Lyratzopoulos, H. Wabinga, and M. Roland, "Awareness of cervical cancer risk factors and symptoms: Cross-sectional community survey in post-conflict northern Uganda," *Health Expectations*, vol. 19, no. 4, pp. 854–867, 2016.

[18] L. Bruni, L. Barrionuevo-Rosas, G. Albero, B. Serrano, M. Mena, D. Gómez et al., "Human Papillomavirus and Related Diseases Report," Tech. Rep., 2017, http://www.hpvcentre.net/statistics/reports/MYS.pdf.

13

Reduced Risk of Parkinson's Disease in Users of Calcium Channel Blockers

Kapil Gudala, Raju Kanukula, and Dipika Bansal

Department of Pharmacy Practice, National Institute of Pharmaceutical Education and Research, SAS Nagar, Punjab 160062, India

Correspondence should be addressed to Dipika Bansal; dipikabansal079@gmail.com

Academic Editor: Koji Kawakami

Aim. To pool the data currently available to determine the association between calcium channel blockers (CCBs) and risk of Parkinson's disease (PD). *Methods.* Literature search in PubMed, EBSCO, and Cochrane library was undertaken through March 2014, looking for observational studies evaluating the association between CCBs use and PD. Pooled relative risk (RR) estimates and 95% confidence intervals (CIs) were calculated using random-effects model. Subgroup analyses, sensitivity Analysis, and cumulative meta-analysis were also performed. *Results.* Six studies were included in our meta-analysis according to the selection criteria, including three cohort studies and three case-control studies involving 27,67,990 subjects including 11,941 PD cases. We found CCBs use was associated with significant decreased risk of PD, compared with not using CCBs (random effects model pooled RR, 0.81 (95% CI, 0.69–0.95)); a significant heterogeneity was found between studies ($P = 0.031$; I^2 54.6%). Both the classes of CCB, that is, dihydropyridine calcium channel blockers (DiCCB) (0.80 (95% CI, 0.65–0.98) $P = 0.032$) and non-DiCCB (0.70 (95% CI, 0.53–0.92) $P = 0.013$), were found to be reducing the risk of PD. *Conclusion.* In our analysis, we found that CCBs use was associated with a Significantly decreased risk of PD compared with non-CCB use.

1. Introduction

Approximately 1% of the population over 60 years of age suffers from Parkinson's disease (PD) which is a second most common chronic progressive neurodegenerative disorder in the elderly after Alzheimer's disease [1]. It has been characterized clinically by three motor symptoms, which includes resting tremors, rigidity, and bradykinesia [2]. Pathology involved in PD is the loss or degeneration of dopaminergic neurons in the substantia nigra of the midbrain and neuronal lewy bodies development. The results in the experimental therapies for treating PD were very limited [3]. A systematic review suggests that the centrally acting calcium channel blockers (CCBs) may have disease-modifying effects, and there were no drugs to prevent the disease or slow its progression [4].

Recent interest in antihypertensive drugs, especially CCBs, has been triggered by the belief that these medications, which inhibit nitric oxide, tumor necrosis factor-alpha, and interleukin-1 beta synthesis, thus reduce oxidative stress and the inflammatory response, which might be neuroprotective [5]. Experiments in animal models indicated that the voltage-gated calcium channel subtype Ca (V) 1.3 has a function in making neurons vulnerable to neurodegeneration [6].

Several observational studies have been conducted to examine the association between CCBs use and PD risk and have generated mixed results. Until now, no definite conclusion on this topic has been established. In the present meta-analysis, we examined the CCB use in relation to risk of PD.

2. Materials and Methods

2.1. Literature Search. Two authors independently performed the literature search by using MedLine (PubMed), EBSCO, and the Cochrane library databases up to March 2014. Search terms include "((((calcium channel blockers) OR antihypertensive agents) OR calcium antagonists) OR dihydropyridine calcium channel blockers) AND parkinson disease" with limits of humans and English language. Titles and abstracts of the resulting articles had been examined to exclude irrelevant studies. Full texts of remaining articles were read to extract information on the topic of interest. Bibliographies and citation sections of retrieved articles had been reviewed for additional pertinent studies.

2.2. Inclusion and Exclusion Criteria. The studies considered in this meta-analysis were all observational (cohort or case-control) studies that evaluated exposure to CCBs and risk of PD. Articles were excluded if they were reviews, letters to the editor without original data, editorials, case reports, or clinical trials. When there were multiple publications from the same population, only data from the most recent report were included in the meta-analysis and the remaining was excluded. Any discrepancies were addressed by a joint reevaluation of the original article.

2.3. Data Extraction. Two authors independently reviewed the primary studies to assess the appropriateness for inclusion in the present meta-analysis and data which has been extracted. The following information was extracted from each study: (i) first author's last name, year of publication, and country of the population studied; (ii) study design; (iii) number of subjects and number of PD cases; (iv) effect estimates and 95% confidence intervals (CIs); (v) assessment of CCB exposure; (vi) PD assessment; and (vii) control for confounding factors by matching or adjustments, if applicable. We extracted the effect estimates that reflected the greatest degree of control for potential confounder.

2.4. Quality Assessment. Two authors using the Newcastle-Ottawa Scale (NOS) [7] assessed the quality of each study independently. The NOS consists of three parameters of quality: selection, comparability, and outcome/exposure and it assigns a maximum of four points for selection, two points for comparability, and three points for exposure/outcome. Therefore, 9 points altogether reflect the high quality and 7-8 points reflect medium quality and six or less points reflect low quality. Any discrepancies were addressed by a joint revaluation of the original article with a third author.

2.5. Data Synthesis and Analysis. Because the risk of PD is low, the risk ratio (RR) in prospective cohort studies mathematically approximates the odds ratio [8], therefore permitting the combination of cohort and case-control studies. Publication bias was assessed using Egger's regression asymmetry test [9, 10]. To assess the heterogeneity among studies, we used the Cochran Q and I^2 statistics; for the Q statistic, a P value <0.10 and for I^2, a value >50% was considered statistically significant for heterogeneity [11]. The primary measure pooled RR of PD from individual studies, calculated using the random-effects model (DerSimonian and Laird method) [12, 13], which accounts for heterogeneity among studies. All analyses were performed using Comprehensive Meta-Analysis software version 2. All statistical tests were two-sided and $P < 0.05$ was considered statistically significant, except otherwise specified.

The primary outcome in this meta-analysis was reported as RR with 95% CI of developing PD in CCB users. Subgroup analyses were performed according to (i) dihydropyridine calcium channel blockers (DiCCBs) versus non-DiCCBs; (ii) individual type of CCB; (iii) dose; (iv) duration; (v) study design (cohort and case-control); (vi) gender; and (vii) age group to examine the impact of these factors on the association. To evaluate the stability of our results, we also performed a one-way sensitivity analysis. The present work was performed in this meta-analysis as per the guidelines for the meta-analysis PRISMA [14].

3. Results

3.1. Search Results. A total of 626 articles were identified during the initial search (Figure 1). After screening the titles of 626 articles, 575 articles were excluded, as they were found irrelevant. Full text of 51 articles was collected and read. After detailed evaluation, 45 articles were found to be ineligible as there were reviews, editorials, case reports, and others which did not meet the inclusion criteria (Figure 1). A total of 6 studies were included for final analysis [15–20].

3.2. Study Characteristics. Six relevant studies were identified, including three cohort [15–17] and three case-control [18–20] studies involving a total of 27,67,990 subjects including 11,941 PD cases.

Three cohort studies involve [15–17] (Table 1) 27,48,578 participants with more than 2,06,000 CCB users out of which 6,182 were incident PD cases. Participants were followed up for 4 to 16 years and the studies have been published between 2009 and 2012. Pasternak et al. [15] study is a historical cohort study in being the biggest cohort among the three studies. Simon et al. [17] have done analysis by combining both the Nurses Health Study (NHS) and Health Professionals Follow-Up Study (HPFS). Louis et al. have reported the results of both cross-sectional and prospective analysis. However, present analysis has included only the prospective results of Louis et al. [16].

Three population-based case-control studies [18–20] (Table 2) involving 5,759 PD cases and 13,653 controls were published in between 2007 and 2010. All three studies are population-based studies, which assessed PD or CCB usage from national database or medical records or from pharmacy database.

3.3. Main Results. As a significant heterogeneity was found ($P = 0.031$; I^2 54.6%), random-effects model was chosen over a fixed effects model. We found CCB use was associated significantly with decreased risk of PD compared with not using CCB (pooled RR, 0.81 (95% CI, 0.69–0.96)). The multivariable adjusted RRs of use of CCB and risk of PD for each study and grouped data of all studies are shown in Figure 2. Visual examination of the funnel plot revealed minimal asymmetry (data not shown), further confirmed by Egger's test ($P = 0.68$) indicating little or no publication bias in our analysis.

3.4. Subgroup Analysis. Table 3 presents the results of subgroup analyses straitened by characteristics of study designs

Table 1: Characteristics of cohort studies included in meta-analysis.

Author, year (country)[a]	Cohort name	Cohort size	Follow-up period (start–end year)	Assessment of CCB use	Number of CCB users	Assessment of PD	Number of PD cases	Quality rating (NOC)
Pasternak et al. [15] 2012 (Denmark)[a]	NR	25,73,281	8 (1998–2006)	Prescription drug registry	2,02,836	National patient registry	5,711	9[b]
Simon et al. [17] 2010 (USA)[a]	Nurses Health study & Health Professionals Follow-Up Study	1,71,355	16 (1986–2002)	Self-reported through structured questionnaire	3,826	Self-reported and after confirmed by medical records and physician	421	7[c]
Louis et al. [16] 2009 (Spain)[a]	Neurological Disorder in Central Spain	3,942	4 (1994–1998)	Self-reported	NR	Presence of any two cardinal signs and physician confirmed PD	NR	8[c]

[a]Country of study conducted.
[b]High quality.
[c]Medium quality.
USA: United States of America, NR: not reported, CCB: calcium channel blockers, PD: Parkinson's disease, and NOC: Newcastle-Ottawa Scale.

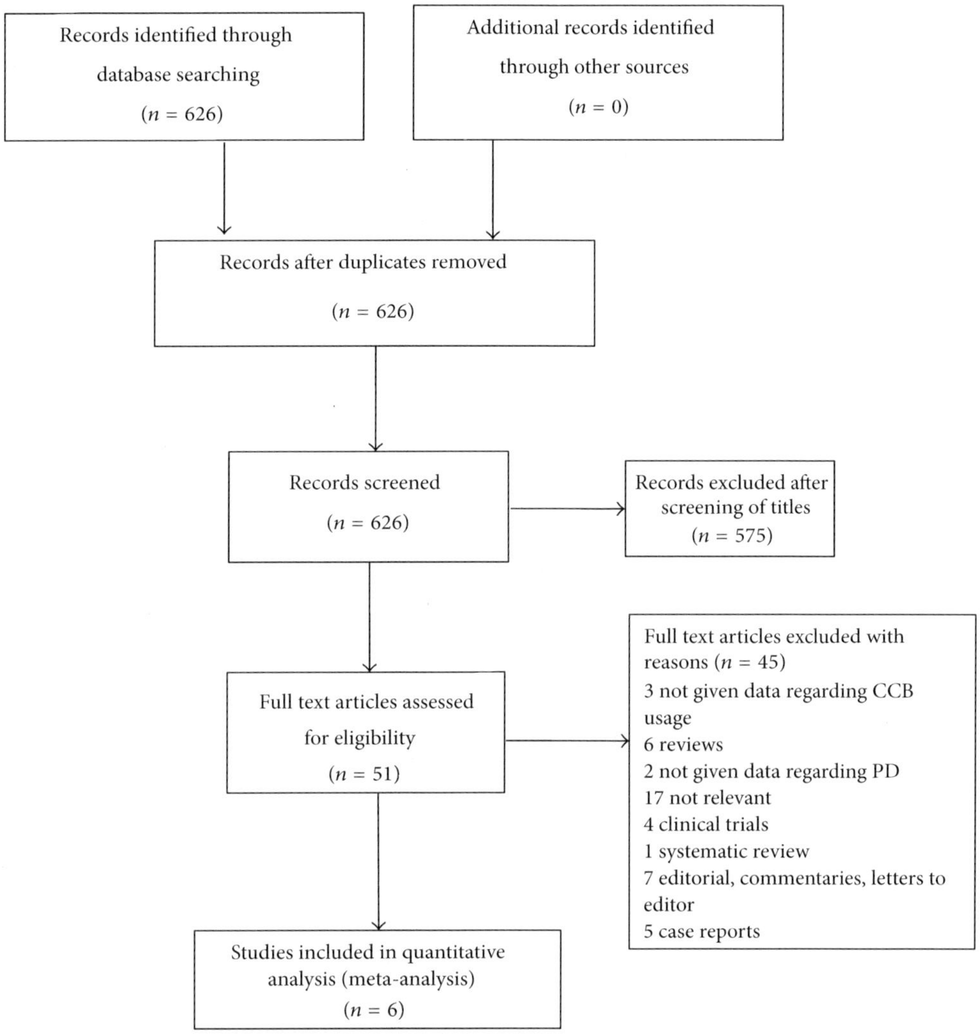

FIGURE 1: Flowchart representing the selection process.

TABLE 2: Characteristics of case-control studies included in meta-analysis.

Author, year (country)[a]	Period of recruitment	Source of study population	Study size	Number of PD patients	Assessment of CCB usage	Assessment of PD	Quality rating (NOC)
Ritz et al. [18] 2010 (Denmark)	2001–2006	Population based	11,582	1,931	National pharmacy database	Hospital register	8[c]
Becker et al. [19] 2008 (UK)	1994–2005	Population based	7,274	3,637	General practice research database	General practice research database	8[c]
Ton et al. [20] 2007 (USA)	1992–2002	Population based	556	191	Medical records	Medical records and cardinal signs	9[b]

[a]Country of study conducted.
[b]High quality.
[c]Medium quality.
UK: United Kingdom, USA: United States of America, CCB: calcium channel blockers, PD: Parkinson's disease, and NOC: Newcastle-Ottawa Scale.

Table 3: Overall effect estimates for Parkinson's disease and calcium channel blockers use according to study characteristics.

Characteristic	n	Risk ratio (95% CI)	P value	Heterogeneity	
				I^2 (%)	Cochrane Q
All studies	6	0.81 (0.69–0.96)	0.014[a]	54.6	0.031
Study design					
Cohort	3	0.73 (0.64–0.84)	<0.001[a]	42.6	0.156
Case-control	3	0.84 (0.68–1.04)	0.111	58.1	0.06
Class of CCB					
DiCCB	4	0.80 (0.65–0.98)	0.032[a]	72.9	0.011
Non-DiCCB	2	0.70 (0.53–0.92)	0.013[a]	0	0.546
Gender					
Men	3	0.85 (0.66–1.12)	0.243	53.1	0.118
Women	3	0.67 (0.55–0.81)	<0.001[a]	0	0.919
Sensitivity analysis					
All studies except Pasternak et al. [15]	—	0.85 (0.71–1.01)	0.080[a]	NA	NA
All studies except Becker et al. [19]	—	0.83 (0.68–1.01)	0.071[a]	NA	NA
Quality					
High	2	0.70 (0.61–0.81)	<0.001[a]	0	0.774
Medium	4	0.89 (0.72–1.09)	0.272	55.3	0.062

[a]P value representing significant inverse association between CCBs use and Parkinson's disease.
CCB: calcium channel blockers, DiCCB: dihydropyridine calcium channel blockers, and NA: not available.
CI: confidence interval.

Study name	Risk ratio	Lower limit	Upper limit
Ton et al., 2007	0.85	0.43	1.67
Becker et al., 2008	0.77	0.63	0.95
Louis et al., 2009	1.24	0.43	3.59
Simon et al., 2010	1.18	0.73	1.91
Ritz et al., 2010 (L-type DiCCB)	0.70	0.52	0.94
Ritz et al., 2010 (amlodipine)	1.04	0.87	1.25
Pasternak et al., 2012 (DiCCB)	0.71	0.61	0.83
Pasternak et al., 2012 (non-DiCCB)	0.64	0.42	0.97
Pooled risk ratio	0.82	0.70	0.96

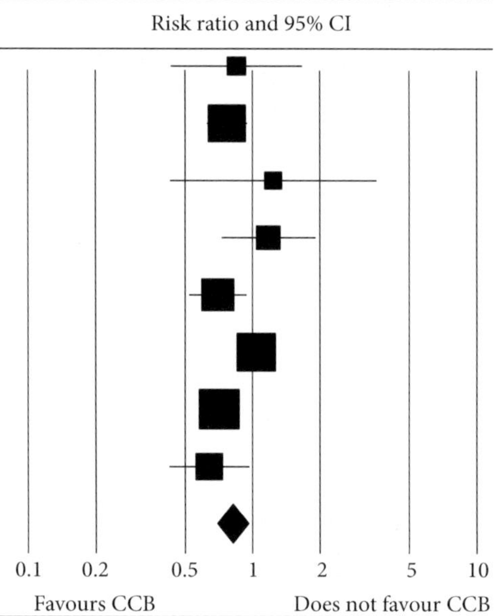

Figure 2: Combined estimate of risk ratio and 95% confidence intervals of Parkinson's disease associated with calcium channel blockers use based on six studies (three case-control and three cohort) of 27,67,990 subjects including 11,941 PD cases. Squares indicate RR in each study. The square size is proportional to the weight of the corresponding study in the meta-analysis; the length of horizontal lines represents the 95% CI. The shaded diamond indicates the combined RR and 95% CI (random-effects model).

and populations. When cohort studies were analyzed alone [15–17], the pooled RR was found to be 0.73 (95% CI, 0.64–0.84). Using case-control studies alone [18–20], we found that the pooled RR was 0.84 (95% CI, 0.68–1.04). We found a significant difference between studies according to study design, where cohort studies significantly showed decreased risk of PD in CCB users. Although the RR of case-control studies is nonsignificant but still the effect estimate is on lower side.

Both the classes of CCB, that is, DiCCB (0.80 (95% CI, 0.65–0.98) $P = 0.032$) and non-DiCCB (0.70 (95% CI, 0.53–0.92) $P = 0.013$), were found to be reducing the risk of PD.

We found a significant reduced risk of PD in females 0.67 (95% CI, 0.55–0.81) $P = 0.243$, in contrary to males 0.85 (95% CI, 0.66–1.12) $P < 0.001$.

To test the robustness of our findings, we also performed a sensitivity analysis. To do this, the overall effect size was calculated by removing one study at a time. This analysis showed no significance variation when excluding the Pasternak et al. [15] study 0.85 (95% CI, 0.71–1.01) $P = 0.080$ and Becker et al. [19] study 0.83 (95% CI, 0.68–1.01) $P = 0.07$.

Subgroup of studies having high quality [15, 19] presented significant inverse association (RR 0.70 95% CI, (0.61–0.81), $P < 0.001$) compared to studies having medium quality [16–18, 20] (RR 0.89 95% CI, (0.72–1.09) $P = 0.272$) (Table 3). Studies having better-quality scores (NOS score 9) showed a significant decreased risk of PD (0.70 95% CI, (0.61–0.81), $P < 0.001$).

4. Discussion

In the past decade, the role of CCBs in reduction of PD has been understood increasingly. With the present pooled analysis of 6 observational studies, a 19% reduction in PD risk among CCBs users as compared to nonusers was observed. CCBs are one of the most important antihypertensive drugs. The present analysis demonstrated the potential neuroprotective role of CCBs in reducing the risk of PD.

The etiopathogenesis of PD is complex. It involves α-synuclein deposition, dysfunction of protein turnover, and mitochondrial dysfunction leading to neuronal loss via excitotoxicity, calcium overload, and apoptosis [21]. Factors that potentiate pathological α-synuclein aggregation include posttranslational modifications, oxidative stress, and raised intracellular calcium ion [22, 23]. *In vitro* culture models showed that transient increases of intracellular calcium induce cytoplasmic α-synuclein aggregates [23, 24]. In addition to the intracellular calcium overload, oxidative stress cooperatively promotes α-synuclein aggregation. By blocking the influx of calcium, CCBs can prevent or stop the progression of PD [23]. Dopaminergic neurons in substantia nigra possess L-type voltage gated calcium channels 1.3 for their pacemaker activity [25]. Kang et al. reported that, by selectively antagonizing Ca (V) 1.3 L-type channels, one could provide a solution for diminishing cell loss in PD with minimal side effects [26]. This provides a potential therapeutic target, by using drugs that modulate the amount of free Ca^{+2} in the cell. An array of CCBs are approved by USFDA to treat hypertension which could be tried to lessen the increase in intracellular Ca^{+2} seen in aged neurons in patients at high risk of developing PD based on family history.

Evidence on association between hypertension and risk of PD is conflicting. Prospective studies [27–29] showed an increased risk of PD in hypertensive patients. Some speculative mechanisms include untreated chronic hypertension which may lead to ischemic cerebrovascular lesions, increased oxidative stress, and modulation of central renin-angiotensin system (RAS) leading to PD [27]. It is not clear that whether lowering blood pressure has any role in reducing the risk of PD. The observed effect of decreased risk of PD in CCB users is assumed primarily by its neuroprotection action and not due to reduction of blood pressure in patients with hypertension.

Other antihypertensive drugs were also studied as potential agents to prevent or to stop progression of PD. *In vitro* and few *in vivo* studies have shown the role of agents modulating the RAS such as angiotensin converting enzyme inhibitors (ACEIs) and angiotensin receptor blockers (ARBs) [30]. Angiotensin type II when binds to the angiotensin type 1 receptor (AT1) activates the nicotinamide adenine dinucleotide phosphate oxidase complex, thus providing a major source of oxidative stress. In addition, activation of the AT_1 receptor stimulates the NF-B signal transduction pathway which facilitates the synthesis of inflammatory mediators, which cause inflammation and later cell death. Thus ARBs and ACEIs act by modulating the oxidative stress and inflammation at the level of dopaminergic neurons in substansia nigra and basal ganglia. This makes them potential future targets to prevent or to stop progression of PD [30].

In our subgroup analysis, we found more pronounced reduced risk in women among CCBs users 0.67 (0.55–0.81, $P = 0.243$) as compared to men 0.85 (0.66–1.12, $P < 0.001$). These results are well coincided with the results published by Becker et al. [19]. Our study results were found to be significantly affected by study design, which might possibly be due to large sample size in cohort studies [15–17] as compared to case-control studies [18–20]. The definition of CCBs use in cohort and case-control studies is different. Moreover, none of the studies except study by Pasternak et al. [15] provided data regarding individual type of CCBs, duration, and dose. They emphasized on the protective association of amlodipine and felodipine with reduced risk of PD. They also concluded that individuals using high doses of amlodipine were at lower risk compared to those using standard dose. However, similar correlation was not observed in case of felodipine and nifedipine. Moreover, the results were nonconclusive because of low sample size.

Subgroup analysis revealed that use of nondihydropyridine CCBs was reported in only two studies [15, 19]. We found a significant reduced risk of PD in subgroup of nondihydropyridine CCBs users. The observed effect may explain that the protective role of CCBs in PD may not be limited to inhibition of voltage gated calcium channels [15].

A word of caution is necessary in interpretation of the analysis because sensitivity analysis by excluding study by Pasternak et al. [15] or Becker et al. [19] resulted in nonsignificant decrease in the RR of PD. The reason for this can be that these are two large well-conducted studies, which reported a decreased risk of PD in CCB users. These have a major contribution while pooling of effect estimates. Moreover subgroup analysis of high quality studies [15, 20] further suggested decreased risk of PD in CCB users, which further helps to conclude the usefulness of CCBs use in prevention of PD.

Several limitations of our study need to be addressed. Our analysis was restricted to articles in English language, which may have led to somewhat biased results. All the studies included were observational studies with different follow-up periods, and no standard definition of CCBs usage was there.

The specific role of individual drugs and doses was also not possible because of nonreporting in the studies.

Our analysis suggests that CCBs may have protective role in PD. However, future prospective studies with larger sample size are required to understand the effect of individual CCBs at various dose and duration of use.

References

[1] L. M. de Lau and M. M. Breteler, "Epidemiology of Parkinson's disease," *The Lancet Neurology*, vol. 5, no. 6, pp. 525–535, 2006.

[2] M. Göttlich, T. F. Münte, M. Heldmann, M. Kasten, J. Hagenah, and U. M. Krämer, "Altered resting state brain networks in Parkinson's disease," *PLoS ONE*, vol. 8, no. 10, Article ID e77336, 2013.

[3] J. M. Beitz, "Parkinson's disease: a review," *Frontiers in Bioscience (Scholar Edition)*, vol. 6, pp. 65–74, 2014.

[4] K. Rees, R. Stowe, S. Patel et al., "Anti-hypertensive drugs as disease-modifying agents for Parkinson's disease: evidence from observational studies and clinical trials," *Cochrane Database of Systematic Reviews*, no. 11, Article ID CD008535, 2011.

[5] Y. Li, X. Hu, Y. Liu, Y. Bao, and L. An, "Nimodipine protects dopaminergic neurons against inflammation-mediated degeneration through inhibition of microglial activation," *Neuropharmacology*, vol. 56, no. 3, pp. 580–589, 2009.

[6] M. J. Hurley, B. Brandon, S. M. Gentleman, and D. T. Dexter, "Parkinson's disease is associated with altered expression of Ca_V1 channels and calcium-binding proteins," *Brain*, vol. 136, no. 7, pp. 2077–2097, 2013.

[7] Ottawa Hospital Research Institute, "The Newcastle-Ottawa Scale (NOS) for assessing the quality of nonrandomised studies in meta-analyses," 2011, http://www.ohri.ca/programs/clinical_epidemiology/oxford.asp.

[8] J. Zhang and K. F. Yu, "What's the relative risk? A method of correcting the odds ratio in cohort studies of common outcomes," *The Journal of the American Medical Association*, vol. 280, no. 19, pp. 1690–1691, 1998.

[9] F. Song, T. A. Sheldon, A. J. Sutton, K. R. Abrams, and D. R. Jones, "Methods for exploring heterogeneity in meta-analysis," *Evaluation and the Health Professions*, vol. 24, no. 2, pp. 126–151, 2001.

[10] M. Egger, G. D. Smith, M. Schneider, and C. Minder, "Bias in meta-analysis detected by a simple, graphical test," *British Medical Journal*, vol. 315, no. 7109, pp. 629–634, 1997.

[11] J. P. T. Higgins, S. G. Thompson, J. J. Deeks, and D. G. Altman, "Measuring inconsistency in meta-analyses," *British Medical Journal*, vol. 327, no. 7414, pp. 557–560, 2003.

[12] R. DerSimonian and N. Laird, "Meta-analysis in clinical trials," *Controlled Clinical Trials*, vol. 7, no. 3, pp. 177–188, 1986.

[13] R. DerSimonian and R. Kacker, "Random-effects model for meta-analysis of clinical trials: an update," *Contemporary Clinical Trials*, vol. 28, no. 2, pp. 105–114, 2007.

[14] "PRISMA check list," http://www.prisma-statement.org/2.1.2%20-%20PRISMA%202009%20Checklist.pdf.

[15] B. Pasternak, H. Svanström, N. M. Nielsen, L. Fugger, M. Melbye, and A. Hviid, "Use of calcium channel blockers and Parkinson's disease," *American Journal of Epidemiology*, vol. 175, no. 7, pp. 627–635, 2012.

[16] E. D. Louis, J. Benito-León, and F. Bermejo-Pareja, "Antihypertensive agents and risk of Parkinson's disease, essential tremor and dementia: a population-based prospective study (NEDICES)," *Neuroepidemiology*, vol. 33, no. 3, pp. 286–292, 2009.

[17] K. C. Simon, X. Gao, H. Chen, M. A. Schwarzschild, and A. Ascherio, "Calcium channel blocker use and risk of Parkinson's disease," *Movement Disorders*, vol. 25, no. 12, pp. 1818–1822, 2010.

[18] B. Ritz, S. L. Rhodes, L. Qian, E. Schernhammer, J. H. Olsen, and S. Friis, "L-type calcium channel blockers and Parkinson disease in Denmark," *Annals of Neurology*, vol. 67, no. 5, pp. 600–606, 2010.

[19] C. Becker, S. S. Jick, and C. R. Meier, "Use of antihypertensives and the risk of Parkinson disease," *Neurology*, vol. 70, no. 16, pp. 1438–1444, 2008.

[20] T. G. N. Ton, S. R. Heckbert, W. T. Longstreth Jr. et al., "Calcium channel blockers and β-blockers in relation to Parkinson's disease," *Parkinsonism & Related Disorders*, vol. 13, no. 3, pp. 165–169, 2007.

[21] J. B. Schulz, "Mechanisms of neurodegeneration in idiopathic Parkinson's disease," *Parkinsonism and Related Disorders*, vol. 13, no. 3, pp. S306–S308, 2007.

[22] V. M.-Y. Lee and J. Q. Trojanowski, "Mechanisms of Parkinson's disease linked to pathological alpha-synuclein: new targets for drug discovery," *Neuron*, vol. 52, no. 1, pp. 33–38, 2006.

[23] K. Vekrellis and L. Stefanis, "Targeting intracellular and extracellular alpha-synuclein as a therapeutic strategy in Parkinson's disease and other synucleinopathies," *Expert Opinion on Therapeutic Targets*, vol. 16, no. 4, pp. 421–432, 2012.

[24] C. Lo Bianco, J.-L. Ridet, B. L. Schneider, N. Déglon, and P. Aebischer, "α-synucleinopathy and selective dopaminergic neuron loss in a rat lentiviral-based model of Parkinson's disease," *Proceedings of the National Academy of Sciences of the United States of America*, vol. 99, no. 16, pp. 10813–10818, 2002.

[25] C. S. Chan, J. N. Guzman, E. Ilijic et al., "'Rejuvenation' protects neurons in mouse models of Parkinson's disease," *Nature*, vol. 447, no. 7148, pp. 1081–1086, 2007.

[26] S. Kang, G. Cooper, S. F. Dunne et al., "CaV1.3-selective L-type calcium channel antagonists as potential new therapeutics for Parkinson's disease," *Nature Communications*, vol. 3, p. 1146, 2012.

[27] C. Qiu, G. Hu, M. Kivipelto et al., "Association of blood pressure and hypertension with the risk of parkinson disease: the national FINRISK study," *Hypertension*, vol. 57, no. 6, pp. 1094–1100, 2011.

[28] K. C. Simon, H. Chen, M. Schwarzschild, and A. Ascherio, "Hypertension, hypercholesterolemia, diabetes, and risk of Parkinson disease," *Neurology*, vol. 69, no. 17, pp. 1688–1695, 2007.

[29] A. Paganini-Hill, "Risk factors for Parkinson's disease: the Leisure world cohort study," *Neuroepidemiology*, vol. 20, no. 2, pp. 118–124, 2001.

[30] B. Mertens, P. Vanderheyden, Y. Michotte, and S. Sarre, "The role of the central renin-angiotensin system in Parkinson's disease," *Journal of the Renin-Angiotensin-Aldosterone System*, vol. 11, no. 1, pp. 49–56, 2010.

14

Prevalence and Predictors of Metabolic Syndrome in Young Asymptomatic Gujarati Population

Sharad R. Jain,[1] Komal H. Shah,[2] Himanshu N. Acharya,[2] Kaushik Barot,[1] and Kamal H. Sharma[1]

[1] *Department of Cardiology, U. N. Mehta Institute of Cardiology and Research Center, BJ Medical College and Civil Hospital Campus, Asarwa, Ahmedabad, Gujarat 380 016, India*

[2] *Department of Research, U. N. Mehta Institute of Cardiology and Research Center, BJ Medical College and Civil Hospital Campus, Asarwa, Ahmedabad, Gujarat 380 016, India*

Correspondence should be addressed to Sharad R. Jain; drsharadrjain@gmail.com

Academic Editor: Hasan Korkaya

Background. Metabolic syndrome is a cluster of risk factors leading to the development of atherosclerotic cardiovascular diseases. We aimed to evaluate the prevalence of metabolic syndrome (MS) and its predictors in young and apparently healthy Gujarati individuals. *Methods.* This population based cross-sectional study involved a total of 1500 healthy adults of 20–40 years of age. Demographic details and clinical data such as body mass index (BMI), waist circumference (WC), and blood pressure were measured along with the estimations of lipoprotein (a), total cholesterol (TC), triglyceride (TG), total lipid, LDL/HDL ratio, TC/HDL ratio, and fasting blood glucose (FBS). *Results.* Overall in young Gujarati population (20–40 years) prevalence rates of MS were 16.0% (male: 21.5%; female: 10.8%) where the metabolic abnormalities increased with advanced age as 9.56% of the young population (20–30 years) had MS, in contrast to the 24.57% in the old (31–40 years). Odds ratio analysis had indicated BMI (1.120; 95% CI: 1.077–1.163; $P < 0.0001$) as the strongest risk factor for MS closely followed by advancing age (1.100; 95% CI: 1.061–1.139; $P < 0.0001$) levels. *Conclusion.* Prevalence of metabolic syndrome in young Gujarati population reinforces the need for early life style intervention and awareness programs in this ethnic group.

1. Introduction

The metabolic syndrome (MS) is a cluster of metabolic abnormalities possessing complex pathogenesis. The most widely documented metabolic risk factors are atherogenic dyslipidemia, hypertension, and diabetes. Atherogenic dyslipidemia is a combination of lipoprotein abnormalities including a reduced level of high-density lipoprotein cholesterol (HDL-C) and increased level of serum triglyceride (TG), apolipoprotein B, and low-density lipoprotein cholesterol (LDL-C). These characteristic abnormalities provide evidence of a prothrombotic and a proinflammatory state of an individual. Recently it was documented that about one-third of the urban Indians are suffering from MS clearly indicating the role of urbanization and mechanization in the disease onset. The overall prevalence of MS in Indian population is 31.4% where females (48.2%) are more affected than their male counterparts (16.3%) [1, 2]. The age-wise MS prevalence had increased from 2.9% in those aged 18–30 years to 31.0% in those aged 60–69 years in Asians [3].

The metabolic factors causative of MS are highly associated with cardiovascular diseases (CVD) and diabetes. These factors often lead to a 2-fold elevation in CVD risk and a 5-fold elevation in risk of diabetes (if not already present) within 5 years, with an even higher long-term risk. In urban India, nearly 77.2% of the diabetic patients had MS which was significantly higher in women (87.71%) as compared to men (69.33%), whereas in coronary artery disease (CAD) patients, the prevalence of MS was reported to be 60.06%. However, the epidemiological assessment of MS prevalence and the individual components contributing to its development in young and apparently healthy Indians is less studied [4].

In this state of affairs, the aim of the study was to assess the prevalence of MS in young and apparently healthy Gujarati

Asian Indians and look for its predictors in this ethnic group of population [5].

2. Material and Method

2.1. Study Design. This observational and randomized screening study was conducted by U. N. Mehta Institute of Cardiology and Research Center. The protocol was approved and cleared by Institutional Ethics Committee. Total 1500 individuals of both genders (729 males and 1006 females), who were apparently healthy, asymptomatic, disease-free, and ranging in age from 20 to 40 years, were included in the study. The subjects taking any medications and with abnormal stress test were excluded from the investigation. The details of demographic data, ethnicity, family history of CAD, and smoking were collected for each individual.

2.2. Metabolic Syndrome Risk Factors Assessment. Laboratory assessments included obtaining venous blood samples in a fasted state for the determination of lipid components (total cholesterol (TC), HDL-C, LDL-C and TG, and total lipid) and blood glucose. Serum glucose and lipids were measured by International Federation of Clinical Chemistry (IFCC) approved enzymatic methods using commercially available kit on autoanalyzer (ARCHITECH PLUS ci4100, Germany). Blood pressure was measured using a sphygmomanometer and hypertension was diagnosed if the systolic blood pressure (SBP) was higher than 140 mmHg or the diastolic blood pressure (DBP) was above 90 mmHg. Waist circumference (WC) was evaluated at midway between the iliac crest and the last rib.

2.3. Definition and Preferred Cutoff Values. The MS was defined according to the NCEP-ATPIII guidelines with an anthropometric modification of WC value that is specifically applicable to South Asians [5]. Patients were defined as having the MS when they met at least 3 of 5 criteria: (1) elevated WC > 90 cm in men and >80 cm in women, (2) elevated blood pressure (SBP > 130 mmHg and/or DBP > 85 mmHg), (3) reduced HDL-C < 40 mg/dL in men and <50 mg/dL in women, (4) elevated fasting glucose > 110 mg/dL or drug treatment for elevated glucose, and (5) elevated TG ≥ 150 mg/dL or drug treatment for elevated TG.

2.4. Statistical Analysis. Statistical analysis was performed using SPSS, Version 20.0 (Chicago, IL, USA). Qualitative data were expressed as proportions whereas the quantitative data was expressed as mean ± SD. As the data follows non-Gaussian distribution the variables were compared using Mann-Whitney U test. The level of significance was accepted at $P < 0.05$. Binary logistic regression test was used to assess the predictors contributing to the development of MS in this population.

3. Result

The demographic characteristics of the study population are presented in Table 1. Out of 1500 healthy young subjects, 771 were females (51.4%) and 729 were males (48.6%) showing the overall mean age of 29.88 (±5.97) years. According to modified NCEP-ATPIII criteria, 240 (16.0%) individuals were suffering from MS. The lipid profile of the overall population showed mean value of Lp. (a), TC, TG, HDL-C, LDL-C, VLDL, and total lipid as 28.16 ± 25.81, 171.48 ± 34.76, 103.72 ± 61.82, 43.82 ± 9.93, 106.91 ± 29.28, 20.74 ± 12.36, and 619.02±84.13 mg/dL, respectively. The levels of other risk factors such as blood sugar, SBP, DBP, BMI, and WC were 80.39 ± 14.24 mg/dL, 124.09 ± 16.23 mm/Hg, 79.5 mm/Hg, 23.12 ± 4.82 (kg/m^2), and 86.80 ± 25.16 cm correspondingly. Among study participants, 155 (10.3%) had family history of premature CAD and 123 (8.2%) had addiction.

Comparison of various risk factors according to the presence or absence of MS is shown in Table 2. The population affected with MS was mostly male (65.4% versus 45.4%) and older (33.00 ± 5.33 versus 29.29 ± 5.91 years). The levels of blood sugar (89.00 ± 20.30 versus 78.75 ± 12.00), blood pressure (SBP: 137.96 ± 16.91 versus 121.45 ± 14.69, DBP: 86.60 ± 9.18 versus 78.15 ± 9.18), TC (192.75 ± 40.00 versus 167.42 ± 32.11), TG (157.37 ± 99.30 versus 93.50 ± 45.04), LDL-C (120.49 ± 32.77 versus 104.32 ± 27.85), BMI (2598 ± 3.80 versus 22.66 ± 4.82), and WC (95.63 ± 10.92 versus 85.09 ± 26.78) were significantly (<0.0001) higher in the population having MS as compared to the population not having MS. The low HDL-C (40.80 ± 9.40) level was highly prevalent in individuals detected with MS. However,

Table 1: Demographic data of the study population.

Study variable	Mean ± SD, N (%)
Gender	
Male	729 (48.6%)
Female	771 (51.4%)
Age (year)	29.88 ± 5.97
Lp. (a) (mg/dL)	28.16 ± 25.81
Blood sugar (mg/dL)	80.39 ± 14.24
TC (mg/dL)	171.48 ± 34.76
TG (mg/dL)	103.72 ± 61.82
HDL-C (mg/dL)	43.82 ± 9.93
LDL-C (mg/dL)	106.91 ± 29.28
VLDL (mg/dL)	20.74 ± 12.36
Total lipid (mg/dL)	619.02 ± 84.13
LDL-C/HDL-C	2.59 ± 1.13
TC/HDL-C	4.12 ± 1.52
Premature CAD	155 (10.3%)
Addiction	123 (8.2%)
SBP (mm/hg)	124.09 ± 16.23
DBP (mm/hg)	79.50 ± 9.79
BMI (kg/m^2)	23.12 ± 4.82
WC (cm)	86.80 ± 25.16
Metabolic syndrome	240 (16.0%)

Lp. (a): lipoprotein; TC: total cholesterol; TG: triglyceride; HDL-C: high-density lipoprotein cholesterol; LDL-C: low-density lipoprotein cholesterol; VLDL: very low-density lipoprotein; SBP: systolic blood pressure; DBP: diastolic blood pressure; BMI: body mass index; WC: waist circumference.

TABLE 2: Profile comparison of population with and without metabolic syndrome.

Variable	With MS, $N = 240$ Mean ± SD, N (%)	Without MS, $N = 1260$ Mean ± SD, N (%)	P value
Gender			
Male	157 (65.4%)	572 (45.4%)	<0.0001
Female	83 (34.6%)	688 (54.6%)	<0.0001
Age (year)	33.00 ± 5.33	29.29 ± 5.91	<0.0001
Lp. (a) (mg/dL)	26.86 ± 24.45	28.40 ± 26.83	0.3970
Blood sugar (mg/dL)	89.00 ± 20.30	78.75 ± 12.10	<0.0001
TC (mg/dL)	192.75 ± 40.00	167.42 ± 32.11	<0.0001
TG (mg/dL)	157.37 ± 99.30	93.50 ± 45.06	<0.0001
HDL-C (mg/dL)	40.80 ± 9.40	44.39 ± 9.92	<0.0001
LDL-C (mg/dL)	120.49 ± 32.77	104.32 ± 27.85	<0.0001
VLDL (mg/dL)	31.46 ± 19.88	18.71 ± 09.00	<0.0001
Total lipid (mg/dL)	690.92 ± 123.13	605.32 ± 66.16	<0.0001
LDL-C/HDL-C	3.10 ± 1.05	2.50 ± 1.17	<0.0001
TC/HDL-C	4.93 ± 1.37	3.96 ± 1.49	<0.0001
Premature CAD	32 (13.3%)	123 (9.8%)	0.1211
Addiction	25 (10.4%)	98 (7.8%)	0.2160
SBP (mm/hg)	137.96 ± 16.91	121.45 ± 14.69	<0.0001
DBP (mm/hg)	86.60 ± 9.81	78.15 ± 9.18	<0.0001
BMI (kg/m^2)	25.98 ± 3.80	22.66 ± 4.74	<0.0001
WC (cm)	95.63 ± 10.92	85.09 ± 26.78	<0.0001

MS: metabolic syndrome; Lp. (a): lipoprotein; TC: total cholesterol; TG: triglyceride; HDL-C: high-density lipoprotein cholesterol; LDL-C: low-density lipoprotein cholesterol; VLDL: very low-density lipoprotein; SBP: systolic blood pressure; DBP: diastolic blood pressure; BMI: body mass index; WC: waist circumference.

no statistical significance was obtained between the values of Lp. (a), premature CAD, and addiction of both groups.

The population being affected by MS were further categorized according to their gender and the data is presented in Table 3. Results showed that females had better risk factor profile as most of the risk factors were considerably higher in males as compared to females. The risk factors associated with male gender were elevated TG (177.20 ± 108.34), HDL-C (37.45 ± 7.04), VLDL (35.45 ± 21.70), total lipid (710.24 ± 135.24), LDL/HDL ratio (3.32 ± 1.03), TC/HDL ratio (5.33 ± 1.27), SBP (139.90 ± 16.46), and increased WC (96.73 ± 10.03) along with greater incidence of premature CAD (13.4%) and addiction (11.5%). However, the level of lipoprotein (a) (34.30 ± 27.78 versus 22.92 ± 21.56) was significantly higher in females.

The distribution of risk factors causing MS according to age is indicated in Table 4. An increase in frequency of MS was observed with increasing age (20–30 years: 9.57%; 31–40 years: 24.57%). The associated risk factors of metabolic syndrome in comparatively older age group (31–40 years) were male gender (65.8%) and increased levels of TC (198.35 ± 42.06), TG (173.56 ± 111.99), VLDL (34.69 ± 22.42), total lipid (712.44 ± 135.43), TC/HDL-C ratio (5.09 ± 1.39), and DBP (87.49 ± 8.80).

The incidence of MS in individuals having diabetes, hypertension, hypertriglyceridemia, low HDL-C, and abnormal WC was also assessed. Out of 1500 patients, included in the study, 6.3%, 36.4%, 24.86.%, 15.3%, 56.5%, 47.5%, and 10.3% of the population were detected with the abnormalities of sugar, SBP, DBP, TG, HDL-C, WC, and positive history of premature CAD, respectively. From this the prevalence of MS was the highest in individuals having diabetes (51.6%) followed by TG (48.9%). These patients were further categorized according to age and gender and the results are shown in Table 5. The strength of various risk factors in the development of MS was assessed using multivariate logistic regression analysis and the results are presented in Table 6. We have found that BMI (odds ratio: 1.120; 95% CI: 1.077 to 1.163; $P < 0.0001$) and age (odds ratio: 1.100; 95% CI: 1.061 to 1.139; $P < 0.0001$) are two prime contributors of MS in this ethnic group.

4. Discussion

The process of MS may start in very early stage of life which continues to progress during childhood and adolescence, reaching almost 50% in prevalence in severally obese youngster [6–10]. However, this process is subjected to variation according to the region, urbanization, lifestyle patterns, and socioeconomic and cultural factors in Asian Indian community. The prevalence of metabolic syndrome is increasing exponentially in India, in both the urban and rural areas showing the prevalence range from 11% to 41% [11]. In the current study for the first time the prevalence of MS in healthy and young Gujarati Asian Indians has been reported. We found that 16.0% of the young Gujaratis who are below

TABLE 3: Influence of gender on prevalence and profile of metabolic syndrome.

Variable	Males having MS $N = 157$	Females having MS $N = 83$	P value
Age (year)	32.78 ± 5.27	33.40 ± 5.45	0.3925
Lp. (a) (mg/dL)	22.92 ± 21.56	34.30 ± 27.78	0.0005
Blood sugar (mg/dL)	91.10 ± 20.27	85.02 ± 19.89	0.0271
TC (mg/dL)	195.59 ± 42.56	187.40 ± 34.54	0.1325
TG (mg/dL)	177.20 ± 108.34	119.84 ± 65.06	<0.0001
HDL-C (mg/dL)	37.45 ± 7.04	47.13 ± 10.07	<0.0001
LDL-C (mg/dL)	122.69 ± 34.43	116.34 ± 29.10	0.1537
VLDL (mg/dL)	35.45 ± 21.70	23.93 ± 12.96	<0.0001
Total lipid (mg/dL)	710.24 ± 135.24	654.37 ± 85.57	0.0007
LDL-C/HDL-C	3.32 ± 1.39	2.66 ± 0.95	<0.0001
TC/HDL-C	5.33 ± 1.27	4.17 ± 1.23	<0.0001
Premature CAD	21 (13.4%)	11 (13.3%)	0.011
Addiction	18 (11.5%)	7 (8.4%)	0.032
SBP (mm/hg)	139.9 ± 16.46	134.29 ± 17.26	0.0142
DBP (mm/hg)	86.92 ± 10.69	85.99 ± 7.94	0.4864
BMI (kg/m^2)	26.15 ± 3.52	25.66 ± 4.28	0.3429
WC (cm)	96.73 ± 10.03	91.83 ± 11.84	0.0009

MS: metabolic syndrome; Lp. (a): lipoprotein; TC: total cholesterol; TG: triglyceride; HDL-C: high-density lipoprotein cholesterol; LDL-C: low-density lipoprotein cholesterol; VLDL: very low-density lipoprotein; SBP: systolic blood pressure; DBP: diastolic blood pressure; BMI: body mass index; WC: waist circumference.

TABLE 4: Influence of age on prevalence and profile of metabolic syndrome.

Variable	Age group (20–30) $N = 82$	Age group (31–40) $N = 158$	P value
Gender			
Male	53 (64.6%)	104 (65.8%)	0.0026
Female	29 (35.4%)	54 (34.2%)	0.0026
Lp. (a) (mg/dL)	26.89 ± 22.99	26.84 ± 25.24	0.9880
Blood sugar (mg/dL)	83.04 ± 13.16	92.09 ± 22.59	0.0010
TC (mg/dL)	181.96 ± 33.66	198.35 ± 42.06	0.0025
TG (mg/dL)	126.17 ± 57.34	173.56 ± 111.99	0.0004
HDL-C (mg/dL)	41.33 ± 10.04	40.53 ± 9.07	0.5329
LDL-C (mg/dL)	115.39 ± 28.01	123.14 ± 34.77	0.0822
VLDL (mg/dL)	25.24 ± 11.49	34.69 ± 22.42	0.0004
Total lipid (mg/dL)	649.46 ± 80.85	712.44 ± 135.43	0.0001
LDL-C/HDL-C	2.95 ± 1.06	3.17 ± 1.04	0.1239
TC/HDL-C	4.62 ± 1.29	5.09 ± 1.39	0.0116
Premature CAD	7 (8.5%)	25 (15.5%)	0.0884
Addiction	9 (11.0%)	16 (10.1%)	0.0012
SBP (mm/hg)	137.18 ± 15.57	138.37 ± 17.61	0.6063
DBP (mm/hg)	84.88 ± 11.38	87.49 ± 8.80	0.0505
BMI (kg/m^2)	25.93 ± 4.15	26.01 ± 3.62	0.8775
WC (cm)	94.28 ± 9.27	95.42 ± 11.69	0.4441

Lp. (a): lipoprotein; TC: total cholesterol; TG: triglyceride; HDL-C, high-density lipoprotein cholesterol; LDL-C: low-density lipoprotein cholesterol; VLDL: very low-density lipoprotein; SBP: systolic blood pressure; DBP: diastolic blood pressure; BMI: body mass index; WC: waist circumference.

Table 5: Prevalence of metabolic syndrome in population having diabetes, blood pressure, dyslipidemia, and abnormal waist circumference.

Variable	Total affected population	MS present	MS present in males & females	P value	MS present in different age groups	P value
DM (mg/dL)	95 (6.3%)	49 (51.6%)	M = 38 (77.6%) F = 11 (22.4%)	<0.0001	20–30 = 5 (10.2%) 31–40 = 44 (89.8%)	<0.0001
SBP (mm/hg)	546 (36.4%)	188 (34.3%)	M = 128 (68.1%) F = 60 (31.9%)	<0.0001	20–30 = 67 (35.6%) 31–40 = 121 (64.4%)	<0.0001
DBP (mm/hg)	373 (24.86%)	146 (39.5%)	M = 97 (66.4%) F = 49 (33.6%)	<0.0001	20–30 = 43 (29.5%) 31–40 = 103 (70.5%)	<0.0001
TG (mg/dL)	229 (15.3%)	112 (48.9%)	M = 88 (78.6%) F = 24 (21.4%)	<0.0001	20–30 = 29 (25.9%) 31–40 = 83 (74.1%)	<0.0001
HDL-C (mg/dL)	847 (56.5%)	145 (17.1%)	M = 100 (69.0%) F = 45 (31.0%)	<0.0001	20–30 = 51(35.2%) 31–40 = 94 (64.8%)	<0.0001
WC (cm)	712 (47.5%)	216 (30.3%)	M = 135 (62.5%) F = 81 (37.5%)	<0.0001	20–30 = 75 (34.7%) 31–40 = 141 (65.3%)	<0.0001
Premature CAD	155 (10.3%)	32 (20.6%)	M = 21 (65.6%) F = 11 (34.4%)	0.024	20–30 = 7 (21.9%) 31–40 = 25 (78.1%)	<0.0001

MS: metabolic syndrome; DM: diabetes mellitus; SBP: systolic blood pressure; DBP: diastolic blood pressure; TG: triglyceride, HDL-C: high-density lipoprotein cholesterol; WC: waist circumference; CAD: coronary artery disease.

Table 6: Multiple logistic regression analysis using metabolic syndrome as dependent variable.

Variables	B	Wald	Sig.	Adjusted odds ratio	95% CI for EXP(B)
Male gender	0.6853	18.9230	0.0000	1.9844	1.4572–2.7022
Age	0.0809	35.7508	0.0000	1.0842	1.0559–1.1134
Lp. (a)	−0.0017	0.3256	0.5683	0.9983	0.9924–1.0042
Premature CAD	0.0679	0.0901	0.7640	1.0703	0.6869–1.6677
Addiction	−0.0172	0.0047	0.9452	0.9830	0.6024–1.6040
BMI	0.1145	49.9796	0.0000	1.1213	1.0863–1.1575
Constant	−7.2995	169.9954	0.0000	0.0007	

CI: confidence interval; CAD: coronary artery disease; BMI: body mass index.

the age of 40 are suffering from MS. The mean blood sugar, TG, TC, LDL-C, SBP, and DBP were significantly higher and HDL-C levels were significantly lower in this population. These findings were similar to those obtained in the studies on Chennai urban population by Kota et al. and on US adult population by Chen et al. [12, 13].

We have observed that the occurrence of MS varies according to the gender as more young males (21.50%; n = 157) were having MS as compared to females (10.8%; n = 83). The higher prevalence of diabetes, dyslipidemia, and hypertension was found to be the contributor of MS in male gender, whereas young females had fairer risk factor profile due to premenopausal estrogenic protection. We have observed that male gender itself provides strong prediction of MS development in this ethnic group as maximum odds were observed with this subset of population. However as reported by others the level of Lp. (a), a factor possessing genetic association, was highly prevalent in females as matched to their males counterparts. This pattern of lipid abnormality was documented in a recent Nigerian study [14] and Roshni et al. [15] studies also. The family history of premature CAD and addiction were also significantly higher in females which may play a role in the development of the MS especially in younger woman [16].

We found that the prevalence of MS is highly associated with advancing age in both genders. It is noteworthy that the frequency of MS increases from 9.56% in 20–30-year individuals to 24.57% in 30–40-year individuals. Hildrum et al. [17] found increase in prevalence of metabolic syndrome with increasing age that 6.7% of subjects in the age group of 20–29 years are increased to 29.3% of subjects in the age group of 30–39 years. Hildrum et al. [17] findings were almost similar to this study on Norwegian population. Total cholesterol, TG, VLDL, total lipid, and TC/HDL-C had significantly higher prevalence in comparatively older group of 31–40 years compared to age group of 20–30 years.

Though the factors of MS are multifactorial, distribution of these risk factors is subjected to ethnic and racial variations. Asian Indians have higher rates of diabetes and hence are more prone to develop MS as compared to their Caucasian counterparts [18]. Diabetes mellitus is characterized by disorders of insulin action or insulin secretion, either of which may be a predominant feature. Hyperinsulinemia appears to be a compensatory mechanism that responds to increased levels of circulating glucose and hence development of MS. People who develop diabetes usually pass through the phases of excessive adipogenesis (obesity), insulin resistance, hyperinsulinemia, pancreatic beta cells stress, and damage leading to progressive decrease of insulin secretion, impaired glucose postprandial, and fasting levels [19, 20]. The second key contributor of MS development in Gujarati Asians was TG (48.9% and odds) which has long been identified as "obesity epidemic" contributing to the rising prevalence of MS in Indians. This phenomenon refers to the fact that despite the relatively lower prevalence rates of generalized obesity, Indians tend to have a greater degree of central body obesity and increased body fat, particularly increased visceral fat, and have lower cutoffs for BMI in comparison to their Caucasian counterparts [21]. Obesity contributes significantly to the development of MS, especially in presence of increased WC, as it induces insulin resistance and exerts highly deleterious impact on metabolism [22].

Collectively, diabetes and obesity are risk predictors of both venous thrombosis and an occlusive arterial disease most likely due to existence of an atherothrombotic syndrome secondary to insulin resistance and defective fibrinolysis. Patients with MS were found to have significantly more atherosclerosis compared with the patients without MS, independent of their diabetes status [23].

5. Conclusion

In conclusion, prevalence of metabolic syndrome in young Gujarati Asian Indian population reinforces the need for a comprehensive noncommunicable disease prevention and control program. This study has shown the unacceptably high prevalence rate of MS in males (65.4%) compared to females (34.6%) showing an accelerating trend with ageing. Increasing awareness and early identification of these clusters of risk factors should be emphasized in designing population-wide prevention strategies for Gujarati Asian Indians, in particular.

References

[1] K. Pandit, S. Goswami, S. Ghosh, P. Mukhopadhyay, and S. Chowdhury, "Metabolic syndrome in South Asians," *Indian Journal of Endocrinology and Metabolism*, vol. 16, no. 1, pp. 44–55, 2012.

[2] M. Das, S. Pal, and A. Ghosh, "Association of metabolic syndrome with obesity measures, metabolic profiles, and intake of dietary fatty acids in people of Asian Indian origin," *Journal of Cardiovascular Disease Research*, vol. 1, no. 3, pp. 130–135, 2010.

[3] C.-E. Tan, S. Ma, D. Wai, S.-K. Chew, and E.-S. Tai, "Can we apply the national cholesterol education program adult treatment panel definition of the metabolic syndrome to Asians?" *Diabetes Care*, vol. 27, no. 5, pp. 1182–1186, 2004.

[4] V. Achari, A. K. Thakur, and A. K. Sinha, "The metabolic syndrome-its prevalence and association with coronary artery disease in type 2 diabetes," *Journal, Indian Academy of Clinical Medicine*, vol. 7, no. 1, pp. 32–38, 2006.

[5] A. Misra, J. S. Wasir, and R. M. Pandey, "An evaluation of candidate definitions of the metabolic syndrome in adult Asian Indians," *Diabetes Care*, vol. 28, no. 2, pp. 398–403, 2005.

[6] C. S. Yensel, D. Preud'Homme, and D. M. Curry, "Childhood obesity and insulin-resistant syndrome," *Journal of Pediatric Nursing*, vol. 19, no. 4, pp. 238–246, 2004.

[7] M. I. Goran and B. A. Gower, "Abnormal obesity and cardiovascular risk in children," *Coronary Artery Disease*, vol. 9, pp. 427–436, 1998.

[8] R. Weiss, J. Dziura, T. S. Burgert et al., "Obesity and the metabolic syndrome in children and adolescents," *The New England Journal of Medicine*, vol. 350, no. 23, pp. 2362–2374, 2004.

[9] R. Sinha, G. Fisch, B. Teague et al., "Prevalence of impaired glucose tolerance among children and adolescents with marked obesity," *The New England Journal of Medicine*, vol. 346, no. 11, pp. 802–810, 2002.

[10] R. S. Strauss and H. A. Pollack, "Epidemic increase in childhood overweight, 1986–1998," *The Journal of the American Medical Association*, vol. 286, no. 22, pp. 2845–2848, 2001.

[11] A. Misra and L. Khurana, "Obesity and the metabolic syndrome in developing countries," *The Journal of Clinical Endocrinology & Metabolism*, vol. 93, no. 11, pp. s9–s30, 2008.

[12] S. Kota, J. Sarangi, S. Jali, L. Meher, and S. Raveendranathan, "Prevalence of hypothyroidism in patients with metabolic syndrome," *Thyroid Research and Practice*, vol. 10, no. 2, p. 60, 2013.

[13] J. Chen, P. Muntner, L. L. Hamm et al., "The metabolic syndrome and chronic kidney disease in US adults," *Annals of Internal Medicine*, vol. 140, no. 3, pp. 167–139, 2004.

[14] K. W. Wahab, M. Sani, M. Gbadamosi, and M. Yandutse, "Frequency and determinants of the metabolic syndrome in apparently healthy adult Nigerians," *Tropical Doctor*, vol. 38, no. 4, pp. 224–226, 2008.

[15] M. Roshni, R. Chandni, and P. Bhagyanathan, "Metabolic syndrome and the frequency of occurrence of its components in urban south Indian population," *British Journal of Medicine and Medical Research*, vol. 4, no. 29, pp. 4855–4867, 2014.

[16] H. Cai, J. Huang, G. Xu et al., "Prevalence and determinants of metabolic syndrome among women in Chinese rural areas," *PLoS ONE*, vol. 7, no. 5, Article ID e36936, 2012.

[17] B. Hildrum, A. Mykletun, T. Hole, K. Midthjell, and A. A. Dahl, "Age-specific prevalence of the metabolic syndrome defined by the International Diabetes Federation and the National Cholesterol Education Program: the Norwegian HUNT 2 study," *BMC Public Health*, vol. 7, article 220, 2007.

[18] R. Oza-Frank, M. K. Ali, V. Vaccarino, and K. M. V. Narayan, "Asian Americans: diabetes prevalence across U.S. and World Health Organization weight classifications," *Diabetes Care*, vol. 32, no. 9, pp. 1644–1646, 2009.

[19] M. R. Hayden and S. C. Tyagi, "Intimal redox stress: accelerated atherosclerosis in metabolic syndrome and type 2 diabetes mellitus. Atheroscleropathy," *Cardiovascular Diabetology*, vol. 1, no. 1, article 3, 2002.

[20] D. Porte Jr. and S. E. Kahn, "β-Cell dysfunction and failure in type 2 diabetes: potential mechanisms," *Diabetes*, vol. 50, supplement 1, p. S160, 2001.

[21] R. Unnikrishnan, R. M. Anjana, and V. Mohan, "Diabetes in South Asians: is the phenotype different?" *Diabetes*, vol. 63, no. 1, pp. 53–55, 2014.

15

Female Sex Hormones Pattern and Its Relation to Disease Severity and Treatment in Pre- and Postmenopausal Patients with Chronic Hepatitis C Virus (Genotype 4) Infection

Nora H. Ahmed,[1] Taghrid B. El-Abaseri,[1] Hesham F. El-Sayed,[2] and Taher I. El-Serafi[1]

[1] *Department of Medical Biochemistry, Faculty of Medicine, Suez Canal University, Ismailia 41111, Egypt*
[2] *Department of Pediatrics and Unit of Clinical Epidemiology, Faculty of Medicine, Suez Canal University, Ismailia 41511, Egypt*

Correspondence should be addressed to Nora H. Ahmed; nour_fomscu@hotmail.com

Academic Editor: Tadeusz Robak

Chronic hepatitis C (CHC) course revealed differences between men and women. Male gender and postmenopausal women are thought to be of the critical factors affecting HCV infection progression. The study aimed to assess female sex hormones and their relation to disease severity and treatment in HCV infected females. Subjects were divided to 2 groups: 44 CHC female patients and 44 controls. Both groups were classified to premenopausal and postmenopausal females. Serum estradiol (E2), progesterone (PRG), and total testosterone (TT) were assessed using chemiluminescent immunoassay. Our results showed that menopausal patients had significantly higher levels of estradiol, total testosterone, and progesterone compared to controls ($P < 0.001$). Reproductive aged patients had lower level of total testosterone compared to menopausal patients ($P < 0.001$). HCV infected females of reproductive age had higher level of progesterone compared to menopausal HCV infected females ($P = 0.0014$). Indicators of disease severity and treatment response were significantly worse in menopausal women compared to reproductive aged women (fibrosis: $P < 0.001$, activity: $P = 0.045$, and treatment: $P < 0.001$). We observed that lower estradiol level may be related to fibrosis severity in CHC females. Higher total testosterone and progesterone levels may be related to fibrosis severity and poor response to treatment in CHC menopausal females only.

1. Introduction

Hepatitis C is caused by HCV infection. It is estimated that about 3% of the world's population has been infected with HCV and 170 million are chronic carriers at risk of developing liver cirrhosis and/or liver cancer [1]. Prevalence of HCV in Egypt is 14.7% [2].

The clinical course of chronic hepatitis C revealed several differences between men and women. Male gender is thought to be one of the critical factors in the progression of HCV infection [3]. Besides, the development of hepatic fibrosis is faster in postmenopausal than in premenopausal women [4]. In addition, serum total testosterone is associated with increased risk of both advanced hepatic fibrosis and advanced hepatic inflammatory activity in HCV infected men [5].

Sex differences are believed to be one of the factors affecting response to therapy. Female sex correlated positively with sustained virological response (SVR) [6]. However, early menopause associated with lack of SVR among women with genotype 1 hepatitis C virus infection [7].

2. Materials and Methods

2.1. Type of Study and Selection of Patients. Descriptive analytical study included 44 female patients, proven to have chronic hepatitis C infection [8] by polymerase chain reaction (PCR) and 44 control females, age matched to the patients, were selected from healthy blood donors, proven to be negative for HCV on hepatitis C antibody test.

Patients were recruited from Virology Center in Ismailia Fever Hospital, a referral center for treatment of HCV in Ismailia under the supervision of the Ministry of Health as part of the national project for combating viral hepatitis. Patients were subjected to thorough history taking, clinical examination, and routine workup including complete blood picture (CBC), serum transaminases (AST, ALT), total bilirubin, albumin, International Normalized Ratio (INR), alpha fetoprotein (AFP), and HCV quantitative PCR. Histopathological examination of histological activity and degree of hepatic fibrosis, of ultrasound guided percutaneous liver biopsy, was performed according to Metavir's score. Blood samples were included in the study between May 2013 and October 2013.

2.2. Serum Estradiol, Progesterone, and Total Testosterone Assay. Serum estradiol, progesterone, and total testosterone were assessed using IMMULITE 1000 (Siemens, IMMULITE, catalog number LKE21 for estradiol, LKTW1 for total testosterone, and LKPW1 for progesterone), a solid-phase enzyme-labeled, chemiluminescent immunoassay. Chemiluminescence generates electromagnetic radiation as light. The light intensity depends on a chemical reaction using a labeled enzyme and a chemiluminescent compound supplied as the enzyme substrate in excess to assure saturation kinetics. Light intensity is measured using stored master curves based on manufacturer's instructions.

2.3. Patients' Classification. Patients were classified according to their reproductive status to 22 premenopausal and 22 postmenopausal females in each group (patients and controls). Further grouping of female patients according to (1) treatment (combined interferon and ribavirin therapy) response (nonresponders: patients who had detectable HCV RNA at weeks 12, 24, and 48; relapsers: patients who had detectable HCV RNA 24 weeks after stopping treatment; and responders: patients with sustained virological response (SVR) with undetectable HCV RNA six months after stopping treatment), (2) viral load (<600,000 and ≥600,000), and (3) fibrosis stage (≤F2 and >F2) was done to compare between groups.

2.4. Patients Characteristics. Females included were nonsmokers, of reproductive age group (i.e., with regular menses, not pregnant or lactating), ≥18 years, and postmenopausal females (i.e., no menstrual period for 12 consecutive months).

CHC females having hepatocellular carcinoma (HCC), coinfection with human immunodeficiency virus (HIV), coinfection with hepatitis B virus (HBV), other causes of liver disease (alcoholic, autoimmune, and Wilson disease), previous liver transplant, hormone replacement therapy, hormonal contraception, and history of active substance or alcohol consumption were excluded.

2.5. Patients Consent. All regulations adopted by the ethics committee in Faculty of Medicine, Suez Canal University, including patient consent were considered and approved.

2.6. Statistical Analysis. Quantitative parametric variables were presented by mean and standard deviation (SD) and compared by Student's t-test. Qualitative variables were compared by the chi-square test. In all tests, P value was considered significant if <0.05.

3. Results

The demographic, clinical, biochemical, and histopathological data of the studied subjects are shown in Table 1. Similar distributions were noted for age, BMI, age at menarche, marital status, reproductive status and the presence of diabetes and/or hypertension in HCV female patients, at reproductive age and menopausal group, and their respective healthy controls. Among the baseline laboratory data platelets count and albumin levels were significantly lower ($P = 0.007$ and 0.03, resp.), while INR level was significantly higher ($P = 0.005$) in the menopausal patients compared to the reproductive aged patients. Menopausal women had worse indicators of disease severity (fibrosis: $P < 0.001$; activity: $P = 0.045$) and reduced response to treatment ($P < 0.001$) compared to reproductive aged women.

Hormonal levels in the studied subjects showed that estradiol level is higher in menopausal patients compared to their healthy controls ($P < 0.001$) (Table 1). Similarly, menopausal HCV infected females have significantly higher level of total testosterone than controls ($P < 0.001$). Total testosterone level is lower in reproductive aged HCV infected females than menopausal HCV infected females ($P < 0.001$). Progesterone level in HCV infected females of reproductive age group was higher than in menopausal HCV infected females ($P = 0.0014$).

The relation between fibrosis and hormonal levels in reproductive aged and menopausal patients is shown in Table 2. Estradiol level appeared to be higher in the group with fibrosis stage ≤F2 than the group of fibrosis stage >F2 ($P = 0.005$) for reproductive aged patients. In menopausal patients total testosterone and progesterone levels were significantly lower (TT: $P = 0.002$; PRG: $P = 0.023$), while estradiol level was significantly higher ($P = 0.003$) in group with fibrosis stage ≤F2 than the group of fibrosis stage >F2.

The relation between virological response and hormonal levels in the studied groups is shown in Table 3. While the majority of the reproductive aged women responded to HCV therapy, only 13.6% appeared to be nonresponders and 9.1% were relapsers. In menopausal patients, total testosterone and progesterone levels were higher in the nonresponder group than in the responder group (TT: $P < 0.001$; PRG: $P < 0.001$). No t-test was done for reproductive aged patients as there were great differences in numbers of each group, which cannot be compared statistically. The study of menopausal patients included one patient who showed relapse in response to treatment with hormonal levels (E2 = 97.3, TT = 29.00, and PRG = 0.60).

Table 4 showed that the comparative relationship of hormonal levels and viral load in both groups (reproductive aged and menopausal females) appeared with no statistically significant value in all variables. Table 5 showed the correlations between hormonal levels in reproductive aged and menopausal patients and the fibrosis stage, activity grade, and virological response.

Table 6 showed the relation between estradiol level and fibrosis in reproductive aged and menopausal patients; lower estradiol level was associated with significant increase of fibrosis level in reproductive aged patients between 35 and

TABLE 1: Demographic, clinical, biochemical, and histopathological data of patients and healthy controls.

Variables	Controls (RA)	Cases (RA)	Controls (M)	Cases (M)
N	22	22	22	22
Age (yrs)	34.32 ± 8.39	38.27 ± 7.38	57.09 ± 3.73^{B}	55.32 ± 3.80^{C}
BMI (kg/m^2)	24.45 ± 3.17	25.14 ± 3.63	27.45 ± 3.23^{B}	26.27 ± 3.31
AAM (yrs)	11.41 ± 1.50	12.18 ± 1.62	11.41 ± 1.84	11.18 ± 1.74
Married (%)	14 (63.6%)	18 (81.1%)	21 (95.4%)^{B}	21 (95.4%)
Parity	2.29 ± 1.27	2.78 ± 1.11	3.33 ± 1.39^{B}	3.38 ± 1.20
DM (%)	3 (13.6%)	3 (13.6%)	10 (45.5%)^{B}	7 (31.8%)
HTN (%)	3 (13.6%)	5 (22.7%)	9 (40.9%)^{B}	10 (45.5%)
Hemoglobin (12–16 g/dL)	12.43 ± 0.96	12.6 ± 1.2	12.37 ± 1.05	12.52 ± 1.47
TLC (4.000–11.000/mm^3)	7543.63 ± 2432.9	7081.82 ± 2194.56	7140.45 ± 2241.4	6215.0 ± 2279.34
Platelets (150.000–400.000/mm^3)	233000 ± 66960.5	214954.5 ± 86489.46	226136.4 ± 59978.8	154818.2 ± 46953.5^{A,C}
ALT (40) IU/L	23.68 ± 5.07	51.99 ± 31.93^{A}	24.4 ± 3.87	57.86 ± 29.3^{A}
AST (40) IU/L	23.18 ± 4.97	48.6 ± 19.87^{A}	25 ± 3.48	61.90 ± 27.8^{A}
Bilirubin (0–2 mg/dL)	0.63 ± 0.32	0.563 ± 0.22	0.66 ± 0.28	0.66 ± 0.25
Albumin (3.5–5 g/dL)	3.96 ± 0.21	3.9 ± 0.49	3.87 ± 0.28	3.56 ± 0.58^{A,C}
INR (0.9–1.1)	0.95 ± 0.2	1.09 ± 0.12	0.91 ± 0.27	1.26 ± 0.24^{A,C}
AFP (10 ng/dL)	—	3.56 ± 3.04	—	5.56 ± 3.7
HCV RNA (IU/mL) [baseline before treatment]	—	577340 ± 293440	—	587400 ± 230269
Histological parameters				
≤F2 number (%)	—	16 (72.7%)	—	9 (40.9%)^{C}
>F2 number (%)	—	6 (27.3%)	—	13 (59.1%)
<A2 number (%)	—	11 (50%)	—	8 (36.4%)^{C}
≥A2 number (%)	—	11 (50%)	—	14 (63.6%)
Response to treatment				
Responders number (%)	—	17 (77.3%)	—	9 (40.9%)^{C}
Nonresponders number (%)	—	3 (13.6%)	—	12 (54.4%)
Relapsers number (%)	—	2 (9.1%)	—	1 (4.5%)
Hormonal levels				
E2 (pg/mL)	106.5 ± 50.85	120.0 ± 56.74	20.43 ± 2.12^{B}	94.91 ± 46.82^{A}
TT (ng/dL)	19.9 ± 0.85	20.51 ± 2.88	19.97 ± 1.02	31.6 ± 13.0^{A,C}
PRG (ng/mL)	1.15 ± 0.76	1.21 ± 0.76	0.30 ± 0.133^{B}	0.60 ± 0.32^{A,C}

A, activity; AAM, age at menarche; ALT, alanine aminotransferase; AFP, alpha fetoprotein; AST, aspartate aminotransferase; BMI, body mass index; DM, diabetes mellitus; E2, estradiol; F, fibrosis; HTN, hypertension; INR, International Normalized Ratio; M, menopausal group; N, number of individuals; PRG, progesterone; RA, reproductive age group; TLC, total leucocytic count; TT, total testosterone. t-test: ^{A}statistically significant difference between corresponding *controls and cases* groups "menopausal or reproductive aged women"; ^{B}statistically significant difference between control group reproductive aged women and menopausal women; ^{C}statistically significant difference between *HCV infected group* reproductive aged women and menopausal women.

TABLE 2: The relation between fibrosis and hormonal levels in reproductive aged and menopausal patients.

Hormones	Fibrosis stage (RA) ≤F2	Fibrosis stage (RA) >F2	Activity grade (RA) <A2	Activity grade (RA) ≥A2	Fibrosis stage (M) ≤F2	Fibrosis stage (M) >F2	Activity grade (M) <A2	Activity grade (M) ≥A2
N (%)	16 (72.7%)	6 (27.3%)	11 (50%)	11 (50%)	9 (40.9%)	13 (59.1%)	8 (36.4%)	14 (63.6%)
E2 (pg/mL)	139.4 ± 50.72	68.25 ± 37.25*	142.67 ± 49.31	97.3 ± 56.54	127.6 ± 44.3	72.3 ± 34.17*	113.96 ± 52.29	84.04 ± 41.47
TT (ng/dL)	19.95 ± 1.55	22.0 ± 4.89	21.6 ± 3.67	19.4 ± 1.18	22.1 ± 3.67	38.23 ± 13.09*	21.13 ± 3.18	37.64 ± 12.68*
PRG (ng/mL)	1.30 ± 0.82	0.97 ± 0.54	1.5 ± 0.8	0.90 ± 0.51	0.407 ± 0.18	0.717 ± 0.34*	0.33 ± 0.14	0.74 ± 0.30*

*Statistically significant difference ($P < 0.05$).

TABLE 3: The relation between virological response and hormonal levels in reproductive aged and menopausal patients.

Hormones	Responders (RA)	Nonresponders (RA)	Relapsers (RA)	Responders (M)	Nonresponders (M)	Relapsers (M)
N (%)	17 (77.3%)	3 (13.6%)	2 (9.1%)	9 (40.9%)	12 (54.4%)	—
E2 (pg/mL)	120.01 ± 58.49	148.33 ± 38.83	77.35 ± 61.73	106.4 ± 54.4	86.13 ± 42.9	—
TT (ng/dL)	19.6 ± 1.14	22.14 ± 1.67	25.85 ± 8.27	20.21 ± 0.64	40.42 ± 11.43*	—
PRG (ng/mL)	1.14 ± 0.77	1.46 ± 0.82	1.41 ± 0.90	0.30 ± 0.11	0.81 ± 0.27*	—

*Statistically significant difference ($P < 0.05$).

TABLE 4: The relation between viral load and hormonal levels in reproductive aged and menopausal patients.

Hormones	HCV RNA (IU/mL) [baseline before treatment] (RA) <600,000	(RA) ≥600,000	(M) <600,000	(M) ≥600,000
N (%)	10 (45.5%)	12 (54.5%)	10 (36.4%)	12 (63.6%)
E2 (pg/mL)	135.38 ± 58.13	107.18 ± 54.65	106.71 ± 52.69	85.09 ± 41.02
TT (ng/dL)	20.25 ± 1.66	20.73 ± 3.67	29.11 ± 9.99	33.73 ± 15.18
PRG (ng/mL)	1.02 ± 0.64	1.37 ± 0.83	0.55 ± 0.24	0.62 ± 0.38

TABLE 5: The correlations between hormonal levels in reproductive aged and menopausal patients and the fibrosis stage, activity grade, and virological response.

Hormones	Fibrosis stage (RA)	Activity grade (RA)	Treatment (RA)	Fibrosis stage (M)	Activity grade (M)	Treatment (M)
E2 (pg/mL)	−0.68	−0.43	−0.29	−0.60	−0.21	0.18
TT (ng/dL)	0.37	−0.35	0.20	0.69	0.74	−0.66
PRG (ng/mL)	−0.04	−0.23	−0.04	0.46	0.62	−0.63

TABLE 6: The relation between fibrosis and estradiol level in reproductive aged and menopausal patients.

Age	(RA) 20–35 yrs N (= 9)	(RA) 35–50 yrs N (= 13)	(M) 47–55 yrs N (= 13)	(M) 55–60 yrs N (= 9)
	E2 (pg/mL)			
Fibrosis stage				
≤F2	152.1 ± 43.57 N (= 7)	129.6 ± 56.11 N (= 9)	147.22 ± 23.13 N (= 5)	103.15 ± 55.6 N (= 4)
>F2	83.0 ± 36.77 N (= 2)	60.88 ± 40.56* N (= 4)	54.15 ± 13.48* N (= 8)	101.26 ± 38.46 N (= 5)
Activity grade				
<A2	148.28 ± 51.51 N (= 5)	138.00 ± 51.8 N (= 6)	129.18 ± 48.78 N (= 6)	68.30 ± 41.01 N (= 2)
≥A2	122.25 ± 51.78 N (= 4)	83.1 ± 57.8 N (= 7)	56.31 ± 12.97* N (= 7)	111.8 ± 41.01 N (= 7)

*Statistically significant difference ($P < 0.05$).

TABLE 7: The relation between virological response and estradiol level in reproductive aged and menopausal patients.

Age	(RA) 20–35 yrs N (= 9)	(RA) 35–50 yrs N (= 13)	(M) 47–55 yrs N (= 13)	(M) 55–60 yrs N (= 9)
	E2 (pg/mL)			
Responders	137.91 ± 55.68 N (= 7)	107.48 ± 59.92 N (= 10)	116.7 ± 55.4 N (= 7)	70.15 ± 43.63 N (= 2)
Nonresponders	132.5 ± 38.89 N (= 2)	180.00 ± 00.00 N (= 1)	58.7 ± 12.4* N (= 6)	113.55 ± 45.7 N (= 6)
Relapsers	— N (= 0)	77.35 ± 61.73 N (= 2)	— N (= 0)	97.3 ± 00.0 N (= 1)

*Statistically significant difference ($P < 0.05$).

50 years and menopausal patients between 47 and 55 years (RA: $P = 0.037$; M: $P < 0.001$). The relation between estradiol level and virological response in reproductive aged and menopausal patients (Table 7) showed that estradiol level was significantly lower with nonresponders in menopausal patients between 47 and 55 years ($P = 0.03$).

4. Discussion

The findings of our study reveal that CHC infection is associated with elevated levels of estradiol, total testosterone, and progesterone in both pre- and postmenopausal females when compared to their healthy controls. This may be explained by the impaired metabolism of these hormones as a result of the defective liver function in chronic liver disease patients [9–13].

Menopausal HCV infected women had higher levels of estradiol, total testosterone, and progesterone when compared to their healthy controls ($P < 0.001$, <0.001, and <0.001, resp.). On the other hand reproductive aged women had statistically nonsignificant increased levels of these hormones when compared to their healthy controls ($P < 0.28$, <0.346, and <0.80, resp.). Menopausal Greek females with HCC females had also higher levels regarding estradiol and testosterone compared to their healthy controls [13]. To our knowledge this is the first study to evaluate progesterone level in women with HCV infection.

There were higher significant level of total testosterone and lower significant level of progesterone in menopausal women with CHC compared to females of reproductive age with CHC, and this was not the case for estradiol level that showed a slight, however, nonsignificant decrease ($P = 0.093$). On the other hand the comparison between the same groups (menopausal and reproductive aged females) in control women showed higher significant levels regarding estradiol and progesterone levels in reproductive age females ($P < 0.001$, <0.001, resp.) and nonsignificant difference in testosterone level between both groups.

HCV infection is associated with increased hormonal levels of estradiol, total testosterone, and progesterone in both groups reproductive aged and menopausal women; moreover estradiol and progesterone levels decreased with age, while total testosterone level increased with age in HCV group. In addition, although hormonal levels in reproductive aged group were higher than their healthy controls they are of statistically nonsignificant values and appeared to be minimally affected by hepatitis C, while menopausal group had hormonal levels high enough to be statistically significant in all variables compared to their healthy controls, providing evidence that this group was highly affected by hepatitis C.

Our study revealed that women of reproductive age had lower disease severity as measured by the liver necroinflammation activity and fibrosis compared to older menopausal women. The observed changes in the studied hormonal levels could be implicated in these findings. The high estradiol and progesterone levels and low total testosterone level in the reproductive aged patients may in part have protected against the development of severe liver injury. In contrast, menopausal women exhibited greater disease severity, probably due to the decline in estradiol and progesterone levels and the rise in total testosterone level that occurs with menopause development, supporting the concept that the progression of fibrosis in women is not on the same pace: mild during reproductive age and severe after menopause. Similar to our findings, Villa et al. 2012 conducted a study on four groups of women divided according to their reproductive stage (fully reproductive, premenopausal, early menopausal, and late menopausal) in addition to four age-matched groups of men serving as controls [14]. According to this study they found that liver fibrosis was advanced in the early menopausal HCV infected women compared to fully reproductive or premenopausal women. In addition, late menopausal women had higher liver fibrosis compared with younger women [14]. The favorable role of estrogens in liver disease has also been suggested by Shimizu et al., 2001, and Maffei et al., 2004, two case reports, in which different pathological conditions required prolonged estrogen treatment in two young men, one with hepatitis C and the other with nonalcoholic steatohepatitis. In the first case, the addition of estradiol reduced disease activity and maintained viral loads at lower levels than those observed before treatment. In the second case, it reversed hepatic steatosis and insulin resistance [15, 16].

A number of molecular mechanisms could explain the protective role of E2; for example, E2 inhibits the transforming growth factor- (TGF-) b1 expression and hepatic stellate cell (HSC) activation, thereby suppressing the induction of hepatic fibrosis [15–17]. In addition, E2 also downregulates tumor necrosis factor (TNF) alpha, interleukin-6 (IL-6), and IL-1b, mediators contributing to hepatic necroinflammation and the activation of HSCs [18–20]. Moreover, E2 possesses antioxidant, antiapoptotic activities in fibrotic liver and cultured hepatocytes [21, 22] that prevented the accumulation of monocytes-macrophages and inhibits proinflammatory cytokine production, whereas progesterone may counteract the favorable E2 effects [23, 24].

The total testosterone level was significantly higher in menopausal HCV infected females compared to reproductive aged HCV infected females. This finding is in agreement with the recently reported positive correlation between testosterone level and increased risk of both advanced hepatic fibrosis and advanced hepatic inflammatory activity in HCV infected men [5], in which higher unopposed level of testosterone related to higher severity of the disease and increased risk of HCC in men [25]. Other studies did not correlate high testosterone levels to hepatic fibrosis [26]. Potential explanations for the discordant findings of our study and those studies may include differences in underlying target populations, host factors, or difference in viral genotype.

Our findings of excess testosterone-associated risk in HCV positive females are consistent with the findings of increased liver cancer risk in males who abuse anabolic steroids, in androgen-treated Fanconi anemia patients [27], in women with hyperandrogenemia secondary to polycystic ovarian disease [28], and in HBV positive Taiwanese males with higher serum testosterone level [29–31].

To our knowledge no studies addressing the changes in progesterone level have been conducted yet. Our study showed that menopausal patients had poorer responses to combined therapy than reproductive aged patients (menopause versus reproductive age: $P < 0.001$). Previous studies including genotype 1 (most common genotype in Japan and Italy) highlighted the same findings [7, 32, 33].

The relationship between hormonal parameters in menopausal women and virological response showed that higher total testosterone and progesterone levels were significantly associated with unfavorable outcomes ($P < 0.001$ and <0.001, resp.). Estradiol level appeared to be of no significant relationship. A number of previous studies suggested, however, a potential link to estrogen secretion [32, 33]. Another nonconcordant study, the study of Furusyo et al. 2012, used raloxifene hydrochloride (RLX) (oral selective estrogen receptor modulator) plus SOC (standard of care) treatment in postmenopausal women with genotype 1b chronic hepatitis C; the SVR rate was significantly higher for RLX plus SOC patients (61.3%) than for SOC only patients (34.4%) ($P = 0.0051$) [34]. These inconsistent results may be explained by the difference in host genetic factors, viral genotype (Egypt common genotype 4 versus Japan common genotype 1), or ethnicity. Impairments in humoral, cellular, and innate immunity in the elderly and modulation of inflammatory factors, such as IL-6 and TNF-α, at menopause may be another important factor which are responsible for decreasing successful responses to treatment in menopausal patients [7, 35].

Our study revealed that there was a statistically nonsignificant difference regarding viral load values between the two groups. Besides, the comparative relationship of hormonal levels and viral load appeared to be of statistically nonsignificant value in all variables of both groups (menopausal and reproductive aged females). This finding is supported by one in vitro study that treated human hepatoma-derived cell line (Huh-7.5 cells) with E2 and PRG and found inhibition of HCV virion production (in case of E2 only) but not HCV RNA replication or HCV protein synthesis [36]. On the other hand, to our knowledge, no studies were found addressing its relation to total testosterone level.

5. Conclusion

The present study explored the possible involvement of female sex hormones in the pathogenesis and/or progression of liver disease in HCV infected Egyptian females. We observed that lower estradiol level is significantly related to fibrosis severity in CHC females, while higher total testosterone and progesterone levels are significantly related to fibrosis severity in CHC menopausal females only. Besides, higher total testosterone and progesterone levels are related to poorer treatment response in CHC menopausal females, while estradiol level is not. Additionally, the detected higher hormonal levels did not have significant relation to viral load in both groups. We suggest that screening of progesterone and total testosterone levels should selectively target females with high grade fibrosis. Our findings underscore the potential favorable effects of antitestosterone treatment to target HCV infected females. We assume that giving hormone replacement therapy to infected menopausal females would not have a beneficial effect regarding HCV course or treatment response.

References

[1] National Institutes of Health Consensus Development Conference Statement, "Management of hepatitis C," *Gastroenterology*, vol. 123, no. 6, pp. 2082–2099, 2002.

[2] F. W. A. El-Zanaty, *Egypt Demographic and Health Survey 2008*, Ministry of Health, El-Zanaty and Associates, Macro International, Cairo, Egypt, 2009, http://www.measuredhs.com/pubs/pdf/fr220/fr220.pdf.

[3] T. Poynard, V. Ratziu, F. Charlotte, Z. Goodman, J. McHutchison, and J. Albrecht, "Rates and risk factors of liver fibrosis progression in patients with chronic hepatitis C," *Journal of Hepatology*, vol. 34, no. 5, pp. 730–739, 2001.

[4] V. Di Martino, P. Lebray, R. P. Myers et al., "Progression of liver fibrosis in women infected with hepatitis C: long-term benefit of estrogen exposure," *Hepatology*, vol. 40, no. 6, pp. 1426–1433, 2004.

[5] D. L. White, S. Tavakoli-Tabasi, J. Kuzniarek, R. Pascua, D. J. Ramsey, and H. B. El-Serag, "Higher serum testosterone is associated with increased risk of advanced hepatitis C-related liver disease in males," *Hepatology*, vol. 55, no. 3, pp. 759–768, 2012.

[6] M. H. Ling, J. Albrecht, T. Poynard, J. McHutchison, and Z. Goodman, "Is an 'a la carte' combination interferon alfa-2b plus ribavirin regimen possible for the first line treatment in patients with chronic hepatitis C. The algovirc project group," *Hepatology*, vol. 31, pp. 211–218, 2000.

[7] E. Villa, A. Karampatou, C. Cammà et al., "Early menopause is associated with lack of response to antiviral therapy in women with chronic hepatitis C," *Gastroenterology*, vol. 140, no. 3, pp. 818–829, 2011.

[8] "EASL International Consensus Conference on hepatitis C. Paris, 26-27 February 1999. Consensus statement," *Journal of Hepatology*, vol. 31, pp. 3–8, 1999.

[9] B. Zumoff, J. Fishman, T. F. Gallagher, and L. Hellman, "Estradiol metabolism in cirrhosis," *The Journal of Clinical Investigation*, vol. 47, no. 1, pp. 20–25, 1968.

[10] S. J. Glass, H. A. Edmondson, and S. N. Soll, "Sex hormone changes associated with liver disease," *Endocrinology*, vol. 27, no. 5, pp. 749–752, 1940.

[11] P. Bannister, J. Oakes, P. Sheridan, and M. S. Losowsky, "Sex hormone changes in chronic liver disease: a matched study of alcoholic versus non-alcoholic liver disease," *Quarterly Journal of Medicine*, vol. 63, no. 240, pp. 305–313, 1987.

[12] Y. Maruyama, Y. Adachi, N. Aoki, Y. Suzuki, H. Shinohara, and T. Yamamoto, "Mechanism of feminization in male patients with non-alcoholic liver cirrhosis: role of sex hormone-binding globulin," *Gastroenterologia Japonica*, vol. 26, no. 4, pp. 435–439, 1991.

[13] L. A. Mucci, H. E. Kuper, R. Tamimi, P. Lagiou, E. Spanos, and D. Trichopoulos, "Age at menarche and age at menopause in relation to hepatocellular carcinoma in women," *British Journal of Obstetrics and Gynaecology*, vol. 108, no. 3, pp. 291–294, 2001.

[14] E. Villa, R. Vukotic, C. Cammà et al., "Reproductive status is associated with the severity of fibrosis in women with hepatitis C," *PLoS ONE*, vol. 7, no. 9, Article ID e44624, 2012.

[15] I. Shimizu, T. Omoya, Y. Kondo et al., "Estrogen therapy in a male patient with chronic hepatitis c and irradiation-induced testicular dysfunction," *Internal Medicine*, vol. 40, no. 2, pp. 100–104, 2001.

[16] L. Maffei, Y. Murata, V. Rochira et al., "Dysmetabolic syndrome in a man with a novel mutation of the aromatase gene: effects of testosterone, alendronate, and estradiol treatment," *Journal of Clinical Endocrinology and Metabolism*, vol. 89, no. 1, pp. 61–70, 2004.

[17] I. Shimizu, Y. Mizobuchi, M. Yasuda et al., "Inhibitory effect of oestradiol on activation of rat hepatic stellate cells in vivo and in vitro," *Gut*, vol. 44, no. 1, pp. 127–136, 1999.

[18] A. Rogers and R. Eastell, "The effect of 17β-estradiol on production of cytokines in cultures of peripheral blood," *Bone*, vol. 29, no. 1, pp. 30–34, 2001.

[19] S. L. Friedman, "Hepatic stellate cells: protean, multifunctional, and enigmatic cells of the liver," *Physiological Reviews*, vol. 88, no. 1, pp. 125–172, 2008.

[20] R. A. Kireev, A. C. F. Tresguerres, C. Garcia et al., "Hormonal regulation of pro-inflammatory and lipid peroxidation processes in liver of old ovariectomized female rats," *Biogerontology*, vol. 11, no. 2, pp. 229–243, 2010.

[21] Y. Liu, I. Shimizu, T. Omoya, S. Ito, and X.-S. Gu, "Protective effect of estradiol on hepatocytic oxidative damage," *World Journal of Gastroenterology*, vol. 8, no. 2, pp. 363–366, 2002.

[22] G. Lu, I. Shimizu, X. Cui et al., "Antioxidant and antiapoptotic activities of idoxifene and estradiol in hepatic fibrosis in rats," *Life Sciences*, vol. 74, no. 7, pp. 897–907, 2004.

[23] Y. Yuan, I. Shimizu, M. Shen et al., "Effects of estradiol and progesterone on the proinflammatory cytokine production by mononuclear cells from patients withchronic hepatitis C," *World Journal of Gastroenterology*, vol. 14, no. 14, pp. 2200–2207, 2008.

[24] H. Huang, J. He, Y. Yuan et al., "Opposing effects of estradiol and progesterone on the oxidative stress-induced production of chemokine and proinflammatory cytokines in murine peritoneal macrophages," *Journal of Medical Investigation*, vol. 55, no. 1-2, pp. 133–141, 2008.

[25] K. Tanaka, H. Sakai, and M. Hashizume, "Serum testosterone: estradiol ratio and the development of hepatocellular carcinoma among male cirrhotic patients," *Cancer Research*, vol. 60, no. 18, pp. 5106–5110, 2000.

[26] H. V. Nguyen, L. C. Mollison, T. W. Taylor, S. A. P. Chubb, and B. B. Yeap, "Chronic hepatitis C infection and sex hormone levels: effect of disease severity and recombinant interferon-α therapy," *Internal Medicine Journal*, vol. 36, no. 6, pp. 362–366, 2006.

[27] I. Velazquez and B. P. Alter, "Androgens and liver tumors: Fanconi's anemia and non-Fanconi's conditions," *American Journal of Hematology*, vol. 77, no. 3, pp. 257–267, 2004.

[28] E. Vassilatou, S. Lafoyianni, A. Vryonidou et al., "Increased androgen bioavailability is associated with non-alcoholic fatty liver disease in women with polycystic ovary syndrome," *Human Reproduction*, vol. 25, no. 1, pp. 212–220, 2010.

[29] M.-W. Yu and C.-J. Chen, "Elevated serum testosterone levels and risk of hepatocellular carcinoma," *Cancer Research*, vol. 53, no. 4, pp. 790–794, 1993.

[30] M.-W. Yu, S.-W. Cheng, M.-W. Lin et al., "Androgen-receptor gene CAG repeats, plasma testosterone levels, and risk of hepatitis B-related hepatocellular carcinoma," *Journal of the National Cancer Institute*, vol. 92, no. 24, pp. 2023–2028, 2000.

[31] M.-W. Yu, Y.-C. Yang, S.-Y. Yang et al., "Hormonal markers and hepatitis B virus-related hepatocellular carcinoma risk: a nested case-control study among men," *Journal of the National Cancer Institute*, vol. 93, no. 21, pp. 1644–1651, 2001.

[32] J. Hoyoshi, Y. Kishihara, K. Ueno et al., "Age-related response to interferon alfa treatment in women vs men with chronic hepatitis C virus infection," *Archives of Internal Medicine*, vol. 158, no. 2, pp. 177–181, 1998.

[33] H. Sezaki, F. Suzuki, Y. Kawamura et al., "Poor response to pegylated interferon and ribavirin in older women infected with hepatitis C virus of genotype 1b in high viral loads," *Digestive Diseases and Sciences*, vol. 54, no. 6, pp. 1317–1324, 2009.

[34] N. Furusyo, E. Ogawa, M. Sudoh et al., "Raloxifene hydrochloride is an adjuvant antiviral treatment of postmenopausal women with chronic hepatitis C: a randomized trial," *Journal of Hepatology*, vol. 57, no. 6, pp. 1186–1192, 2012.

[35] L. Ginaldi, M. F. Loreto, M. P. Corsi, M. Modesti, and M. De Martinis, "Immunosenescence and infectious diseases," *Microbes and Infection*, vol. 3, no. 10, pp. 851–857, 2001.

[36] K. Hayashida, I. Shoji, L. Deng, D.-P. Jiang, Y.-H. Ide, and H. Hotta, "17β-estradiol inhibits the production of infectious particles of hepatitis C virus," *Microbiology and Immunology*, vol. 54, no. 11, pp. 684–690, 2010.

16

Age and Sex Specific Reference Intervals for Modifiable Risk Factors of Cardiovascular Diseases for Gujarati Asian Indians

Sibasis Sahoo,[1] Komal H. Shah,[2] Ashwati R. Konat,[2] Kamal H. Sharma,[1] and Payal Tripathi[3]

[1]*Department of Cardiology, U. N. Mehta Institute of Cardiology and Research Centre (UNMICRC), Asarwa, Ahmedabad 380016, India*
[2]*Research Department, U. N. Mehta Institute of Cardiology and Research Centre (UNMICRC), Asarwa, Ahmedabad 380016, India*
[3]*Pathology Department, U. N. Mehta Institute of Cardiology and Research Centre (UNMICRC), Asarwa, Ahmedabad 380016, India*

Correspondence should be addressed to Sibasis Sahoo; shasikant_sahoo@yahoo.com

Academic Editor: Jose Tellez-Zenteno

Objective. We aimed to establish age and sex specific percentile reference data for cardiovascular risk factors such as lipids, sugar, blood pressure, and BMI in apparently healthy and disease-free Gujarati population. *Methods.* In this cross-sectional study, we enrolled 3265 apparently healthy and disease-free individuals of both genders residing in Gujarat state. Fasting samples of blood were used for biochemical estimations of lipids and sugar. The measurement of BMI and blood pressure was also done according to the standard guidelines. Age and gender specific 5th, 25th, 50th, 75th, 90th, and 95th percentiles were obtained. *Results.* The mean values of lipids, sugar, blood pressure, and BMI were significantly ($p < 0.001$) higher in males as compared to female population. Age-wise distribution trends showed increase in the risk factors from the 2nd decade until the 5th to 6th decade in most of the cases, where loss of premenopausal protection in females was also observed. Specific trends according to gender and age were observed in percentile values of various parameters. *Conclusion.* The outcome of current study will contribute significantly to proposing clinically important reference values of various lipids, sugar, blood pressure, and BMI that could be used to screen the asymptomatic Gujarati Indian population with a propensity of developing dyslipidemia, diabetes, blood pressure, and obesity.

1. Introduction

South Asians, especially Indians, are group of communities bearing genetically diverse ethnic characteristics and are passing through epidemic health shift due to urbanization [1]. This leads to a marked increase in the incidence of noncommunicable diseases such as cardiovascular diseases (CVDs), which are subjected to race-ethnic diversity and are longitudinally related to the classical risk profile of the particular community [2]. Mortality and morbidity statistics of the last few decades had reported substantial increase and regional variation in cardiovascular epidemic trends in India [3]. Hence, it is noteworthy that despite similar risk factor profile the prediction and interpretation of mortality and morbidity in Indians are prone to ethnic and geographic variations. Socioeconomic status and presence of modifiable risk factors such as individual life style factors, lipid levels, diabetes, and hypertension are noted as the proximate/primordial determinants of CVDs [4].

The circulating lipid levels provide substantially good evidence of progressive atherosclerosis in asymptomatic individuals [5, 6]. Reports from various individual studies have documented steep rise in mean values of Total Cholesterol (TC), Low Density Lipoprotein Cholesterol (LDL-C) and non-High Density Lipoprotein Cholesterol (non-HDL-C), and Triglyceride (TG) and fall in HDL-C in Indians [7]. A population based survey had reported a great degree of variation in lipid associated allele frequencies across multiple racial and ethnic population [8]. Moreover, the evaluation of ethnicity based factors on lipid levels in various communities was recommended by Third Report of the National Cholesterol Education Program Expert Panel on Detection, Evaluation, and Treatment of High Blood Cholesterol in Adults (NCEP-ATP III) also [9]. Hence, expert panels from various regions of world have established well-defined guidelines for reference values of lipids, and following this in India also various states have proposed the reference ranges for lipids exclusive for particular geographic and ethnic population [10–12]. In the same manner, racial disparities in diabetes, hypertension, and obesity are reported by many.

Gujarat is a rich state located in the western region of India. Numerous studies conducted on native and migrated Gujarati populations have reported that this community possesses different cardiovascular risk factor profile as compared to other ethnic groups [13, 14]. Apart from the fact that it has the highest number of newly diagnosed diabetic population, it also has considerably high incidence of smokeless tobacco consumption, obesity, and dyslipidemias [15–17]. The earlier attempt of comparing the mean values of lipid profile components of healthy Gujaratis with other Indian communities showed a great degree of variations between these groups [18]. Moreover, the age and sex specific representative percentile reference data for lipids, sugar, hypertension, and Body Mass Index (BMI) of Gujarati population is lacking. Keeping in mind the lacuna of research, current study was designed to establish the percentile values for serum lipids and sugar, blood pressure, and BMI in healthy Gujarati male and female in order to provide reference data of clinical relevance.

2. Methods

2.1. Design and Data Collection. This cross-sectional study was conducted in September 2013 at U. N. Mehta Institute of Cardiology and Research Center which was approved and cleared by institutional ethics committee. In the current investigation, 3265 individuals of both genders, who were apparently healthy, free from any illness and major complications or surgery for the last three months with normal BP, ECG, ECHO, and stress test, were selected. The sample was taken from the self-reported healthy population who visited the hospital during awareness camp. The population was from various regions of Gujarat state. The demographic details of the population such as age, sex, and disease history were recorded for all the individuals. The subjects were asked to relax and then the blood pressure was measured for three times and the average was taken into account. All clinical investigations were conducted according to the principles expressed in the Declaration of Helsinki.

2.2. Laboratory Tests. Fasting serum lipids and glucose concentrations were measured by International Federation of Clinical Chemistry (IFCC) approved enzymatic methods using commercially available kit on autoanalyzer (ARCHITECT PLUS ci4100, Germany). Lipids levels were classified according to the National Cholesterol Education Program (NCEP) and Adult Treatment Panel III (ATP III) guidelines. Blood pressure of the population was measured according to earlier reported guidelines [19]. Individuals having BMI greater than 30 were considered to be obese as per WHO standards [20].

2.3. Quality Control. The accuracy and precision of laboratory parameters were achieved by participating in the external and internal quality control programs of CMC, Vellore, and Bio-Rad. To maintain the reproducibility and reliability of the test, the quality assessment programs were routinely practiced and accordingly the values were standardized for mean ± 1 standard deviation (SD). For internal quality control, the accuracy of reports was tested by retesting the same sample within the hospital. Performance of all results was done following quality control program based on west grade QC rule like 1-2s as warning rule and 2-2s, 1-3s, and 1-4s as rejection rule. Test performance was started with acceptable QC range. In case of rejection (QC outlier), recalibration and use of fresh control analysis were done. For external quality control, the sample was sent to reputed NABL accredited laboratories for interlab comparison and verification of accuracy of the reports. In addition, the participation in periodic EQAS Programs for Haematology, Clinical Chemistry and Immunoassay was done on the basis of AIIMS, Delhi, Bio-Rad, USA, respectively. The data obtained from everyday quality control check was expressed in terms of SD and Coefficient of Variation (CV) and is presented in Table 1.

2.4. Statistical Analysis. All collected data were analyzed by SPSS v. 20 (Chicago, IL, USA). Distribution analysis showed that most of the parameters follow non-Gaussian distribution. Mean, median, and percentile data of 5th, 25th, 50th, 75th, and 95th were calculated for the values of lipids, glucose, blood pressure, and BMI.

3. Results

The overall results obtained from the current investigation are presented in Table 2 as mean ± SD and median of lipid profile, glucose, blood pressure, and BMI in Gujarati Indian population.

Our results showed mean ± SD of cholesterol to be 185.33 ± 39.24 mg/dL and Triglyceride in the studied population was found to be 115.59 ± 63.47 mg/dL. The mean ± SD was 118.5 ± 33.45 mg/dL for LDL-C and 43.7 ± 9.87 mg/dL for HDL-C and 23.11 ± 12.69 mg/dL for VLDL. The mean reference values obtained for TL, LDL-C/HDL-C, and TC/HDL-C were 644.62 ± 88.02, 2.84 ± 1.02, and 4.42 ± 1.4 mg/dL, respectively. In the current study cohort females showed superior lipid profile (TC: 181.55 ± 38.93 versus 188.48±39.2; TG: 100.63±48.18 versus 127.91±71.44; HDL-C: 47.52±9.68 versus 40.56±8.81; LDL-C: 113.89±33.54 versus 122.34±32.89; VLDL: 20.12±9.63 versus 25.58±14.28; TL: 629.72 ± 75.45 versus 656.96 ± 95.46; LDL-C/HDL-C: 2.49 ± 0.88 versus 3.12 ± 1.01; TC/HDL-C: 3.94 ± 1.07 versus 4.81 ± 1.46), glucose (83.08 ± 21.49 versus 88.64 ± 25.12), blood pressure (SBP: 126.47 ± 18.87 versus 133.74 ± 17.97;

Table 1: Comparison of quality control material at levels I and II from Bio-Rad with the mean and percentage of Coefficient of Variations obtained from laboratory.

Analyte	Reference mean		Mean obtained		% of CV	
	Level I	Level II	Level I	Level II	Level I	Level II
TC (mg/dL)	249.6	104.4	250.1	103.9	3.4	0.92
TG (mg/dL)	182.5	95.9	182.3	95.2	1.4	1.06
HDL-C (mg/dL)	65.4	26.9	65.2	26.5	2.5	1.96
Blood sugar (mg/dL)	297.9	81.8	297.6	81.5	3.3	3.3

Level I: Bio-Rad control (abnormal); level II: Bio-Rad control (normal); CV: Coefficient of Variation; TC: Total Cholesterol; TG: Triglyceride; HDL-C: High Density Lipoprotein Cholesterol.

Table 2: Mean and median values of lipid profile, sugar, blood pressure, and BMI in Gujarati population.

Variable	Total	Male	Female
TC (mg/dL)			
Mean ± SD	185.33 ± 39.24	188.48 ± 39.20	181.55 ± 38.93
Median	182	187	178
TG (mg/dL)			
Mean ± SD	115.59 ± 63.47	127.91 ± 71.44	100.63 ± 48.18
Median	99	110	88
HDL-C (mg/dL)			
Mean ± SD	43.7 ± 9.87	40.56 ± 8.81	47.52 ± 9.68
Median	43	40	47
LDL-C (mg/dL)			
Mean ± SD	118.5 ± 33.45	122.34 ± 32.89	113.89 ± 33.54
Median	116	121.2	110
LDL-C/HDL-C			
Mean ± SD	2.84 ± 1.02	3.12 ± 1.01	2.49 ± 0.88
Median	2.71	3.05	2.37
TC/HDL-C			
Mean ± SD	4.42 ± 1.40	4.81 ± 1.46	3.94 ± 1.07
Median	4.26	4.68	3.77
VLDL (mg/dL)			
Mean ± SD	23.11 ± 12.69	25.58 ± 14.28	20.12 ± 9.63
Median	19.8	22	17.6
TL (mg/dL)			
Mean ± SD	644.62 ± 88.02	656.96 ± 95.46	629.72 ± 75.45
Median	629	641.5	617
Blood sugar (mg/dL)			
Mean ± SD	86.13 ± 23.71	88.64 ± 25.12	83.08 ± 21.49
Median	83	85	81
SBP (mm/Hg)			
Mean ± SD	130.45 ± 18.73	133.74 ± 17.97	126.47 ± 18.87
Median	130	130	122
DBP (mm/Hg)			
Mean ± SD	82.57 ± 10.61	84.14 ± 10.55	80.67 ± 10.37
Median	80	82	80
BMI (kg/m^2)			
Mean ± SD	26.87 ± 66.52	27.09 ± 44.67	26.61 ± 85.88
Median	24.12	24.16	24.05

TC: Total Cholesterol; TG: Triglycerides; LDL-C: Low Density Lipoprotein Cholesterol; HDL-C: High Density Lipoprotein Cholesterol; VLDL: Very Low Density Lipoprotein; TL: Total Lipid; SBP: Systolic Blood Pressure; DBP: Diastolic Blood Pressure; BMI: Body Mass Index.

Data was expressed as mean ± SD. Significance was obtained between males and females using Mann-Whitney *U* Test. Level of significance was accepted at $p < 0.05$ level.

TABLE 3: Percentile values of lipid profile, sugar, blood pressure, and BMI in population.

		n	5th percentile	25th percentile	50th percentile	75th percentile	95th percentile	97th percentile
TC (mg/dL)	Men	1789	128	161	187	213.5	255	268.3
	Women	1476	127	154.25	178	204	250	262
TG (mg/dL)	Men	1789	59	83	110	152	257.5	293.5
	Women	1476	50.85	68	88	119	194.3	214
HDL-C (mg/dL)	Men	1789	29	35	40	45	55	58.3
	Women	1476	33	41	47	53	65	67
LDL-C (mg/dL)	Men	1789	71	99	121	142	178	188.3
	Women	1476	66.85	89	110	134	174	183
LDL-C/HDL-C	Men	1789	1.64	2.4	3.05	3.76	4.8	5.04
	Women	1476	1.25	1.83	2.37	3.02	4.08	4.39
TC/HDL-C	Men	1789	2.97	3.87	4.68	5.58	7.05	7.47
	Women	1476	2.5	3.16	3.77	4.6	5.91	6.26
VLDL (mg/dL)	Men	1789	12	17	22	30	51.5	58.3
	Women	1476	10	14	18	24	39	43
TL (mg/dL)	Men	1789	540	592	641	701	830	865
	Women	1476	531	577	617	672	772.15	799.69
Blood sugar (mg/dL)	Men	1789	65	76	85	94	120	139
	Women	1476	62	73	81	89	108	115
SBP (mm/Hg)	Men	1789	110	120	130	142	168	176
	Women	1476	100	112	122	136	162	176
DBP (mm/Hg)	Men	1789	70	80	82	90	100	100.6
	Women	1476	70	70	80	88	100	100
BMI (kg/m^2)	Men	1789	17	22	24	27	32	34
	Women	1476	17	20	24	27	33	35

TC: Total Cholesterol; TG: Triglycerides; HDL-C: High Density Lipoprotein Cholesterol; LDL-C: Low Density Lipoprotein Cholesterol; VLDL: Very Low Density Lipoprotein; TL: Total Lipid; SBP: Systolic Blood Pressure; DBP: Diastolic Blood Pressure; BMI: Body Mass Index. Data are expressed as the 5th to 97th percentile of median.

DBP: 80.67 ± 10.37 versus 84.14 ± 10.55), and BMI (26.61 ± 85.88 versus 27.09 ± 44.67) as compared to males, which was highly significant ($p < 0.001$; Table 2).

The percentile limits from 5th to 95th for various lipids, glucose, and blood pressure according to gender tabulated in Table 3 show higher cutoff values of all the variables in males as compared to females except for slight elevation in BMI levels in higher percentile values. Age-wise distribution trends analysis showed steep increase in the levels of lipids, glucose, blood pressure, and obesity from the 2nd decade till the 5th to 6th decade in most of the cases (Table 4), indicating natural ageing itself as one of the risk factors. In contrast to others, the level of HDL-C was found to increase with the advancing of age. The 5th to the 95th percentile values of lipids, glucose, SBP, DBP, and BMI in various age groups were also analyzed (Table 5). Most of the variables achieved stable levels after the 5th decade and in some cases a decline was observed after the 6th decade of life.

Comparative examination of reference values established for various communities based on the population mean has been presented in Table 6. We have observed that the TC of Gujarati population had the third highest (185.33 ± 39.245 mg/dL) mean value in comparison to other Indian populations, whereas LDL-C had the third highest (118.5 ± 33.46) mean value amongst all including Venezuelan and Nepali populations. The level of good cholesterol, HDL-C, was lowest (43.70 ± 9.870) in Gujarati population.

4. Discussion

The need for establishment of different reference intervals of lipids, sugar, blood pressure, and obesity in various community could be justified by the fact that these risk factors are subjected to racial and geographic variations with life style changes, demographic shifts, epidemiological transition, and urbanization playing a prime role. Moreover, Indians possess some of the unique characteristics such as higher predisposition to the development of type 2 diabetes mellitus, excess visceral fat and centripetal obesity, and smaller body size, which needs to be considered before screening the patients with any guidelines formerly standardized on western population [21]. Along with the "genetically deformed life style," other modifiable risk factors of CVD such as dyslipidemia, diabetes, hypertension, and obesity are increasing in Gujarati population [22, 23]. A physically inactive life style and diet rich in oil and sugar have made Gujarat the second largest contributor of Indian diabetic population. This ethnic group is highly prone to develop and suffer from premature vascular ageing as their heart age is 6.7 years higher than their chronological age with dyslipidemia,

TABLE 4: Decade-wise percentile values of lipid profile, sugar, blood pressure, and BMI in Gujarati population.

		20–29	30–39	40–49	50–59	60–69	>70
TC (mg/dL)	Total	161.29 ± 30.64	181.18 ± 178	193.10 ± 37.01	201.40 ± 38.81	201.31 ± 41.98	197.98 ± 37.94
	Male	165.93 ± 32.64	187.38 ± 37.99	193.43 ± 38.89	197.94 ± 38.69	195.83 ± 40.28	193.91 ± 33.42
	Female	158.15 ± 28.83	172.89 ± 30.15	192.70 ± 34.64	206.90 ± 38.51	213.04 ± 43.49	219.22 ± 53.58
TG (mg/dL)	Total	89.7 ± 42.60	116.05 ± 71.59	122.85 ± 66.11	131.56 ± 65.81	127.38 ± 58.36	128.28 ± 60.26
	Male	106.09 ± 50.87	131.09 ± 82.10	133.23 ± 76.71	138.90 ± 73.11	124.34 ± 40.28	124.65 ± 61.63
	Female	78.63 ± 31.50	95.95 ± 47.68	110.30 ± 47.54	119.87 ± 50.27	134.21 ± 62.95	147.22 ± 51.47
HDL-C (mg/dL)	Total	45.43 ± 10.56	42.18 ± 8.72	43.37 ± 9.34	43.44 ± 9.24	43.93 ± 11.93	44.12 ± 10.39
	Male	40.30 ± 8.22	39.56 ± 7.62	40.15 ± 7.89	40.87 ± 8.49	42.58 ± 12.88	43.08 ± 9.91
	Female	48.98 ± 10.57	45.69 ± 8.89	47.26 ± 9.48	47.51 ± 8.95	46.97 ± 8.75	49.55 ± 11.72
LDL-C (mg/dL)	Total	97.91 ± 26.15	115.78 ± 29.61	125.16 ± 31.80	131.64 ± 33.89	131.72 ± 35.81	128.2 ± 30.16
	Male	104.41 ± 27.69	121.59 ± 31.38	126.63 ± 32.55	129.28 ± 33.62	128.38 ± 33.81	125.89 ± 26.86
	Female	93.52 ± 24.12	108.01 ± 25.09	123.37 ± 30.83	135.41 ± 34.13	139.22 ± 39.11	140.22 ± 43.72
LDL-C/HDL-C	Total	2.28 ± 0.87	2.85 ± 2.71	3.00 ± 0.94	3.15 ± 1.06	3.13 ± 3.04	3.0 ± 0.82
	Male	2.70 ± 0.90	3.16 ± 0.95	3.24 ± 0.95	3.28 ± 1.13	3.17 ± 1.03	3.04 ± 0.87
	Female	2.00 ± 0.74	2.44 ± 0.70	2.70 ± 0.84	2.94 ± 0.91	3.04 ± 0.94	2.82 ± 0.53
TC/HDL-C	Total	3.72 ± 1.08	4.45 ± 1.19	4.62 ± 1.20	4.84 ± 1.77	4.76 ± 1.24	4.64 ± 1.11
	Male	4.26 ± 1.12	4.87 ± 1.22	4.95 ± 1.22	5.06 ± 2.06	4.81 ± 1.29	4.68 ± 1.19
	Female	3.35 ± 0.88	3.89 ± 0.88	4.21 ± 1.02	4.48 ± 1.08	4.65 ± 1.12	4.44 ± 0.60
VLDL (mg/dL)	Total	17.94 ± 8.52	23.21 ± 14.31	24.571 ± 13.22	26.31 ± 13.16	25.74 ± 11.67	25.65 ± 12.05
	Male	21.21 ± 10.17	26.21 ± 16.42	26.64 ± 15.34	27.78 ± 14.62	24.86 ± 11.21	24.93 ± 12.32
	Female	15.72 ± 6.30	19.19 ± 9.53	22.06 ± 9.50	23.97 ± 10.05	26.84 ± 12.59	29.44 ± 10.29
TL (mg/dL)	Total	596.42 ± 63.56	639.4 ± 93.55	659.33 ± 86.84	676.40 ± 85.69	672.44 ± 85.32	670.39 ± 82.16
	Male	612.33 ± 72.96	658.04 ± 105.79	666.82 ± 99.99	677.72 ± 92.57	662.75 ± 82.91	661.65 ± 79.75
	Female	585.68 ± 53.84	614.5 ± 66.55	650.26 ± 66.62	674.30 ± 73.77	694.23 ± 87.09	716.00 ± 83.97
Blood sugar (mg/dL)	Total	76.93 ± 11.06	82.80 ± 15.86	88.816 ± 23.10	93.49 ± 30.84	94.55 ± 36.14	89.39 ± 16.43
	Male	79.23 ± 11.02	85.16 ± 17.77	87.00 ± 17.68	95.61 ± 33.78	92.48 ± 26.06	90.85 ± 17.15
	Female	75.37 ± 10.81	79.64 ± 12.20	87.00 ± 17.68	90.12 ± 25.27	99.21 ± 52.04	81.77 ± 9.29
SBP (mm/Hg)	Total	120.5 ± 14.72	127.14 ± 16.49	133.28 ± 18.13	137.85 ± 19.06	139.53 ± 36.14	138.25 ± 16.36
	Male	128.23 ± 15.42	129.95 ± 15.85	134.44 ± 18.36	137.59 ± 18.35	139.76 ± 20.43	137.31 ± 15.28
	Female	115.28 ± 11.62	123.37 ± 16.60	131.87 ± 17.77	138.27 ± 20.20	139.01 ± 20.91	143.11 ± 21.61
DBP (mm/Hg)	Total	77.40 ± 9.04	81.70 ± 9.90	84.30 ± 9.92	86.25 ± 11.07	85.62 ± 11.66	83.28 ± 8.75
	Male	80.77 ± 8.46	83.02 ± 10.02	84.90 ± 9.83	86.31 ± 11.88	85.98 ± 12.13	83.06 ± 8.95
	Female	75.12 ± 8.71	79.94 ± 9.47	83.58 ± 9.99	86.15 ± 9.68	84.80 ± 10.54	84.44 ± 7.98
BMI (kg/m^2)	Total	24.78 ± 42.60	24.40 ± 5.00	27.52 ± 44.00	30.98 ± 131.38	25.42 ± 6.32	36.99 ± 94.84
	Male	29.48 ± 66.63	24.33 ± 4.64	28.94 ± 59.24	25.23 ± 4.46	24.81 ± 4.20	39.40 ± 103.51
	Female	21.60 ± 4.55	24.50 ± 5.46	25.82 ± 5.70	40.12 ± 211.5	26.79 ± 9.39	24.39 ± 4.70

TC: Total Cholesterol; TG: Triglycerides; HDL-C: High Density Lipoprotein Cholesterol; LDL-C: Low Density Lipoprotein Cholesterol; VLDL: Very Low Density Lipoprotein; TL: Total Lipid; SBP: Systolic Blood Pressure; DBP: Diastolic Blood Pressure; BMI: Body Mass Index.
Data are expressed as mean ± SD.

hypertension, increased waist circumference, and diabetes as the involved factors [17]. Hence, it is of utmost importance to standardize the reference range of CVD contributing risk factor in Gujaratis. The first attempt to establish normal percentile values of serum lipid levels in healthy, vegetarian Gujarati population was done by Jhala et al. in 1998 [18]. The study showed natural ageing and gender specific disturbance in lipid profile. The author had reappraised the lipid values of the same community in 2009 [24] and compared the data with other populations from different states of India showing variation in lipid profile of Gujaratis as compared to others. In spite of the significant contribution of both studies in lipid reference range establishment, the findings lacked percentile values specific to various age groups and gender. Moreover, none of the studies has established reference range for blood glucose, blood pressure, and BMI in healthy, adult Gujarati population.

To the best of our knowledge, this is the first ever large study providing representative age and gender specific percentile values for serum lipids, glucose, blood pressure, and BMI in healthy Gujarati Indians. Contrary to earlier reports where no substantial sex specific difference was noted

TABLE 5: Decade-wise percentile values of lipid profile, sugar, blood pressure, and BMI in Gujarati population.

	Age in years	n	5th percentile	25th percentile	50th percentile	75th percentile	95th percentile	97th percentile
TC (mg/dL)	20–29	796	118	140.25	157	179.75	216	228.09
	30–39	653	128	157.5	178	201	242.3	254.38
	40–49	844	138	169	190	213	256.5	276.3
	50–59	627	140	175	200	226	270	278
	60–69	289	132.5	174	198	228.5	274	288.5
	>70	56	127.85	173.5	202.5	220.25	254.3	275.43
TG (mg/dL)	20–29	796	47.85	63	77	102.75	178.15	202.09
	30–39	653	52	72	98	141	230.3	278
	40–49	844	62	83	106	142.75	231.75	264.3
	50–59	627	63.4	88	115	153	271	292.8
	60–69	289	62.5	89	112	154	241.5	274.5
	>70	56	59	74.75	116.5	172.75	240.1	284.66
HDL-C (mg/dL)	20–29	796	30	38	44	52	65	67.09
	30–39	653	29	36	42	47	58	60
	40–49	844	31	37	42	49	61	63
	50–59	627	30	38	42	49	61	63
	60–69	289	30	37	42	49.5	60	63.3
	>70	56	30.85	36.25	41.5	51.25	64.15	66.74
LDL-C (mg/dL)	20–29	796	60	81	93	113	146	158
	30–39	653	71	94	114	133	169	178.38
	40–49	844	77.25	104	123	143	179	185
	50–59	627	77	109	131	153	185.6	200
	60–69	289	72.5	107.5	131	155	195	203
	>70	56	80.25	111	127	146.75	177.35	196.6
LDL-C/HDL-C	20–29	796	1.184	1.645	2.109	2.747	3.979	4.311
	30–39	653	1.573	2.185	2.717	3.414	4.498	4.792
	40–49	844	1.626	2.327	2.89	3.603	4.63	4.976
	50–59	627	1.719	2.476	3.045	3.711	4.871	5.249
	60–69	289	1.707	2.316	3.047	3.882	4.956	5.037
	>70	56	1.692	2.399	2.975	3.429	4.686	4.913
TC/HDL-C	20–29	796	2.359	2.924	3.474	4.31	5.74	6.195
	30–39	653	2.842	3.562	4.315	5.164	6.78	7.395
	40–49	844	2.935	3.729	4.477	5.353	6.61	7.276
	50–59	627	3.116	3.914	4.666	5.468	7	7.302
	60–69	289	3.008	3.805	4.738	5.602	6.88	7.278
	>70	56	2.974	3.868	4.361	5.373	6.91	7.52
VLDL (mg/dL)	20–29	796	9.85	13	15	20.75	36	40.09
	30–39	653	10	14.5	20	28	46	55.76
	40–49	844	12	17	21	28.75	46	53
	50–59	627	13	18	23	31	54.6	58.16
	60–69	289	12.5	18	22	31	48	55.3
	>70	56	12	15	23.5	34.75	48.05	57.19
TL (mg/dL)	20–29	796	520	555	585	623	722	763.09
	30–39	653	533	579	623	677	791.9	849.9
	40–49	844	560	605.25	646	691	799.75	848.3
	50–59	627	563.4	618	665	714	846.6	868.8
	60–69	289	555.5	614	662	714	839	895
	>70	56	544.55	598.75	677.5	729.75	831.65	859.45

TABLE 5: Continued.

	Age in years	n	5th percentile	25th percentile	50th percentile	75th percentile	95th percentile	97th percentile
Blood sugar (mg/dL)	20–29	796	60	70	77	84	95	98.09
	30–39	652	64	74	81	89	102	112
	40–49	844	67	78	85	94	116	137.95
	50–59	627	66	79	88	98	134.2	178.96
	60–69	289	65	78	89	99.5	146	155.9
	>70	56	69.7	79	86.5	94	130.65	143.77
SBP (mm/Hg)	20–29	796	100	110	120	130	148	152
	30–39	653	104	116	126	136	154	164
	40–49	844	110	120	130	142	169.75	176
	50–59	627	110	126	138	150	170	180
	60–69	289	110	126	140	150	179	182.6
	>70	56	109.1	128	140	150	164.7	180
DBP (mm/Hg)	20–29	796	68	70	80	80	90	96
	30–39	653	70	76	80	90	100	100
	40–49	844	70	80	84	90	100	102
	50–59	627	70	80	86	90	100	100.32
	60–69	289	70	80	84	90	100	105.8
	>70	56	67.4	80	82	90	100	100
BMI (kg/m^2)	20–29	796	15.93	18.42	21.35	24.82	30.43	31.96
	30–39	653	17.45	21.35	23.93	26.65	32.11	33.92
	40–49	844	17.88	22.37	25	28.14	33.69	35.3
	50–59	627	19.22	22.78	25.51	28.22	33.33	34.66
	60–69	289	18.45	22.28	25.06	27.51	32.34	34.25
	>70	56	17.86	21.11	23.44	26.75	33.67	35.54

TC: Total Cholesterol; TG: Triglycerides; HDL-C: High Density Lipoprotein Cholesterol; LDL-C: Low Density Lipoprotein Cholesterol; VLDL: Very Low Density Lipoprotein; TL: Total Lipid; SBP: Systolic Blood Pressure; DBP: Diastolic Blood Pressure; BMI: Body Mass Index. Data are expressed as the 5th to 97th percentile of median.

TABLE 6: Comparison between mean lipid values of different studies.

	N	TC (mg/dL)	TG (mg/dL)	HDL-C (mg/dL)	LDL-C (mg/dL)	LDL/HDL	TC/HDL	VLDL (mg/dL)
Our study	3265	185.33 ± 39.245	115.6 ± 33.460	43.70 ± 9.870	118.50 ± 33.460	2.843 ± 1.028	4.429 ± 1.405	23.12 ± 12.70
Rajasthan	1527	168.13 ± 31.40	113 ± 47.44	45.10 ± 10.75	100.50 ± 27.71	—	—	—
Andhra Pradesh	1922	175.3 ± 34.6	132 ± 60.9	47.2 ± 10.4	101.1 ± 3.0	2.4 ± 1	4.15 ± 1.13	—
Bengal	1396	189.7 ± 33.3	132 ± 42.2	52.9 ± 10.1	115.6 ± 29.8	—	—	21.1 ± 6.5
Maharashtra	751	198 ± 37.16	119 ± 53.27	47 ± 11.13	121 ± 29.39	—	4.4 ± 1.13	—
Venezuela	434	191.96 ± 46	130.50 ± 102.53	44.27 ± 12.12	122.10 ± 38.40	—	—	26.10 ± 20.50
Nepal	454	184.0 ± 50.7	147.4 ± 88.7	45.0 ± 11.7	111.9 ± 42.0	—	—	—

TC: Total Cholesterol; TG: Triglycerides; HDL-C: High Density Lipoprotein Cholesterol; LDL-C: Low Density Lipoprotein Cholesterol; VLDL: Very Low Density Lipoprotein. Data are expressed as mean ± SD.

in the lipid profile [11, 25], we had obtained significant difference between the risk profiles of males and females of the study population. The females were having superior CVD risk factor profile due to the estrogenic protective effect, which was found to be lost in the 5th to the 6th decade of life.

Natural ageing induced elevation in CVD risk factors was observed in the study population; however, surprisingly, the mean value of HDL was found to increase steadily after the 3rd decade with the increasing age in both genders which is in accordance with other studies (Andhra Pradesh). A significant finding reflected from decade-wise analysis is the loss of premenopausal protection in females in the 5th to 6th decade of life as the mean values of serum Total Cholesterol, LDL-C, SBP, and BMI were higher in females of 50–59 age group as compared to their male counterpart of the same age group [11, 12]. Several epidemiological studies have shown the interplay between multiple risk factors of CVD such as dyslipidemia, diabetes, BMI, and hypertension [26, 27]. In concordance with our study, the coexistence of these risk factors in Gujarati population has been reported by others also [28]. One of the most striking outcomes of the study is the relatively low level of HDL-C in Gujaratis compared to Rajasthani, Andhra Pradesh, Bengali, Maharashtrian, Venezuelan, and Nepalese population [10, 12, 29–32]. All of these studies were undertaken on apparently healthy population similar to ours. Prajapati et al. had shown great degree of association between higher carotid intima thickness and low HDL-C [33] levels in Gujarati children, making HDL-C one of the strongest predictors of CAD in the studied community. We have observed the alarmingly high proportion of population being unaware of the CVD risk factors prevalence.

Representative percentile reference data of modifiable risk factors of CVD are highly required for the framing of appropriate diagnostic and preventive policies. The values provided in the current study could be effectively used as reference values that are specific for Gujarati population. The strengths of the study are the well-defined percentile values of modifiable risk factors, larger population size, standard laboratory techniques, and participants from different regions of Gujarat state. However, the study also possesses some limitations such as lack of information regarding the history of genetics, diet, and stress, daily consumption of alcohol and tobacco of the study population.

5. Conclusion

The outcome of the current study will contribute significantly to standardization of the reference values of various lipids, glucose, blood pressure, and BMI which are of clinical importance and will help in the designing of better diagnostic strategies.

References

[1] K. S. Reddy and S. Yusuf, "Emerging epidemic of cardiovascular disease in developing countries," *Circulation*, vol. 97, no. 6, pp. 596–601, 1998.

[2] K. E. North, B. V. Howard, T. K. Welty et al., "Genetic and environmental contributions to cardiovascular disease risk in American Indians the strong heart family study," *American Journal of Epidemiology*, vol. 157, no. 4, pp. 303–314, 2003.

[3] R. Gupta, S. Guptha, K. K. Sharma, A. Gupta, and P. Deedwania, "Regional variations in cardiovascular risk factors in India: India heart watch," *World Journal of Cardiology*, vol. 4, no. 4, pp. 112–120, 2012.

[4] H. Zeljko, T. Škarić-Jurić, N. S. Narančić et al., "Traditional CVD risk factors and socio-economic deprivation in Roma minority population of Croatia," *Collegium Antropologicum*, vol. 32, no. 3, pp. 667–676, 2008.

[5] R. Carmena, P. Duriez, and J.-C. Fruchart, "Atherogenic lipoprotein particles in atherosclerosis," *Circulation*, vol. 109, no. 23, supplement 3, pp. III-2–III-7, 2004.

[6] I. Shai, E. B. Rimm, S. E. Hankinson et al., "Multivariate assessment of lipid parameters as predictors of coronary heart disease among postmenopausal women: potential implications for clinical guidelines," *Circulation*, vol. 110, no. 18, pp. 2824–2830, 2004.

[7] R. Gupta, S. Guptha, A. Agrawal, V. Kaul, K. Gaur, and V. P. Gupta, "Secular trends in cholesterol lipoproteins and triglycerides and prevalence of dyslipidemias in an urban Indian population," *Lipids in Health and Disease*, vol. 7, no. 1, article 40, 2008.

[8] A. S. Foulkes, D. A. Wohl, I. Frank et al., "Associations among race/ethnicity, ApoC-III genotypes, and lipids in HIV-1-infected individuals on antiretroviral therapy," *PLoS Medicine*, vol. 3, no. 3, pp. 337–347, 2006.

[9] National Heart, Lung, and Blood Institute, "Third report of the National Cholesterol Education Program (NCEP) expert panel on detection, evaluation, and treatment of high blood cholesterol in adults (Adult Treatment Panel III) final report," *Circulation*, vol. 106, no. 25, pp. 3143–3421, 2002.

[10] D. Yadav, M. Gupta, S. Mishra, and P. Sharma, "Reference interval for lipid profile in North Indian population from Rajasthan according to various partitioning criteria," *Clinica Chimica Acta*, vol. 426, pp. 145–151, 2013.

[11] M. Das and M. Saikia, "Stimation of reference interval of lipid profile in Assamese population," *Indian Journal of Clinical Biochemistry*, vol. 24, no. 2, pp. 190–193, 2009.

[12] T. Malati and M. R. U. Mahesh, "Reference intervals for serum total cholesterol, HDL-cholesterol, LDL-cholesterol, triglycerides, Lp (a), apolipoprotein A-I, A-II, B, C-II, C-III, and E in healthy South Indians from Andhra Pradesh," *Indian Journal of Clinical Biochemistry*, vol. 24, no. 4, pp. 343–355, 2009.

[13] M. P. M. de Maat, F. Green, P. de Knijff, J. Jespersen, and C. Kluft, "Factor VII polymorphisms in populations with different risks of cardiovascular disease," *Arteriosclerosis, Thrombosis, and Vascular Biology*, vol. 17, no. 10, pp. 1918–1923, 1997.

[14] J. K. Cruickshank, J. Cooper, M. Burnett, J. Macduff, and U. Drubra, "Ethnic differences in fasting plasma C-peptide and insulin in relation to glucose tolerance and blood pressure," *The Lancet*, vol. 338, no. 8771, pp. 842–847, 1991.

[15] S. R. Joshi, B. Saboo, M. Vadivale et al., "Prevalence of diagnosed and undiagnosed diabetes and hypertension in India—results from the Screening India's Twin Epidemic (SITE) study," *Diabetes Technology and Therapeutics*, vol. 14, no. 1, pp. 8–15, 2012.

[16] D. V. Bala, I. L. A. N. Bodiwala, D. D. Patel, and P. M. Shah, "Epidemiological determinants of tobacco use in Gujrat State, India," *Indian Journal of Community Medicine*, vol. 31, no. 3, pp. 173–176, 2006.

[17] P. M. McKeigue, B. Shah, and M. G. Marmot, "Relation of central obesity and insulin resistance with high diabetes prevalence and cardiovascular risk in South Asians," *The Lancet*, vol. 337, no. 8738, pp. 382–386, 1991.

[18] C. I. Jhala, U. V. Shah, T. K. Shah, B. K. Naik, and J. D. Dafda, "A study of serum lipid profile part—1: establishment of normal reference values of serum lipid levels in healthy vegetarian population of Gujarat," *Indian Journal of Clinical Biochemistry*, vol. 13, no. 1, pp. 1–7, 1998.

[19] Indian Consensus Group, "Indian consensus for prevention of coronary artery disease: a joint scientific statement of Indian society of hypertension and International College of Nutrition," *Journal of Nutritional and Environmental Medicine*, no. 6, pp. 309–318, 1996.

[20] World Health Organization, *The World Health Report: 2002: Reducing Risks, Promoting Healthy Life: Overview*, World Health Organization, Geneva, Switzerland, 2002.

[21] S. Kanjilal, J. Shanker, V. S. Rao et al., "Prevalence and component analysis of metabolic syndrome: an Indian atherosclerosis

research study perspective," *Vascular Health and Risk Management*, vol. 4, no. 1, pp. 189–197, 2008.

[22] H. Pandya, J. D. Lakhani, and N. Patel, "Obesity is becoming synonym for diabetes in rural areas of india also an alarming situation," *International Journal of Biological and Medical Research*, vol. 2, no. 2, pp. 556–560, 2011.

[23] A. Joshi, P. Bhugra, J. Lakhani, and S. Desai, "Body mass index and central obesity in hypertensive patients," *Gujarat Medical Journal*, vol. 61, no. 3, pp. 33–36, 2004.

[24] C. Jhala, P. Joshi, T. Shah, and B. Naik, "Establishment of normal lipid reference values in healthy vegetarian population of rural western & northern Gujarat and comparison with available similar data of other parts of India," *Gujarat Medical Journal*, vol. 64, no. 2, pp. 25–31, 2009.

[25] V. Kaur, M. Verma, A. Kaur, S. Gupta, and K. Singh, "To establish the reference intervals of lipid profile in Punjab," *Indian Journal of Clinical Biochemistry*, vol. 27, no. 3, pp. 290–295, 2012.

[26] J. F. Price, P. I. Mowbray, A. J. Lee, A. Rumley, G. D. O. Lowe, and F. G. R. Fowkes, "Relationship between smoking and cardiovascular risk factors in the development of peripheral arterial disease and coronary artery disease; Edinburgh Artery study," *European Heart Journal*, vol. 20, no. 5, pp. 344–353, 1999.

[27] D. Betteridge, "The interplay of cardiovascular risk factors in the metabolic syndrome and type 2 diabetes," *European Heart Journal Supplements*, vol. 6, supplement G, pp. G3–G7, 2004.

[28] K. H. Sharma, S. Sahoo, K. H. Shah et al., "Are Gujarati Asian Indians 'older' for their 'vascular age' as compared to their 'chronological age'?" *Quarterly Journal of Medicine*, vol. 105, no. 2, pp. 105–112, 2014.

[29] T. F. Ashavaid, A. A. Kondkar, S. P. Todur, A. J. Dherai, J. Morey, and R. Raghavan, "Lipid, lipoprotein, apolipoprotein and lipoprotein (a) levels: reference intervals in a healthy Indian population," *Journal of Atherosclerosis and Thrombosis*, vol. 12, no. 5, pp. 251–259, 2005.

[30] K. Goswami and A. Bandyopadhyay, "Lipid profile in middle class Bengali population of Kolkata," *Indian Journal of Clinical Biochemistry*, vol. 18, no. 2, pp. 127–130, 2003.

[31] V. J. Bermúdez, L. M. Bello, A. Naguib et al., "Lipid profile reference intervals in individuals from Maracaibo, Venezuela: an insight from the Maracaibo City Metabolic Syndrome prevalence study," *Revista Latinoamericana de Hipertension*, vol. 7, no. 2, pp. 24–34, 2011.

[32] Y. R. Limbu, S. K. Rai, K. Ono et al., "Lipid profile of adult Nepalese population," *Nepal Medical College Journal*, vol. 10, no. 1, pp. 4–7, 2008.

[33] J. Prajapati, S. Dani, S. Jain et al., "AS-209: risk factor profile for coronary artery disease in very young gujarati population," *The American Journal of Cardiology*, vol. 103, no. 9, supplement, p. 90B, 2009.

17

Metabolic Syndrome in Apparently "Healthy" Ghanaian Adults

Richard Ofori-Asenso,[1] Akosua Adom Agyeman,[1] and Amos Laar[2]

[1] *Research Unit, Health Policy Consult, Weija, Accra, Ghana*
[2] *Department of Population, Family and Reproductive Health, School of Public Health, University of Ghana, Legon, Accra, Ghana*

Correspondence should be addressed to Richard Ofori-Asenso; asensox215@gmail.com

Academic Editor: Jochen G. Schneider

Background. Metabolic syndrome (MetS) is a major public health problem in Sub-Saharan Africa. We systematically reviewed the literature towards estimating the prevalence of MetS among apparently "healthy" Ghanaian adults. *Methods.* We searched PubMed, Web of Science, Scopus, Africa Journals Online, African Index Medicus, and Google scholar as well as the websites of the Ministry of Health and Ghana Health service through September 2016. Only studies conducted among apparently "healthy" (no established disease, e.g., diabetes and hypertension) adults aged ≥ 18 years were considered. Only studies that utilised the National Cholesterol Education Program Adult Treatment Panel (NCEP-ATP), World Health Organization (WHO), or International Diabetes Federation (IDF) classifications for MetS were included. *Results.* Data from nine studies involving 1,559 individuals were pooled. The prevalence of MetS based on NCEP-ATP, WHO, and IDF classifications was 12.4% (95% confidence interval [CI] = 8.3–17.4%), 6.0% (95% CI = 1.4–13.1%), and 21.2% (95% CI = 12.4–30.9), respectively. Prevalence of MetS was higher among women than men. *Conclusion.* Among a population of adult Ghanaians deemed "healthy," there is a high prevalence of MetS. Preventive measures are required to address the risk components of MetS such as obesity and hypertension which are rapidly rising in Ghana.

1. Background

Metabolic syndrome (MetS)—a cluster of conditions—that is, increased blood pressure, high blood sugar, excess body fat around the waist, and abnormal cholesterol or triglyceride levels that occur together and increase the risk of heart disease, stroke, and diabetes, is recognised to be of significant global public health importance [1, 2]. Evidence suggests that the combined effects of the individual MetS disorders raise the risk of further disease and mortality much more than the sum of the individual risk components [3]. Subsequently, persons suffering from MetS have been found to be about two times more likely to die from and three times likely to experience heart attacks or stroke compared to persons without the condition [4]. Individuals with MetS are also about five times more likely to develop type 2 diabetes [4].

While the increased risk of type 2 diabetes and cardiovascular diseases (CVDs) consequent to MetS is widely recognised, the definition and contributions of the underlying components of MetS have been subject of debate [5]. This has sometimes been a source of confusion for clinicians regarding how MetS should be diagnosed; estimating the true prevalence of MetS in any setting is equally a challenge [5, 6]. Since 1988 when metabolic syndrome was first described [7], several definitional perspectives have emerged. The most widely used definitions/classification for MetS are those provided by World Health Organization (WHO) [8], The US National Cholesterol Education Program Adult Treatment Panel (NCEP-ATP, 2001 and 2004 revision) [9, 10], and International Diabetes Federation (IDF) [11] (Supplemental Table S1 in Supplementary Material.

The underlying cause of MetS is not entirely understood but insulin resistance and central obesity are considered to be major players [11, 12]. Prevalence of MetS increases along with body mass index (BMI) and age. Genetics, sedentary lifestyle, a proinflammatory state, and hormonal changes may also have a causal effect, but the individual contributions of these factors may vary widely according to ethnicity [11, 13].

In spite of the challenges in the determination of MetS prevalence due to the different classifications, the IDF estimates that nearly a quarter of the world's population suffers from MetS [4]. Grundy et al. [10] reports that around 20–30% of the adult population in most countries suffer from MetS. Kaur [14] on the other hand indicates that the prevalence of MetS can vary widely across countries in the range 10–84% depending on a number of factors such as ethnicity, gender, age, and race of population under consideration.

MetS is considered to be of significant public health importance in many African countries with prevalence deemed to be on the rise and more frequent in women and urban dwellers [15]. The individual risk factors of MetS have frequently been reported among Ghanaians [16–18]. Ghana is experiencing rapid epidemiological transition which has been linked to factors such as increasing sedentary lifestyle and nutrition changes as a consequence of globalization and urbanization [19, 20]. There is concern among public health practitioners that the ongoing changes in lifestyle among Ghana's population could result in an escalation of metabolic disorders [19]. However, the burden of MetS among Ghanaian adults has not been comprehensively reviewed, although such information is critical to inform clinical practice and the design of appropriate public health preventive measures.

In this study, we sought to systematically review the available evidence of MetS among apparently "healthy" Ghanaians towards providing an estimate of the prevalence. To our knowledge, this is believed to be the first published systematic review that has attempted to estimate the national prevalence of MetS in Ghana.

2. Methods

This systematic review was conducted in accordance with the Preferred Reporting Items for Systematic Reviews and Meta-Analyses PRISMA guidelines [21].

2.1. Search Strategy. Searches for studies reporting prevalence of MetS among Ghanaians were conducted by RO in PubMed, Web of Science, Scopus, Africa Journals Online (AJOL), African Index Medicus, and Google scholar databases for entries up to 25th September 2016. The keywords used were "metabolic syndrome or dysmetabolic syndrome or syndrome X or insulin resistance syndrome or cardiovascular syndrome or cardio-metabolic syndrome" and "Ghana OR Ghanaian." We also searched the websites of the Ministry of Health (http://www.moh.gov.gh/) and the Ghana Health Service (http://www.ghanahealthservice.org/) for nonindexed studies. The online searches were supplemented by reference screening of selected publications to identify additional studies not captured through the online searches.

2.2. Studies Selection. We included only studies published in English conducted on apparently healthy adults aged ≥ 18 years. Studies carried out on persons with known health disorders were excluded. Studies that mixed healthy adults and persons with known diseases were excluded unless separate prevalence was reported for the healthy population. For a study to be included, the prevalence of MetS should have been established based on an internationally recognised guideline/classification (WHO, IDF, etc., as indicated in Supplemental table S1). The quality of each study was assessed using a 12-point scoring system as adopted from the Downs and Black checklist [22]. The quality assessment focused on variables related to study objectives, characteristics of the study participants, description of inclusion/exclusion criteria, data collection methods, and appropriate data analysis techniques (e.g., whether confounders reported) and whether the discussion of the findings was appropriate and any limitations acknowledged. Individual study information and data were independently extracted by RO and AAA and crosschecked. Any discrepancies were resolved via consensus-based discussions.

2.3. Data Analysis. Data analysis was carried out using MetaXL and Open Meta (analyst). As adopted in similar reviews [32, 33], we conducted a meta-analysis proportion to estimate the prevalence of MetS among Ghanaians with no established disease. Individual study prevalence and pooled estimates were assessed at 95% confidence interval (CI). The level of heterogeneity was assessed based on Cohran's Q statistic test and degree of inconsistency (I^2) [34]. As we anticipated some level of heterogeneity across studies for multiple reasons we opted to use the random effect model over the fixed effect model in the analysis of pooled effects [34]. The presence of publication bias was assessed by direct observation of funnel plots and confirmed with an egger statistic test [35]. A metaregression analysis was also carried out to assess the effects of age of participants and sampling period as possible sources of heterogeneity among the study finding. Statistical significance was set at $p < 0.05$.

3. Results

3.1. Studies Characteristics. Figure 1 is a summary of the steps in retrieving appropriate studies for the review. Out of 197 citations retrieved from the database searches, 18 were subjected to full text analysis following removal of duplicates and exclusion of studies based on titles and abstracts. Of the 18 studies, nine (9) met the overall inclusion criteria for addition into the review (Table 1). The nine studies excluded at this stage were mainly because they reported MetS prevalence in a group of people with known diseases (HIV, diabetes, hypertension, etc.). The 9 selected studies [23–31] were published between 2011 and 2016, although the sampling occurred during 2005–2011. The nine studies altogether included a total population of 1,559 sampled across 4 regions of Ghana. Six studies were conducted in Ashanti region [23, 25, 26, 28, 30, 31], one was conducted in Eastern region [27], one was conducted in Greater Accra [24], and one study involved participants sampled from two regions (Northern and Ashanti) [29]. Five studies had a cross-sectional design and 4 were case-control studies. The mean age of study participants across the nine studies was within the range 30.2–54.9 years. Most (89%, $n = 8$) of the studies were conducted among urban dwellers. Four studies adopted NCEP-ATP, WHO, and IDF criteria concurrently, three studies used only NCEP-ATP classification, one study used

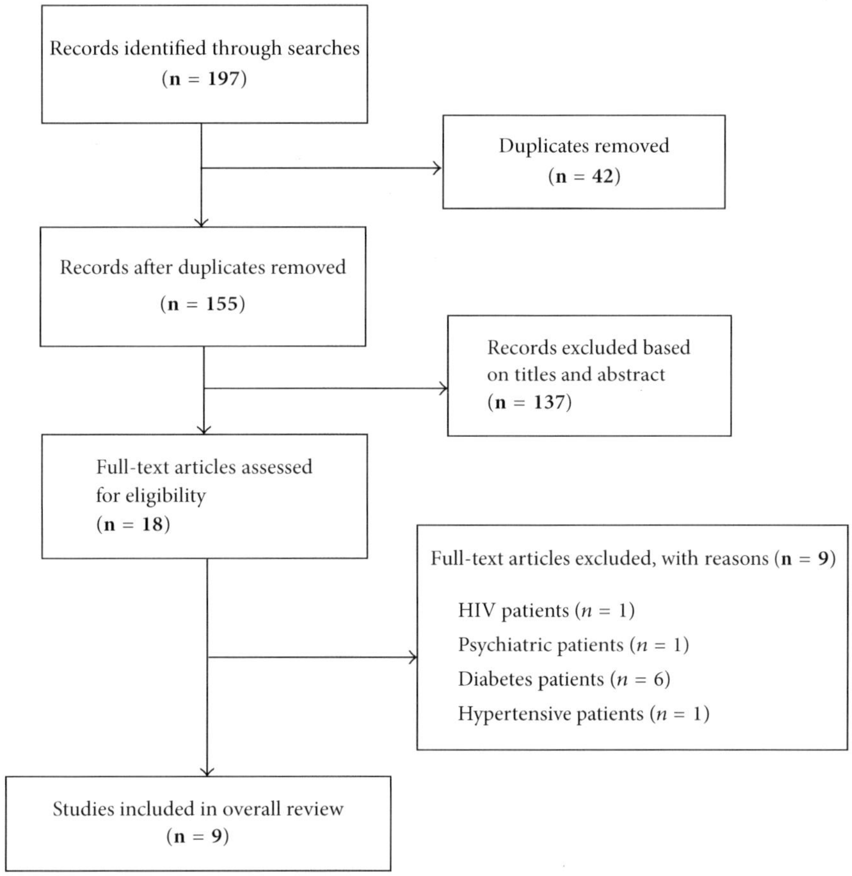

FIGURE 1: Flow chart of studies retrieval process.

the NCEP-ATP along with the IDF classification, and another study adopted the WHO and NCEP-ATP classifications. Of the nine (9) studies that presented prevalence based on NCEP-ATP classification only six (6) studies [24, 25, 28–31] explicitly stated that the 2001 definition had been used whereas the remaining three studies did not specify if the 2001 classification or its revised version had been adopted [23, 26, 27]. In view of this, we combined all studies that used NCEP-ATP irrespective of version. Per the quality appraisal criteria, 67% of studies included in the review were graded as of high quality and 33% were graded to be of medium quality.

3.2. Prevalence of MetS Based on NCEP-ATP. MetS prevalence based on NCEP-ATP classification was retrieved from 9 studies. The reported prevalence of MetS based on NCEP-ATP definition was within the range 3.75–25.6%. The pooled prevalence of MetS based on NCEP-ATP classification was estimated as 12.4% (95% CI = 8.3–17.4%, $I^2 = 0.86$) (Figure 2). MetS prevalence for males based on the NCEP-ATP classification was estimated as 8.1% (3.4–14.6%, $I^2 = 0.87$). Among females, the prevalence of MetS using the NCEP-ATP classification was 19.2% (95% CI = 12.7–26.8%, $I^2 = 0.82$). The difference (11.2%, 95% CI = 7.7–14.7%) in prevalence of MetS among male and females based on the NCEP-ATP classification was statistically significant ($p < 0.001$).

3.3. Prevalence of MetS Based on IDF Criteria. The prevalence of MetS based on IDF classification was retrieved from 5 studies. The reported prevalence of MetS based on IDF definition was within the range 13.0–35.9%. The pooled prevalence of MetS among apparently healthy Ghanaian adults based on IDF classification was estimated as 21.2% (95% CI = 12.4–30.9, $I^2 = 0.92$) (Figure 2). MetS prevalence for males based on the IDF classification was estimated as 12.3% (95% CI = 7.74–17.6%, $I^2 = 0.47$). Among females, the prevalence of MetS using the IDF guideline was 37.2% (95% CI = 20.2–56.1%, $I^2 = 0.91$). The gender difference (24.9%, 95% CI = 18.7–30.8%) in prevalence of MetS according to the IDF classification among male and females was statistically significant ($p < 0.001$).

3.4. Prevalence of MetS Based on WHO Criteria. MetS prevalence based on the WHO classification was retrieved from 5 studies. The reported prevalence of MetS based on WHO definition was within the range 0–16%. The pooled (Figure 2) prevalence of MetS based on WHO classification was estimated as 6.0% (95% CI = 1.4–13.1%, $I^2 = 0.92$). MetS prevalence for males based on the IDF classification was estimated

TABLE 1: Descriptive characteristics of studies.

S/N	Author, year	Study design	Sampling period	Population	Mean age (years)	Sample size (n)	Region	Setting	Quality grade
(1)	Adamu et al., 2014 [23]	Cross-sectional	2005	Christians (population-based)	41.36 ± 13.59	387 120 (m) 267 (f)	Ashanti	Urban	Medium
(2)	Akpalu et al., 2011 [24]	Case-control	n.s	Healthy controls (no CVD)	54.9 ± 11.0	100 54 (m) 46 (f)	Greater Accra	Urban	Medium
(3)	Amidu et al., 2012 [25]	Cross-sectional	2009	Garage workers (males)	30.2 ± 7.8	200	Ashanti	Urban	High
(4)	Arthur et al., 2013 [26]	Cross-sectional	2011	Pre- + postmenopausal women	44.23 ± 0.90	250	Ashanti	Urban	High
(5)	Gyakobo et al., 2012 [27]	Cross-sectional	2007	General population	44.4 ± 6.9	206 102 (m) 104 (f)	Eastern	Rural	High
(6)	Owiredu et al., 2011 [28]	Cross-sectional	2010	Active sports individuals + sedentary persons	43.56 ± 1.06	186	Ashanti	Urban	Medium
(7)	Owiredu et al., 2012 [29]	Case-control	2007–09	Healthy matched cohorts (no CKD)	46.3 ± 1.9	80	Ashanti and Northern	Urban	High
(8)	Owiredu et al., 2016 [30]	Cross-sectional	2009-10	Healthy control (normotensive)	49.32 ± 10.10	100 55 (m) 45 (f)	Ashanti	Urban	High
(9)	Turpin et al., 2008 [31]	Case-control	2006-07	Healthy female control (no PIH)	30.22 ± 0.57	50	Ashanti	Urban	High

S/N: study number; n.s: not specified; m: male; f: female; CVD: cardiovascular disease; CKD: chronic kidney disease; PIH: pregnancy induced hypertension; WHO: World Health Organization; IDF: International Diabetes Federation; NCEP-ATP: The National Cholesterol Education Program Adult Treatment Panel.

as 12.3% (95% CI = 7.7–17.6%). There were no statistically significant differences between MetS prevalence among males and females using the WHO criteria ($p = 0.7768$).

3.5. Assessment of Heterogeneity and Bias. There was no evidence of publication bias as depicted by egger regression tests which were not statistically significant, NCEP-ATP III ($p = 0.2193$), WHO ($p = 0.1512$), and IDF ($p = 0.4111$). The results of the metaregression also did not reveal any effect of mean participant age on the prevalence of MetS ($p = 0.798$). However, with each year increase in sampling period, the prevalence of MetS increased by 0.022% (coefficient: 0.022, $p = 0.04$).

4. Discussion

The current study aimed to systematically review the available evidence towards providing an estimate of the burden of MetS among apparently healthy adult Ghanaians. To our knowledge, this is the first systematic review that has attempted to provide an estimate of the national prevalence of MetS in Ghana.

The prevalence of MetS among Ghanaians was estimated to be in the range 6–21.2% based on three guidelines, NCEP-ATP, WHO, and IDF. The mean prevalence of MetS among adult Ghanaians is low when compared to estimates for other countries such as Iran (37.7%) [32], US (33%) [36], Australia (22.0%) [37], and Brazil (29.6%) [38] and across multiple countries in central America (30.3%) [39]. Nonetheless, comparison of the MetS prevalence across countries should be made with some caution as the condition is known to increase with age and as such countries experiencing an ageing population are likely to have higher prevalence [5]. For countries with demographic profile similar to Ghana, Oguoma et al. [40] reported a higher mean prevalence (29.2%) of MetS among Nigerians. However, their analysis included persons with established diseases like type 2 diabetes which may have contributed to the higher prevalence.

Prevalence of MetS among Ghanaians was highest with the use of the IDF classification (21.2%), followed by the NCEP-ATP guideline (12.6%) and the lowest prevalence reported with the WHO definition (6.2%). In a similar systematic review conducted among South Asians, Aryal and Wasti [41] found highest prevalence of MetS using IDF definition compared to NCEP-ATP and WHO classifications. There are at times wide discrepancies in MetS prevalence based on the guideline adopted. For instance, in the study by Turpin et al. [31], none (0%) of the participants was deemed to have MetS when the WHO definition was used, although 10% were diagnosed to have MetS per the NCEP-ATP classification. Similarly, Gyakobo et al. found an over 2-fold increase in MetS prevalence when the IDF definition was applied as opposed to the NCEP-ATP classification [27]. Obviously, the existence of multiple classifications makes precise estimation of MetS prevalence a difficult task. As expected, many researchers have called for a standardized

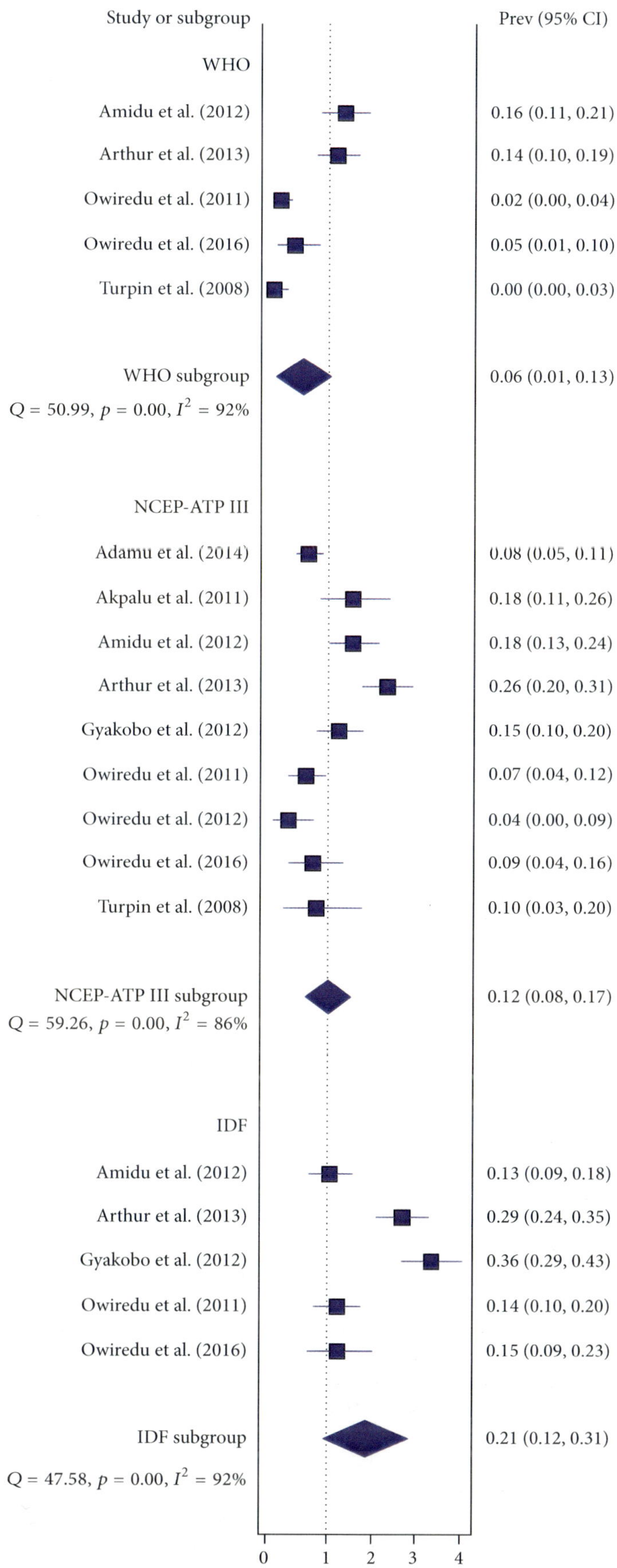

FIGURE 2: Pooled prevalence of MetS among apparently "healthy" Ghanaian adults based on different guideline classifications.

international definition accepted by all to allow for consistency in estimation of the burden of MetS and to minimise the confusion among clinical practitioners [5, 40, 42].

The 2001 NCEP-ATP definition was revised in 2004 by lowering the thresholds for central obesity and fasting glucose as well as including patients being treated for dyslipidemia, hyperglycemia, or systemic hypertension [10]. However, the majority of studies that used the NCEP-ATP guidelines resorted to the 2001 classification. Of note a systematic review and meta-analysis by Mottillo et al. [43] that compared estimates of CVD risk associated with the metabolic syndrome using both the NCEP and revised NCEP (rNCEP) definitions in the general population and among patients without type 2 diabetes mellitus concluded that little variation exists in risk between the NCEP and rNCEP definitions of the metabolic syndrome.

Among the available classifications, it appears that the NCEP-ATP guideline is the most frequently used among Ghanaian researchers, although how this translates into clinical practice is not known. The frequent use of the NCEP-ATP guideline may be as a result of its relative simplicity. Within other countries such as Australia with advanced health systems, Cameron et al. found that the WHO definition was not practical for clinical use as compared to other definitions and suggested that the IDF definition may be better suited for CVD prevention in their country [37]. Further research will however need to focus on assessing the efficiency of the different classifications within the Ghanaian health system context.

Only one study by Gyakobo et al. was conducted among Ghanaian rural dwellers and this reported a very high prevalence of MetS [35.9% (IDF) and 15.0% (NCEP-ATP)] [27]. Earlier studies in other West African countries found much lower prevalence of MetS in rural settings [44, 45]. Although high prevalence of MetS and its associated noncommunicable diseases (NCDs) are usually blamed on Western diets, Gyakobo et al. argue that the high prevalence recorded in their study could not be easily attributed to a presumed westernization of diet and lifestyle, as these data emerged from a rural, agrarian community with traditional reliance on home-cooked foods, and a high burden of physical labour [27]. Preventive measures must therefore target both urban and rural dwellers focusing on the appropriate risk factors within these settings which are likely to vary.

As in previous reviews [32, 39, 41, 46], we observed a higher prevalence of MetS among females compared with males. Gyakobo et al. reported almost four times higher prevalence of MetS in Ghanaian females than males [27]. The authors guessed that the difference was due to the significant and higher prevalence of overweight and obesity among females (55.0%) than males (29.0%) study participants [27]. Even among women, it has been previously reported that the prevalence of MetS varies and depends on the characteristics of the population as well as the diagnostic criteria applied. Arthur et al. reported a higher prevalence of MetS among Ghanaian postmenopausal women [(43.0% IDF)] than premenopausal women [(18.9% IDF)] [26]. This observation is similar to results reported by Pandey et al. that showed higher prevalence of MetS among postmenopausal Indian women [(55% IDF)] compared to their premenopausal [(45% IDF)] counterparts [47]. Just as in other gendered health conditions, preventive efforts will need to identify sociodemographic and environmental correlates particularly those influencing women.

Prominent among suggested interventions to address MetS is lifestyle modification. A systematic review and meta-analysis published in 2012 by Yamaoka and Tango concluded that such interventions were effective in resolving MetS and reducing the severity of related abnormalities (fasting blood glucose, waist circumference, SBP and DBP, and triglycerides) in subjects with MetS [48].

Given the established association between MetS and increased risk of developing CVD [49], the findings from the current review have both clinical and public health implications. While NCDs are currently equally prevalent in developed and developing countries, their impact is far more devastating in developing countries [50]. A 2002 WHO report identified CVDs as accounting for 9.2% of total deaths in the African region in 2001, and it is estimated that by the year 2020 the number of deaths in Africa due to NCDs in general will exceed that due to communicable diseases [51]. This looming epidemic is enough reason for the early institution of appropriate interventions to reduce the risk factors for CVD, including that related to MetS [24]. In Ghana, and in other countries in the subregion, the prevalence of hypertension [16], diabetes mellitus [52], hyperlipidemia, and obesity [17, 53], which are individual components of MetS, is on the increase. To curtail the rising trend, primary prevention strategies that focus on reducing absolute CVD risk through a comprehensive risk assessment and management approach should be adopted rather than focusing on addressing isolated individual risk factors [54].

Our systematic review makes a unique contribution to knowledge regarding the burden of MetS in apparently healthy individuals. Previous studies and reviews have dwelled predominantly on persons with NCDs and other ailments. To our knowledge, this is the first systematic review and meta-analysis of studies on the subject of MetS in Ghana. The strengths of our study include the absence of publication bias and the fact that all included studies were conducted over the last decade. The MetS prevalence presented should serve as a useful starting point for understanding the burden of MetS in Ghana and for informing future research directions, design of preventive measures, and resource allocation and planning.

The following limitations of the study are worth noting. This analysis was confined to English-language articles, which could also introduce some bias as Moher et al. found language-restricted meta-analyses to overestimate treatment effect by only 2% on average compared with language-inclusive meta-analyses [21]. Considering that English is the official language of Ghana, we expect this to have a minimal effect. The studies included in this review involved participants sampled across 4 of the 10 regions of Ghana and hence the MetS prevalence estimate presented is likely to shift when more information from the other regions become available. We included only population-based studies conducted in apparently healthy adults aged $\geq$ 18 years;

studies carried out in persons with known health disorders were excluded. A total of nine studies were excluded because they reported MetS prevalence in a group of people with known diseases (HIV, diabetes, hypertension, etc.). Given the established relationship between MetS and other conditions as diabetes and hypertension, it is possible that ours was an underestimate of the burden of MetS in Ghana.

5. Conclusion

Among a population of adult Ghanaians deemed to be "healthy," there is a high prevalence of MetS. Nonetheless, the existence of multiple classifications makes precise estimation of MetS prevalence a difficult task. The efficiency of the various guidelines needs to be assessed within the Ghanaian context and efforts must be made towards defining a standard criteria for the local population. Preventive measures are required to address the risk components of MetS such as obesity and hypertension which are rapidly rising in Ghana.

Authors' Contributions

Richard Ofori-Asenso carried out the literature search, conducted the analysis, and drafted the manuscript. Akosua Adom Agyeman contributed to data extraction and manuscript revision. Amos Laar provided critical inputs into the manuscript revision. All authors read and approved the final manuscript.

References

[1] D. W. Lam and D. LeRoith, "Metabolic syndrome," in *Endotext*, L. J. De Groot, Ed., MDText.com, Inc., South Dartmouth, Mass, USA, 2000, Metabolic Syndrome.

[2] A. Misra and L. Khurana, "The metabolic syndrome in South Asians: epidemiology, determinants, and prevention," *Metabolic Syndrome and Related Disorders*, vol. 7, no. 6, pp. 497–514, 2009.

[3] A. S. Gami, B. J. Witt, D. E. Howard et al., "Metabolic syndrome and risk of incident cardiovascular events and death: a systematic review and meta-analysis of longitudinal studies," *Journal of the American College of Cardiology*, vol. 49, no. 4, pp. 403–414, 2007.

[4] International Diabetes Federation, *IDF Worldwide Definition of the Metabolic Syndrome*, IDF, 2015.

[5] S. O'Neill and L. O'Driscoll, "Metabolic syndrome: a closer look at the growing epidemic and its associated pathologiess," *Obesity Reviews: An Official Journal of the International Association for the Study of Obesity*, vol. 16, pp. 1–12, 2015.

[6] K. G. Alberti, R. H. Eckel, S. M. Grundy et al., "Harmonizing the metabolic syndrome: a joint interim statement of the international diabetes federation task force on epidemiology and prevention; National heart, lung, and blood institute; American heart association; World heart federation; International atherosclerosis society; and international association for the study of obesity," *Circulation*, vol. 120, no. 16, pp. 1640–1645, 2009.

[7] G. M. Reaven, "Role of insulin resistance in human disease," *Diabetes*, vol. 37, no. 12, pp. 1595–1607, 1988.

[8] K. G. M. M. Alberti and P. Z. Zimmet, "Definition, diagnosis and classification of diabetes mellitus and its complications. Part 1: diagnosis and classification of diabetes mellitus. Provisional report of a WHO consultation," *Diabetic Medicine*, vol. 15, no. 7, pp. 539–553, 1998.

[9] Expert Panel on Detection Evaluation and Treatment of High Blood Cholesterol in Adults, "Executive summary of the third report of the National Cholesterol Education Program (NCEP) expert panel on detection, evaluation, and treatment of high blood cholesterol in adults (adult treatment panel III)," *Journal of the American Medical Association*, vol. 285, no. 19, pp. 2486–2497, 2001.

[10] S. M. Grundy, H. B. Brewer, J. I. Cleeman, S. C. Smith, and C. Lenfant, "Definition of metabolic syndrome: report of the national heart, lung, and blood institute/American heart association conference on scientific issues related to definition," *Arteriosclerosis, Thrombosis, and Vascular Biology*, vol. 24, no. 2, pp. e13–e18, 2004.

[11] International Diabetes Federation, *The IDF Consensus Worldwide Definition of the Metabolic Syndrome*, IDF, Brussels, Belgium, 2006.

[12] D. B. Carr, K. M. Utzschneider, R. L. Hull et al., "Intra-abdominal fat is a major determinant of the National Cholesterol Education Program Adult Treatment Panel III criteria for the metabolic syndrome," *Diabetes*, vol. 53, no. 8, pp. 2087–2094, 2004.

[13] P. J. Anderson, J. A. J. H. Critchley, J. C. N. Chan et al., "Factor analysis of the metabolic syndrome: Obesity vs insulin resistance as the central abnormality," *International Journal of Obesity*, vol. 25, no. 12, pp. 1782–1788, 2001.

[14] J. Kaur, "A comprehensive review on metabolic syndrome," *Cardiology Research and Practice*, vol. 2014, Article ID 943162, 21 pages, 2014.

[15] C. I. Okafor, "The metabolic syndrome in Africa: current trends," *Indian Journal of Endocrinology and Metabolism*, vol. 16, no. 1, pp. 56–66, 2012.

[16] W. K. Bosu, "Epidemic of hypertension in Ghana: a systematic review," *BMC Public Health*, vol. 10, article 418, 2010.

[17] R. Ofori-Asenso, A. A. Agyeman, A. Laar, and D. Boateng, "Overweight and obesity epidemic in Ghana - a systematic review and meta-analysis," *BMC Public Health*, vol. 16, no. 1, article 1239, 2016.

[18] M. L. Doherty, E. Owusu-Dabo, O. S. A. Kantanka, R. O. Brawer, and J. D. Plumb, "Type 2 diabetes in a rapidly urbanizing region of Ghana, West Africa: a qualitative study of dietary preferences, knowledge and practices," *BMC Public Health*, vol. 14, article 1069, 2014.

[19] R. Ofori-Asenso and D. Garcia, "Cardiovascular diseases in Ghana within the context of globalization," *Cardiovascular Diagnosis and Therapy*, vol. 6, no. 1, pp. 67–77, 2016.

[20] S. Agyei-Mensah and A. de-Graft Aikins, "Epidemiological transition and the double burden of disease in Accra, Ghana," *Journal of Urban Health: Bulletin of the New York Academy of Medicine*, vol. 87, no. 5, pp. 879–897, 2010.

[21] D. Moher, D. G. Altman, A. Liberati, and J. Tetzlaff, "PRISMA statement," *Epidemiology*, vol. 22, article 128, p. 128, 2011.

[22] S. H. Downs and N. Black, "The feasibility of creating a checklist for the assessment of the methodological quality both of

randomised and non-randomised studies of health care interventions," *Journal of Epidemiology and Community Health*, vol. 52, no. 6, pp. 377–384, 1998.

[23] M. Adamu, W. Owiredu, and J. Plange-Rhule, "Metabolic syndrome in relation to body mass index and waist to hip ratio; a study in kumasi metropolis," *Obesity & Weight Loss Therapy*, vol. 4, 2014.

[24] J. Akpalu, A. Akpalu, and F. Ofei, "The metabolic syndrome among patients with cardiovascular disease in Accra, Ghana," *Ghana Medical Journal*, vol. 45, no. 4, pp. 161–166, 2011.

[25] N. Amidu, W. Owiredu, E. Mireku, and C. Agyemang, "Metabolic syndrome among garage workers in the automobile industry in Kumasi, Ghana," *Journal of Medical and Biomedical Sciences*, vol. 1, pp. 29–36, 2012.

[26] F. K. Arthur, M. Adu-Frimpong, J. Osei-Yeboah, F. O. Mensah, and L. Owusu, "he prevalence of metabolic syndrome and its predominant components among pre-and postmenopausal Ghanaian women," *BMC Research Notes*, vol. 6, article 446, 2013.

[27] M. Gyakobo, A. G. B. Amoah, D.-A. Martey-Marbell, and R. C. Snow, "Prevalence of the metabolic syndrome in a rural population in Ghana," *BMC Endocrine Disorders*, vol. 12, article 25, 2012.

[28] W. Owiredu, N. Amidu, E. Gockah-Adapoe, and R. Ephraim, "The prevalence of metabolic syndrome among active sportsmen/sportswomen and sedentary workers in the Kumasi metropolis," *Journal of Science and Technology*, vol. 31, pp. 23–36, 2011.

[29] W. Owiredu, R. Ephraim, B. Eghan Jnr, N. Amidu, and E. Laing, "Metabolic syndrome among Ghanaian patients presenting with chronic kidney disease," *Journal of Medical and Biomedical Sciences*, vol. 1, pp. 1–12, 2012.

[30] W. Owiredu, C. Nkrumah, G. Bedu-Addo, L. Quaye, and H. Alidu, "Co-existence of syndrome X and hypertension among Ghanaians," *Journal of Medical and Biomedical Sciences*, vol. 5, pp. 8–16, 2016.

[31] C. Turpin, L. Ahenkorah, W. Owiredu, E. Laing, and N. Amidu, "The prevalence of the metabolic syndrome among ghanaian pregnancy-induced hypertensive patients using the world health organisation and the national cholesterol education program III Criteria," *Journal of Medical Sciences*, vol. 8, no. 5, pp. 443–451, 2008.

[32] B. Amirkalali, H. Fakhrzadeh, F. Sharifi et al., "Prevalence of metabolic syndrome and its components in the Iranian adult population: A systematic review and meta-analysis," *Iranian Red Crescent Medical Journal*, vol. 17, no. 12, Article ID e24723, 2015.

[33] R. Li, W. Li, Z. Lun et al., "Prevalence of metabolic syndrome in mainland China: A meta-analysis of published studies," *BMC Public Health*, vol. 16, no. 1, article no. 296, 2016.

[34] J. P. Higgins, S. G. Thompson, J. J. Deeks, and D. G. Altman, "Measuring inconsistency in meta-analyses," *British Medical Journal*, vol. 327, no. 7414, pp. 557–560, 2003.

[35] M. Egger, G. D. Smith, M. Schneider, and C. Minder, "Bias in meta-analysis detected by a simple, graphical test," *British Medical Journal*, vol. 315, pp. 629–634, 1997.

[36] M. Aguilar, T. Bhuket, S. Torres, B. Liu, and R. J. Wong, "Prevalence of the metabolic syndrome in the United States, 2003-2012," *Jama*, vol. 313, pp. 1973-1974, 2015.

[37] A. J. Cameron, D. J. Magliano, P. Z. Zimmet, T. Welborn, and J. E. Shaw, "The metabolic syndrome in Australia: prevalence using four definitions," *Diabetes Research and Clinical Practice*, vol. 77, no. 3, pp. 471–478, 2007.

[38] F. de Carvalho Vidigal, J. Bressan, N. Babio, and J. Salas-Salvado, "Prevalence of metabolic syndrome in Brazilian adults: a systematic review," *BMC Public Health*, vol. 13, article 1198, 2013.

[39] R. A. Wong-McClure, E. W. Gregg, A. Barceló, K. Lee et al., "Prevalence of metabolic syndrome in Central America: a cross-sectional population-based study," *Pan American journal of public health*, vol. 38, pp. 202–208, 2015.

[40] V. M. Oguoma, E. U. Nwose, and R. S. Richards, "Prevalence of cardio-metabolic syndrome in Nigeria: a systematic review," *Public Health*, vol. 129, pp. 413–423, 2015.

[41] N. Aryal and S. P. Wasti, "The prevalence of metabolic syndrome in South Asia: A systematic review," *International Journal of Diabetes in Developing Countries*, vol. 36, no. 3, pp. 255–262, 2016.

[42] A. Patel, K.-C. Huang, E. D. Janus et al., "Is a single definition of the metabolic syndrome appropriate? - A comparative study of the USA and Asia," *Atherosclerosis*, vol. 184, no. 1, pp. 225–232, 2006.

[43] S. Mottillo, K. B. Filion, J. Genest et al., "The metabolic syndrome and cardiovascular risk: a systematic review and meta-analysis," *Journal of the American College of Cardiology*, vol. 56, no. 14, pp. 1113–1132, 2010.

[44] O. O. Oladapo, L. Salako, O. Sodiq, K. Shoyinka, K. Adedapo, and A. O. Falase, "A prevalence of cardiometabolic risk factors among a rural Yoruba south-western Nigerian population: a population-based survey," *Cardiovascular Journal of Africa*, vol. 21, no. 1, pp. 26–31, 2010.

[45] L. Fezeu, B. Balkau, A.-P. Kengne, E. Sobngwi, and J.-C. Mbanya, "Metabolic syndrome in a sub-Saharan African setting: Central obesity may be the key determinant," *Atherosclerosis*, vol. 193, no. 1, pp. 70–76, 2007.

[46] R. M. Mabry, M. M. Reeves, E. G. Eakin, and N. Owen, "Gender differences in prevalence of the metabolic syndrome in Gulf Cooperation Council Countries: a systematic review," *Diabetic Medicine : A Journal of the British Diabetic Association*, vol. 27, no. 5, pp. 593–597, 2010.

[47] S. Pandey, M. Srinivas, S. Agashe et al., "Menopause and metabolic syndrome: a study of 498 urban women from western India," *Journal of Mid-Life Health*, vol. 1, no. 2, pp. 63–69, 2010.

[48] K. Yamaoka and T. Tango, "Effects of lifestyle modification on metabolic syndrome: a systematic review and meta-analysis," *BMC Medicine*, vol. 10, article 138, 2012.

[49] B. Isomaa, P. Almgren, T. Tuomi et al., "Cardiovascular morbidity and mortality associated with the metabolic syndrome," *Diabetes Care*, vol. 24, no. 4, pp. 683–689, 2001.

[50] K. S. Reddy and S. Yusuf, "Emerging epidemic of cardiovascular disease in developing countries," *Circulation*, vol. 97, pp. 596–601, 1998.

[51] World Health Organization, *World Health Report ;2002; Reducing Risk, Promoting Healthy Life*, WHO, Geneva, Switzerland, 2002.

[52] "Diabetes in Ghana: a review of research on prevalence, experiences and healthcare," in *Chronic Non Communicable Diseases in Ghana: Multidisciplinary Perspectives*, A. D. Aikins, E. Owusu-Dabo, and C. Agyemang, Eds., Sub-Saharan Publishers, Accra, Ghana, 2013.

[53] A. R. Abubakari, W. Lauder, C. Agyemang, M. Jones, A. Kirk, and R. S. Bhopal, "Prevalence and time trends in obesity among adult West African populations: a meta-analysis," *Obesity Reviews*, vol. 9, no. 4, pp. 297–311, 2008.

18

The Microbial Hypothesis: Contributions of Adenovirus Infection and Metabolic Endotoxaemia to the Pathogenesis of Obesity

Amos Tambo, Mohsin H. K. Roshan, and Nikolai P. Pace

Centre for Molecular Medicine and Biobanking, University of Malta, Msida, Malta

Correspondence should be addressed to Amos Tambo; amos.tambo.13@um.edu.mt

Academic Editor: Jochen G. Schneider

The global obesity epidemic, dubbed "globesity" by the World Health Organisation, is a pressing public health issue. The aetiology of obesity is multifactorial incorporating both genetic and environmental factors. Recently, epidemiological studies have observed an association between microbes and obesity. Obesity-promoting microbiome and resultant gut barrier disintegration have been implicated as key factors facilitating metabolic endotoxaemia. This is an influx of bacterial endotoxins into the systemic circulation, believed to underpin obesity pathogenesis. Adipocyte dysfunction and subsequent adipokine secretion characterised by low grade inflammation, were conventionally attributed to persistent hyperlipidaemia. They were thought of as pivotal in perpetuating obesity. It is now debated whether infection and endotoxaemia are also implicated in initiating and perpetuating low grade inflammation. The fact that obesity has a prevalence of over 600 million and serves as a risk factor for chronic diseases including cardiovascular disease and type 2 diabetes mellitus is testament to the importance of exploring the role of microbes in obesity pathobiology. It is on this basis that Massachusetts General Hospital is sponsoring the Faecal Microbiota Transplant for Obesity and Metabolism clinical trial, to study the impact of microbiome composition on weight. The association of microbes with obesity, namely, adenovirus infection and metabolic endotoxaemia, is reviewed.

1. Introduction

Obesity is a chronic multifactorial pathology driven by the complex interaction between various factors. Extensive research has implicated a number of genetic, epigenetic, nutritional, and lifestyle factors. Furthermore, the composition of the gut microbiome has also been implicated in the development of obesity. Irrespective of the specific causes leading to obesity, it is a strong risk factor for the development of cardiometabolic diseases, including insulin resistance, type 2 diabetes, and hypertension. The clinical consequences of obesity extend further to include a spectrum of other diseases such as malignancies, osteoarthritis, and obstructive sleep apnoea [1, 2]. Moreover, obesity exerts a heavy toll in terms of social and economic consequences [3, 4]. The rising prevalence of both childhood and adult obesity is strongly linked to caloric excess and the sedentary urban lifestyle typical of "Westernised" countries [5]. There is, however, growing evidence for a robust physiological process that restricts the voluntary mechanisms to reduce body weight by drastic changes in lifestyle. In this respect, obesity is increasingly recognised as a disease rather than as a wilful choice [6, 7].

Viral infection has been implicated as a contributing factor in the aetiology of obesity in both animal and human studies [8]. In addition, the gastrointestinal tract is home to over 10^{14} bacteria that collectively form the intestinal microbiome, with a joint genetic repertoire that is larger than the human genome [9]. These symbiotic bacteria establish and maintain the gut immune system and contribute to the breakdown of complex nondigestible plant-derived polysaccharides [10, 11]. Recent evidence links the gut microbiome to the development of obesity and metabolic disease [12]. The aim of this review is to present the epidemiological evidence for the association between microbes and obesity, and discuss the cellular and molecular mechanisms underpinning the inflammatory response that is central to adipocyte dysfunction in obesity pathobiology.

2. Conventional Perspective of Adipocyte Dysfunction in Obesity Pathogenesis

2.1. Adipocyte Stress Response. Increased circulating levels of triglycerides and glucose perturb metabolic homeostasis and stimulate compensatory adipocyte hypertrophy and hyperplasia [13]. Persistently elevated triglyceride and glucose levels overwhelm the physiological response such that decompensation (so-called adipocyte stress response) arises, and thus adipocyte dysfunction ensues [14–16].

2.2. Chronic Low Grade Inflammation in Adipocyte Dysfunction. Adipocyte dysfunction is epitomised by a low grade chronic inflammatory response, which is an integral feature of obesity [20, 21]. It has been hypothesised that increased caloric intake triggers inflammation leading to adipocyte dysfunction [16]. Adipose tissue is infiltrated with bone marrow-derived macrophages, and the density of these adipose tissue macrophages (ATMs) is dependent on the degree of obesity. The number of ATMs correlates with the degree of insulin resistance [22]. Adipose tissue macrophages exhibit different phenotypes depending on the degree of adiposity. ATMs in lean nonobese individuals are anti-inflammatory (M2 macrophages) as opposed to ATMs in obese individuals that express proinflammatory genes (M1 "classically-activated" macrophages) [23].

In nonobese, insulin sensitive conditions, adipocytes secrete factors that trigger alternative activation of macrophages. The obesity-induced changes in adipocyte gene expression trigger release of proinflammatory cytokines (TNF-α, MCP1) that lead to recruitment and activation of macrophages. The activated M1 macrophages produce and secrete other proinflammatory mediators, including IL-6, TNF-α, IL-1β, and resistin. These mediators establish a positive feedback loop that further enhances insulin resistance and inflammation [23]. Cytokines such as TNFα, IL-6, and IL-1β exert paracrine effects to activate inflammatory pathways. This leads to activation of Jun N-terminal kinase (JNK), inhibitor of κ B kinase β (IKK), and other serine kinases, which activate transcription factor targets (c-Fos/c-Jun) and nuclear factor-kB (NF-kB) that stimulate transcription of inflammatory pathway genes [24, 25].

IL-6 secreted by adipose tissue macrophages is considered a major inflammatory mediator. Primarily, IL-6 triggers subclinical inflammation by instituting a vicious cycle that includes the downregulation of lipoprotein transport to peripheral tissues. This in turn increases plasma lipid levels and promotes triglyceride release into the circulation. The result is development of overt hypertriglyceridemia and hyperlipidaemia, which serves to perpetuate the obesity phenotype by presenting a constitutive signal for adipocyte hypertrophy and hyperplasia. Adipocyte dysfunction thus ensues. It has also been shown that IL-6 expression is more pronounced in metabolically active visceral rather than peripheral adipocytes [26].

2.3. Adipokine Secretion. The adipocyte plays a key endocrine role in the secretion of adipokines. This topic has been extensively reviewed by Ouchi et al. [27]. Adipokine secretion is dysregulated in obesity with increased levels of obesity-promoting adipokines. The expression of proinflammatory proteins, particularly TNF-α, may lead to a reduction in anti-inflammatory adipokines, such as adiponectin which plays a pivotal anti-inflammatory role [28]. Despite the extensive research on adipose tissue inflammation, the direct causal link between the events that trigger chronic inflammation and the final metabolic outcome is still not clearly determined. This review will focus on presenting the evidence linking microbes to adipose tissue dysfunction in the setting of obesity.

3. Viral Infection and Obesity

3.1. Animal Viruses and Obesity. The first association between viruses and obesity in animals was reported by Lyons et al. Mice infected with canine distemper virus (CDV) demonstrated adipocyte hypertrophy and hyperplasia in the absence of CNS pathology [29]. CDV does not infect humans but is antigenically related to the *Paramyxoviridae* family that includes the measles virus. Subsequently other investigators had demonstrated that the virus targets specific hypothalamic regions and is associated with alteration of various neuropeptide-signalling pathways, including leptin, neuropeptide Y, and melanin-concentrating hormone [30–33]. Rous-associated virus 7 (RAV-7) has also been associated with a syndrome of obesity, stunted growth, hypercholesterolaemia, fatty liver, and thyroid dysfunction in chickens [34]. Borna disease virus (BDV) has similarly been implicated in rat obesity. This RNA virus causes a lymphomonocytic inflammation of the hypothalamus, pancreatic islet cell hyperplasia, and elevations of serum glucose and triglyceride levels [35, 36]. BDV is neurotropic and has a wide range of animal hosts. Seroepidemiological studies have implicated BDV in neuropsychiatric diseases including schizophrenia and depression in some populations, though the associations have not been consistent [37–39].

Another animal model of virus-induced obesity implicated the SMAM-1 avian adenovirus in chickens. SMAM-1 was shown to lead to increased adiposity independent of food intake [40]. Subsequently, Dhurandhar et al. demonstrated that body weight and BMI were higher in human subjects positive for anti-SMAM-1 antibodies compared to those negative for anti-SMAM-1 antibodies [41]. This was the first reported association of viral infection with human obesity. The transmissible spongiform encephalopathy scrapie that infects cattle has also been linked to obesity. Kim et al. showed that inoculation of mice with the ME7 strain of scrapie results in obesity that is dependent on the hypothalamic-pituitary-adrenal axis [42].

The few associations between viral infection and animal obesity described above are clearly limited in translational terms, yet are still crucial in demonstrating a strong association between viral infection and obesity. Human adenovirus 36 (Ad-36) is a common human pathogen that has been linked to human obesity and adipocyte function through different mechanisms and is discussed next.

3.2. Adenovirus 36 and Obesity—In Vivo Studies. The adenoviruses are an important group of widely prevalent human pathogens that have been extensively studied. They are non-enveloped icosahedral DNA viruses with a linear double stranded genome that can infect a wide range of species and tissues. Fifty-two human adenovirus serotypes have been described. Their structural biology, genome, evolution, and host cell immune response has been reviewed elsewhere [43–45]. Clinically, they are responsible for a wide array of self-limiting infections, primarily of the respiratory and gastrointestinal tracts. Furthermore, they are effective vectors for gene-based immunotherapy and gene replacement strategies [46]. Ad-36 has been associated with obesity in both animal and human studies.

Ad-36 was first isolated from the faeces of a girl with enteritis [47]. Genomic characterisation of the virus revealed several unique features compared to other human adenoviruses that could possibly account for its unique tissue tropism [48]. The first reported link between Ad-36 and obesity was described in the year 2000 in animal models, where chicken and mice inoculated with Ad-36 demonstrated increased adipose tissue and decreased cholesterol and triglyceride levels in the absence of CNS histopathological changes [49]. Ad-36 DNA was detected in adipose tissue but not in skeletal muscle of the inoculated animals. Subsequently, other studies reproduced the adiposity-promoting effects of Ad-36 in two non-human primate models [50]. It was also shown that horizontal transmission of Ad-36 from infected to control animals produces adiposity and is accompanied by a paradoxical reduction in serum lipids [51]. Rats infected with Ad-36 demonstrate an increase in weight and insulin sensitivity, visceral adipose tissue expression of glycerol 3-phosphate dehydrogenase, and peroxisome proliferator-activated receptor gamma (PPAR-γ). CCAAT/enhancer-binding protein (C/EBP) alpha and beta were greater in infected animals compared to controls [52]. Kapila et al. reported that in a hamster model Ad-36 infection altered lipoprotein metabolism to produce a more atherogenic profile, with diminished HDL-C and increased LDL-C [53]. Viral DNA as a result of acute Ad-36 infection is detected in multiple tissues early following inoculation [54].

3.3. Adenovirus and Adipocyte Biology. Vangipuram et al. provided the first insight into the molecular mechanisms underpinning Ad-36-induced adipogenesis. The authors demonstrated that viral infection in 3T3-L1 murine preadipocytes induces differentiation and an increase in total cell lipid content [55]. These features are not shared with human adenovirus 2. Subsequently, Rathod et al. showed that transient Ad-36 mRNA expression, but not viral DNA replication, is required for preadipocyte differentiation [56]. The increased expression of PPAR-γ and C/EBP reported in animal studies is related to the proadipogenic effects observed *in vitro*, as these genes are key transcription factors that regulate adipocyte differentiation [52, 57]. A detailed analysis of the cellular pathways involved in Ad-36-induced adipogenesis showed that the viral E4 orf-1 gene stimulates proadipogenic differentiation in both 3T3-L1 and human adipose stem cells [58]. Furthermore, Ad-36 E4 orf-1 modulates insulin sensitivity via activation of the phosphatidylinositol 3-kinase (PI3 K) pathway. This accounts for the observed reduction in fasting insulin levels [52]. Studies also showed that Ad-36 suppresses the expression of leptin mRNA and improves glucose uptake in adipocytes [59]. The role of Ad-36 in human adipose tissue was further reinforced by studies that demonstrated that the virus induces commitment, differentiation, and lipid accumulation in human adipose-derived stem cells [60]. Adipocyte differentiation and lipid accumulation were observed in the absence of inducers of adipogenesis and in osteogenic culture media. They were accompanied by expression of the adipocyte-specific transcription factors PPAR-γ and C/EBPβ. Wang et al. also demonstrated that Ad-36 significantly reduced fatty acid oxidation and increased de novo lipogenesis in cultured human muscle cells [61]. Bouwman et al. further demonstrated *in vitro* that incubating preadipocytes and adipocytes with adenovirus (subtypes 2 and 36), amongst other viruses, was responsible for increased production of IL-6 which might contribute to chronic low grade inflammation [62].

4. Adenovirus and Obesity—Epidemiological Links

A number of investigators have studied the epidemiologic association between Ad-36 infection and human obesity. These investigations were carried out in different age groups and population ethnicities and utilised various methodologies for viral detection. The salient findings of these human seroepidemiologic studies have been recently described by Ponterio and Gnessi [63]. The unique genomic and proteomic structure of Ad-36 limits antibody cross reactivity in serum neutralization assays and further strengthens the reported associations between Ad-36 and human obesity. The majority, though not all studies, showed greater seropositivity for Ad-36 in obesity, with extensive variation in seroprevalence rates between countries. Three meta-analyses also showed an association between Ad-36 infection and obesity in both adults and children and are summarized in Table 1.

5. Gut Microbiome, Gut Barrier Integrity, and Their Role in Obesity Pathogenesis

The role of bacteria and their associated products in the pathogenesis of obesity has recently attracted considerable interest. Moreover, it has been proposed that the composition of the gut microbiome may contribute to obesity through their effects on the gut barrier and beyond.

5.1. Gut Microbiome. The relatively recent technological advances in genomics have revolutionized the study of the intestinal microbiome. It is now possible to sequence mixed microbial genetic material directly extracted from environmental samples without prior laboratory culture of individual

TABLE 1: Meta-analyses on the relationship between human adv-36 infection and obesity development in humans.

Study	Number of cases	Population size	Study end points	Major findings
Xu et al. [17]	(i) 9 cross-sectional studies, 9 case-control studies, and 6 cohort studies	(i) 10191 study subjects including adults and children	(i) HAdV-36 infection rate in obese and lean groups (ii) BMI level and BMI z-score in HAdV-36 positive and negative groups	(i) HAdV-36 infection increased the risk of obesity (ii) HAdV-36 also increased the risk of weight gain in adults, which was not observed in children
Shang et al. [18]	(i) 11 case control studies	(i) 5739 study subjects including adults and children	(i) HAdV-36 infection and obesity risk	(i) HAdV-36 infection is associated with an increased risk of obesity development (ii) Risk is increased in children and those with a BMI of ≥30 kg/cm^2
Yamada et al. [19]	(i) 10 cross-sectional studies	(i) 2870 study subjects including adults and children	(i) Evaluating the association between HAdV-36 infection and obesity/metabolic markers	(i) HAdV-36 infection is associated with the risk of obesity and weight gain, but not with abnormal metabolic markers including waist circumference

species. This emerging field, known as metagenomics, enables a survey of the different microorganisms present in a specific environment [64]. Several large-scale projects such as the Human Microbiome Project have characterised microbial genomes from hundreds of isolated human symbionts and have shed light on the complex interplay between the human host and its microbial populace. The implications of compositional changes in health and disease have also been elucidated (http://hmpdacc.org/). Butyrate along with propionate and acetate are short-chain fatty acids (SCFAs) derived from the bacterial degradation of complex polysaccharides in the gut [65]. They have important metabolic roles with butyrate acting as a metabolic substrate for colonic epithelial cells. The functions mediated by butyrate that are pertinent to the pathogenesis of obesity include its role in the maintenance of intestinal epithelial integrity, thereby preventing the translocation of endotoxins produced by intestinal Gram-negative bacteria across the gut barrier [66].

5.2. The Gut Barrier. Maintaining the integrity of the gut barrier is critical in preventing contact between materials originating from the nonsterile external environment (gut lumen) with the sterile systemic circulation [67]. Immunoprotection is conferred by means of the gut-associated lymphoid tissue (GALT) that is present on the mucosal surface and contains antigen presenting cells capable of processing and presenting exogenous antigens. The purpose of antigen presentation is primarily to activate adaptive immunity [68]. The gut barrier is composed primarily of enterocytes which adhere to one another by means of tight junctions, desmosomes, and adherens junctions [69]. This is important in order for discriminative transport of material to occur effectively between the gut lumen and the systemic circulation. Moreover, the gut barrier's role as a physical barrier to infection is key in preventing dissemination of bacteria and their associated products from the lumen into the systemic circulation [69]. The integral membrane proteins claudins and occludin, along with cytoskeletal adaptor proteins ZO-1, ZO-2, and ZO-3, have been demonstrated to facilitate paracellular transport between enterocytes [70]. Disruption of the gut barrier at any of these points results in indiscriminate dysregulated paracellular transport [67, 71]. Furthermore, it has been suggested that the integrity of the tight junction barrier is under strict regulation of proinflammatory and anti-inflammatory signalling. Proinflammatory cytokines implicated in promoting tight junction leakage include TNF-α and IFN-γ. Contrarily, anti-inflammatory cytokines including TGF-β and IL-10 have been suggested to maintain the integrity of tight junctions by downregulating proinflammatory signalling [72–76].

5.3. Dysbiosis. Failure to maintain a robust gut barrier, termed gut barrier dysfunction, may lead to an altered microbiome composition, resulting in microbiome imbalance. This is known as dysbiosis [67, 77]. The underlying causes of dysbiosis are diverse, and a high fat diet poor in prebiotic-containing nutrients has also been highlighted as a leading cause [78]. A high fat diet has been shown to increase the ratio of obesity-promoting bacteria in the microbiome [79].

In vivo studies have been conducted to demonstrate the importance of gut microbiome composition. Widely used models include the obesity mouse model *ob/ob* (leptin deficient) and the *db/db* (leptin receptor mutant) mouse. In a study conducted by Turnbaugh et al. it was shown that transfecting sterile laboratory mice with microbiota from *ob/ob* resulted in the expression of the obesity phenotype akin to *ob/ob* mice [80]. Moreover, sequencing studies performed by Ley et al. compared the microbiome of *ob/ob* mice and lean wild type mice. This revealed changes in two dominant bacterial divisions: Bacteriodetes and Firmicutes. Firmicutes levels were found to be increased in comparison to Bacteriodetes in *ob/ob* mice [81].

The situation is parallel in humans. Ley et al. extended their study to human subjects who adopted either a low-carbohydrate or a low-fat diet for weight control purposes, during a one-year period. Follow-up during this period demonstrated that a change in Bacteriodetes and Firmicutes levels had occurred in study subjects compared to controls. The change was such that from an initial elevated baseline

Firmicutes : Bacteriodetes ratio, the ratio had normalised in those subjects who lost weight and maintained a lean body weight after a year, matching that of controls [82]. Furthermore, faecal microbiome studies in lean and obese monozygotic and dizygotic twins established that the microbiome is shared between relatives, though bacterial lineages were individual-specific. A single dominant bacterial species was not identified and it was concluded that the core microbiome is shared in terms of genetic similarity rather than at a dominant organismal level [83]. Certain studies in humans have revealed beneficial commensal bacteria that strive to maintain the integrity of enterocytes and thus the gut barrier. These include *Akkermansia muciniphila* found in the mucosal mucus coating as well as *Faecalibacterium prausnitzii* [84, 85]. In dysbiosis such beneficial organisms are lost, and this is coupled with endotoxin secretion by other harmful bacteria that promote gut barrier breakdown, precipitating metabolic endotoxaemia.

5.4. Metabolic Endotoxaemia. Central to the paradigm of bacteria as contributors to the pathogenesis of obesity is the concept of "metabolic endotoxaemia." Put simply, this is increased plasma bacterial lipopolysaccharide (LPS) levels which are believed to originate from Gram-negative gut microbiome that spill into the systemic circulation as a direct result of gut barrier dysfunction [67, 77, 78]. A number of systems have been implicated in mediating the "gut-to-adipocyte axis" signalling, a term that we have coined to describe the communication between the gut microbiome and their associated endotoxins with adipocytes. Some systems have been proposed to function as gatekeepers and others as mediators of toxin spillage in the setting of gut barrier dysfunction. These systems include the endocannabinoid system, the apelinergic system, and the enteroendocrine system [78, 86].

5.4.1. Endocannabinoid System. The endocannabinoid system is a key mediator of molecular signalling between LPS (chiefly originating from Gram-negative organisms) and adipocytes [78, 87]. The two most studied bioactive lipids are N-arachidonoylethanolamine (AEA) and 2-arachidonoylglycerol (2-AG) which activate the G protein-coupled receptors CB1 and CB2 [88]. Though the expression of CB1 and CB2 was traditionally believed to be limited to the central nervous system, recent evidence suggests that gastrointestinal expression also occurs [89]. *In vivo* and *ex vivo* studies have implicated the CB1 receptor in gut-to-adipocyte signalling. The exact molecular signalling pathway that mediates metabolic endotoxaemia has not yet been elucidated [88, 90]. However, CB1 receptor activation has been shown to modulate ion channels and activate different mitogen-activated protein kinase (MAPK) pathways (p42/p44 MAPK, p38 MAPK, and c-Jun N-terminal kinase). It has also been implicated in the inhibition of adenylyl cyclase in tissues and cells. The aforementioned actions have been attributed to $G_{i/o}$ proteins. In the case of MAPK pathways, aside from $G_{i/o}$ proteins, PI3 K also mediates CB1 receptor activation [91]. Furthermore, CB1 receptor stimulation results in activation of inwardly rectifying K^+ channels [92]. Similarly, L-type voltage-gated calcium channel activity was also shown to be targeted by CB1 receptor activation in cat cerebral arterial muscle and neonatal rat nucleus tractus solitarius. The effects here were primarily inhibitory [93, 94].

Among the wide array of physiological effects mediated by the endocannabinoid system, the one most pertinent to obesity is mainly increased energy intake and storage [95, 96]. Interestingly, the administration of the CB1 antagonist SR141716 in humans is accompanied by decreased body weight and anorexigenic effects [78]. Furthermore, to investigate the manner in which CB1 receptor agonist treatment or LPS treatment gives rise to the metabolic features of diet-induced obesity, mice were chronically treated with low-dose LPS before and during a high fat challenge. The plasma LPS levels were significantly increased (metabolic endotoxaemia) as well as mRNA levels of the macrophage markers *F4/80* and *CD11c* in adipose tissue. The increased macrophage mRNA markers suggested macrophage infiltration in adipose tissue [90]. This study clearly demonstrates a cause and effect relationship between LPS inoculation and mediators of inflammation.

It is therefore believed that one of the manners by which endotoxaemia promotes obesity is through the upregulation of the endocannabinoid system, thereby indirectly promoting adipogenesis [97]. Endotoxaemia has also been implicated in setting up chronic low grade inflammation in obesity, which is in keeping with experimental evidence in animal models [78].

5.4.2. Apelinergic System. Apelin is a peptide involved in the regulation of the central nervous, gastrointestinal, cardiovascular, and immune systems. It is also an adipokine secreted by mature adipocytes in mice and humans and mediates its effects via the APJ receptor [98]. It has been suggested as a negative regulator of obesity, though its precise mechanisms in this capacity are yet to be unravelled [87]. A myriad of signalling cascades are triggered upon activation of APJ receptor, the endpoint of which is the activation or repression of a number of transcription factors. Coupling of the APJ receptor to $G_{q/11}$ stimulates PLC-β signalling and subsequent hydrolysis of phosphatidylinositol 4,5-bisphosphate (PIP_2) to IP_3 and diacylglycerol (DAG). DAG activates PKC which then activates the Ras protein. The Ras cascade can proceed by activating either the MAPK or JNK pathways. An alternative signalling pathway also exists, where the APJ receptor is coupled to $G_{i/o}$. This pathway activates the MAPK cascade via PKC and it can also activate PI3K, which in turn activates Akt and mammalian target of rapamycin (mTOR). mTOR activates both p70S6K and endothelial nitric oxide synthase (eNOS). In addition, adenylate cyclase is inhibited by $G_{i/o}$, whereas G_s increases cyclic AMP synthesis from ATP and activates the PKA pathway [99].

A hyperactive endocannabinoid system in the pathogenic setting of obesity, along with low grade chronic inflammation, has been suggested as the culprits for the augmentation in apelin levels observed in obese animal models and humans [87]. The mechanisms of communication between the endocannabinoid and apelinergic systems are poorly understood. It has been previously shown that inflammation regulates both apelin and APJ mRNA expression [87]. Intraperitoneal administration of apelin in obese and normal mice over a 14-day period induced weight loss independent of food intake [100]. In addition, it was demonstrated in *db/db* mice that apelin and APJ mRNA levels showed twofold and threefold respective increase [87]. Possibly, a hyperactive endocannabinoid system and low grade inflammation may directly or indirectly trigger activation of the apelinergic system as a homeostatic mechanism to counteract obesity.

5.4.3. Enteroendocrine System. The L-cells of the enteroendocrine system are neuroendocrine cells expressed from the duodenum to the rectum and produce glucagon-like peptides 1 and 2 (GLP-1 and GLP-2) [101, 102]. GLP-1 is an incretin hormone known for its role in glucose homeostasis and energy balance. It also inhibits glucagon secretion, reduces food intake, and delays gastric emptying. Its role extends beyond glucose homeostasis [102]. GLP-1 may be implicated in antagonising the effects of metabolic endotoxaemia by regulating epithelial cell proliferation, thus sustaining the gut barrier [103]. In order to determine the mechanisms through which intestinal proliferation is promoted by GLP-1, C57BL/6 WT mice were treated with the GLP-1 receptor agonist exenatide (EX-4: exendin-4) for a period of one week. Increased weight, length, and weight per unit length of small bowel and large were noted. These effects were also observed with chronic (1 month) treatment of C57BL/6 WT mice. However, this effect was not evident in *Glp1r*$^{-/-}$ mice who were subjected to the same treatment over the same period of time. Upregulated gene expression profiles included *IGF1*, *IGF1R*, and *areg*. A conditional deletion of the *IGF1R* gene from intestinal epithelial cells and subsequent Liraglutide and Exenatide administration increased both small bowel and colon weight and length. Activation of GLP-1 receptor signalling in *Fgf7*$^{-/-}$ mice failed to increase small bowel and colon mass in the absence of Fgf7. It was therefore deduced that GLP-1 receptor agonists activate components of IGF-1 and ErbB signalling pathways and that the proliferative actions of GLP-1 receptor agonists are selectively mediated through mechanisms requiring Fgf7 [102].

Similarly, GLP-2 has been shown to induce proliferation *in vitro* in Caco-2 cells. The cells were subcultured in the presence or absence of GLP-2 as well as different kinase antagonist concentrations. These included Genistein (global tyrosine kinase inhibitor), LY294002 (PI3K) inhibitor, and PD 098059 (mitogen-activated/extracellular signal-regulated kinase (MEK) inhibitor). Cells which were administered GLP-2 exhibited more than 10-fold increase in proliferation, a response which was blunted by Genistein, LY294002, and PD 098059 in a dose-dependent fashion. Such a response was attributed at least in part to both the PI 3-kinase and the MAPK pathways [104].

Further studies in humans are warranted in order to elucidate the underlying mechanisms pertinent in gut proliferation mediated by both GLP-1 and GLP-2. However, the experimental models provide clear evidence of the involvement of the enteroendocrine system in intestinal proliferation.

6. The "Microbial Hypothesis" in Inflammation of Adipocyte Dysfunction

6.1. Limitations of the Classical Hypothesis of Adipocyte Dysfunction. In light of the previously discussed viral infection and bacterial endotoxaemia, the conventional perspective of adipocyte dysfunction in the pathogenesis of obesity clearly exhibits a number of limitations in substantially explaining adipocyte inflammation as a feature of obesity pathogenesis. Firstly, the trigger for inflammatory cell recruitment and secretion of inflammatory cytokines in adipose tissue is poorly accounted for, with no experimental evidence in existence to the best of our knowledge [105–107]. Secondly, inflammation in obesity is described as being "sterile" in nature [105]. No consideration has therefore been given to the contributory role of microbes or microbial endotoxins such as bacterial LPS in initiating and perpetuating chronic low grade inflammation.

6.2. Postulated Inflammatory Triggers of Adipocyte Dysfunction. The physiological goal of inflammation is primarily to eliminate an insult which the body deems alien and noxious. This is often employed via the innate and subsequently the adaptive immune responses should the insult persist. The acute inflammatory response is therefore converted to chronic inflammation in the setting of a persistent insult [107]. It is therefore not unreasonable to propose that viral infection and metabolic endotoxaemia may serve as triggers of inflammation that underpin adipocyte dysfunction. Mechanistically, we have subdivided possible triggers of inflammation into "transient" and "persistent" factors on the basis of chronicity.

6.2.1. Transient Inflammatory Triggers. In the case of viral infection, it is plausible to suggest that acute repetitive infections may serve as a transient factor that regularly initiates acute inflammation. This is later converted to chronic inflammation by background persistent factors. The infective situation may be described as a repetitive acute-on-chronic scenario. Repetitive infections may be explained by the fact that obesity is associated with an increased susceptibility to infection due to impaired systemic immune function [108].

6.2.2. Persistent Inflammatory Triggers. The chronic nature of dysbiosis and subsequent metabolic endotoxaemia is in keeping with the chronicity of inflammation observed in obesity and may qualify as persistent factors. This may therefore suggest a critical role for dysbiosis and endotoxaemia in initiating and perpetuating chronic inflammation via the persistent presence of bacterial LPS in the systemic circulation. The repetitive acute-on-chronic viral infections along with chronic dysbiosis and metabolic endotoxaemia may therefore possibly act in a concerted manner to promote chronic inflammation.

6.3. Determinants of Low Grade Inflammatory Tone. The characteristically low grade "subclinical" tone of inflammation in obesity can also be accounted for. The resident gut microflora is an essential component of gastrointestinal physiology and its myriad role is beyond the scope of this review. A degree of immunological tolerance is exerted so as not to instigate an immune response against them, in order to preserve their critical function [109, 110]. It has been suggested that the gut microbiome regulates not only local intestinal immunity but also systemic immunity [111]. It is therefore logical to suggest that the impaired systemic immune function that occurs in obesity may at least in part be attributed to dysbiosis and metabolic endotoxaemia, therefore resulting in subclinical inflammation.

6.4. The Adipocyte as an Immune Cell. It has been demonstrated that immature haematopoietic stem cells are present in adipocytes, and mature adipocytes express membrane-bound NADPH oxidase similar to that of phagocytic neutrophils [112]. It has also been suggested that the fact that adipocytes and their progenitors share a common embryonic origin with cells of the immune system rationalises the adipogenic response to endotoxaemia (i.e., adipocyte expansion) [108]. It is therefore plausible to propose that adipocyte hypertrophy and hyperplasia (i.e., the obesity response) are akin to an immune response mounted against an exogenous antigen, in terms of immune cell replication and phagocytosis. Therefore, perhaps the effects of the often recommended healthy diet and exercise extend far beyond lipolysis and weight loss. The beneficial effects of such measures may in addition restore a healthy microbiome and thus eliminate dysbiosis and endotoxaemia as triggers of obesity. Exercise-induced hyperaemia and angiogenesis may serve to increase circulatory transport of repair factors to regions of gut barrier damage, promoting repair and resolution.

The "microbial hypothesis" attempts to address the limitations of the classical hypothesis in explaining the trigger of inflammation in adipocyte dysfunction, and the possible role that microbes and microbial endotoxins may play in the process. Rather than refute the classical hypothesis altogether, this hypothesis acts to supplement the classical hypothesis. It does so in terms of filling in the missing link in the chain of events, taking into account the aforementioned recent experimental data that have undoubtedly suggested a critical role for microbes and microbial products in obesity pathobiology.

7. Conclusion

Taken together, there is undoubtedly an association between viral infection and metabolic endotoxaemia in the pathogenesis of obesity. However, proof of association, no matter how appealing or robust, does not necessarily imply causation. Since the obesity epidemic is recognised as being multifactorial in origin, a multifaceted approach to management is therefore warranted. Infection treatment and prevention do not formally feature in clinical practice guidelines given the fact that basic science research in "infectobesity" is still at its infancy, yet very promising. However, one should make no mistake to undermine the overwhelming evidence in both animal models and humans that suggest an important role for infection and endotoxaemia in the development of obesity. In fact, this is gaining prominence so much so that Massachusetts General Hospital is sponsoring the Faecal Microbiota Transplant for Obesity and Metabolism clinical trial, the first clinical trial to study the impact of gut bacteria on weight (https://clinicaltrials.gov/ct2/show/NCT02530385). The trial is currently at recruitment stage and due to commence soon. The results of this trial are awaited anxiously by the scientific community, as it could possibly cause a paradigm shift in our understanding of obesity and alter the management course of this epidemic.

Competing Interests

The authors declare that there is no conflict of interests regarding the publication of this paper.

References

[1] G. A. Bray, "Medical consequences of obesity," *The Journal of Clinical Endocrinology & Metabolism*, vol. 89, no. 6, pp. 2583–2589, 2004.

[2] G. De Pergola and F. Silvestris, "Obesity as a major risk factor for cancer," *Journal of Obesity*, vol. 2013, Article ID 291546, 11 pages, 2013.

[3] A. M. Rissanen, "The economic and psychosocial consequences of obesity," *Ciba Foundation Symposium*, vol. 201, pp. 194–206, 1996.

[4] C. M. Apovian, "The clinical and economic consequences of obesity," *The American Journal of Managed Care*, vol. 19, no. 11, supplement, pp. S219–S228, 2013.

[5] A. Berghöfer, T. Pischon, T. Reinhold, C. M. Apovian, A. M. Sharma, and S. N. Willich, "Obesity prevalence from a European perspective: a systematic review," *BMC Public Health*, vol. 8, article 200, 2008.

[6] M. J. Müller, A. Bosy-Westphal, and S. B. Heymsfield, "Is there evidence for a set point that regulates human body weight?" *F1000 Medicine Reports*, vol. 2, no. 1, article 59, 2010.

[7] J. M. Friedman, "Modern science versus the stigma of obesity," *Nature Medicine*, vol. 10, no. 6, pp. 563–569, 2004.

[8] N. V. Dhurandhar, "Infectobesity: obesity of infectious origin," *Journal of Nutrition*, vol. 131, no. 10, pp. 2794S–2797S, 2001.

[9] B. Zhu, X. Wang, and L. Li, "Human gut microbiome: the second genome of human body," *Protein and Cell*, vol. 1, no. 8, pp. 718–725, 2010.

[10] Y. K. Lee and S. K. Mazmanian, "Has the microbiota played a critical role in the evolution of the adaptive immune system?" *Science*, vol. 330, no. 6012, pp. 1768–1773, 2010.

[11] H. J. Flint, E. A. Bayer, M. T. Rincon, R. Lamed, and B. A. White, "Polysaccharide utilization by gut bacteria: potential for new insights from genomic analysis," *Nature Reviews Microbiology*, vol. 6, no. 2, pp. 121–131, 2008.

[12] J. K. DiBaise, H. Zhang, M. D. Crowell, R. Krajmalnik-Brown, G. A. Decker, and B. E. Rittmann, "Gut microbiota and its possible relationship with obesity," *Mayo Clinic Proceedings*, vol. 83, no. 4, pp. 460–469, 2008.

[13] J. Jo, O. Gavrilova, S. Pack et al., "Hypertrophy and/or hyperplasia: dynamics of adipose tissue growth," *PLoS Computational Biology*, vol. 5, no. 3, Article ID e1000324, 2009.

[14] M. M. Avram, A. S. Avram, and W. D. James, "Subcutaneous fat in normal and diseased states. 3. Adipogenesis: from stem cell to fat cell," *Journal of the American Academy of Dermatology*, vol. 56, no. 3, pp. 472–492, 2007.

[15] N. Hosogai, A. Fukuhara, K. Oshima et al., "Adipose tissue hypoxia in obesity and its impact on adipocytokine dysregulation," *Diabetes*, vol. 56, no. 4, pp. 901–911, 2007.

[16] G. Ghigliotti, C. Barisione, S. Garibaldi et al., "Adipose tissue immune response: novel triggers and consequences for chronic inflammatory conditions," *Inflammation*, vol. 37, no. 4, pp. 1337–1353, 2014.

[17] M.-Y. Xu, B. Cao, D.-F. Wang et al., "Human adenovirus 36 infection increased the risk of obesity: a meta-Analysis update," *Medicine*, vol. 94, no. 51, Article ID e2357, 2015.

[18] Q. Shang, H. Wang, Y. Song et al., "Serological data analyses show that adenovirus 36 infection is associated with obesity: a meta-analysis involving 5739 subjects," *Obesity*, vol. 22, no. 3, pp. 895–900, 2014.

[19] T. Yamada, K. Hara, and T. Kadowaki, "Association of adenovirus 36 infection with obesity and metabolic markers in humans: a meta-analysis of observational studies," *PLoS ONE*, vol. 7, no. 7, Article ID e42031, 2012.

[20] L. K. Heilbronn and L. V. Campbell, "Adipose tissue macrophages, low grade inflammation and insulin resistance in human obesity," *Current Pharmaceutical Design*, vol. 14, no. 12, pp. 1225–1230, 2008.

[21] G. S. Hotamisligil, "Inflammation and metabolic disorders," *Nature*, vol. 444, no. 7121, pp. 860–867, 2006.

[22] P. Mathieu, I. Lemieux, and J.-P. Després, "Obesity, inflammation, and cardiovascular risk," *Clinical Pharmacology and Therapeutics*, vol. 87, no. 4, pp. 407–416, 2010.

[23] D. Patsouris, P.-P. Li, D. Thapar, J. Chapman, J. M. Olefsky, and J. G. Neels, "Ablation of CD11c-positive cells normalizes insulin sensitivity in obese insulin resistant animals," *Cell Metabolism*, vol. 8, no. 4, pp. 301–309, 2008.

[24] J. M. Olefsky and C. K. Glass, "Macrophages, inflammation, and insulin resistance," *Annual Review of Physiology*, vol. 72, pp. 219–246, 2010.

[25] P. Nikolai, "Inflammation and insulin resistance: evolution, pathology, and therapy Malta: the Synapse," 2014, http://213.175.193.245/index.php/explore/network-updates/18-netann-members/2412-inflammation-and-insulin-resistance-evolution-pathology-and-therapy.

[26] K. Eder, N. Baffy, A. Falus, and A. K. Fulop, "The major inflammatory mediator interleukin-6 and obesity," *Inflammation Research*, vol. 58, no. 11, pp. 727–736, 2009.

[27] N. Ouchi, J. L. Parker, J. J. Lugus, and K. Walsh, "Adipokines in inflammation and metabolic disease," *Nature Reviews Immunology*, vol. 11, no. 2, pp. 85–97, 2011.

[28] J. Hector, B. Schwarzloh, J. Goehring et al., "TNF-α alters visfatin and adiponectin levels in human fat," *Hormone and Metabolic Research*, vol. 39, no. 4, pp. 250–255, 2007.

[29] M. J. Lyons, I. M. Faust, R. B. Hemmes, D. R. Buskirk, J. Hirsch, and J. B. Zabriskie, "A virally induced obesity syndrome in mice," *Science*, vol. 216, no. 4541, pp. 82–85, 1982.

[30] K. Nagashima, J. B. Zabriskie, and M. J. Lyons, "Virus-induced obesity in mice: association with a hypothalamic lesion," *Journal of Neuropathology and Experimental Neurology*, vol. 51, no. 1, pp. 101–109, 1992.

[31] A. Bernard, R. Cohen, S.-T. Khuth et al., "Alteration of the leptin network in late morbid obesity induced in mice by brain infection with canine distemper virus," *Journal of Virology*, vol. 73, no. 9, pp. 7317–7327, 1999.

[32] B. Griffond, O. Verlaeten, M.-F. Belin, P.-Y. Risold, and A. Bernard, "Specific alteration of the expression of selected hypothalamic neuropeptides during acute and late mouse brain infection using a morbillivirus: relevance to the late-onset obesity?" *Brain Research*, vol. 1022, no. 1-2, pp. 173–181, 2004.

[33] O. Verlaeten, C. Casery, S. Cavagna et al., "Identification of Urop11, a novel leptin-modulated gene that is upregulated in the hypothalamus of mice with virus-induced obesity," *Journal of Molecular Endocrinology*, vol. 38, no. 1-2, pp. 3–17, 2007.

[34] J. K. Carter, C. L. Ow, and R. E. Smith, "Rous-associated virus type 7 induces a syndrome in chickens characterized by stunting and obesity," *Infection and Immunity*, vol. 39, no. 1, pp. 410–422, 1983.

[35] J. A. Richt, S. VandeWoude, M. C. Zink et al., "Infection with Borna disease virus: molecular and immunobiological characterization of the agent," *Clinical Infectious Diseases*, vol. 14, no. 6, pp. 1240–1250, 1992.

[36] C. Herden, S. Herzog, J. A. Richt et al., "Distribution of Borna disease virus in the brain of rats infected with an obesity-inducing virus strain," *Brain Pathology*, vol. 10, no. 1, pp. 39–48, 2000.

[37] C.-H. Chen, Y.-L. Chiu, C.-K. Shaw, M.-T. Tsai, A.-L. Hwang, and K.-J. Hsiao, "Detection of Borna disease virus RNA from peripheral blood cells in schizophrenic patients and mental health workers," *Molecular Psychiatry*, vol. 4, no. 6, pp. 566–571, 1999.

[38] K. Kubo, T. Fujiyoshi, M. M. Yokoyama et al., "Lack of association of Borna disease virus and human T-cell leukemia virus type 1 infections with psychiatric disorders among Japanese patients," *Clinical and Diagnostic Laboratory Immunology*, vol. 4, no. 2, pp. 189–194, 1997.

[39] K.-S. Na, S.-H. Tae, J.-W. Song, and Y.-K. Kim, "Failure to detect Borna disease virus antibody and RNA from peripheral blood mononuclear cells of psychiatric patients," *Psychiatry Investigation*, vol. 6, no. 4, pp. 306–312, 2009.

[40] N. V. Dhurandhar, P. Kulkarni, S. M. Ajinkya, and A. Sherikar, "Effect of adenovirus infection on adiposity in chicken," *Veterinary Microbiology*, vol. 31, no. 2-3, pp. 101–107, 1992.

[41] N. V. Dhurandhar, P. R. Kulkarni, S. M. Ajinkya, A. A. Sherikar, and R. L. Atkinson, "Association of adenovirus infection with human obesity," *Obesity Research*, vol. 5, no. 5, pp. 464–469, 1997.

[42] Y. S. Kim, R. I. Carp, S. M. Callahan, and H. M. Wisniewski, "Adrenal involvement in scrapie-induced obesity," *Proceedings of the Society for Experimental Biology and Medicine*, vol. 189, no. 1, pp. 21–27, 1988.

[43] A. J. Davison, M. Benko, and B. Harrach, "Genetic content and evolution of adenoviruses," *Journal of General Virology*, vol. 84, no. 11, pp. 2895–2908, 2003.

[44] W. C. Russell, "Adenoviruses: update on structure and function," *Journal of General Virology*, vol. 90, no. 1, pp. 1–20, 2009.

[45] Q. Liu and D. A. Muruve, "Molecular basis of the inflammatory response to adenovirus vectors," *Gene Therapy*, vol. 10, no. 11, pp. 935–940, 2003.

[46] W. S. M. Wold and K. Toth, "Adenovirus vectors for gene therapy, vaccination and cancer gene therapy," *Current Gene Therapy*, vol. 13, no. 6, pp. 421–433, 2013.

[47] R. Wigand, H. Gelderblom, and G. Wadell, "New human adenovirus (candidate adenovirus 36), a novel member of subgroup D," *Archives of Virology*, vol. 64, no. 3, pp. 225–233, 1980.

[48] J. Arnold, M. Jánoska, A. E. Kajon et al., "Genomic characterization of human adenovirus 36, a putative obesity agent," *Virus Research*, vol. 149, no. 2, pp. 152–161, 2010.

[49] N. V. Dhurandhar, B. A. Israel, J. M. Kolesar, G. F. Mayhew, M. E. Cook, and R. L. Atkinson, "Increased adiposity in animals due to a human virus," *International Journal of Obesity and Related Metabolic Disorders*, vol. 24, no. 8, pp. 989–996, 2000.

[50] N. V. Dhurandhar, L. D. Whigham, D. H. Abbott et al., "Human adenovirus Ad-36 promotes weight gain in male rhesus and marmoset monkeys," *Journal of Nutrition*, vol. 132, no. 10, pp. 3155–3160, 2002.

[51] N. V. Dhurandhar, B. A. Israel, J. M. Kolesar, G. Mayhew, M. E. Cook, and R. L. Atkinson, "Transmissibility of adenovirus-induced adiposity in a chicken model," *International Journal of Obesity*, vol. 25, no. 7, pp. 990–996, 2001.

[52] M. Pasarica, A. C. Shin, M. Yu et al., "Human adenovirus 36 induces adiposity, increases insulin sensitivity, and alters hypothalamic monoamines in rats," *Obesity*, vol. 14, no. 11, pp. 1905–1913, 2006.

[53] M. Kapila, P. Khosla, and N. V. Dhurandhar, "Novel short-term effects of adenovirus Ad-36 on hamster lipoproteins," *International Journal of Obesity*, vol. 28, no. 12, pp. 1521–1527, 2004.

[54] M. Pasarica, S. Loiler, and N. V. Dhurandhar, "Acute effect of infection by adipogenic human adenovirus Ad36," *Archives of Virology*, vol. 153, no. 11, pp. 2097–2102, 2008.

[55] S. D. Vangipuram, J. Sheele, R. L. Atkinson, T. C. Holland, and N. V. Dhurandhar, "A human adenovirus enhances preadipocyte differentiation," *Obesity Research*, vol. 12, no. 5, pp. 770–777, 2004.

[56] M. Rathod, S. D. Vangipuram, B. Krishnan, A. R. Heydari, T. C. Holland, and N. V. Dhurandhar, "Viral mRNA expression but not DNA replication is required for lipogenic effect of human adenovirus Ad-36 in preadipocytes," *International Journal of Obesity*, vol. 31, no. 1, pp. 78–86, 2007.

[57] J. M. Ntambi and K. Young-Cheul, "Adipocyte differentiation and gene expression," *Journal of Nutrition*, vol. 130, no. 12, pp. 3122S–3126S, 2000.

[58] P. M. Rogers, K. A. Fusinski, M. A. Rathod et al., "Human adenovirus Ad-36 induces adipogenesis via its E4 orf-1 gene," *International Journal of Obesity*, vol. 32, no. 3, pp. 397–406, 2008.

[59] S. D. Vangipuram, M. Yu, J. Tian et al., "Adipogenic human adenovirus-36 reduces leptin expression and secretion and increases glucose uptake by fat cells," *International Journal of Obesity*, vol. 31, no. 1, pp. 87–96, 2007.

[60] M. Pasarica, N. Mashtalir, E. J. McAllister et al., "Adipogenic human adenovirus ad-36 induces commitment, differentiation, and lipid accumulation in human adipose-derived stem cells," *Stem Cells*, vol. 26, no. 4, pp. 969–978, 2008.

[61] Z. Q. Wang, Y. Yu, X. H. Zhang, E. Z. Floyd, and W. T. Cefalu, "Human adenovirus 36 decreases fatty acid oxidation and increases de novo lipogenesis in primary cultured human skeletal muscle cells by promoting Cidec/FSP27 expression," *International Journal of Obesity*, vol. 34, no. 9, pp. 1355–1364, 2010.

[62] J. J. M. Bouwman, F. L. J. Visseren, K. P. Bouter, and R. J. A. Diepersloot, "Infection-induced inflammatory response of adipocytes in vitro," *International Journal of Obesity*, vol. 32, no. 6, pp. 892–901, 2008.

[63] E. Ponterio and L. Gnessi, "Adenovirus 36 and obesity: an overview," *Viruses*, vol. 7, no. 7, pp. 3719–3740, 2015.

[64] E. R. Mardis, "Next-generation DNA sequencing methods," *Annual Review of Genomics and Human Genetics*, vol. 9, pp. 387–402, 2008.

[65] W. Scheppach, "Effects of short chain fatty acids on gut morphology and function," *Gut*, vol. 35, no. 1, pp. S35–S38, 1994.

[66] L. Peng, Z.-R. Li, R. S. Green, I. R. Holzman, and J. Lin, "Butyrate enhances the intestinal barrier by facilitating tight junction assembly via activation of AMP-activated protein kinase in Caco-2 cell monolayers," *The Journal of Nutrition*, vol. 139, no. 9, pp. 1619–1625, 2009.

[67] P. D. Cani, "Crosstalk between the gut microbiota and the endocannabinoid system: impact on the gut barrier function and the adipose tissue," *Clinical Microbiology and Infection*, vol. 18, no. 4, pp. 50–53, 2012.

[68] I. Koboziev, F. Karlsson, and M. B. Grisham, "Gut-associated lymphoid tissue, T cell trafficking, and chronic intestinal inflammation," *Annals of the New York Academy of Sciences*, vol. 1207, supplement 1, pp. E86–E93, 2010.

[69] K. R. Groschwitz and S. P. Hogan, "Intestinal barrier function: molecular regulation and disease pathogenesis," *Journal of Allergy and Clinical Immunology*, vol. 124, no. 1, pp. 3–20, 2009.

[70] S. Prasad, R. Mingrino, K. Kaukinen et al., "Inflammatory processes have differential effects on claudins 2, 3 and 4 in colonic epithelial cells," *Laboratory Investigation*, vol. 85, no. 9, pp. 1139–1162, 2005.

[71] M. T. DeMeo, E. A. Mutlu, A. Keshavarzian, and M. C. Tobin, "The small intestine and nutrition: intestinal permeation and gastrointestinal disease," *Journal of Clinical Gastroenterology*, vol. 34, no. 4, pp. 385–396, 2002.

[72] R. Al-Sadi, M. Boivin, and T. Ma, "Mechanism of cytokine modulation of epithelial tight junction barrier," *Frontiers in Bioscience*, vol. 14, no. 7, pp. 2765–2778, 2009.

[73] J. Matricon, M. Meleine, A. Gelot et al., "Review article: associations between immune activation, intestinal permeability and the irritable bowel syndrome," *Alimentary Pharmacology and Therapeutics*, vol. 36, no. 11-12, pp. 1009–1031, 2012.

[74] G. R. Martin and J. L. Wallace, "Gastrointestinal inflammation: a central component of mucosal defense and repair," *Experimental Biology and Medicine*, vol. 231, no. 2, pp. 130–137, 2006.

[75] M. Camilleri, "Peripheral mechanisms in irritable bowel syndrome," *The New England Journal of Medicine*, vol. 367, no. 17, pp. 1626–1635, 2012.

[76] M. Camilleri, K. Lasch, and W. Zhou, "Irritable bowel syndrome: methods, mechanisms, and pathophysiology. the confluence of increased permeability, inflammation, and pain in irritable bowel syndrome," *American Journal of Physiology—Gastrointestinal and Liver Physiology*, vol. 303, no. 7, pp. G775–G785, 2012.

[77] G. L. Klein, B. W. Petschow, A. L. Shaw, and E. Weaver, "Gut barrier dysfunction and microbial translocation in cancer cachexia: a new therapeutic target," *Current Opinion in Supportive and Palliative Care*, vol. 7, no. 4, pp. 361–367, 2013.

[78] L. Geurts, A. M. Neyrinck, N. M. Delzenne, C. Knauf, and P. D. Cani, "Gut microbiota controls adipose tissue expansion, gut barrier and glucose metabolism: novel insights into molecular targets and interventions using prebiotics," *Beneficial Microbes*, vol. 5, no. 1, pp. 3–17, 2014.

[79] M. A. Hildebrandt, C. Hoffmann, S. A. Sherrill-Mix et al., "High-fat diet determines the composition of the murine gut microbiome independently of obesity," *Gastroenterology*, vol. 137, no. 5, pp. 1716.e2–1724.e2, 2009.

[80] P. J. Turnbaugh, R. E. Ley, M. A. Mahowald, V. Magrini, E. R. Mardis, and J. I. Gordon, "An obesity-associated gut microbiome with increased capacity for energy harvest," *Nature*, vol. 444, no. 7122, pp. 1027–1031, 2006.

[81] R. E. Ley, F. Bäckhed, P. Turnbaugh, C. A. Lozupone, R. D. Knight, and J. I. Gordon, "Obesity alters gut microbial ecology," *Proceedings of the National Academy of Sciences of the United States of America*, vol. 102, no. 31, pp. 11070–11075, 2005.

[82] R. E. Ley, P. J. Turnbaugh, S. Klein, and J. I. Gordon, "Microbial ecology: human gut microbes associated with obesity," *Nature*, vol. 444, no. 7122, pp. 1022–1023, 2006.

[83] P. J. Turnbaugh, M. Hamady, T. Yatsunenko et al., "A core gut microbiome in obese and lean twins," *Nature*, vol. 457, no. 7228, pp. 480–484, 2009.

[84] A. Everard, C. Belzer, L. Geurts et al., "Cross-talk between Akkermansia muciniphila and intestinal epithelium controls diet-induced obesity," *Proceedings of the National Academy of Sciences of the United States of America*, vol. 110, no. 22, pp. 9066–9071, 2013.

[85] H. Sokol, B. Pigneur, L. Watterlot et al., "Faecalibacterium prausnitzii is an anti-inflammatory commensal bacterium identified by gut microbiota analysis of Crohn disease patients," *Proceedings of the National Academy of Sciences of the United States of America*, vol. 105, no. 43, pp. 16731–16736, 2008.

[86] P. D. Cani, H. Plovier, M. Van Hul et al., "Endocannabinoids—at the crossroads between the gut microbiota and host metabolism," *Nature Reviews Endocrinology*, vol. 12, no. 3, pp. 133–143, 2016.

[87] L. Geurts, V. Lazarevic, M. Derrien et al., "Altered gut microbiota and endocannabinoid system tone in obese and diabetic leptin-resistant mice: impact on apelin regulation in adipose tissue," *Frontiers in Microbiology*, vol. 2, article 149, 2011.

[88] G. G. Muccioli, D. Naslain, F. Bäckhed et al., "The endocannabinoid system links gut microbiota to adipogenesis," *Molecular Systems Biology*, vol. 6, article 392, 2010.

[89] K. L. Wright, M. Duncan, and K. A. Sharkey, "Cannabinoid CB_2 receptors in the gastrointestinal tract: a regulatory system in states of inflammation," *British Journal of Pharmacology*, vol. 153, no. 2, pp. 263–270, 2008.

[90] L. Geurts, G. G. Muccioli, N. M. Delzenne, and P. D. Cani, "Chronic endocannabinoid system stimulation induces muscle macrophage and lipid accumulation in type 2 diabetic mice independently of metabolic endotoxaemia," *PLoS ONE*, vol. 8, no. 2, Article ID e55963, 2013.

[91] G. Turu and L. Hunyady, "Signal transduction of the CB1 cannabinoid receptor," *Journal of Molecular Endocrinology*, vol. 44, no. 2, pp. 75–85, 2010.

[92] D. J. Henry and C. Chavkin, "Activation of inwardly rectifying potassium channels (GIRK1) by co-expressed rat brain cannabinoid receptors in Xenopus oocytes," *Neuroscience Letters*, vol. 186, no. 2-3, pp. 91–94, 1995.

[93] T. Endoh, "Pharmacological characterization of inhibitory effects of postsynaptic opioid and cannabinoid receptors on calcium currents in neonatal rat nucleus tractus solitarius," *British Journal of Pharmacology*, vol. 147, no. 4, pp. 391–401, 2006.

[94] D. Gebremedhin, A. R. Lange, W. B. Campbell, C. J. Hillard, and D. R. Harder, "Cannabinoid CB1 receptor of cat cerebral arterial muscle functions to inhibit L-type Ca^{2+} channel current," *American Journal of Physiology—Heart and Circulatory Physiology*, vol. 276, no. 6, pp. H2085–H2093, 1999.

[95] I. Matias and V. Di Marzo, "Endocannabinoids and the control of energy balance," *Trends in Endocrinology and Metabolism*, vol. 18, no. 1, pp. 27–37, 2007.

[96] U. Pagotto, G. Marsicano, D. Cota, B. Lutz, and R. Pasquali, "The emerging role of the endocannabinoid system in endocrine regulation and energy balance," *Endocrine Reviews*, vol. 27, no. 1, pp. 73–100, 2006.

[97] M. Blüher, S. Engeli, N. Klöting et al., "Dysregulation of the peripheral and adipose tissue endocannabinoid system in human abdominal obesity," *Diabetes*, vol. 55, no. 11, pp. 3053–3060, 2006.

[98] R. Ladeiras-Lopes, J. Ferreira-Martins, and A. F. Leite-Moreira, "The apelinergic system: the role played in human physiology and pathology and potential therapeutic applications," *Arquivos Brasileiros de Cardiologia*, vol. 90, no. 5, pp. 343–349, 2008.

[99] A.-M. O'Carroll, S. J. Lolait, L. E. Harris, and G. R. Pope, "The apelin receptor APJ: journey from an orphan to a multifaceted regulator of homeostasis," *Journal of Endocrinology*, vol. 219, no. 1, pp. R13–R35, 2013.

[100] K. Higuchi, T. Masaki, K. Gotoh et al., "Apelin, an APJ receptor ligand, regulates body adiposity and favors the messenger ribonucleic acid expression of uncoupling proteins in mice," *Endocrinology*, vol. 148, no. 6, pp. 2690–2697, 2007.

[101] A. R. Gunawardene, B. M. Corfe, and C. A. Staton, "Classification and functions of enteroendocrine cells of the lower gastrointestinal tract," *International Journal of Experimental Pathology*, vol. 92, no. 4, pp. 219–231, 2011.

[102] J. A. Koehler, L. L. Baggio, B. Yusta et al., "GLP-1R agonists promote normal and neoplastic intestinal growth through mechanisms requiring Fgf7," *Cell Metabolism*, vol. 21, no. 3, pp. 379–391, 2015.

[103] P. E. Dubé and P. L. Brubaker, "Frontiers in glucagon-like peptide 2: multiple actions, multiple mediators," *American Journal of Physiology—Endocrinology and Metabolism*, vol. 293, no. 2, pp. E460–E465, 2007.

[104] J. Jasleen, N. Shimoda, E. R. Shen et al., "Signaling mechanisms of glucagon-like peptide 2-induced intestinal epithelial cell proliferation," *Journal of Surgical Research*, vol. 90, no. 1, pp. 13–18, 2000.

[105] R. Medzhitov, "Origin and physiological roles of inflammation," *Nature*, vol. 454, no. 7203, pp. 428–435, 2008.

[106] F. P. de Heredia, S. Gómez-Martínez, and A. Marcos, "Obesity, inflammation and the immune system," *Proceedings of the Nutrition Society*, vol. 71, no. 2, pp. 332–338, 2012.

[107] G. Cildir, S. C. Akıncılar, and V. Tergaonkar, "Chronic adipose tissue inflammation: all immune cells on the stage," *Trends in Molecular Medicine*, vol. 19, no. 8, pp. 487–500, 2013.

[108] V. Hegde and N. V. Dhurandhar, "Microbes and obesity—interrelationship between infection, adipose tissue and the immune system," *Clinical Microbiology and Infection*, vol. 19, no. 4, pp. 314–320, 2013.

[109] A. Iwasaki and B. L. Kelsall, "Freshly isolated peyer's patch, but not spleen, dendritic cells produce interleukin 10 and induce the differentiation of T helper type 2 cells," *Journal of Experimental Medicine*, vol. 190, no. 2, pp. 229–239, 1999.

[110] L. E. Smythies, M. Sellers, R. H. Clements et al., "Human intestinal macrophages display profound inflammatory anergy despite avid phagocytic and bacteriocidal activity," *Journal of Clinical Investigation*, vol. 115, no. 1, pp. 66–75, 2005.

19

Prevalence of Osteoporosis and Its Risk Factors in Men with COPD in Qazvin

Mahnaz Abbasi,[1] Mohammadali Zohal,[2] Banafsheh Atapour,[3] and Zohreh Yazdi[4]

[1]*Rheumatology, Metabolic Diseases Research Center, Qazvin University of Medical Sciences, Qazvin, Iran*
[2]*Pulmonary Diseases, Metabolic Diseases Research Center, Qazvin University of Medical Sciences, Qazvin, Iran*
[3]*Metabolic Diseases Research Center, Qazvin University of Medical Sciences, Qazvin, Iran*
[4]*Occupational Medicine, Social Determinants of Health Research Center, Qazvin University of Medical Sciences, Qazvin, Iran*

Correspondence should be addressed to Mohammadali Zohal; mzohal@qums.ac.ir

Academic Editor: Mariano Bizzarri

Introduction. Chronic obstructive pulmonary disease (COPD) is a major cause of morbidity and mortality worldwide. Proper diagnosis of osteoporosis as a systemic adverse effect of COPD is of significant importance. The present study aimed at evaluating the prevalence of osteoporosis and its risk factors in men suffering from COPD in Qazvin (2014). *Methods*. This descriptive-analytical study was conducted on 90 patients with COPD using random sampling. Anthropometric data and results from physical examination were collected. Pulmonary function test and bone mineral densitometry were done for all participants as well. *Results*. The prevalence of osteopenia and osteoporosis in COPD patients was 31.5 and 52.8 percent, respectively. Bone mineral density (BMD) at the femoral neck was associated significantly with body mass index (BMI), increased severity of COPD, and use of oral corticosteroid ($P < 0.05$). *Conclusion*. The results showed that patients' BMI and severity of COPD are two valuable risk factors for osteoporosis screening in COPD patients.

1. Introduction

Chronic obstructive pulmonary disease (COPD) is a progressive lung disease with prevalence rate of 5–13 percent [1, 2]. COPD is characterized by inflammation in the lung parenchyma and airways and irreversible obstruction in airflow. Patients suffering from COPD present with shortness of breath, dyspnea on exertion, cough, and sputum production [3]. It is a multisystem disorder that affects many organs such as bones causing osteopenia and osteoporosis [4, 5].

Osteopenia is a condition in which bone mineral density is reduced. Likewise, osteoporosis is a more severe condition, where decreased bone density increases the risk of fracture. The most common sites of fracture are wrist, spine, ribs, and hip. These fractures can result in pain, disability, reduced mobility, and other serious injuries [6].

Recent evidences suggest that osteoporosis in COPD patients is debilitating. Osteoporosis can cause multiple vertebral fractures in spine which result in a loss of at least 15–20% of its height. These fractures often result in patients' height loss, chronic pain, and kyphosis which ultimately damage respiratory function. The complications can lead to death if they are left untreated [7, 8].

Researchers are investigating further to clarify the relationship between osteoporosis and COPD. Most researchers, however, believe that the two diseases have a number of risk factors in common including smoking, older age, low level of vitamin D, long-term treatment with corticosteroids, excessive weight loss, and low body mass index in patients. Moreover, 22 to 69 percent of men with COPD may develop hypogonadism that has been associated with other systemic manifestations including osteoporosis and depression [4, 9, 10].

Since osteoporosis is a chronic disease similar to COPD and tends to deteriorate with age, it is crucial to pay more attention to its risk factors so as to enable its prevention, early diagnosis, and treatment. Thus, estimating the prevalence of risk factors for osteoporosis in patients with COPD is important. For example, it is possible to use bisphosphonates for prophylaxis and treatment of osteoporosis, if corticosteroids are recognized as the main culprit in COPD patients [11, 12]. Proper protective effect of bisphosphonates has been reported in glucocorticoid-induced osteoporosis in previous studies [11–13].

Since most COPD patients are old men with risk factors for osteoporosis, the present study aimed to evaluate the prevalence of osteoporosis and detect its risk factors in men with COPD in Qazvin (2014).

2. Methods

This cross-sectional study was performed in lung clinic of Bouali Hospital in Qazvin in 2014. Ninety men with COPD aged from 60 to 86 years were enrolled. The study was approved by the ethics committee of Qazvin University of Medical Sciences (QUMS). Inclusion criteria were diagnosis of COPD by pulmonologist and obtaining informed consent from patients, whereas exclusion criteria included history of asthma or any chronic pulmonary disorders except COPD, history of bone disease, and patients who had been treated for osteoporosis or used diuretics. In addition, patients with chronic diseases affecting the bone mineral density (e.g., hyperthyroidism) or patients with a history of thoracic surgery and malignancy were excluded. Diagnosis of COPD in the patients was considered according to criteria provided by American Thoracic Society (ATS) and European Respiratory Society (ERS) [14].

For this purpose, pulmonologist used the patients' medical records, current symptoms, and the results of pulmonary function test. Lung function was assessed by trained technicians (SPM300 spirometer). The forced expiratory volume 1 (FEV1) and forced vital capacity (FVC) were measured by spirometer, and the FEV1/FVC ratio was calculated. COPD was diagnosed for the patients through spirometry, where postbronchodilatory FEV1/FVC was lower than 70%.

Using FEV1, according to GOLD guideline, the COPD patients were then classified into four groups of severity [15].

Having calculated the body mass index (BMI) by dividing weight (in kilograms) by the square of the weight, the patients were categorized as underweight (BMI $< 17\,kg/m^2$), normal weight ($17–25\,kg/m^2$), overweight ($25.1–30\,kg/m^2$), and obese ($>30\,kg/m^2$) [16].

The bone mineral density was measured by using dual-energy X-ray absorptiometry at lumbar spine and femoral neck (Hologic QDR 2000, Bedford, MA, USA, model). The results of BMD were categorized according to the WHO criteria. Therefore, subjects with spine or femur neck T-score of −2.5 or below were considered as having osteoporosis. Subjects with T-score between −1 and −2.5 and more than −1 were considered as having osteopenia and normal people, respectively [17].

Data were presented using frequency and percentage for categorical variables. Chi-square test was used to compare qualitative variables. All statistical analyses were performed using SPSS software version 19 and P values less than 0.05 were considered statistically significant.

3. Results

A total of 90 patients with COPD aged from 60 to 86 years (mean age: 69 ± 6) participated in this study. The majority of patients (61.8%) were between 60 and 69 years, and 30.3% and 7.9% of patients were between 70 and 79 years and between 80 and 89 years, respectively. The mean body mass index (BMI) was $22.2 \pm 4.17\,kg/m^2$, and 44.9% of patients had normal BMI.

Based on GOLD criteria, 14 (15.7%) patients had GOLD II, 27 (30.3%) patients had GOLD III, and 31 (34.8%) patients had GOLD IV. The mean lumbar spine and neck of femur BMD of the patients were 0.85 ± 0.15 and 0.7 ± 0.12, respectively.

According to WHO criteria, 47 patients (52.8%) had osteoporosis. Results for relationship between variables and bone mineral density in the lumbar spine and neck of femur are shown in Table 1.

As shown in the table, only BMI and severity of COPD were significantly associated with osteoporosis. This relationship was not found in other risk factors. The statistically significant relationship was observed only between severity of COPD and osteoporosis in neck of femur ($P = 0.042$). As seen in Figure 1, with increasing the severity of COPD in patients, severity of bone loss (osteoporosis) increased significantly.

Figure 2 shows the relationship between patients' BMI and osteoporosis based on T-score of femoral neck. As illustrated in Figure 2, reduction in patients' BMI leads to significant increase in osteoporosis.

Statistical analyses did not show any significant relationship between oral corticosteroid use and osteoporosis based on lumbar spine T-score. Other results, however, showed that there was a significant correlation between dose of oral corticosteroid and patients' osteoporosis based on femoral neck T-score ($r = 0.26$; P value $= 0.015$).

4. Discussion

In this study, the prevalence of osteopenia and osteoporosis in COPD patients was 31.5% and 52.8%, respectively. In a study conducted by Abu-Bakr and his colleagues, the prevalence of osteopenia and osteoporosis was observed in 50 and 30 percent of COPD patients [8]. The results were consistent with those of another study conducted by Mansour and his colleagues. They reported the prevalence of osteoporosis and osteopenia in COPD patients as a range of 9–69% and a range of 27–76%, respectively. Their explanation for the differences observed in the studies was using different diagnostic methods, different study population, and different severity in the underlying respiratory disease [8, 18].

In the present study, severity of osteoporosis according to femoral neck T-score increased with the increase of the severity of COPD. In other words, reduction of FEV1 in subjects was associated with low levels of bone mineral density. Nuti and his colleagues also found similar results and showed that bone mineral density in COPD patients was low and decreased with increasing disease severity [19]. Nevertheless, the relationship between lung function parameters and osteoporosis is complex and ambiguous. Cellular

Table 1: Frequency of different risk factors of osteoporosis in COPD patients.

Variable	Spine Normal	Spine Osteopenia	Spine Osteoporosis	P value	Femur Normal	Femur Osteopenia	Femur Osteoporosis	P value
Age (year)								
60–69	10 (11.2%)	19 (21.3%)	26 (29.2%)		13 (14.6%)	28 (31.5%)	14 (15.7%)	
70–79	8 (9%)	8 (9%)	11 (12.4%)	0.49	7 (7.9%)	9 (10.1%)	11 (12.4%)	0.52
80–89	0 (0%)	3 (3.4%)	4 (4.5%)		1 (1.1%)	3 (3.4%)	3 (3.4%)	
Smoking (pack/year)								
<20	2 (2.2%)	8 (9%)	8 (9%)		5 (5.6%)	9 (10.1%)	4 (4.5%)	
21–40	7 (7.9%)	10 (11.2%)	16 (18%)	0.76	7 (7.9%)	16 (18%)	10 (11.2%)	0.82
>40	9 (10.1%)	12 (13.5%)	17 (19.1%)		9 (10.1%)	15 (16.9%)	14 (15.7%)	
Severity of COPD								
Mild (grade I)	6 (6.7%)	4 (4.5%)	7 (7.9%)		5 (5.6%)	9 (10.1%)	3 (3.4%)	
Moderate (grade II)	1 (1.1%)	6 (6.7%)	7 (7.9%)	0.38	6 (6.7%)	3 (3.4%)	5 (5.6%)	0.042
Severe (grade III)	3 (3.4%)	11 (12.4%)	13 (14.6%)		3 (3.4%)	17 (19.1%)	7 (7.9%)	
Very severe (grade IV)	8 (9%)	9 (10.1%)	14 (15.7%)		7 (7.9%)	11 (12.4%)	13 (14.6%)	
BMI								
Low	19 (21.3%)	13 (14.6%)	8 (9%)		4 (4.5%)	21 (23.6%)	15 (16.9%)	
Moderate	10 (11.2%)	15 (16.9%)	5 (5.6%)	0.79	13 (14.6%)	11 (12.4%)	6 (6.7%)	0.034
Overweight	8 (9%)	3 (3.4%)	2 (2.2%)		2 (2.2%)	8 (9%)	3 (3.4%)	
Obese	2 (2.2%)	4 (4.5%)	0 (0%)		2 (2.2%)	0 (0%)	4 (4.5%)	
Corticosteroid								
Budesonide	2 (2.2%)	4 (4.5%)	4 (4.5%)	0.89	3 (3.4%)	5 (5.6%)	2 (2.2%)	0.69
Inhaled corticosteroid	17 (19.1%)	30 (33.7%)	40 (44.9%)	0.45	20 (22.5%)	40 (44.9%)	27 (30.3%)	0.42

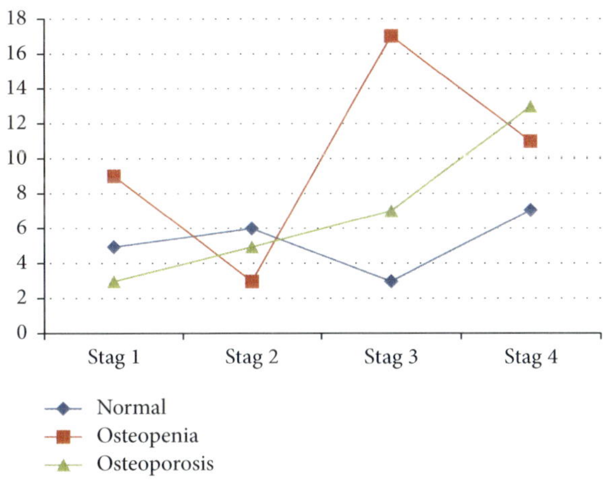

Figure 1: Interaction between osteoporosis in the femoral neck and severity of COPD.

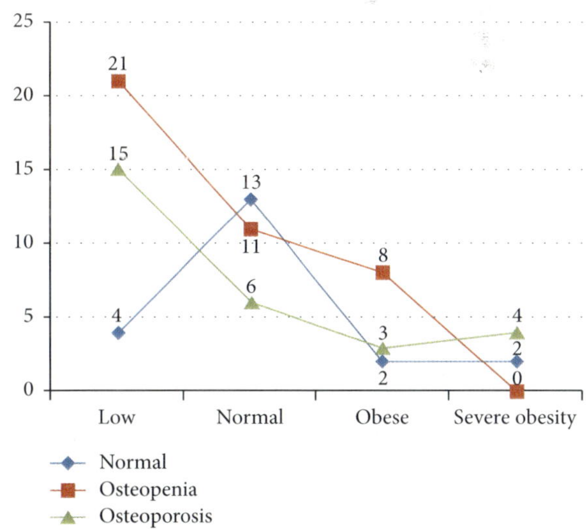

Figure 2: Interaction between osteoporosis in the femoral neck and patients' BMI.

microstructural defects in COPD are not well understood as well [20].

An experimental study of transbone biopsy in COPD patients showed that microstructure skeletal disorders (both cancellous and cortical bones) are more in COPD patients compared to control groups [21]. It is very likely that an underlying reason for the disorders is the increased levels of cytokines and production of catalytic enzymes. It has been shown that there is a continuous systemic inflammatory state in patients with COPD, which results in the release of inflammatory cytokines such as TNF-α, IL-1, and IL-6. On the other hand, production of catalytic enzymes, for example, matrix metalloproteinases, increases during the course of COPD. Protein catabolic process and the inflammatory cytokines induce bone resorption and inhibit bone formation [21–24].

The use of corticosteroids in these patients is also considered as another cause of low bone density [22, 25]. This was examined in the present study as well, and a significant relationship was observed between the osteoporosis in femoral neck based on T-score and the use of oral corticosteroid. In other words, by increasing the oral corticosteroid use, an increased risk for osteoporosis was observed. Almost all patients were given inhaled corticosteroids in the present study, and no significant relationship was observed between the osteoporosis in lumbar spine based on T-score and the use of oral corticosteroid. Similarly, no association was found between inhaled corticosteroid and budesonide use with osteoporosis in both regions. The treatment, however, can be strongly confusing in the interpretation of the results concerning the relevance of COPD and low BMI (at least in this specific sample) as a risk factor for osteoporosis. Israel et al. found a reduced bone density after long-term treatment with triamcinolone [26], but studies on the effects of budesonide and fluticasone did not eventuate in the same results. In the TORCH study carried out by Ferguson et al., no significant effect on bone mineral density for inhaled corticosteroids was found [27]. In another study by Johnell et al., effects of long-term treatment with budesonide on fracture rates and bone mineral density were not found to be clinically significant [28]. In contrast, Nuti et al. showed that both severity of COPD and using inhaled oral glucocorticoid therapy increase the risk of vertebral fractures [19]. Casadp and his colleagues also found that patient's treatment with glucocorticoid and severity of COPD are correlated [29]. In a similar study, Dam et al. found that patients with COPD or asthma using corticosteroid had the lowest amount of BMD, and the risk of osteoporosis in their bones was two times more compared to those without COPD and asthma [30].

In this study, a significant relationship was found between BMI and osteoporosis in femoral neck based on T-score, such that a reduction in BMI was shown to be associated with increased severity of osteoporosis. However, no association was observed between BMI and osteoporosis based on T-score of lumbar spine. Bone mass is directly associated with BMI and patients with a higher BMI have higher BMD [31, 32]. This is partly due to the effect of weight bearing on bones and the higher levels of estrogen in obese people. Aromatization and the conversion of testosterone to estrogen increase in obese people [33]. The effect of BMI on BMD is reportedly dependent on the bone place in body. Accordingly, hip would be the first to be affected followed by lumbar spine and distal radius, respectively. It has also been suggested that this order may be due to differences in body fat percentage and weight bearing condition in different areas [34]. The mechanism of the relationship between low BMI and osteoporosis is not fully clear in patients with COPD. It is probably due to the increase in inflammatory processes, the decrease in physical activity, and other mechanisms of proteolysis [35–38]. Therefore, osteoporosis is considered as a major problem in men with COPD. It can cause multiple fractures in spines and reduce forced vital capacity (FVC) in COPD patients and, consequently, can exacerbate the adverse effects of COPD in patients. Therefore, identifying and controlling the common risk factors for COPD and osteoporosis are essential in any society [8].

5. Conclusion

The results showed that an increase in severity of COPD, using oral corticosteroid, and decrease of BMI are three risk factors for high prevalence of osteoporosis in COPD patients in Qazvin province. Given the importance of osteoporosis in COPD, it is recommended that all COPD patients be screened for osteoporosis so as to prevent serious complications such as but not limited to fractures.

Disclosure

This study was officially registered as Internal Medicine specialty thesis at the School of Medicine in Qazvin University of Medical Sciences.

Competing Interests

The authors declare that they have no competing interests.

Acknowledgments

The authors wish to thank the staff of the Metabolic Disease Research Center, Qazvin University of Medical Sciences, for their help in preparing this paper.

References

[1] P. Lou, Y. Zhu, P. Chen et al., "Prevalence and correlations with depression, anxiety, and other features in outpatients with chronic obstructive pulmonary disease in China: a cross-sectional case control study," *BMC Pulmonary Medicine*, vol. 12, article 53, 2012.

[2] R. A. Pauwels, A. S. Buist, P. M. A. Calverley, C. R. Jenkins, and S. S. Hurd, "Global strategy for the diagnosis, management, and prevention of chronic obstructive pulmonary disease. NHLBI/WHO Global Initiative for Chronic Obstructive Lung Disease (GOLD) Workshop summary," *American Journal of Respiratory and Critical Care Medicine*, vol. 163, no. 5, pp. 1256–1276, 2001.

[3] J. Vestbo, S. S. Hurd, A. G. Agustí et al., "Global strategy for the diagnosis, management, and prevention of chronic obstructive pulmonary disease: GOLD executive summary," *American Journal of Respiratory and Critical Care Medicine*, vol. 187, no. 4, pp. 347–365, 2013.

[4] L. Graat-Verboom, F. W. J. M. Smeenk, B. E. E. M. van den Borne et al., "Risk factors for osteoporosis in Caucasian patients with moderate chronic obstructive pulmonary disease: a case control study," *Bone*, vol. 50, no. 6, pp. 1234–1239, 2012.

[5] N. Cielen, K. Maes, and G. Gayan-Ramirez, "Musculoskeletal disorders in chronic obstructive pulmonary disease," *BioMed Research International*, vol. 2014, Article ID 965764, 17 pages, 2014.

[6] J. H. M. Driessen, L. Hansen, S. A. Eriksen et al., "The epidemiology of fractures in Denmark in 2011," *Osteoporosis International*, vol. 27, no. 6, pp. 2017–2025, 2016.

[7] Z. Ciric, I. Stankovic, T. Pejcic, L. Ristic, M. Rancic, and M. Radovic, "Osteoporosis in patients with chronic obstructive pulmonary disease," *Medical Archives*, vol. 66, no. 6, pp. 385–387, 2012.

[8] S. M. Abu-Bakr, M. M. Galal Eldin, M. R. Hafez, S. M. Salem, and H. T. Qandeel, "Assessment of osteoporosis in patients with chronic obstructive pulmonary disease," *Egyptian Journal of Chest Diseases and Tuberculosis*, vol. 63, no. 3, pp. 597–602, 2014.

[9] C.-W. Lin, Y.-Y. Chen, Y.-J. Chen, C.-Y. Liang, M.-S. Lin, and W. Chen, "Prevalence, risk factors, and health-related quality of life of osteoporosis in patients with COPD at a community hospital in Taiwan," *International Journal of Chronic Obstructive Pulmonary Disease*, vol. 10, no. 1, pp. 1493–1500, 2015.

[10] S. J. Lee, K. A. Kong, Y. J. Ryu, J. H. Lee, and J. H. Chang, "Late-breaking abstract: risk factors for osteoporosis in patients with COPD: 2008–2010 Korean NHANES," *European Respiratory Journal*, vol. 44, supplement 58, Article ID P3590, 2014.

[11] S. A. Aljubran, G. J. Whelan, M. C. Glaum, and R. F. Lockey, "Osteoporosis in the at-risk asthmatic," *Allergy*, vol. 69, no. 11, pp. 1429–1439, 2014.

[12] D. H. Solomon, S. J. Diem, K. Ruppert et al., "Bone mineral density changes among women initiating proton pump inhibitors or H2 receptor antagonists: a SWAN cohort study," *Journal of Bone and Mineral Research*, vol. 30, no. 2, pp. 232–239, 2015.

[13] M. Sarkar, R. Bhardwaj, I. Madabhavi, and J. Khatana, "Osteoporosis in chronic obstructive pulmonary disease," *Clinical Medicine Insights: Circulatory, Respiratory and Pulmonary Medicine*, vol. 9, pp. 5–21, 2015.

[14] B. R. Celli, W. MacNee, A. Agusti et al., "Standards for the diagnosis and treatment of patients with COPD: a summary of the ATS/ERS position paper," *European Respiratory Journal*, vol. 23, no. 6, pp. 932–934, 2004.

[15] K. F. Rabe, S. Hurd, A. Anzueto et al., "Global strategy for the diagnosis, management, and prevention of chronic obstructive pulmonary disease: GOLD executive summary," *American Journal of Respiratory and Critical Care Medicine*, vol. 176, no. 6, pp. 532–555, 2007.

[16] E. Anuurad, K. Shiwaku, A. Nogi et al., "The new BMI criteria for asians by the regional office for the western pacific region of WHO are suitable for screening of overweight to prevent metabolic syndrome in elder Japanese workers," *Journal of Occupational Health*, vol. 45, no. 6, pp. 335–343, 2003.

[17] M. Sahmani, S. Omidian, A. Javadi, M. Sirati Sabet, and M. Abbasi, "Association between the serum levels of zinc, copper and lipid profile with osteoporosis in iranian postmenopausal women," *Biotechnology and Health Sciences*, vol. 1, no. 1, Article ID e19190, 2014.

[18] O. F. Mansour, R. M. Bakr, R. A. Elwahsh, and A. M. Zanfal, "Osteoporosis in patients with chronic obstructive pulmonary disease," *Menoufia Medical Journal*, vol. 28, no. 2, pp. 521–524, 2015.

[19] R. Nuti, P. Siviero, S. Maggi et al., "Vertebral fractures in patients with chronic obstructive pulmonary disease: the EOLO study," *Osteoporosis International*, vol. 20, no. 6, pp. 989–998, 2009.

[20] B. M. Misof, P. Roschger, V. Jorgetti et al., "Subtle changes in bone mineralization density distribution in most severely affected patients with chronic obstructive pulmonary disease," *Bone*, vol. 79, pp. 1–7, 2015.

[21] C. A. M. Kulak, V. C. Borba, V. Jorgetti et al., "Skeletal microstructural abnormalities in postmenopausal women with chronic obstructive pulmonary disease," *Journal of Bone and Mineral Research*, vol. 25, no. 9, pp. 1931–1940, 2010.

[22] N. R. Jørgensen and P. Schwarz, "Osteoporosis in chronic obstructive pulmonary disease patients," *Current Opinion in Pulmonary Medicine*, vol. 14, no. 2, pp. 122–127, 2008.

[23] H. Fujimoto, K. Fujimoto, A. Ueda, and M. Ohata, "Hypoxemia is a risk factor for bone mass loss," *Journal of Bone and Mineral Metabolism*, vol. 17, no. 3, pp. 211–216, 1999.

[24] C. E. Bolton, A. A. Ionescu, K. M. Shiels et al., "Associated loss of fat-free mass and bone mineral density in chronic obstructive pulmonary disease," *American Journal of Respiratory and Critical Care Medicine*, vol. 170, no. 12, pp. 1286–1293, 2004.

[25] K. Panday, A. Gona, and M. B. Humphrey, "Medication-induced osteoporosis: screening and treatment strategies," *Therapeutic Advances in Musculoskeletal Disease*, vol. 6, no. 5, pp. 185–202, 2014.

[26] E. Israel, T. R. Banerjee, G. M. Fitzmaurice, T. V. Kotlov, K. LaHive, and M. S. LeBoff, "Effects of inhaled glucocorticoids on bone density in premenopausal women," *The New England Journal of Medicine*, vol. 345, no. 13, pp. 941–947, 2001.

[27] G. T. Ferguson, P. M. A. Calverley, J. A. Anderson et al., "Prevalence and progression of osteoporosis in patients with COPD: results from the towards a revolution in COPD health study," *Chest*, vol. 136, no. 6, pp. 1456–1465, 2009.

[28] O. Johnell, R. Pauwels, C. G. Löfdahl et al., "Bone mineral density in patients with chronic obstructive pulmonary disease treated with budesonide Turbuhaler®," *European Respiratory Journal*, vol. 19, no. 6, pp. 1058–1063, 2002.

[29] E. Casado, M. Larrosa, E. Naval et al., "Osteoporosis in men with chronic obstructive pulmonary disease. Utility of phalangeal densitometry (AccuDEXA) as a screening method," *Reumatologia Clinica*, vol. 1, no. 1, pp. 7–11, 2005.

[30] T.-T. Dam, S. Harrison, H. A. Fink, J. Ramsdell, and E. Barrett-Connor, "Bone mineral density and fractures in older men with chronic obstructive pulmonary disease or asthma," *Osteoporosis International*, vol. 21, no. 8, pp. 1341–1349, 2010.

[31] S. A. Sternberg, R. Levin, S. Dkaidek, S. Edelman, T. Resnick, and J. Menczel, "Frailty and osteoporosis in older women—a prospective study," *Osteoporosis International*, vol. 25, no. 2, pp. 763–768, 2014.

[32] X. Jiang, L. E. Good, R. Spinka, and P. F. Schnatz, "Osteoporosis screening in postmenopausal women aged 50–64 years: BMI alone compared with current screening tools," *Maturitas*, vol. 83, pp. 59–64, 2016.

[33] D. M. Biskobing, "Copd and osteoporosis," *Chest*, vol. 121, no. 2, pp. 609–620, 2002.

[34] P. Ravn, G. Cizza, N. H. Bjarnason et al., "Low body mass index is an important risk factor for low bone mass and increased bone loss in early postmenopausal women. Early Postmenopausal Intervention Cohort (EPIC) study group," *Journal of Bone and Mineral Research*, vol. 14, no. 9, pp. 1622–1627, 1999.

[35] L. Graat-Verboom, B. E. E. M. van den Borne, F. W. J. M. Smeenk, M. A. Spruit, and E. F. M. Wouters, "Osteoporosis in COPD outpatients based on bone mineral density and vertebral fractures," *Journal of Bone and Mineral Research*, vol. 26, no. 3, pp. 561–568, 2011.

[36] V. P. Balasubramanian and B. Varkey, "Chronic obstructive pulmonary disease: effects beyond the lungs," *Current Opinion in Pulmonary Medicine*, vol. 12, no. 2, pp. 106–112, 2006.

20

An Innovative Approach to Evaluate the Morphological Patterns of Soft Palate in Oral Submucous Fibrosis Patients: A Digital Cephalometric Study

Chintamaneni Raja Lakshmi, Dharmavaram Ayesha Thabusum, and Sujana Mulk Bhavana

Department of Oral Medicine and Radiology, Drs. Sudha & Nageswara Rao Siddhartha Institute of Dental Sciences, Gannavaram Mandal, Krishna District, Andhra Pradesh 521286, India

Correspondence should be addressed to Chintamaneni Raja Lakshmi; lakshmi.chintamaneni@yahoo.com

Academic Editor: Jens Klotsche

Oral submucous fibrosis (OSMF) is a chronic insidious disease affecting mucosa and submucosa of oral cavity and soft palate. The present study aimed to evaluate the morphology of soft palate in normal individuals and OSMF patients using lateral cephalometry and to compare and correlate these variants of soft palate with different stages of OSMF. 100 subjects were included in the study, who were divided into two groups. Group I included 50 subjects with clinical diagnosis of OSMF and Group II included 50 normal subjects (control group). Using digital lateral cephalometry, velar length and width were measured and soft palatal patterns were categorized based on You et al.'s classification. Leaf and rat-tail patterns of soft palate were predominant in control group, whereas butt and crook shaped variants were more in study group. Anteroposterior (A-P) length of soft palate was significantly greater in stage I OSMF, while superoinferior (S-I) width was greater in stage III OSMF. Interestingly, a negative correlation was observed in staging of OSMF and A-P dimensions. As the staging of OSMF advances, the A-P length of soft palate decreases, but S-I width increases.

1. Introduction

The soft palate is the posterior fibrovascular part of the palate that is attached to the posterior edge of the hard palate [1]. It participates in most of the oral functions like speech, swallowing, and respiration [2]. Although continuous research on dimensional analysis of soft palate and its surrounding structures has been made, still there is a gap in the identification of soft palate morphological patterns and configuration. Soft palate plays a very crucial role in velopharyngeal closure, that is, approximation of soft palate with pharyngeal walls. This sphincteric mechanism separates nasal and oral cavity during speech and deglutition [3]. In this context, the study of these soft palate patterns like shape, length, and width offers a clue to evaluate any risk factors for velopharyngeal incompetence. Various authors conducted studies to assess the dimensional changes of soft palate with increasing age and changes in cleft lip and palate and in patients with sleep apnea using cephalometry [4, 5] whereas studies regarding OSMF were very limited.

Oral submucous fibrosis is a chronic progressive disease affecting any part of the oral cavity and sometimes the pharynx. It is always associated with juxtaepithelial inflammatory reaction followed by fibroelastic change of the lamina propria with epithelial atrophy. The clinical manifestations include stomatitis, limited mouth opening, difficulty in speech and swallowing, and even hearing loss [6]. Oral submucous fibrosis is one such pathology that could alter the dimensions of soft tissue components like oral mucosa and soft palate; in this aspect, the present study aimed to evaluate the morphological patterns of soft palate in both normal and oral submucous fibrosis individuals. According to the literature search, to the best of our knowledge, only two studies have been reported to date.

2. Materials and Methods

All the procedures conducted in the present study were in compliance with the declaration of Helsinki (2000) and the study protocol was approved by the institutional ethical committee of Drs. Sudha & Nageswara Rao Siddhartha Institute of Dental Sciences, Gannavaram, India. A total of 100 subjects with age range of 20–70 years were included in this study. The subjects were randomly selected from the outpatient Department of Oral Medicine and Radiology. They were divided into two groups: Group 1 (study group) comprising 50 subjects who were clinically diagnosed with oral submucous fibrosis and Group 2 (control group) requiring lateral cephalograms for a diagnostic purpose.

Exclusion criteria were as follows: patients with history of systemic diseases, syndromes, fractures of head and neck, and cleft palate were excluded from the study.

Clinical diagnosis and staging of oral submucous fibrosis were done based on classification suggested by Nagesh and Bailoor [7].

Characteristics of stage I, early OSMF, included the following: mild blanching, no restriction in mouth opening (normal distance between central incisor tips: males, 35 to 45 mm; females, 30 to 42 mm), and no restriction in tongue protrusion. Characteristics of stage II, moderate OSMF, included the following: moderate to severe blanching, reduced mouth opening by 33%, demonstrably reduced cheek flexibility also, burning sensation also in the absence of stimuli, palpable bands felt, lymphadenopathy either unilateral or bilateral, and demonstrable anemia on hematological examination. Characteristics of stage III, severe OSMF, included the following: very severe burning sensation. The patient was unable to carry out day-to-day work, with more than 66% reduction in the mouth opening, cheek flexibility, and tongue protrusion. The tongue may appear to be fixed. Ulcerative lesions may appear on the cheek, thick palpable bands and lymphadenopathy bilaterally evident.

All lateral cephalograms were taken using digital radiographic machine (Kodak 8000 digital panoramic and cephalometric machine, Italy). A tube potential of 82 kV, a tube current of 10 mA, and an exposure time of 500 ms were used to optimize the contrast of the digital images. The digital radiographs were processed and viewed by using Kodak dental imaging software, version 6.12. Lateral cephalometric analysis was performed to evaluate the different morphological patterns of soft palate by taking the radiographs in standardized position.

All the radiographs were observed and categorized into six types according to the soft palate morphology and were evaluated by two oral and maxillofacial radiologists. The anteroposterior (A-P) length was evaluated by measuring the linear distance from the posterior nasal spine to the tip of the uvula of the resting palate. The superoinferior (S-I) width was measured at the thickest section of the velum. Different patterns of soft palate were recorded, based on classification by You et al. [1], as follows: type 1 (leaf shape), type 2 (rat-tail shape), type 3 (butt-like shape), type 4 (straight line shape), type 5 (S-shape), and type 6 (crook appearance of the soft palate).

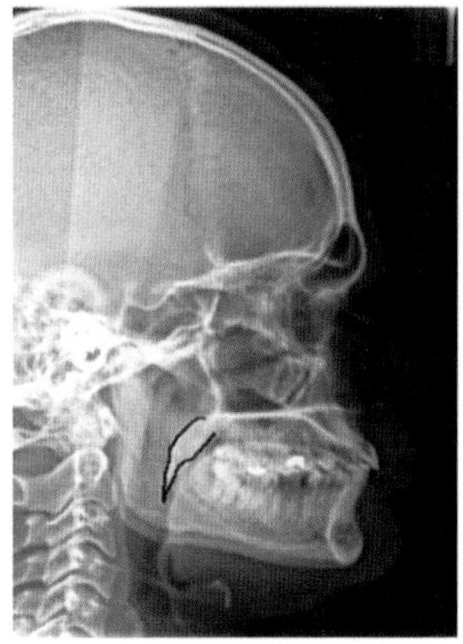

FIGURE 1: Lateral cephalogram with type 1 (leaf shaped) pattern of soft palate.

2.1. Statistical Analysis. All statistical procedures were performed using Statistical Package for the Social Sciences (SPSS) version 16. The significance of the differences between the means and the distribution of various patterns of soft palate were evaluated using Mann-Whitney *U* test and Kruskal Wallis test. Correlation between the considered parameters was performed using Spearman rank correlation test. p value < 0.05 was set to be statistically significant.

3. Results

In the present study, the mean age of the subjects was 39 years. On the basis of the radiographic appearances in the lateral cephalograms, the soft palate patterns were categorized as type 1 ("leaf shape"), which was lanceolate, indicating that the middle portion of the soft palate elevated to both the naso- and the oro-side (Figure 1); type 2 (when the soft palate showed that the anterior portion was inflated and the free margin had an obvious coarctation, the radiographic appearance was described as having a "rat-tail shape") (Figure 2); type 3 ("butt-like" soft palate showed a shorter and fatter velum appearance, and the width had almost no distinct difference from the anterior portion to the free margin) (Figure 3); type 4 (which indicated that the image of the soft palate presented a "straight line shape") (Figure 4); type 5 (the distorted soft palate presented the S-shape); type 6 (which revealed a "crook" appearance of the soft palate, in which the posterior portion of the soft palate crooks anterosuperiorly) (Figure 5) [1]. The highest percentage of rat-tail shaped soft palate was present in control group. Similarly, a high percentage of butt-like and crooked shaped soft palates were present in the study group. Kruskal Wallis test was used for comparing the mean values of A-P length and S-I width in

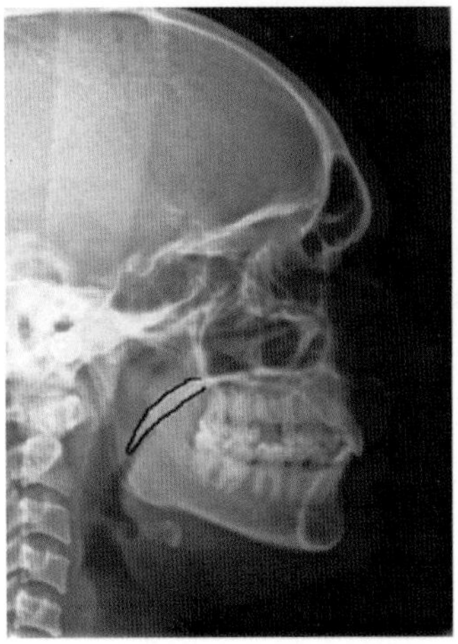

Figure 2: Rat-tail shape seen on lateral cephalogram.

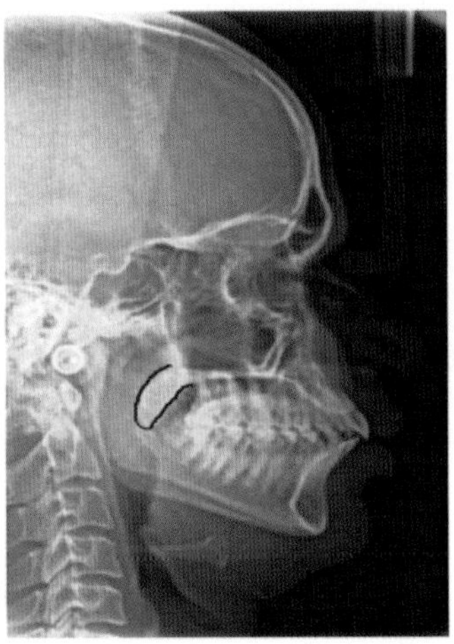

Figure 3: Lateral cephalogram depicting type 3 (butt shape) pattern of soft palate.

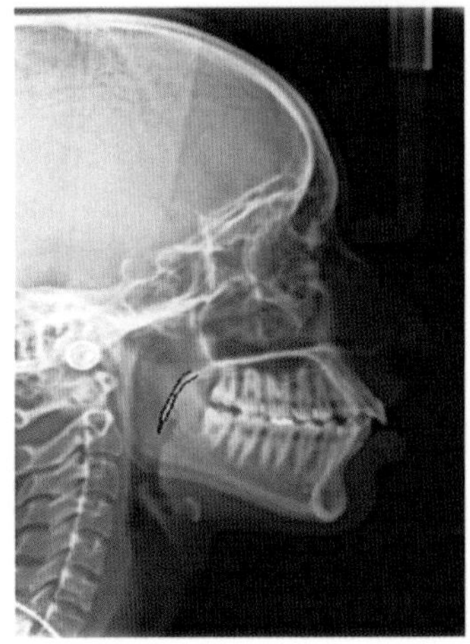

Figure 4: Lateral cephalogram showing type 4 (straight line) pattern of soft palate.

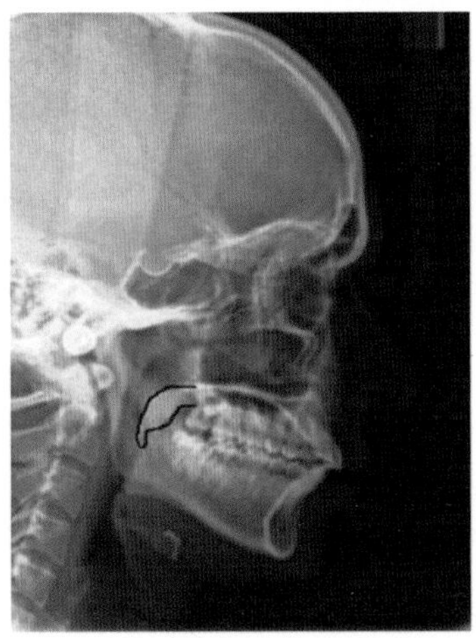

Figure 5: Crook shape seen on lateral cephalogram.

both groups according to type-wise distribution, showing significant difference ($p < 0.05$) in both A-P length and S-I width in type 1 pattern. In type 2 and 3 soft palate patterns, a difference in dimensions was significant only with A-P length and in type 6 with regard to S-I width ($p < 0.05$). No significant difference was observed ($p < 0.05$) between study and control group with respect to S-I width in types 2, 3, and 4 and A-P length in types 4 and 6 ($p > 0.05$). The highest A-P length was observed in leaf shaped soft palate, while the highest S-I width was observed in butt-like soft palate in both groups (Table 1).

Mann-Whitney U test was used to measure the A-P length and S-I width of soft palate showing mean value of A-P length as 32.09 in study group and 35.29 in control group. Mean value of S-I width was 10.19 and 9.23 in study and control groups, respectively, with statistically significant p value of 0.001. This indicates that A-P length was significantly greater in the control group, while S-I width was significantly greater in the study group. This specifies that the soft palate becomes short and stout/bulky in OSMF (Table 2).

Type-wise distribution of soft palate patterns according to staging of OSMF in the study group showed 79.16% of cases with type 1 and 55.56% of cases with type 2 soft palate pattern in stage II OSMF. 66.66% of type 3 and the highest percentage of cases showing type 6 soft palate variant were seen in stage III OSMF. One in each of stage I and II OSMF showed type 4 variant (Table 3).

The mean length and width of soft palate patterns according to stagewise distribution of OSMF revealed that the A-P length of soft palate is significantly greater in stage I than in stage II. The S-I width of stage III palate is significantly greater than of stage I and stage II (Table 4).

Interestingly, a negative correlation was observed in staging of OSMF and A-P dimensions. That is, as the staging increases, the A-P dimension decreases, but the S-I dimension increases along with staging (Table 5).

TABLE 1: Comparison of anteroposterior (A-P) length and superoinferior (S-I) width in the study and control group using Kruskal Wallis test.

Type of soft palate	Length of soft palate	Group	*N* (number) (%)	Mean	Standard deviation	*p* value
Type 1	A-P length	Study group	24 (52.2%)	34.00	2.552	0.001*
		Control group	22 (47.8%)	36.82	1.107	
	S-I width	Study group	24	10.14	.629	0.007*
		Control group	22	9.73	.400	
Type 2	A-P length	Study group	9 (34.6%)	31.80	.993	0.001*
		Control group	17 (65.4%)	35.31	.893	
	S-I width	Study group	9	8.34	.770	0.062
		Control group	17	8.60	.357	
Type 3	A-P length	Study group	10 (66.7%)	28.99	1.382	0.020*
		Control group	5 (33.3%)	30.64	.772	
	S-I width	Study group	10	11.66	.538	0.327
		Control group	5	11.42	.326	
Type 4	A-P length	Study group	2 (40.0%)	28.98	1.202	0.083
		Control group	3 (60.0%)	35.15	.507	
	S-I width	Study group	2	9.80	.778	0.083
		Control group	3	5.62	.195	
Type 6	A-P length	Study group	5 (62.5%)	30.89	1.269	0.230
		Control group	3 (37.5%)	31.90	1.294	
	S-I width	Study group	5	10.95	.325	0.025*
		Control group	3	9.14	.259	

*Statistically significant, $p < 0.05$.

TABLE 2: Mean distribution of anteroposterior (A-P) length and superoinferior (S-I) width in the study group and control group using Mann-Whitney *U* test.

Velar dimensions	Group	*N* (total number)	Mean	Standard deviation	*p* value
A-P length	Study group	50	32.09	2.834	0.001*
	Control group	50	35.29	2.209	
S-I width	Study group	50	10.19	1.220	0.001*
	Control group	50	9.23	1.288	

*Statistically significant, $p < 0.05$.

TABLE 3: Cross tabulation for type of soft palate and staging of OSMF.

Type of soft palate	Stage I	Stage II	Stage III	Total
Type 1	2	19	3	24
	8.33%	79.16%	12.5%	100%
Type 2	4	5	0	9
	44.44%	55.56%	0.00%	100%
Type 3	0	4	6	9
	0.00%	44.44%	66.66%	100%
Type 4	1	1	0	2
	50%	50%	0.00%	100%
Type 6	0	0	5	5
	0.00%	0.00%	100%	100%

4. Discussion

The assessment of the soft tissue elements like soft palate and surrounding structures cephalometry is a comparatively economical method [8]. The dimensional analysis of the soft palate and its surrounding structures, especially the velar length and width, which has been overlooked in the past, is reasonably responsible for the different dimensions of the soft palate [9]. To diagnose varied pathologies of soft palate like neoplastic, neurologic, and inflammatory conditions, radiological investigations were greatly helpful. Morphological variants of soft palate play a very crucial role especially in conditions like cleft palate and obstructive sleep apnea [10]. Velopharyngeal insufficiency and hypernasal speech are still the topic of debate in surgically successful but functionally compromised cases owing to varied morphologies of

Table 4: The mean anteroposterior (A-P) length and superoinferior (S-I) width of soft palate patterns according to stagewise distribution of OSMF using Kruskal Wallis test.

Velar dimensions	OSMF staging	*N*	Mean	Standard deviation	*p* value
A-P length	Stage I	7	32.96	1.844	0.002*
	Stage II	29	32.70	3.055	
	Stage III	14	29.98	1.385	
	Total	50	32.09	2.834	
S-I width	Stage I	7	8.97	1.001	0.001*
	Stage II	29	10.00	1.152	
	Stage III	14	11.18	.592	
	Total	50	10.19	1.220	

*Statistically significant, $p < 0.05$.

Table 5: Correlation of anteroposterior (A-P) length and superoinferior (S-I) width with the staging of OSMF using Spearman rank correlation.

	A-P length	S-I width
Staging of OSMF	−.461*	.619*
p value	0.001	0.000
N (total number)	50	50

*Statistically significant, $p < 0.05$.

soft palate and surrounding structures. Henceforth, proper assessment of soft tissue morphology is mandatory to gain better results.

Oral submucous fibrosis is a chronic insidious disease of the oral cavity affecting mucosa and submucosa of soft palate, anterior faucial pillars, buccal mucosa, tongue, and lips [11, 12]. Gaining meticulous knowledge regarding changes in soft palate morphology due to OSMF will be helpful for proper diagnosis and successful structural and functional outcome. According to literature search, there were only limited studies regarding this aspect; hence, the present study was performed to evaluate morphological changes of soft palate in OSMF patients and comparison was done with normal individuals.

In our study group, 52.2% had leaf shape soft palate which was the most common variant, with straight line variant being the least common type. The S-shape soft palate was not observed in both study and control groups. These findings were consistent with the study conducted by Shankar et al. [13]. In the control group, rat-tail shaped soft palate was predominantly seen, and straight line and crook shaped patterns were the least common. Our results were similar to a study conducted by Praveen et al. [14]. But according to You et al. [1], Kumar and Gopal [15], and Verma et al. [16], leaf shaped soft palate was described as the most common variant and crook shape as the least common variant.

In the current study, stage II OSMF was predominantly seen in 29 cases, in which type 1 pattern was seen in 19 cases (leaf shape), type 2 (rat-tail shape) in 5 cases, type 3 (butt-like shape) in 4 cases, and type 4 (straight line) in 1 case. Stage III OSMF was observed in 14 cases, in which type 1 was shown in 3 cases (leaf shape), type 3 (butt-like shape) in 6 cases, and type 6 (crook shape) in 5 cases. Seven cases were seen in stage I OSMF, among which type 1 (leaf shape) was seen in 2 cases, type 2 (rat-tail shape) in 4 cases, and type 4 (straight line) in 1 case. Based on the above findings, soft palate shows morphological changes with the progression of the disease, that is, long narrow type getting transformed into short thick pattern. These changes were attributed to the fibrosis of the mucosal covering of soft palate and uvula. These findings were in accordance with Shankar et al. and Mohan et al. [13, 17].

The mean length of type 1 (leaf shape) soft palate in the present study was 34 mm whereas for normal individuals it was 36.82 mm. The S-I width in the study group was 10.14 mm and in normal individuals it was 9.73 mm. There is significant reduction in length of the soft palate in the study group when compared with control group. This type of soft palate was seen in 7 cases of stage I, 19 cases of stage II, and 3 cases of stage III OSMF.

Type 2 (rat-tail) soft palate was noted in 4 cases of stage I OSMF and 5 cases of stage II OSMF. The mean A-P length and S-I width in the present study were 31.80 mm and 8.34 mm whereas for normal individuals they were 35.31 mm and 8.60 mm. The difference was statistically significant regarding anteroposterior length ($p < 0.05$). However, Shankar et al. reported no significant difference pertaining to both length and width of type 2 soft palate.

Type 3 (butt-like) soft palate was seen in 4 cases of stage II OSMF and 6 cases of stage III OSMF. The A-P length was 28.99 mm in the study group and 30.64 mm in normal individuals. The S-I width in the study and control group was 11.66 mm and 11.42 mm, respectively. There was a significant difference in A-P length. Even as there was a mild difference observed in S-I width, the difference was not statistically significant ($p > 0.05$). Considering the findings, a slight increase in the width and reduction in the length of soft palate were found. Similar findings were observed in the study conducted by Shankar et al. [13], while contradictory results were obtained according to Verma et al. [16].

Type 4 (straight line) variety of soft palate was seen in one case in each of stage I and II OSMF. The mean A-P length in study and control group was 28.98 mm and 35.15 mm, respectively. The S-I widths between the study group (9.80 mm) and control group (5.62 mm) were compared. Even though the length and width were less in the study group when compared to control group, the results were not statistically significant which may be due to small sample size.

Pépin et al. found the S-shape (type 5) which had hooked appearance of the soft palate in their study, with angulation of about 30° between distal part of uvula and longitudinal axis of soft palate. Therefore, the study concluded that hooked appearance in awake patients indicates a high risk for obstructive sleep apnea syndrome [18]. Kumar and Gopal [15] conducted a study in 100 normal individuals to evaluate the soft palate patterns and found only 2% of the cases showing S-shape (type 5) pattern of soft palate. Praveen et al. [14] reported 2.5% of the cases presented with this pattern. Amusingly, this type of soft palate was not observed in our study.

Type 6 (crook shaped) soft palate was seen in 5 cases of stage III OSMF. The mean A-P length was 30.89 mm whereas for normal individuals it was 31.9 mm and the mean S-I widths were 10.95 mm and 9.14 mm in normal individuals. There was a significant difference concerning the S-I width.

Stage I OSMF was seen in 7 cases where A-P length was 32.96 mm and S-I width was 8.97 mm and where the length is almost comparable with normal individuals, that is, 35.29 mm. In stage II OSMF, A-P length and S-I width were 32.70 mm and 10.00 mm and for stage III they were 29.98 mm and 11.18 mm, respectively. But the change is more pronounced in A-P length than in S-I width. These changes can be attributed to the fact that the length of the soft palate and uvula corresponds to the stage of the disease, that is, gradual shortening of soft palate and uvula with the progression in the staging of OSMF.

In our study, there was a gradual change in the dimensions and patterns of soft palate with advance in staging of OSMF and interestingly a negative correlation was observed in staging of OSMF and anteroposterior dimensions. That is, as the staging advances, the anteroposterior dimension decreases, but the superoinferior dimension increases along with staging. Type 1 and 2 variants of soft palate were predominantly seen in initial stages of OSMF, whereas type 3 and 6 variants were observed in advanced stages of OSMF. There is further scope for validating this field with a larger sample size.

Competing Interests

The authors declare that there is no conflict of interests regarding the publication of this paper.

References

[1] M. You, X. Li, H. Wang et al., "Morphological variety of the soft palate in normal individuals: a digital cephalometric study," *Dentomaxillofacial Radiology*, vol. 37, no. 6, pp. 344–349, 2008.

[2] K. L. Moore and A. M. R. Agur, Eds., *Essential Clinical Anatomy*, Lippincott, Williams and Wilkins, Philadelphia, Pa, USA, 2nd edition, 2002.

[3] D. F. Johns, R. J. Rohrich, and M. Awada, "Velopharyngeal incompetence: a guide for clinical evaluation," *Plastic and Reconstructive Surgery*, vol. 112, no. 7, pp. 1890–1898, 2003.

[4] Š. Bejdová, V. Krajíček, M. Peterka, P. Trefný, and J. Velemínská, "Variability in palatal shape and size in patients with bilateral complete cleft lip and palate assessed using dense surface model construction and 3D geometric morphometrics," *Journal of Cranio-Maxillofacial Surgery*, vol. 40, no. 3, pp. 201–208, 2012.

[5] K. Shimomatsu, E. Nozoe, K. Ishihata, T. Okawachi, and N. Nakamura, "Three-dimensional analyses of facial soft tissue configuration of Japanese females with jaw deformity—a trial of polygonal view of facial soft tissue deformity in orthognathic patients," *Journal of Cranio-Maxillo-Facial Surgery*, vol. 40, no. 7, pp. 559–567, 2012.

[6] J. J. Pindborg and S. M. Sirsat, "Oral submucous fibrosis," *Oral Surgery, Oral Medicine, Oral Pathology*, vol. 22, no. 6, pp. 764–779, 1966.

[7] D. Gupta, M. Gupta, and B. Golher, "Oral submucous fibrosis: clinical study and management by physiofibrolysis," *Journal of Indian Dental Association*, vol. 52, pp. 375–378, 1980.

[8] I. Kollias and O. Krogstad, "Adult craniofacial and pharyngeal changes—a longitudinal cephalometric study between 22 and 42 years of age. Part II: morphological uvulo-glossopharyngeal changes," *European Journal of Orthodontics*, vol. 21, no. 4, pp. 345–355, 1999.

[9] M. A. Bitar, A. T. Macari, and J. G. Ghafari, "Correspondence between subjective and linear measurements of the palatal airway on lateral cephalometric radiographs," *Archives of Otolaryngology—Head and Neck Surgery*, vol. 136, no. 1, pp. 43–47, 2010.

[10] T. E. Nelson, J. B. Mulliken, and B. L. Padwa, "Effect of midfacial distraction on the obstructed airway in patients with syndromic bilateral coronal synostosis," *Journal of Oral and Maxillofacial Surgery*, vol. 66, no. 11, pp. 2318–2321, 2008.

[11] F. Tanwir and H. Akhlaq, "Oral submucous fibrosis: a chronic deliberating disease of oral cavity," *Iranian Journal of Pathology*, vol. 6, no. 4, pp. 165–172, 2011.

[12] W. M. Tilakaratne, M. F. Klinikowski, T. Saku, T. J. Peters, and S. Warnakulasuriya, "Oral submucous fibrosis: review on aetiology and pathogenesis," *Oral Oncology*, vol. 42, no. 6, pp. 561–568, 2006.

[13] V. N. Shankar, K. Hegde, N. S. Ashwini, V. Praveena, and S. M. Ravi Prakash, "Morphometric evaluation of soft palate in oral submucous fibrosis—a digital cephalometric study," *Journal of Cranio-Maxillofacial Surgery*, vol. 42, no. 1, pp. 48–52, 2014.

[14] B. N. Praveen, S. Amrutesh, S. Pal, A. K. Shubashini, and S. Vaseemuddin, "Various shapes of soft palate. A lateral cephalometric study," *World Journal of Dentistry*, vol. 2, no. 3, pp. 207–210, 2011.

[15] D. K. Kumar and K. S. Gopal, "Morphological variants of soft palate in normal individuals: a digital cephalometric study," *Journal of Clinical and Diagnostic Research*, vol. 5, no. 6, pp. 1310–1313, 2012.

[16] P. Verma, K. G. Verma, K. L. Kumaraswam, S. Basavaraju, S. K. Sachdeva, and S. Juneja, "Correlation of morphological variants of the soft palate and need's ratio in normal individuals—a digital cephalometric study," *Imaging Science in Dentistry*, vol. 44, no. 3, pp. 193–198, 2014.

[17] R. P. Mohan, S. Verma, U. Singh, and N. Agarwal, "Morphometric evaluation of soft palate in oral submucous fibrosis—a digital cephalometric analysis," *West African Journal of Radiology*, vol. 21, no. 1, pp. 7–11, 2014.

[18] J. L. D. Pépin, D. Veale, G. R. Ferretti, P. Mayer, and P. A. Levy, "Obstructive sleep apnea syndrome: hooked appearance of the soft palate in awake patients—cephalometric and CT findings," *Radiology*, vol. 210, no. 1, pp. 163–170, 1999.

21

COPD in a Population-Based Sample of Never-Smokers: Interactions among Sex, Gender, and Race

Esme Fuller-Thomson,[1] Rachel S. Chisholm,[1] and Sarah Brennenstuhl[2]

[1]*Factor-Inwentash Faculty of Social Work, University of Toronto, Toronto, ON, Canada*
[2]*Lawrence Bloomberg Faculty of Nursing, University of Toronto, Toronto, ON, Canada*

Correspondence should be addressed to Esme Fuller-Thomson; esme.fuller.thomson@utoronto.ca

Academic Editor: Sreekumar Pillai

This observational epidemiological study investigates sex/gender and racial differences in prevalence of COPD among never-smokers. Data were derived from the 2012 Center for Disease Control's Behavioral Risk Factor Surveillance System. The sample consisted of 129,535 non-Hispanic whites and blacks 50 years of age and older who had never smoked. Descriptive and multivariable analyses were conducted, with the latter using a series of logistic regression models predicting COPD status by sex/gender and race, adjusting for age, height, socioeconomic position (SEP), number of household members, marital status, and health insurance coverage. Black women have the highest prevalence of COPD (7.0%), followed by white women (5.2%), white men (2.9%), and black men (2.4%). Women have significantly higher odds of COPD than men. When adjusting for SEP, black and white women have comparably higher odds of COPD than white men (black women OR = 1.66; 99% CI = 1.46, 1.88; white women OR = 1.49; 99% CI = 1.37, 1.63), while black men have significantly lower odds (OR = 0.62; 99% CI = 0.49, 0.79). This research provides evidence that racial inequalities in COPD (or lack thereof) may be related to SEP.

1. Introduction

Chronic Obstructive Pulmonary Disease (COPD) is the third leading cause of death in the US [1] and a principal cause of disability [2, 3]. Primary smoking is the largest, single risk factor for COPD; however, it is estimated that more than half of COPD cases can be attributed to other causes [4]. With smoking rates decreasing in the US [5], there is an increasing need to identify, among never-smokers, groups that have higher odds of COPD to target prevention.

1.1. Sex, Gender, and COPD. COPD prevalence has been higher among women than men in most age groups for more than two decades [6–8]. As women's smoking rates peaked later than men's, this trend may be explained by the long-latency period of COPD [6, 9]. Other biological explanations may also be relevant [10]. For instance, women have narrower thoracic width and shorter height than men, potentially causing cigarette smoke to be more concentrated in their overall smaller lungs [11]. Women may also have heightened bronchial responsiveness, resulting in particles being deposited more deeply within their lungs [10]. Other biological mechanisms include greater lung growth impairment among female adolescents exposed to cigarette smoke than among similarly-exposed males [12], sex differences in cigarette metabolism resulting in increased production of airway-toxic molecules in women [10], and interactions between hormones and genetic factors that interfere with normal lung functioning [13]. Women's heightened biological vulnerability to COPD is relevant to never-smokers exposed to secondhand smoke and other airborne toxins. Approximately 11% and 7% of COPD cases can be attributed to environmental smoke exposure at home and work, respectively [14]. Low income and poverty increase rates of contact with secondhand smoke, and women are more likely than men to live below the poverty line [9, 15]. Importantly, people with low income, who are disproportionately women, also have a higher chance of being exposed to air pollution, another suspected risk factor for COPD [16]. That is, vulnerabilities relating to sex (i.e., biological differences between women and men) and gender (i.e., social differences between women and men) may contribute to never-smoking women's higher risk of COPD.

1.2. Race and COPD. Another group experiencing detrimental trends surrounding COPD is black Americans, whose mortality from the disease has been increasing faster than other racial groups [17]. Higher rates of smoking among black men can only partially explain the trend, as black women have one of the lowest rates of smoking [5]. Another possible biological explanation is that black Americans have lower sitting heights, on average, than whites, which is linked to lower lung function [18]. Metabolism of cigarette smoke may also vary by race, with cotinine half-life shown to be more elevated in blacks compared to whites [19]. These biological vulnerabilities are relevant to never-smokers, especially because black Americans are disproportionately exposed to higher levels of secondhand smoke [20]. This can be attributed, in part, to higher levels of poverty among black than white Americans [21] and higher likelihood of living in multiunit dwellings [22, 23]. People living in these residences are found to have higher levels of cotinine in their system than those living in single-family dwellings, even if no household member smokes [20].

The purpose of the current study is to investigate sex/gender and racial inequalities in COPD among never-smokers, in a large, representative sample of black and white Americans over the age of 50. We hypothesize that women and black Americans will have higher odds of COPD and that height (a proxy for lung size) and socioeconomic position (SEP) will help explain the association. We also expect a significant interaction between sex and race, such that black never-smoking women will have the highest odds of COPD compared to other groups.

2. Methods

2.1. Sample. Data for the current study are drawn from the 2012 Behavioural Risk Surveillance System. The BRFSS collects ongoing data assessing state-specific behavioral risk factors in the adult population [24]. On a monthly basis, trained interviewers administer a standardized questionnaire over the phone (landline and cellular) to a representative sample of noninstitutionalized adults, aged 18 or older, who are living in households. The BRFSS uses a disproportionate-stratified sample design, which involves dividing all possible phone numbers into high- and medium-density groups, which are then sampled separately. In the current study, we restrict the sample to non-Hispanic white and non-Hispanic black respondents over the age of 50 (i.e., the age over which COPD is most likely to be present) who have never smoked (n = 129,535). Our final sample contained 8,674 black women, 2,708 black men, 80,317 white women, and 37,836 white men.

2.2. Measures. Self-report of a medical diagnosis of COPD was the outcome measure. It was ascertained by positive response to the question of whether a "doctor, nurse or another health professional" ever told the respondent that they had "Chronic Obstructive Pulmonary Disease or COPD, emphysema or chronic bronchitis." There were very little missing data for this question (<0.5% of full sample).

While gender was not measured per se, sex was assessed by self-report using two categories of male and female. Race was also determined by self-report. We included in the analysis those who are identified as non-Hispanic and either white or black/African American (herein referred to as white and black, resp.). There were no missing data on sex and 1.4% missing on race.

Based on a review of the literature, we included height and SEP in the modeling as theoretically important explanatory factors. Height was self-reported (in inches) and entered into the models as a continuous variable (missing = 1.2%). SEP was measured by highest level of education (missing = 0.4%) and net annual household income (missing = 14%). Both were included in the modeling as categorical variables. To prevent losing a large amount of data on household income, a missing category was included.

We controlled for a number of variables in the modeling, including age (by decade, missing = 0.96%) and health care coverage (i.e., whether the respondent reported having health insurance, missing = 0.3%). Also, as an attempt to account for whether the respondent was living or married to a smoker, we adjusted for the number of people in the household (1, 2, ≥3) and marital status (missing = 0.5%). A missing category is included for household size as it was only asked among those sampled over a landline.

2.3. Statistical Analyses. All analyses were undertaken using IBM SPSS version 23. The prevalence of COPD was estimated and differences in COPD status across study variables were tested using the chi-square test for ordinal/categorical variables and t-test for continuous variables. To test our primary hypothesis, we undertook a series of logistic regression models. First, we tested for an interaction between sex/gender and race for predicting COPD status using a likelihood ratio test that compared a model with the main effects and age only with one that also included the interaction terms. Consistent with our initial hypothesis, a significant interaction was found ($\Delta\chi^2$ = 27.16, Δdf = 1, and p < 0.001). To increase its interpretability, we created a four-level variable representing the combination of sex/gender and race as follows: black women, white women, black men, and white men (the reference group). In the first and each subsequent model, we predicted COPD status using this 4-level variable, while controlling for age. In the second model, we also included height. The third model included SEP. The final model included all variables simultaneously (i.e., age, height, and SEP, plus the control variables described above). As group comparisons in this model are all relative to white men, we also conducted contrasts that compare black and white women. To account for the multiple comparisons required to test our hypothesis, we used an adjusted p value of <0.01 to establish statistical significance. All data were weighted to account for selection and nonresponse bias.

3. Results

As shown in Table 1, less than one in 20 (4.4%) never-smokers over the age of 50 reported having a diagnosis of COPD (95% confidence interval (CI) = 4.3–4.5). Black women have the highest prevalence of COPD at 7.0% (95% CI = 6.5–7.5), followed by white women at 5.2% (95% CI = 5.0, 5.4), white men at 2.9% (95% CI = 2.7–3.0), and black men at 2.4% (95% CI = 2.1, 2.9). COPD prevalence increases significantly with age ($p < 0.001$) and with decreasing education and income levels (both $p < 0.001$). Those with COPD are significantly shorter than those without this condition (65.3 versus 66.5 inches; $p < 0.001$). A higher prevalence of COPD is found among those who live alone ($p < 0.001$) and who have a health insurance plan ($p = 0.001$).

Table 2 presents the series of logistic regression models predicting COPD status with the four-level sex/race variable as the focal independent variable. In the first model controlling only for age, both black (OR = 2.51) and white (OR = 1.70) women have higher odds of COPD than white men. Although the odds of COPD among black women are significantly higher than that of white women ($p < 0.001$), there is no difference between black and white men. When height is added to model 2, the relationships are attenuated, but the difference between black and white women remains (black women OR = 2.16; white women OR = 1.45; $p < 0.001$). When SEP is included in model 3, black and white women continue to have significantly higher odds of COPD than white men; however, two important changes happen. First, the odds of COPD for black women are attenuated much more than they are for white women (whose odds actually slightly increase), which results in the elimination of difference in the odds of COPD between black and white women using the adjusted p value (black women OR = 1.66; white women OR = 1.49; $p = 0.02$). Second, the odds of COPD among black men become significantly lower than those among white men (OR = 0.62; $p < 0.001$). Finally, in the fully adjusted model, both black and white women have significantly higher odds of COPD compared to white men and there is no difference between black and white women using the adjusted p value (black women OR = 1.55; white women OR = 1.41; $p = 0.03$). Also, consistent with the model including SEP, black men have significantly lower odds of COPD than white men (OR = 0.62; $p < 0.001$).

4. Discussion

The objective of this study was to investigate sex/gender and racial inequalities in COPD among never-smokers in a population-based sample of Americans. Consistent with our hypotheses, we find that sex/gender and race are associated with COPD prevalence but that the relationships are uniquely influenced by SEP. Specifically, we show that women (both black and white) have higher odds of COPD than men. This finding is consistent with prior research [8] and the hypothesis that females have an increased susceptibility to COPD due to an interaction of sex-related biological causes (e.g., poorer lung function [11]) and gender-associated structural factors (e.g., higher exposure to risk factors, such as secondhand smoke and air pollution [9]). We provide further support for this model by showing that controlling for height (an indicator of smaller lungs) and SEP each reduce the size of difference in odds of COPD among women versus men. Not surprisingly, neither factor individually (nor both together) entirely explains the relationship, suggesting that it is likely a complicated interplay of several biological factors along with a number of gender-related vulnerabilities that fully explain never-smoking women's increased prevalence of COPD.

Importantly, the current study also demonstrates that, among never-smokers, black women have higher odds of COPD than white women but that SEP appears to explain the difference. This finding contradicts an earlier study using the NHANES that found no age-adjusted black/white differences in the odds of self-report of physician-diagnosed COPD among never-smoking women [8]. The latter study, however, is comprised of an earlier cohort of adults, having been interviewed between the early 1970s and early 1980s, of whom only a small proportion were over the age of 50 and, thus, may differ from the BRFSS sample in important ways. It is well accepted that SEP is an important risk factor for lung function and COPD among nonsmokers [4, 25]. Our study finding that socioeconomic factors may be crucial in shaping racial inequalities in COPD, among women in particular, is consistent with knowledge that black women in the US are more likely to live in poverty than white women [26] and, thus, face increased exposure to toxins, such as secondhand smoke and air pollution. Multiple inequalities stemming from sex/gender and race, thus, may make black never-smoking women doubly vulnerable to COPD; however, as this study is the first, in our knowledge, to show higher odds among black never-smoking women prior to adjustment for SEP, further research is needed to confirm the finding in other samples.

Another important finding of the current study is that, among never-smoking men, controlling for SEP allows for a racial effect to emerge, such that black men are found to have *lower* odds of COPD than white men. This finding is consistent with prior research on never-smokers [8, 27]. While we hypothesized that the biological factors that increase black smokers' vulnerability to COPD would also elevate risks in never-smokers (e.g., shorter sitting height [18] and/or poorer metabolism of cigarette smoke [19]), it is likely that different factors are in play. An example may be alpha-1 antitrypsin deficiency, a genetic mutation linked to higher risk of COPD, which is more prevalent among white Americans than blacks [28]. However, if alpha-1 antitrypsin deficiency plays a role, it is unclear why the influence would not be comparable for black-white differences in women as well. While future research on never-smokers is needed to understand the mechanisms underlying COPD prevalence, our findings underscore the importance of considering SEP, without which causes for group-level variations (or lack thereof) may be obscured.

This study's findings must be considered in light of several limitations. One is that COPD was based on self-report of a medical diagnosis. Some smaller studies have shown self-report of a diagnosis of COPD to be quite accurate, when compared to medical charts (i.e., 86% [29] to 97% accurate

Table 1: Description of a sample of never-smoking Americans over the age of 50 according to COPD status (n = 129,535)[1].

	No COPD n = 123,389 (95.6%)	COPD n = 6,146 (4.4%)	p value[2]
Sex/gender and race			
White men	97.1%	2.9%	<0.001
Black men	97.6%	2.4%	
White women	94.8%	5.2%	
Black women	93.0%	7.0%	
Age by decade			
50s	97.0%	3.0%	<0.001
60s	95.3%	4.7%	
70s	94.0%	6.0%	
80s	93.5%	6.5%	
90s	93.2%	6.8%	
Height (mean, SD)	66.18 (4.07)	65.28 (3.98)	<0.001
Education			
Did not graduate high school	91.3%	8.7%	<0.001
Graduated high school	95.0%	5.0%	
Attended college or technical school	95.4%	4.6%	
Graduated from college or technical school	97.4%	2.6%	
Household income			
$75,000 or more	98.2%	1.8%	<0.001
$50,000 to less than $75,000	97.1%	2.9%	
$25,000–$49,999	94.5%	5.5%	
$15,000–$24,999	93.1%	6.9%	
<$15,000	90.0%	10.0%	
Missing	95.3%	4.7%	
Marital status			
Married/common-law	95.6%	4.4%	=0.367
Never married	95.4%	4.6%	
Number of adults/households			
1	94.0%	6.0%	<0.001
2	96.1%	3.9%	
≥3	95.7%	4.3%	
Missing	96.0%	4.0%	
Health plan			
Yes	94.9%	5.1%	=0.001
No	95.6%	4.4%	

[1] Sample sizes are presented in their unweighted form. Percentages are weighted to adjust for the probability of selection and nonresponse.
[2] p value is derived from chi-square tests for categorical variables and t-tests for continuous variables. Source: Behavioral Risk Factor Surveillance System 2012.

[30]). However, other larger, population-based studies have found poor correlation between self-report and measured airflow obstruction, with COPD being substantially underreported [31], and may be more so among blacks than whites [32]. With that being said, the prevalence of COPD found in the current study between 2.4% and 7.0% among nonsmokers is consistent with that reported based on measured airflow obstruction in the US among older nonsmoking adults [33] and in other general populations of nonsmokers [31]. Moreover, while underreporting (and underdiagnosis) may be higher in some groups than others due to lack of access to medical care, we found that controlling for medical care coverage had little effect on the relationships between sex and race and COPD. While we could not totally account

TABLE 2: Logistic regression of COPD by sex/gender and race in a sample of never-smoking Americans over the age of 50 (n = 129,535)[1].

	Model 1 OR (99% CI)	Model 2 Model 1 + height OR (99% CI)	Model 3 Model 1 + SEP OR (99% CI)	Model 4 Fully adjusted OR (99% CI)
Sex/gender, and race				
White men (Ref.)	1.00	1.00	1.00	1.00
Black men	0.89 (0.70, 1.13)	0.88 (0.69, 1.11)	0.62 (0.49, 0.79)	0.62 (0.49, 0.79)
Black women	2.51[a] (2.22, 2.84)	2.16[a] (1.87, 2.49)	1.66 (1.46, 1.88)	1.55 (1.34, 1.80)
White women	1.70[a] (1.56, 1.86)	1.45[a] (1.29, 1.63)	1.49 (1.37, 1.63)	1.41 (1.25, 1.59)
Age by decade				
50s (Ref.)	1.00	1.00	1.00	1.00
60s	1.55 (1.42, 1.70)	1.53 (1.40, 1.68)	1.37 (1.25, 1.50)	1.39 (1.27, 1.53)
70s	1.95 (1.77, 2.15)	1.91 (1.73, 2.10)	1.43 (1.29, 1.58)	1.45 (1.30, 1.62)
80s	2.11 (1.88, 2.36)	2.03 (1.81, 2.27)	1.40 (1.24, 1.57)	1.42 (1.25, 1.61)
90s	2.15 (1.66, 2.78)	2.03 (1.56, 2.63)	1.37 (1.05, 1.78)	1.38 (1.05, 1.81)
Height		0.97 (0.96, 0.99)	—	0.99 (0.99, 1.00)
Socioeconomic position				
Education				
Did not graduate high school	—	—	1.70 (1.49, 1.93)	1.67 (1.47, 1.91)
Graduated high school	—	—	1.19 (1.08, 1.34)	1.19 (1.07, 1.32)
Attended college or technical school	—	—	1.30 (1.17, 1.44)	1.29 (1.16, 1.44)
College or technical school graduate	—	—	1.00	1.00
Household income				
$75,000 or more (Ref.)	—	—	1.00	1.00
$50,000 to less than $75,000	—	—	1.46 (1.25, 1.70)	1.48 (1.27, 1.72)
$25,000–$49,999	—	—	2.50 (2.20, 2.84)	2.53 (2.22, 2.88)
$15,000–$24,999	—	—	2.92 (2.54, 3.35)	2.97 (2.57, 3.43)
<$15,000	—	—	4.24 (3.64, 4.92)	4.34 (3.71, 5.08)
Missing	—	—	1.97 (1.71, 2.27)	1.99 (1.73, 2.30)
Controls				
Marital status				
Married at least once	—	—	—	1.00
Never married				1.01 (0.88, 1.16)
Number of adults/households				
1	—	—	—	1.00
2	—	—	—	0.98 (0.89, 1.08)
≥3	—	—	—	1.21 (1.08, 1.36)
Missing	—	—	—	1.02 (0.90, 1.16)

TABLE 2: Continued.

	Model 1 OR (99% CI)	Model 2 Model 1 + height OR (99% CI)	Model 3 Model 1 + SEP OR (99% CI)	Model 4 Fully adjusted OR (99% CI)
Health plan				
Yes (Ref.)	—	—	—	1.00
No	—	—	—	0.94 (0.81, 1.08)
Nagelkerke R square value	0.026	0.027	0.057	0.057
−2 log likelihood	45940.0	45912.3	44716.7	44683.27

Sample sizes are presented in their unweighted form. Odds ratios, p values, and confidence intervals are weighted to adjust for the probability of selection and nonresponse.
[a]Difference is statistically significant at $p < 0.01$.
OR, Odds ratio; CI, confidence interval; SEP, socioeconomic position.
Source: Behavioral Risk Factor Surveillance System 2012.

for underreporting, the tendency to under- as opposed to overreport COPD means that if our results are biased, they would be biased towards the null.

Smoking status was also self-reported, which means that some of those in our selected sample of never-smokers may have had some history of smoking despite reporting otherwise. However, because our sample is older, we do not expect the negative stigma surrounding smoking, which could provoke underreporting, to be nearly as strong as it might be for younger cohorts. Moreover, systematic underreporting by some groups, such as those in higher socioeconomic groups, would have had the effect of reducing inequalities, thus making our results more conservative. It is important to keep in mind also that our sample is based on community-living adults and, thus, does not include those hospitalized or living in long-term care facilities, some of whom may have had the most severe cases of COPD. Future research using administrative data may remediate some of the issues discussed above.

Another limitation relates to how asthma is dealt with in analyses of COPD, especially when race is concerned, given that asthma prevalence is higher in black populations [34]. While it is clear, on one hand, that COPD and asthma represent distinct conditions, it is not clear, on the other hand, that one cannot evolve into another [35]. Furthermore, it is possible that those with concurrent asthma and COPD represent a unique phenotype [36]. Against this background of uncertainly in the causal role asthma plays on the pathway to COPD and how this pathway might vary by race, simply controlling for it in analyses of COPD may be unfounded. Accordingly, our models do not adjust for asthma diagnosis, which may have had an effect on our results. Future research on COPD and race should consider the issue of asthma comorbidity more centrally.

Finally, we were unable to control for country of birth. This is an important factor as exposure to smoke from biomass fuel, which is common for those growing up in low-income countries, and especially women, is a strong risk factor for COPD [4]. It is unlikely, however, that lack of control for birth country would affect our findings greatly, as recent figures suggest that only just over 10% of those living in the US were born elsewhere [37]. Moreover, as 97% of Americans living in poverty have access to stoves, exposure to cooking smoke would be very minimal among the US-born (as well as migrants born in high-income countries) [38].

Surprisingly, a number of factors in the modeling had little effect on the relationship between sex and race and COPD. To try to account for the possibility of living with a smoker, we controlled for marital status and household size, assuming that those living alone and/or never married would have lower exposure to secondhand smoke at home. However, neither factor affected the magnitude of the sex/race-COPD relationship. Future research should consider asking participants to provide a more detailed history of their exposure to secondhand smoke and other air pollutants, by asking questions about ever living with a smoker, in a multiunit dwelling or nearby a highway, as well as current and past occupations. Many of these factors are likely to be highly gendered (e.g., more women have a smoking spouse than men [9]) and, thus, may help provide a better account of how gender, as opposed to sex, contributes to differences in COPD prevalence.

The frequent focus of health research on proximal risk factors obscures the role that more distal causes, such as structural conditions, play in making some groups more vulnerable to illness than others. While biological factors, such as sex, may be critical for understanding COPD prevalence among nonsmokers, our research suggests that structural factors—gender, race, and SEP—may also be important to consider, not only in research but also in policy development.

Competing Interests

The authors declare that they have no competing interests.

References

[1] American Lung Association, Chronic obstructive pulmonary disease (COPD) fact sheet, 2014, http://www.lung.org/lung-disease/copd/resources/facts-figures/COPD-Fact-Sheet.html.

[2] Centers for Disease Control and Prevention, COPD, 2013, http://www.cdc.gov/copd/.

[3] National Heart Lung and Blood Institute, "What is COPD?" https://www.nhlbi.nih.gov/health/health-topics/topics/copd/.

[4] S. S. Salvi and P. J. Barnes, "Chronic obstructive pulmonary disease in non-smokers," *The Lancet*, vol. 374, no. 9691, pp. 733–743, 2009.

[5] American Lung Association, *Trends in Tobacco Use*, 2011.

[6] L. J. Akinbami and X. Liu, "Chronic obstructive pulmonary disease among adults aged 18 and over in the United States, 1998–2009," *NCHS Data Brief*, no. 63, pp. 1–8, 2011.

[7] Centers for Disease Control and Prevention (CDC), "Data and Statistics," http://www.cdc.gov/copd/data.htm.

[8] A. S. Whittemore, S. A. Perlin, and Y. DiCiccio, "Chronic obstructive pulmonary disease in lifelong nonsmokers: results from NHANES," *American Journal of Public Health*, vol. 85, no. 5, pp. 702–706, 1995.

[9] L. J. Greaves and L. A. Richardson, "Tobacco use, women, gender, and chronic obstructive pulmonary disease: are the connections being adequately made?" *Proceedings of the American Thoracic Society*, vol. 4, no. 8, pp. 675–679, 2007.

[10] S. Ben-Zaken Cohen, P. D. Paré, S. F. Man, and D. D. Sin, "The growing burden of chronic obstructive pulmonary disease and lung cancer in women," *American Journal of Respiratory and Critical Care Medicine*, vol. 176, no. 2, pp. 113–120, 2007.

[11] J. E. Connett, R. P. Murray, A. S. Buist et al., "Changes in smoking status affect women more than men: results of the lung health study," *American Journal of Epidemiology*, vol. 157, no. 11, pp. 973–979, 2003.

[12] D. R. Gold, X. Wang, D. Wypij, F. E. Speizer, J. H. Ware, and D. W. Dockery, "Effects of cigarette smoking on lung function in adolescent boys and girls," *The New England Journal of Medicine*, vol. 335, no. 13, pp. 931–937, 1996.

[13] O. Senn, E. W. Russi, C. Schindler et al., "Circulating alpha1-antitrypsin in the general population: determinants and association with lung function," *Respiratory Research*, vol. 9, no. 1, article 35, 2008.

[14] M. D. Eisner, J. Balmes, P. P. Katz, L. Trupin, E. H. Yelin, and P. D. Blanc, "Lifetime environmental tobacco smoke exposure and the risk of chronic obstructive pulmonary disease," *Environmental Health: A Global Access Science Source*, vol. 4, article 7, 2005.

[15] D. M. Homa, L. J. Neff, B. A. King et al., "Vital signs: disparities in nonsmokers' exposure to secondhand smoke—united states, 1999–2012," *Morbidity and Mortality Weekly Report*, vol. 64, no. 4, pp. 103–108, 2015.

[16] T. To, J. Zhu, P. J. Villeneuve et al., "Chronic disease prevalence in women and air pollution—a 30-year longitudinal cohort study," *Environment International*, vol. 80, pp. 26–32, 2015.

[17] D. M. Mannino, D. M. Homa, L. J. Akinbami, E. S. Ford, and S. C. Redd, "Chronic obstructive pulmonary disease surveillance—United States, 1971–2000," *MMWR Surveillance Summaries*, vol. 51, no. 6, pp. 1–16, 2002.

[18] R. I. Harik-Khan, J. L. Fleg, D. C. Muller, and R. A. Wise, "The effect of anthropometric and socioeconomic factors on the racial difference in lung function," *American Journal of Respiratory and Critical Care Medicine*, vol. 164, no. 9, pp. 1647–1654, 2001.

[19] E. J. Pérez-Stable, B. Herrera, P. Jacob III, and N. L. Benowitz, "Nicotine metabolism and intake in black and white smokers," *The Journal of the American Medical Association*, vol. 280, no. 2, pp. 152–156, 1998.

[20] Centers for Disease Control and Prevention, Secondhand smoke (SHS) facts, 2015, http://www.cdc.gov/tobacco/data_statistics/fact_sheets/secondhand_smoke/general_facts/index.htm.

[21] S. Macartney, A. Bishaw, and K. Fontenot, *Poverty Rates for Selected Detailed Race and Hispanic Groups by State and Place: 2007–2011*, 2013.

[22] B. A. King, S. D. Babb, M. A. Tynan, and R. B. Gerzoff, "National and state estimates of secondhand smoke infiltration among U.S. multiunit housing residents," *Nicotine and Tobacco Research*, vol. 15, no. 7, pp. 1316–1321, 2013.

[23] U.S. Census Bureau, *Annual Estimates of the Resident Population by Sex, Race, and Hispanic Origin for the United States, States, and Counties: April 1, 2010 to July 1, 2013*, 2014.

[24] Centers for Disease Control and Prevention, *BRFSS 2012 Summary Data Quality Report*, 2013.

[25] M. J. Hegewald and R. O. Crapo, "Socioeconomic status and lung function," *Chest*, vol. 132, no. 5, pp. 1608–1614, 2007.

[26] US Census Bureau, *Income, Expenditures, Poverty, and Wealth: Table 713: People below Poverty Level by Selected Characteristics: 2009*, 2012.

[27] C. E. Behrendt, "Mild and moderate-to-severe COPD in nonsmokers: distinct demographic profiles," *Chest*, vol. 128, no. 3, pp. 1239–1244, 2005.

[28] F. J. de Serres, I. Blanco, and E. Fernández-Bustillo, "Ethnic differences in alpha-1 antitrypsin deficiency in the United States of America," *Therapeutic Advances in Respiratory Disease*, vol. 4, no. 2, pp. 63–70, 2010.

[29] R. G. Barr, J. Herbstman, F. E. Speizer, and C. A. Camargo Jr., "Validation of self-reported chronic obstructive pulmonary disease in a cohort study of nurses," *American Journal of Epidemiology*, vol. 155, no. 10, pp. 965–971, 2002.

[30] M. S. Radeos, R. K. Cydulka, B. H. Rowe, R. G. Barr, S. Clark, and C. A. Camargo Jr., "Validation of self-reported chronic obstructive pulmonary disease among patients in the ED," *The American Journal of Emergency Medicine*, vol. 27, no. 2, pp. 191–196, 2009.

[31] J. Evans, Y. Chen, P. G. Camp, D. M. Bowie, and L. McRae, "Estimating the prevalence of COPD in Canada: reported diagnosis versus measured airflow obstruction," *Health Reports*, vol. 25, no. 3, pp. 3–11, 2014.

[32] M. C. Aldrich, H. M. Munro, M. Mumma et al., "Chronic obstructive pulmonary disease and subsequent overall and lung cancer mortality in low-income adults," *PLoS ONE*, vol. 10, no. 3, article e0121805, 2015.

[33] B. Doney, E. Hnizdo, C. F. Dillon et al., "Prevalence of airflow obstruction in U.S. adults aged 40-79 years: NHANES data 1988–1994 and 2007–2010," *COPD: Journal of Chronic Obstructive Pulmonary Disease*, vol. 12, no. 4, pp. 355–365, 2015.

[34] M. McDaniel, C. Paxson, and J. Waldfogel, "Racial disparities in childhood asthma in the United States: evidence from the National Health Interview Survey, 1997 to 2003," *Pediatrics*, vol. 117, no. 5, pp. e868–e877, 2006.

[35] P. G. Gibson and J. L. Simpson, "The overlap syndrome of asthma and COPD: what are its features and how important is it?" *Thorax*, vol. 64, no. 8, pp. 728–735, 2009.

[36] E. Diaz-Guzman, M. Khosravi, and D. M. Mannino, "Asthma, chronic obstructive pulmonary disease, and mortality in the US population," *COPD: Journal of Chronic Obstructive Pulmonary Disease*, vol. 8, no. 6, pp. 400–407, 2011.

[37] E. M. Grieco, Y. D. Acosta, P. G. de la Cruz et al., "The foreign-born population in the united states: 2010," Tech. Rep. ACS-19, American Community Survey, 2012.

[38] J. Siebens, "Extended measures of well-being: living conditions in the United States," Tech. Rep. P70-136, United States Census Bureau, Washington, DC, USA, 2013.

22

The Negligible Influence of Chronic Obesity on Hospitalization, Clinical Status, and Complications in Elective Posterior Lumbar Interbody Fusion

Olaf Suess,[1] Theodoros Kombos,[2] and Frank Bode[3]

[1]*Zentrum fuer Wirbelsaeulenchirurgie und Neurotraumatologie, DRK Kliniken Berlin Westend, Spandauer Damm 130, 14050 Berlin, Germany*
[2]*Neurochirurgische Klinik, Schlosspark Klinik, Heubnerweg 2, 14059 Berlin, Germany*
[3]*Neurochirurgische Klinik, Klinikum Darmstadt, Grafenstrasse 9, 64283 Darmstadt, Germany*

Correspondence should be addressed to Olaf Suess; o.suess@drk-kliniken-berlin.de

Academic Editor: Feng Ru Tang

Background. Posterior lumbar interbody fusion (PLIF) is a common surgical treatment for degenerative spinal instability, but many surgeons consider obesity a contraindication for elective spinal fusion. The aim of this study was to analyze whether obesity has any influence on hospitalization parameters, change in clinical status, or complications. *Methods.* In this prospective study, regression analysis was used to analyze the influence of the body mass index (BMI) on operating time, postoperative care, hospitalization time, type of postdischarge care, change in paresis or sensory deficits, pain level, wound complications, cerebrospinal fluid leakage, and implant complications. *Results.* Operating time increased only 2.5 minutes for each increase of BMI by 1. The probability of having a wound complication increased statistically with rising BMI. Nonetheless, BMI accounted for very little of the variation in the data, meaning that other factors or random chances play a much larger role. *Conclusions.* Obesity has to be considered a risk factor for wound complications in patients undergoing elective PLIF for degenerative instability. However, BMI showed no significant influence on other kinds of peri- or postoperative complications, nor clinical outcomes. So obesity cannot be considered a contraindication for elective PLIF.

1. Introduction

Degeneration of the spine is a leading cause of pain and disability [1–3]. This degeneration alters the discoligamentary structures and often leads to spinal instability. Surgical fusion of the affected spinal segments has long been established as the best available surgical treatment for such instability. Posterior lumbar interbody fusion (PLIF) specifically has been the most common approach to fusion [4, 5].

Obesity is thought to represent a risk factor, or even a contraindication, for spinal surgery, as obese patients often have significant comorbidities. Preoperative imaging may be of lower quality. Anesthesia management may be more difficult. The surgical approach to the bony structures of the spine is made more difficult by the excessive subcutaneous fat deposits. That is why surgeons often have to increase the incision length to allow adequate visualization at the increased depth for obese patients, and it is thought that this may lead to increased complications, especially wound infection.

Several previous studies have reported on the influence of obesity on outcomes and complications for spinal surgery. Most notably, in a prospective study of 150 patients undergoing lumbar spine surgery with one-year follow-up, Andreshak et al. found no significant differences between obese and control patients and concluded that lumbar spine surgery should not be withheld from obese patients who are otherwise appropriate candidates [6]. In a retrospective study of 850 spinal procedures in 521 patients, Wimmer et al. found obesity to be a risk factor for infection, but methodological details on this point were sparse [7]. Similarly, in a retrospective case-control study of 41 cases and 178 controls undergoing laminectomy and/or fusion, Olsen et al. identified morbid obesity (BMI > 35) as a risk factor for surgical site infection and recommended that they receive higher doses of prophylactic antibiotic agents and insulin pumps to maintain serum glucose levels below 200 mg/dL [8]. In analysis of data from a multicenter, prospective, randomized controlled trial involving 75 circumferential fusion patients, Goldstein found that BMI had no effect on functional improvement, pain improvement, or patient satisfaction [9]. In a retrospective study of 84 patients receiving fusion for lumbar or thoracic degeneration, Patel et al. did find that obesity was significantly related to major complications but not to minor ones [10]. In a retrospective review of 497 patients undergoing fusion, Glassman et al. noted that BMI had no influence on physical quality-of-life (SF-36 PCS) or functionality (ODI) at 1 or 2 years post-op [11]. In a retrospective chart review of 43 ICLF patients receiving Worker's Comp, LaCaille et al. found that obesity was significantly related to total worker's compensation received but not to total medical costs [12]. Thus although there is some evidence that obesity is a risk factor for wound infection [7, 8] and other complications [10], the literature mostly shows that obesity does not negatively influence outcomes [6, 9, 11] and usually concurs that obesity is not a contraindication for PLIF [6, 8, 9, 11].

In clinical practice though obesity is often still regarded as a contraindication for elective spinal instrumentation. This may represent more an unacknowledged bias against overweight people rather than best-evidence medicine, though the scientific literature is not yet entirely consistent and conclusive. Considering that obesity is already pandemic in Europe and growing worldwide [13–15], it is crucial to scientifically determine whether or not it really is a contraindication against surgery. So we undertook an analysis of 78 patients who had undergone PLIF at our department over a two-year period. The aim of this study was to search for any evidence that obesity has a negative influence on hospitalization, clinical status, or complications.

2. Methods

2.1. Patients and Surgery. The research was designed as a prospective cohort study. All patients presenting to our department between 06/2006 and 06/2007 were candidates for this study. The inclusion criteria were (1) mono- or bisegmental lumbar instability, confirmed clinically and radiologically and (2) persistence of symptoms despite conservative treatment. The following radiological measurements have been used to establish lumbar instability. Direct signs of instability are as follows: 3 mm or more of anterior translation measured between flexion and extension X-ray and/or abnormal axial rotation in which posterior margin of the vertebral body has a focal double contour during bending. Indirect signs of instability are as follows: disc degeneration with space narrowing, osteosclerosis, and osteophytosis of the vertebral end plates. Furthermore, the presence of traction spur, which is a particular type of osteophyte that is located 2-3 mm from the end plate and has a horizontal orientation, and presence of an intervertebral vacuum phenomenon were considered as indirect signs of instability.

As a clinical sign, aberrant motions such as the instability catch occurring during active ROM testing was used to indicate instability. The instability catch has been described as a sudden acceleration or deceleration of movement or a movement occurring outside of the primary plane of motion (e.g., side bending or rotation occurring during flexion) and is proposed as an indication of segmental lumbar instability. Other clinical tests for the evaluation of instability included Gower's sign (thigh climbing to return from a flexed to an upright position), hypermobility during spring testing (posterior-to-anterior (PA) glide), pain during spring testing, and increased muscle guarding or muscle spasm. The exclusion criteria were (1) previous spinal surgery, (2) improvement of symptoms through conservative treatment, and (3) uncorrelated patient symptom complaints. Underweight patients (BMI < 18.5) were excluded from the present analysis.

The surgery followed standard procedures for PLIF, as described in the literature. In brief, mono- or bisegmental laminectomy was performed (according to the number of levels to be fused). Dural sac and nerve roots were relieved from discoligamentary compression. After localization of the pedicles of the vertebrae to be fused, polyaxial 6.5 mm pedicle screws (XIA Low Profile or XIA Precision, Stryker, USA) were introduced with discontinuous fluoroscopy. The intervertebral space was cleared, olisthesis was corrected by retraction if necessary, and finally bilateral intervertebral PEEK cages (Wave, AMT, Germany) were introduced and filled with autologous bone graft. The pedicle screws were blocked and fixed with lateral rods under mild compression. Finally, the wound was closed in typical manner with multilayer resorbable sutures. Antibiotics (2nd generation cephalosporins) were given as a single shot prophylaxis 20 minutes prior to skin incision.

2.2. Measurements. Standardized questionnaires (including ODI and SF36) were used to document sociodemographic variables and preoperative risk factors. BMI was determined by physical examination and graded as normal ≥ 18.5–25; overweight ≥ 25–30; obese ≥ 30–35, severely obese ≥ 35–40, and morbidly obese ≥ 40. Preoperative spondylolisthesis was assessed radiographically and scored by Meyerding's grade. Operating time and hospitalization duration were recorded by hospital staff. Immediate post-op care (defined as the first 12 hours after surgery) was recorded as neurosurgical ward, intermediate monitoring unit, or intensive care unit (ICU). Postdischarge care was recorded as home/self, outpatient treatment, or rehabilitation clinic. Motor strength was measured on a BMRC grading scale (0/5–5/5), for L3-S1, preoperatively and postoperatively. Dermatome-specific sensory deficits were recorded as absent or present left and right, for L3-S1, preoperatively and postoperatively. Adductor reflexes, patellar tendon reflexes, and Achilles' tendon reflexes were each tested left and right and scored on a scale of 0–3, preoperatively and postoperatively. Urogenital disorders, spinal claudication, and Lasègue's sign were each assessed clinically as present versus absent, preoperatively and postoperatively. Pain symptoms were quantified preoperatively and postoperatively using a 10-point visual analogue scale (VAS) and recorded semiquantitatively as "none" (0), "light" (1–3), "moderate" (4–6), or "severe" (7–10). Complications were recorded individually in the patient records.

2.3. Statistical Analysis. Statistical analysis was performed to test the influence of BMI on hospitalization parameters, clinical outcomes, and complications. In all analyses, the following factors were controlled for sex, age, Meyerding grade, and preoperative risk factors. Hospitalization parameters included operating time, type of immediate post-op care, hospitalization duration, and discharge facility. Multiple linear regression was used to analyze operating time, controlling additionally for the number of spinal levels being fused, and the presence of osteoporosis. Multinomial regression was used to analyze the influence of BMI on post-op care. Cox proportional hazard regression was used for hospitalization duration. Multinomial regression was used to analyze the influence of BMI on postdischarge care.

Clinical outcomes included change in paresis, change in sensory deficits, change in reflexes, and change in pain level. For statistical analysis, the motor strength scores for all levels left and right were summed for each pre-op and post-op, and the change in paresis was calculated as the post-op sum minus the pre-op sum; an identical procedure was used for sensory deficits and to sum the three reflex measurements, left and right. The influence of BMI on each paresis, sensory deficits, and reflexes was analyzed first with multiple regression treating the outcome measures as continuous variables, and then alternatively with logistic regression comparing improvement (post-op score − pre-op score = 1 or greater) to no improvement or deterioration (post-op − pre-op = 0 or less). Logistic regression was used to assess the influence of BMI on change in bladder/colon dysfunction, spinal claudication, and Lasègue's sign, individually. Ordinal regression was used to analyze the influence of BMI on change in pain level.

Complications included wound, implant, and cerebrospinal (CSF) complications. "Wound complications" was the sum of wound healing disorders, wound infections, and surgical revision of wounds; due to the small number of cases with two or more wound complications, this variable was dichotomized as 0 versus 1 or more. Logistic regression was used, controlling here additionally for operating time. "Implant complications" was the sum of device loosening and device breakage; again, this variable was dichotomized as 0 versus 1 or more, and logistic regression was used. "Cerebrospinal (CSF) complications" was the sum of dura injuries, nerve root injuries, cerebrospinal fluid fistulas, and cerebrospinal fluid accumulation; again, this variable was dichotomized as 0 versus 1 or more, and logistic regression was used.

The data met all the necessary assumptions for use of these regression models. Statistical analysis was performed with Stata 10.0 (Stata, College Station, Texas, USA). Statistical graphing was with performed with Stata 10.0 (Stata, College Station, Texas, USA) and Adobe Illustrator 10 (Adobe; San Jose, CA, USA).

3. Results

3.1. Patient Population. The study included 78 patients. The patients' sex and age are shown in Figure 1(a). The distribution of the patients' BMIs is shown in Figure 1(b). The distribution of patients according to spinal level(s) in need of operation and grade of preoperative spondylolisthesis is shown in Table 1. The incidence of risk factors in this patient cohort is shown in Figure 1(c). Twenty-four of the 78 patients (30.8%) had a BMI > 30 and were regarded as being obese (16/24), severely obese (7/24), or morbidly obese (1/24) (for examples, see Figures 2(a)–2(c)).

Table 1: Box chart of spinal levels operated and Meyerding grade.

		Meyerding grade				
		1	2	3	4	Total
Spinal level(s) operated	L2/L3	2	1	0	0	**3**
	L3/L4	4	3	0	0	**7**
	L4/L5	38	11	1	0	**50**
	L5/S1	6	5	1	0	**12**
	L3/L4 + L4/L5	3	0	0	0	**3**
	L4/L5 + L5/S1	2	1	0	0	**3**
	Total	**55**	**21**	**2**	**0**	**78**

3.2. Hospitalization Parameters. The median (range) operating time was 220 (125–350) minutes (Table 2). BMI had a statistically significant influence on operating time, when controlling for age and number of levels operated (Figure 3). Operating time increased by 2.5 minutes for each BMI increase of 1, after controlling for age and levels operated, thus, for example, predicting that operating on a patient with a BMI of 40 would take 50 minutes longer than on a patient with a BMI of 20.

Immediate post-op care was on the neurosurgical ward for 73 (93.6%) patients, whereas 5 patients (6.4%) needed an intermediate monitoring unit for up to 48 hours post-op due to cardiopulmonary complications; no patients were on ICU. BMI had no significant influence on the patients' immediate post-op care. The median (interquartile range and min–max range) hospitalization duration was 15 (12–20; 7–92) days. BMI had no significant influence on the duration of hospitalization. The postdischarge care was home/self for 38 (48.7%) patients, outpatient care for 36 (46.2%) patients, and inpatient rehabilitation for 4 (5.1%) patients. BMI had no significant influence on the patients' type of postdischarge care.

3.3. Clinical Status. The median (interquartile range) change of the sum scores for paresis 0 (0-0), sensory deficits 0 (0-1), and reflex status 0 (0-0) showed that BMI had no significant influence on motor or sensory outcome. Furthermore, BMI had no significant influence on the pre-op to post-op change of urogenital dysfunction, spinal claudication, or Lasègue's sign. The median (interquartile range) change of pain level was 2 (2-3) levels. BMI had no significant influence on change in pain level.

3.4. Complications. There was delayed wound healing in 12 (15%) patients, a bacterial wound infection in 2 (2.6%) patients and a need for surgical wound revision (due to CSF

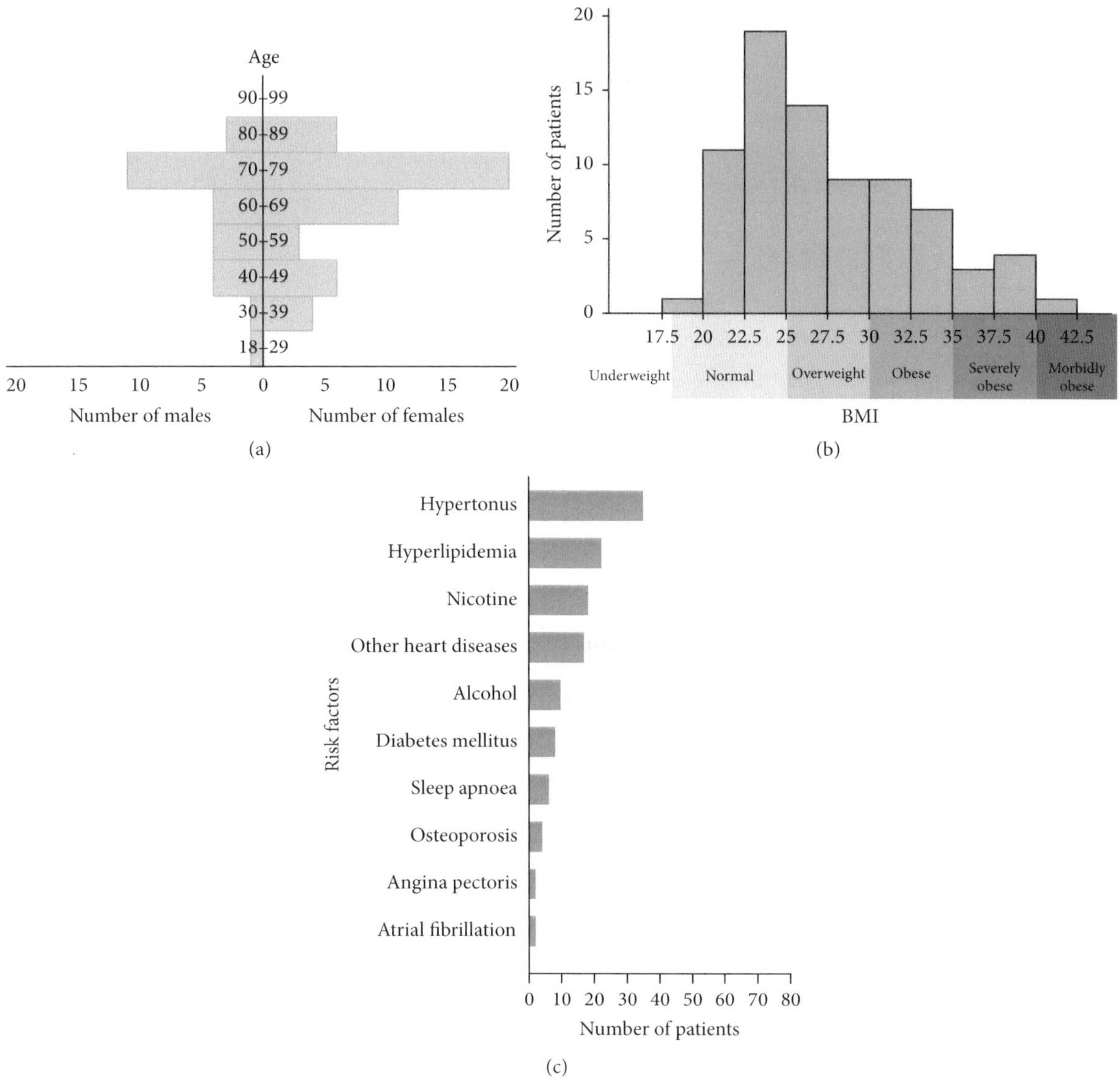

Figure 1: Patient characteristics. (a) Population pyramid, showing the sex and age distribution of the study sample. (b) Histogram of BMI. (c) Bar graph of the incidence of risk factors (see Table 1).

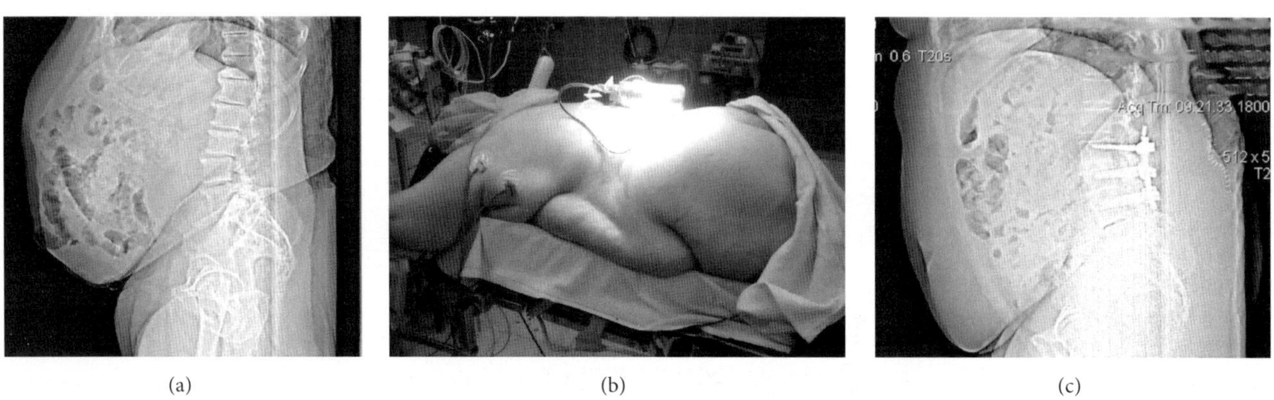

Figure 2: Example of obese patients with BMI > 30. (a) Presurgical CT scout of a 64 y.o. male patient with BMI 34.6. (b) Severely obese 59 y.o. female patient with BMI 37.1 positioned on the OR-table. (c) CT scout of the patient shown in (c) after two-level PLIF.

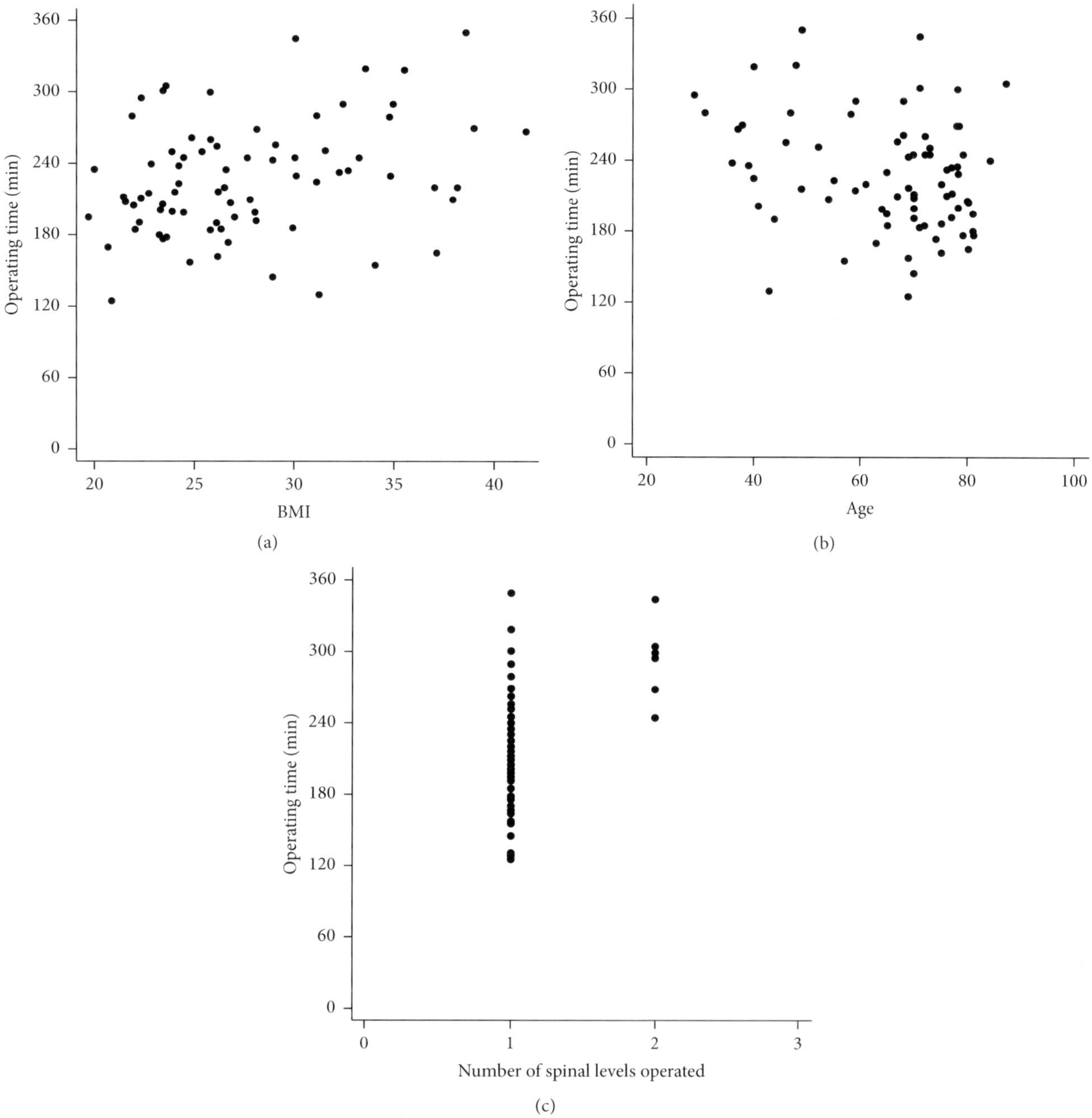

FIGURE 3: Influence of BMI on operating time. The graph shows a scatter-plot of the BMI and operating time data. The thumbnails are similar scatter-plots showing the influence on operating time from age and numbers of levels fused, which were also significant in the overall regression model. It should be kept in mind that each graph shows only the bivariate distribution of operating time and one other variable; the graphs cannot visually adjust or control for the other two significant variables. The statistical parameters for this regression model were as follows: regression slope = 2.56, 95% CI = 0.79 to 4.35, $t = 2.87$, $p = 0.005$, and adjusted $r^2 = 0.31$.

leakage or deep wound infection) in 5 (6.4%) patients; when dichotomized, 15 (19.2%) patients had one or more wound complications. BMI had a statistically significant influence on wound complications (Figure 4). In addition to being statistically significant, the actual magnitude of the influence of BMI on the risk for a wound complication was clinically substantial (as can be seen by the large rise in the probability curve in Figure 4). Thus for illustration, the probability of having a wound complication rose from about 8% at a BMI of 20 to about 33% at a BMI of 35. Despite being statistically significant and clinically substantial, BMI had weak explanatory power for the actual occurrence of a wound complication (as can be seen by the fact that the data dots in Figure 4 cluster only weakly as one looks from the bottom left to the top right and by the wideness of the 95% CI above and below the probability curve in Figure 4). BMI accounted for only about 5% of the variance in the data and therefore cannot be regarded as more than a minor factor in explaining which

TABLE 2: Summary of influence of BMI on hospitalization parameters, clinical status, and adverse events. Multinomial regression was used to analyze the influence of BMI (body mass index) on post-op care, Cox proportional hazard regression was used for hospitalization duration, and multinomial regression was used to analyze the influence of BMI on postdischarge care. The influence of BMI on motor and sensory function was analyzed with multiple regression first, as well as logistic regression comparing postsurgical improvement scores. Logistic regression was used to assess the influence of BMI on change in urogenital dysfunction and spinal claudication as well as on the appearance of adverse events. Ordinal regression was used to analyze the influence of BMI on change in pain level.

		Influence of BMI
Hospitalization parameters		
Operating time	220 min (125–350) mean (min–max range)	*Moderate influence*: (+2.5 min for each BMI increase of 1)
Immediate post-op care		No influence
Neurosurgical ward	73 (93.6%)	
Monitoring unit	5 (6.4%)	
Intensive care unit	0 (0%)	
Hospitalization duration	15 days (12–20; 7–92) mean (interquartile range, min–max range)	No influence
Post discharge care		No influence
Home	38 (48.7%)	
Outpatient care	36 (46.2%)	
Inpatient rehabilitation	4 (5.1%)	
Postsurgical clinical status		
Motor function		No influence
Sensory function		No influence
Urogenital function		No influence
Claudication		No influence
Pain level (VAS)		No influence
Complications		
Wound healing problems	12 (15.4%)	*Minor influence*: (Probability 8% at BMI 20, 33% at BMI 35; BMI accounts for only 5% of variance)
Bacterial wound infections	2 (2.6%)	
Surgical wound revisions	5 (6.4%)	
Screw/implant breakage	1 (1.3%)	No influence
Implant loosening/nonfusion	3 (3.8%)	No influence
Dura injuries	6 (7.7%)	No influence
Cerebrospinal fluid fistula	4 (5.1%)	No influence

patients actually have a wound complication. Yet no other control variable in our analysis, including operating time, had a significant influence on wound complications. This implies that random chance or other uncaptured factors account for the other 95% of variance in the data.

There were 1 (1.3%) instance of device breakage and 3 (3.8%) cases with radiological signs of nonfusion and device loosening after 12-month follow-up. BMI had no significant influence on the occurrence of an implant complication. There were 6 (7.7%) cases of intraoperative dura injuries and 4 (5.2%) cases of postoperative cerebrospinal fluid fistulas. BMI had no significant influence on the occurrence of a cerebrospinal complication.

4. Discussion

In this study, we found an influence of BMI only on operating time and wound complications. BMI had no significant influence on any of the other hospitalization parameters, clinical outcomes, or complications analyzed here. Although the operating time increased with rising BMI, the magnitude of additional operating time was small and all patients were still within the range of typical operating time for spinal surgery. Moreover, operating time has not been proven to have any convincing clinical relevance. BMI did substantially increase the probability of having a wound complication. But a higher risk for a wound complication cannot be viewed as sufficient grounds to contraindicate back pain patients for PLIF. As Olsen et al. have explained in greater detail [8], the appropriate response to this finding is simply that surgeons need to take more preventive measures when operating on obese patients, including, for example, doubling the dose of antibiotics used and using an insulin pump to maintain serum glucose levels under 200 mg/dL. Furthermore, obese patients should simply be informed that they have a higher risk of wound complication, so extra preventive measures will

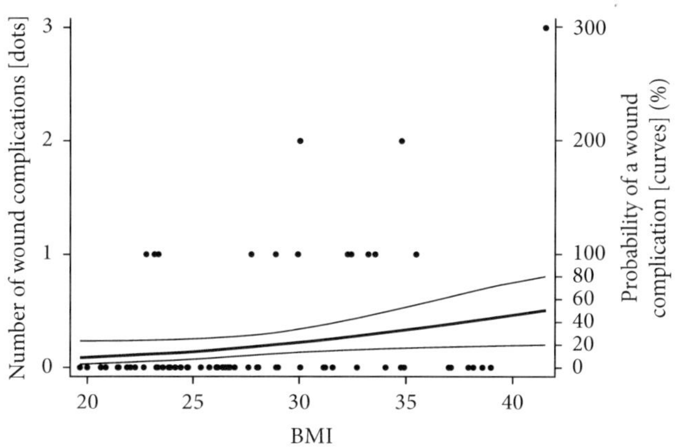

FIGURE 4: Influence of BMI on wound complications. The graph shows a scatter-plot of BMI and the number of wound complications, with the regression curve and 95% CI superimposed using the right-side axis. Dots represent the actual data of BMI and wound complications from this study. The middle curve represents the probability of a wound complication, and the upper and lower curves show the interval within which the probability curve can be assumed with 95% confidence to lie. The statistical parameters for this model were as follows: regression slope = 0.11, 95% CI = 0.005 to 0.217, $z = 2.28$, $p = 0.04$, and pseudo $r^2 = 0.07$.

be taken if they decide to opt for the surgery anyway [16–18]. It should also be emphasized that BMI explained very little of the variation in the data, meaning that other factors are the main explanations of which patients actually have a wound complication. So if our concern is to avoid wound complications, further research is needed on the factors that lead to them [19]. Besides operating time and wound complications, BMI had no significant influence on any of the variables analyzed here.

No one study can single-handedly settle any scientific questions, including whether or not obesity is a contraindication for spinal surgery. Only the overall body of literature can answer the question. The present findings are consistent with most other studies. The only anomalous exception has been the study by Patel et al. [10], which had a study size, sample, and design comparable to our own. They had a much lower rate of wound infection (3 cases in 84 patients versus our 15 cases in 78 patients), but a higher rate of cerebrospinal fluid leakage (8 cases versus our 4 cases of cerebrospinal fluid fistulas or accumulation). They also reported several complications that we never observed, including deep vein thrombosis, cardiac events, pneumonia, prolonged intubation, urological issues, and palsy. The occurrence of all these other complications cannot be due solely to obesity; otherwise, we (and other researchers) would have observed at least some of them too. Instead, these complications are probably due to general health differences in these (American versus German) study populations or differences in the hospital setting. Furthermore, the rate of complications observed by Patel et al. appears to be rather high in comparison to most other previous studies on spine surgery in obese patients. This might be due in part to the broad definition of "complications" that they used, yet it remains difficult to understand why they had so many major complications such as cardiac events and pneumonia. Several other studies have reported no difference in clinical outcomes for obese patients and no such long lists of major complications [6, 8, 9, 11, 12].

5. Conclusions

Obesity is well-known to be a risk factor for heart disease, diabetes, and other medical conditions, and it is associated with higher rates of health care consumption [15, 20–22]. However, according to the results of this study and consistent with the bulk of currently available evidence, obesity is not clearly associated with enough increased risk of complications or poor outcomes to be viewed as a contraindication for PLIF.

Competing Interests

The authors declare that there are no competing interests regarding the publication of this paper.

Acknowledgments

The authors would like to thank Michael Hanna, Ph.D., and Stefan Lhachimi, M.S., M.P.P. (both from Mercury Medical Research & Writing), for providing publication advising (Michael Hanna), statistical analysis (Stefan Lhachimi and Michael Hanna), data graphing (Stefan Lhachimi and Michael Hanna), and medical writing services (Michael Hanna).

References

[1] S. J. Atlas and R. A. Nardin, "Evaluation and treatment of low back pain: an evidence-based approach to clinical care," *Muscle and Nerve*, vol. 27, no. 3, pp. 265–284, 2003.

[2] M. C. Battié, T. Videman, and E. Parent, "Lumbar disc degeneration: epidemiology and genetic influences," *Spine*, vol. 29, no. 23, pp. 2679–2690, 2004.

[3] N. J. Manek and A. J. MacGregor, "Epidemiology of back disorders: prevalence, risk factors, and prognosis," *Current Opinion in Rheumatology*, vol. 17, no. 2, pp. 134–140, 2005.

[4] R. B. Cloward, "Posterior lumbar interbody fusion updated," *Clinical Orthopaedics and Related Research*, vol. 193, pp. 16–19, 1985.

[5] P. Enker and A. D. Steffee, "Interbody fusion and instrumentation," *Clinical Orthopaedics and Related Research*, no. 300, pp. 90–101, 1994.

[6] T. G. Andreshak, H. S. An, J. Hall, and B. Stein, "Lumbar spine surgery in the obese patient," *Journal of Spinal Disorders*, vol. 10, no. 5, pp. 376–379, 1997.

[7] C. Wimmer, H. Gluch, M. Franzreb, and M. Ogon, "Predisposing factors for infection in spine surgery: a survey of 850 spinal procedures," *Journal of Spinal Disorders*, vol. 11, no. 2, pp. 124–128, 1998.

[8] M. A. Olsen, J. Mayfield, C. Lauryssen et al., "Risk factors for surgical site infection in spinal surgery," *Journal of Neurosurgery*, vol. 98, no. 2, pp. 149–155, 2003.

[9] J. A. Goldstein, "Does body mass index (BMI) affect the clinical outcome of 1-level ProDisc-L IDE patients," *The Spine Journal*, vol. 7, no. 5, p. 104S, 2007.

[10] N. Patel, B. Bagan, S. Vadera et al., "Obesity and spine surgery: relation to perioperative complications," *Journal of Neurosurgery: Spine*, vol. 6, no. 4, pp. 291–297, 2007.

[11] S. Glassman, M. F. Gornet, C. Branch et al., "MOS Short form 36 and Oswestry Disability Index outcomes in lumbar fusion: a multicenter experience," *Spine Journal*, vol. 6, no. 1, pp. 21–26, 2006.

[12] R. A. LaCaille, M. S. DeBerard, L. J. LaCaille, K. S. Masters, and A. L. Colledge, "Obesity and litigation predict workers' compensation costs associated with interbody cage lumbar fusion," *Spine Journal*, vol. 7, no. 3, pp. 266–272, 2007.

[13] M. T. Bassett and S. Perl, "Obesity: the public health challenge of our time," *American Journal of Public Health*, vol. 94, no. 9, p. 1477, 2004.

[14] T. Groves, "Pandemic obesity in Europe," *British Medical Journal*, vol. 333, no. 7578, pp. 1081–1082, 2006.

[15] A. D. Woolf, F. C. Breedveld, and T. K. Kvien, "Controlling the obesity epidemic is important for maintaining musculoskeletal health," *Annals of the Rheumatic Diseases*, vol. 65, no. 11, pp. 1401–1402, 2006.

[16] A. Coulter, "Patient information and shared decision-making in cancer care," *British Journal of Cancer*, vol. 89, no. 1, pp. S15–S16, 2003.

[17] W. Godolphin, "The role of risk communication in shared decision making," *British Medical Journal*, vol. 327, no. 7417, pp. 692–693, 2003.

[18] W. W. Weston, "Informed and shared decision-making: the crux of patient-centred care," *Canadian Medical Association Journal*, vol. 165, no. 4, pp. 438–439, 2001.

[19] A. Gawande, "On washing hands," *The New England Journal of Medicine*, vol. 350, no. 13, pp. 1283–1286, 2004.

[20] T. L. Gary and F. L. Brancati, "Strategies to curb the epidemic of diabetes and obesity in primary care settings," *Journal of General Internal Medicine*, vol. 19, no. 12, pp. 1242–1243, 2004.

[21] S. Jarvis, "Obesity and the overworked GP," *British Journal of General Practice*, vol. 56, no. 530, pp. 654–655, 2006.

[22] C. P. Quesenberry Jr., B. Caan, and A. Jacobson, "Obesity, health services use, and health care costs among members of a health maintenance organization," *Archives of Internal Medicine*, vol. 158, no. 5, pp. 466–472, 1998.

23

Medication Noncompliance among Patients with Chronic Diseases Attending a Primary Health Facility in a Periurban District in Ghana

Bright Addo,[1] **Sally Sencherey,**[2] **and Michael N. K. Babayara**[3]

[1] *University of Ghana School of Public Health, Legon, Accra, Ghana*
[2] *Komfo Anokye Teaching Hospital (KATH), Kumasi, Ghana*
[3] *Postgraduate College, 37 Military Hospital, Accra Central, Ghana*

Correspondence should be addressed to Bright Addo; addobright1@gmail.com

Academic Editor: Paola Muti

Background. Despite the growing interest in understanding the aetiology of chronic diseases, limited studies exist on medication noncompliance, especially, among periurban and rural dwellers in Ghana. In this study, we determined the prevalence of medication noncompliance and explored the medication intake behaviour of patients with chronic diseases. The relative influence of cost on medication noncompliance and the risk factors for noncompliance were also assessed. *Methods.* The design was a cross-sectional study of 200 patients from ages below 40 years to ages above 60 years sampled from the Offinso South Municipality, a periurban district of the Ashanti region of Ghana. Data collected through the administration of structured questionnaires was coded, cleaned, and analysed using the SPSS (v20) software programme. Descriptive and multivariate analyses using binary logistic regression were performed. *Results.* Medication noncompliance was high (55.5%), with patients living with HIV/AIDS and those with psychological disorders being the most noncompliant. Majority of patients took at least 2 medications (81.5%), did so twice daily (79.0%), did not experience side effects with intake (67.0%), considered their medication to be effective (88.5%), and were aware of the complications that could arise from noncompliance. The dominant route of medication intake was oral (86.8%) and a lesser proportion of patients (22.5%) took herbal preparation alongside their prescribed medications. The cost of medication did not prevent patients from adhering to their medication regimen as most of these drugs were covered by the National Health Insurance Scheme (NHIS). Age, duration of diagnosis and difficulty in remembering medication instructions were identified as significant predictors of noncompliance. *Conclusion.* Educating patients on the need to be compliant with their medication regimen, the complications that could arise from noncompliance and avoidance of intake of herbal medications during their treatment should form part of the clinical sessions organized for patients with chronic conditions.

1. Introduction

The success of every therapeutic regimen depends on the compliance of the individual involved. The efforts put in by healthcare providers can therefore only yield the desired effect if patients are compliant to their medication regimen. Unfortunately, medication noncompliance with its associated detrimental effects is becoming widespread and has been found to be most prevalent among patients with chronic diseases.

Globally, chronic diseases have been found to be the leading cause of mortality and disability, and the disease rates from these conditions are not only accelerating but advancing across every region and pervading every socioeconomic class [1]. The WHO projects that, by 2020, the incidence of chronic disease will account for almost three-quarters of all death occurring worldwide, and that 71% of deaths due to ischaemic heart disease (IHD), 75% of deaths due to stroke, and 70% of deaths due to diabetes will occur in the developing countries [2]. The WHO further estimates that the number of people in the developing world with diabetes will increase by more than 2.5-fold, with the 1995 number of 84 million sharply rising to 228 million in 2025. On a global scale, 60% of the burden of chronic diseases and 79% of deaths attributed to these diseases are expected to occur in developing countries, of which Ghana is included [2].

In Ghana, hypertension alone is said to have accounted for between 19% and 54.8% of the outpatient morbidity in adults above 45 years in 2012 [3]. Diabetes mellitus also accounted for 6.8% of all adult admissions and also 7.8% of all adult deaths in at the Korle-Bu Teaching Hospital [4].

Among patients with chronic diseases such as hypertension, diabetes, HIV/AIDS, and psychiatric illnesses, medication noncompliance has been found to be very common [5, 6].

Poor adherence to therapy among hypertensive patients contributes to two-thirds of poor blood pressure control [5]. Failure to achieve blood pressure control subsequently leads to development of cardiovascular complications including myocardial infarction and stroke. For patients with psychiatric disorders, not only do they have a challenge following a medical regimen, but they also have the greatest potential for benefiting from compliance [7].

Among patients living with HIV/AIDS, with the advent of antiretroviral drugs, anything less than thorough compliance can result in reduced efficacy of the drugs and later lead to development of resistant viral strains [8].

There is a threefold effect to medication noncompliance, and these effects are manifested in the clinical outcome of the patient, the cost of treatment, and the risk of hospitalizations, all of which have been identified as the main cause of failure to effectively manage chronic diseases [9–11].

Over the last two decades, there have been a plethora of studies that have examined variables that could be demonstrated as predictive of adherence to various medical regimens. The factors most often hypothesized in these studies as powerfully predicting compliance have generally been attributed to characteristics of both the disease and the patients. For example, to explore and evaluate the most common factors causing therapeutic noncompliance, Jin and colleagues found factors that could be categorized into (1) patient-centered factors, (2) therapy-related factors, (3) social and economic factors, (4) healthcare system factors, and (5) disease factors [9]. Factors which relate to patients (e.g., suboptimal health literacy and lack of involvement in the treatment decision-making process), physicians (e.g., prescription of complex drug regimens, communication barriers, ineffective communication of information about adverse effects, and provision of care by multiple physicians), and health care systems (e.g., limited access to care, lack of health information technology, and office visit times limitations) have also been found [12].

In the West African subregion and particularly in Ghana, studies have identified specific factors such as depression, concern about disease medications, formal education, and use of herbal preparations to be associated with nonadherence among hypertensive patients [11] and factors such as educational level and mode of payment to be associated with nonadherence among diabetic patients [10].

In an era where cost-effectiveness is a buzz word in healthcare delivery, these identified factors must be a concern for healthcare providers and health systems [9]. Unfortunately, risk factor studies identifying the proximate determinants of medication noncompliance have generally been inconclusive. Whiles some factors have been identified to significantly associate with noncompliance in one geographical context, same factors have been found to be nonsignificant in others.

With the persistent rise in the prevalence of chronic diseases, medication compliance as an area of research study is gaining much recognition and whiles there is now ample research on the subject, most of these studies have been conducted in developed countries. The extant literatures on medication nonadherence in Ghana have mostly focused on the two chronic diseases, hypertension and diabetes much to the neglect of other chronic conditions such as HIV/AIDS and psychiatric disorders. The plethora of studies which even do exist on medication nonadherence among diabetic and hypertensive patients have mostly been conducted in urban settings of the country, with limited studies conducted among periurban and rural dwellers. On this premise, this study sought to determine the prevalence of medication noncompliance among patients with chronic diseases in a periurban district in Ghana. Medication intake behaviour, the relative influence of cost on medication noncompliance, and the risk factors for medication noncompliance were also assessed.

2. Methods

2.1. Study Area. The study was conducted in the Offinso South Municipality, one of the 30 Municipals in the Ashanti region of Ghana. The 2010 Population and Housing Census put the population of the municipality at 76,895 with a population density of 131 persons per square kilometre. A high percentage (70.0%) of the population in the municipality is economically active, with over 50.0% of the employed being skilled agricultural and fishery workers [13]. More females (16,071) than males (14,348), of the working age population in the municipality, have an occupation. On health, the Municipality Health Services are organized around 5 submunicipalities: namely, Bonsua, Abofour, Offinso Central, Anyinasuso, and Kwagyekrom. There are eleven (11) health facilities with the ownership being government/public, CHAG, and private. Due to the absence of a municipal government or public hospital, St. Patrick's Hospital is earmarked as the municipal hospital. In addition, there are 3 functional CHPS compounds and 42 CHPS zones with the respective CHOs assigned. There are also 76 trained TBAs and 61 CBSVs. The municipality recorded a total of 455 household deaths 12 months prior to the 2010 PHC representing 1.6% of the entire Ashanti region. The crude death rate, which is the number of deaths per 1000 of the population in the Municipality, is 5.9 [13].

2.2. Study Design. This was a cross-sectional descriptive survey using systematic random sampling to collect quantitative data involving multiple variables which were analysed to determine distribution patterns and test relationships.

2.3. Study Population. The sampling population included people aged 18 and above presenting at the special OPD clinic at St. Patrick's Hospital who had been diagnosed of a chronic ailment and consented to participate in the study.

2.3.1. Inclusion Criteria. To be included in the study, patients had to be diagnosed of at least one out of the four chronic diseases of interest, that is, hypertension, diabetes, HIV/AIDS, or psychiatric disorder. The patient should also have been on medication for more than 6 months and must have consented to participate in the study.

2.3.2. Exclusion Criteria. Patients who had been diagnosed of any of the chronic diseases of interest and were yet to start medication or had been on medication for less than 6 months were exempted from the study. Patients below the age of 18 years were also excluded.

2.4. Sample and Sampling Technique. The hospital facility was chosen for the study as it was easier to get access to patients that met the inclusion category. Of the number of health facilities available at the Offinso South Municipality, St. Patrick's Hospital was purposively selected as it was the largest hospital and was frequented by most people in the municipality.

The systematic random sampling technique was used to sample 200 eligible patients. At a particular clinic, the first person was given the chance to participate and every third person was also sampled to participate. Consent was sought from the selected participant before inclusion into the study.

2.5. Instrumentation. Standard questionnaires were used for the study. The study's research questions and objectives informed the design of the questionnaires. Prior to the design, a thorough literature search was conducted to determine and categorize concepts and variables used in studies related to the topic. Information from the literature review focused on issues relating to noncompliance to medication régimen among patient with chronic diseases. The research instrument crafted for this study was a 28-item self-reporting research instrument utilizing closed ended questions with response categories that were precoded which facilitated numerical coding of the data after collection. The entire questionnaire was arranged into content subsections A, B, and C.

Section "A" consisted of nine (9) sociodemographic survey items which distinguished patients in terms of their age, gender, religion, employment status, occupation, marital status, educational attainment, chronic condition(s) suffered, and duration of condition since diagnosis. Section "B" consisted of 14 questionnaire items developed to measure patients' compliance to medication regimen. The questions asked mainly bothered on the different medications patients took for their condition, frequency of daily intake, route of administration of medication, number of tablets/capsules taken daily, adherence to doctor's instructions as to how medication should be taken, side effects experienced if any, etc. (see attached study questionnaire for full details available here).

Section "C" also consisted of 4 questions developed to measure the influence of cost on compliance to medication. The first question ascertained whether patients' medication was covered by the National Health Insurance Scheme (NHIS), whiles the second was a follow-up question for respondents who indicated "No" as a response to indicate how they paid for their drugs. The third and fourth questions requested patients to indicate the cost of their medication(s) and whether they missed their medication for a period of time due to cost.

Additionally, there were standard instructions that requested respondents to select the most suitable answer with the assurance that there was no right or wrong answer in the selection of answers to the questions.

2.6. Validation and Pretesting of Questionnaire. The questionnaire validation process was a two-step one. The first step was the establishment of face validity of the questionnaire which was achieved by consulting two experts: (1) a university professor and (2) a practicing physician. These two experts were tasked to ascertain if the questions asked effectively captured the topic under investigation. Their suggestions and recommendations made were then incorporated.

A pretest was then carried out after the validation to obtain information to improve the questionnaire and to assess the feasibility of the study. The respondents in the pretest were similar to those in the study and it was carried out under similar settings. Conducting the pretest helped to identify problems with the questionnaire, to gauge the time needed to complete the questionnaire and ultimately, and to ensure that the questions were understood by respondents. The feedback obtained helped in fine-tuning the questionnaire. The pretest was conducted among 15 patients at the Komfo Anokye Teaching Hospital (KATH).

2.7. Data Collection. Data was collected over a period of one month, from March to April, 2016 at the St. Patrick's Hospital which doubles as the municipal's hospital after pretesting of the research questionnaire. Quantitative data was primarily sought for the study. The data was obtained through the use of a structured questionnaire specifically designed to suit respondents understanding of the study. The response categories of the various questions or variables were mostly precoded. A word of acknowledgment was rendered to study respondents for their participation in the survey.

2.8. Data Analysis. The data collected was first edited to ensure that all questionnaires were complete and properly filled. In all, 200 complete questionnaires were obtained from the respondents. After editing, the data from the completed questionnaire was coded and entered into the SPSS (v20) programme. Preliminary data analysis was conducted to obtain frequency distribution for all variables. The preliminary analysis also served as a cleaning strategy which helped to identify data entry errors. The validation tool in the SPSS programme which gives information about missing values with their identification numbers and wrong entries made was further utilized to confirm that the data was clean and ready for analysis.

Descriptive analysis was conducted on respondents' background characteristics and reported in frequencies and percentages. Multivariate analysis using binary logistic regression was conducted to determine the factors for noncompliance to medication regimen.

2.9. Ethical Considerations. Ethical approval was obtained from the Ethical Review Committee of the Komfo Anokye Teaching Hospital (KATH) through the School of Medical Sciences, KNUST, Kumasi. Permission for the research was granted from the Administration of St. Patrick's Hospital as well as the head of the special clinic of the hospital. The purpose of the study was explained to every participant. Confidentiality was assured and either verbal or written consent was sought from every individual who participated in the study.

Participation in the study was not compulsory and anonymity of respondents was respected. All respondents voluntarily gave verbal consent to participate in the study after the rationale of the study was explained to them. Couples were interviewed separately and care was taken to ensure privacy and confidentiality.

3. Results

3.1. Background Characteristics of Respondents. A total of 200 patients participated in the study. Patients' ages ranged from below 40 to 60+ years with majority of them being less than 40 years and between 40 and 60 years. Together, these two age cohorts constituted 79% of the entire sample size. Majority of the respondents were females (76%), were in marital unions (57%), had attained basic education, that is primary and up to Junior High School (59%), were into trading, and belonged to the Christian faith (88%). Patients who were diagnosed with diabetes were the most (42.4%), followed by those with hypertension and HIV/AIDS. Patients who had lived with their disease condition between 1 and 5 years constituted a half (which was majority) of the entire sample (see Table 1).

3.2. Prevalence of Medication Noncompliance. Medication noncompliance (assessed by patients indicating whether they always admitted to their doctor's instruction) in the sample of 200 patients was found to be relatively high ($n = 111$, 55.5%) (Table 2(a)). Comparatively, patients with HIV/AIDS and those with psychological disorders were found to be the most noncompliant (61.7%; 55.0%, respectively). Patients who were hypertensive were the least noncompliant (53.3%) (Figure 1).

3.3. Medication Intake Behaviour of Patients. Majority of the patients (81.5%) were found to be taking at least 2 medications. Patients who were on exactly two medications for their disease condition were however the most (38.0%). A higher percentage of the patients (79.0%) took their medication twice daily, with the dominant route of intake being orally (86.8%). More than half (55.8%) of the patients who were on oral medications reported they took less than 5 tablets

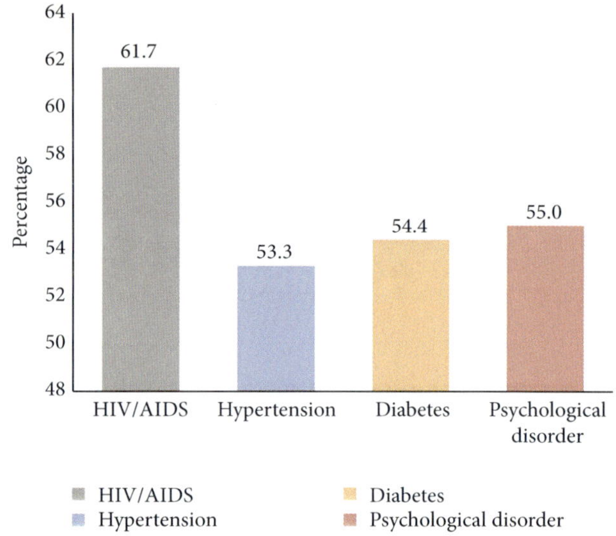

Figure 1: Proportion of patients with chronic diseases who are noncompliant to their medication regimen.

daily. Majority of the patients (67.0%) did not experience side effects with the intake of their drugs and the few who did (33.0%) mostly complained of general body weakness and insomnia. Of those who experienced side effects, most were able to tolerate it (Table 2(a)).

A lesser proportion of patients (22.5%) took herbal preparation alongside their prescribed medications and out of that, 8.0% stopped taking their prescribed medications and 8.5% took it alongside prescribed medications, which is an unhealthy practice. Majority of the patients (93.5%) had no problem with remembering medication instructions and forgetfulness was a problem in only about 16.0%. A higher percentage of the patients considered their medication effective (88.5%), were aware of the complications that could arise from noncompliance (58.0%), and were self-reminded to take their medications (87.5%) (see Table 2(b)).

3.4. Cost and Noncompliance to Medication Regimen. Most of the drugs patients used (71.0%) were covered by the NHIS. Out of the 29.0% of patients who had to pay for their drugs, 15.5% paid from their own income and 13.5% were being supported by family members; however, 12% were missing their medications because they could not at a point in time pay for their drugs (Table 3). The cost of drugs patients had to purchase by themselves mostly ranged from between 10 and 30 Ghana cedis ($2.22–$7.5).

3.5. Factors for Medication Noncompliance. Based on the three main categories of factors (i.e., personality characteristics and disease related and medication related factors) identified in the literature to influence medication compliance, the regression analysis was modelled to contain the variables comprising these three factors. Of the twelve factors (4 personality characteristics and 1 disease related and 7 medication related factors) entered into the regression model, only age, duration of diagnosis, and difficulty remembering

Table 1: Distribution of respondents by background characteristics ($N = 200$).

Characteristic	Frequency (n)	Percent (%)
Age (years)		
<40	80	40.0
40–60	79	39.5
>60	41	20.5
Gender		
Male	48	24.0
Female	152	76.0
Religion		
Christian	176	88.0
Islam	16	8.0
African Traditional	4	2.0
None	4	2.0
Occupation		
Farming	41	20.5
Trading	68	34.0
Artisan	13	6.5
Teacher	5	2.5
Driver	6	3.0
Health worker	1	.5
Mechanic	1	.5
Unemployed	65	32.5
Marital status		
Single	43	21.5
Married	114	57.0
Divorced	14	7.0
Widowed	29	14.5
Educational attainment		
None	45	22.5
Primary	40	20.0
Junior High School	77	38.5
Senior High School	28	14.0
Tertiary	10	5.0
Chronic diseases suffered[a]		
HIV/AIDS	60	22.3
Hypertension	75	27.9
Diabetes	114	42.4
Psychiatric illness	20	7.4
Duration of diagnosis		
Less than a year ago	15	7.5
1–5 years ago	100	50.0
5–10 years ago	38	19.0
More than 10 years ago	47	23.5

[a]Multiple response item.

medication instructions were found to be significant predictors of noncompliance to medication regimen. Patients who were old were more likely to be noncompliant. Those whose disease condition was long diagnosed were found to be 2 times more likely to be noncompliant; likewise those who did not have difficulty remembering medication instructions are 6 times more likely to be noncompliant (see Table 4).

4. Discussion

There has been a dearth in studies to assess the level of noncompliance to medications for chronic diseases over the years, especially among patients with chronic conditions living in rural and periurban districts in sub-Saharan Africa. Taking cognisance of the fact that the success of every

TABLE 2

(a) Medication intake behaviour of patients ($N = 200$)

Characteristic	Frequency (n)	Percent (%)
Number of medications taken for condition		
One	25	12.5
Two	76	38.0
Three	43	21.5
Four	36	18.0
More than 4	20	10.0
Frequency of intake		
Once daily	28	14.0
Twice daily	158	79.0
Thrice daily	14	7.0
Route of intake[a]		
Oral	197	86.8
Injection	30	13.2
Number of tablets taken if oral		
Less than 5	110	55.8
Between 5 and 10	82	41.6
More than 10	5	2.6
Always admit to doctor's instructions		
Yes	89	44.5
No	111	55.5
Notification of side effects of drugs		
Yes	66	33.0
No	134	67.0
Side effects mostly experienced[c]		
Weakness	13	6.5
Insomnia	8	4.0
Dizziness	6	3.0
General malaise	6	3.0
Irritability	4	2.0
Lethargy	4	2.0
Oversleeping	4	2.0
N/A[b]	134	67.0
Able to tolerate side effects		
Yes	40	20.0
No	26	13.0
N/A[b]	134	67.0

[a]Multiple response; [b]N/A = patients who indicated that they did not experience any side effects; [c]predominant side effects experienced by patients.

(b) Medication intake behaviour of patients ($N = 200$)

Characteristic	Frequency (n)	Percent (%)
Use of herbal medication		
Yes	45	22.5
No	155	77.5
Influence of intake on medication compliance		
Doesn't influence it	17	8.5
Stop taking the prescribed medication	16	8.0
Take it alongside prescribed medication	12	8.0
N/A[a]	155	77.5
Difficulty in remembering medication instructions		
Yes	13	6.5
No	187	93.5

(b) Continued.

Characteristic	Frequency (n)	Percent (%)
Medication is effective		
Yes	177	88.5
No	10	5.0
Sometimes	13	6.5
Frequency of forgetting to take medications		
Daily	3	1.5
Frequently	28	14.0
Rarely	104	52.0
Never	65	32.5
Awareness of complications arising from non-compliance		
Yes	116	58.0
No	84	42.0
Ways of being reminded to be compliant with medications		
Doctor's advice	5	2.5
Advice from other health workers	2	1.0
Radio or TV	1	.5
Friends or family	17	8.5
Self	175	87.5

[a]N/A = patients who indicated that they did not use herbal medication.

Table 3: Cost and medication noncompliance ($N = 200$).

Variable	Frequency (n)	Percent (%)
Medication covered by NHIS		
Yes	142	71.0
No	4	2.0
Some of them	54	27.0
Means of paying for drugs		
From income	31	15.5
Support of family members	27	13.5
N/A[a]	142	71.0
Cost of medications		
Less than 10 cedis	7	3.5
10–30 cedis	33	16.5
31–60 cedis	15	7.5
61+ cedis	3	1.5
N/A[a]	142	71.0
Missed medication because of cost		
Yes	24	12.0
No	34	17.0
N/A[a]	142	71.0

[a]N/A = not applicable.

therapeutic regimen depends on the compliance of the individual involved and that medication noncompliance is becoming widespread, we found this study to be crucial and timely. We found the overall prevalence of medication noncompliance among the patients to be 55.5%. This rate is higher than that of a similar study conducted in Northwest Ethiopia (42%) to determine noncompliance in patients with chronic illnesses [14]. The highest level of compliance and in effect the lowest level of noncompliance, was recorded among patients with hypertension, 53.3%. This percentage in hypertension is close to the level, 52.3% obtained in another study at the Korle-Bu Teaching hospital [6] and lower than 93% recorded in a similar study at KATH [15].

We found compliance to antihypertensive drugs to be comparatively better probably because there has been much more education on hypertension leading to interventions to improve compliance among patients with hypertension. The reduced side effects and the NHIS covering some hypertensive medications could also be a contributing factor. Among the four disease conditions, we found the prevalence

TABLE 4: Multivariate analysis of risk factors for medication noncompliance.

Factor	B	S.E.	p-value	OR (95% CI)
Gender				
Male	1			
Female	−.335	.394	.395	.715 (.331–1.547)
Age				
Young	1			
Old	−1.047	.384	.006*	.351 (.165–.745)
Education				
Not educated	1			
Educated	−.567	.411	.168	.567 (.253–1.270)
Marital status				
Single	1			
Married	.137	.324	.673	1.147 (.608–2.163)
Duration of diagnosis				
Short (<6 years)	1			
Long (>5 years)	.794	.336	.018*	2.213 (1.145–4.278)
Number of tablets taken orally				
Less than 5	1			
Between 5 and 10	.452	.368	.219	1.571 (.764–3.232)
More than 10	−.213	1.096	.846	.808 (.094–6.919)
Notification of drugs side effects				
Yes	1			
No	.304	.335	.363	1.356 (.704–2.612)
Use of herbal medication				
Yes	1			
No	−.230	.387	.552	.794 (.372–1.697)
Difficulty remembering medication instructions				
Yes	1			
No	1.715	.736	.020*	5.557 (1.313–23.524)
Efficacy of medication				
Yes	1			
No	.323	.767	.674	1.381 (.307–6.217)
Sometimes	1.304	.793	.100	3.685 (.779–17.433)
Awareness of complications that can arise from non-compliance				
Yes	1			
No	.313	.324	.334	1.367 (.724–2.580)
Medication covered by NHIS				
Yes	1			
No	−.717	1.176	.542	.488 (.049–4.893)
Some of them	.743	.363	.041	2.102 (1.032–4.278)

*$p < .05$.

of medication noncompliance to be the highest among patients living with HIV/AIDS (61.7%). This rate is high compared to a study conducted in Eldoret which revealed a noncompliance prevalence rate of 36.8% [8]. This high rate in noncompliance could be attributed to the stigma attached to the disease. Some patients affected by the disease have to travel distant towns for their medication in order not to be seen by people. They can therefore delay in getting their medications refilled if they are unable to make it to these distant towns. Added to this is the fact that some of these patients have to hide in order to take their medications so that the people around them do not get suspicious of an ailment. This implies that in situations where there is no privacy these patients may miss their medications.

The level of nonadherence to medications for diabetes in our study was found to be 54.4%. Comparatively, the rate is higher than that obtained in a Ugandan study which recorded a prevalence rate of 28.9% nonadherence among patients [16]. Another study in Nigeria however showed a much higher level of nonadherence, 73.6% [17]. The level of noncompliance among patients with psychiatric illnesses was found to be 55.0%. This was the overall level of adherence of the patients reporting at the psychiatric clinic, some of whom had mainly schizophrenia, bipolar disorders, and epilepsy.

Our study reports a medication intake behaviour where a high proportion of patients were on oral medications which was taken twice daily and a lesser proportion taking herbal preparations alongside their prescribed medications. Some patients however stopped the intake of their prescribed medications and resorted to the use of herbal drugs, a practice we find to be unhealthy. There has been a current upsurge in the use of herbal medication to treat chronic diseases in Ghana, especially diabetes. This upsurge has been fueled by the several advertisements aired by most of the mass media houses in the country. Often times, the efficacy of the drugs being advertised is yet to be scientifically proven, though most claim to have received an FDA approval.

On the effect of medication cost on noncompliance, we found that patients who had all or some of their medications covered by the NHIS were generally more compliant. The cost of medications, therefore, to some extent has the potential of influencing patients' compliance which implies that having more medications covered by the NHIS can improve overall adherence. This finding is consistent with the study of Buabeng and colleagues conducted at the Korle-Bu Teaching Hospital (KBTH) in Ghana which found unaffordable drug prices as the major cause of noncompliance among patients with hypertension [15]. Medications such as insulin are not covered by the NHIS, and with the cost of the drug being high, majority of patients could miss their medications because they cannot afford to purchase them.

Variations in the significant factors predicting medication compliance and noncompliance have been observed in numerous studies. While some factors have been found to be significant in some studies, the same factors have been found to be nonsignificant in other studies. In this study we found patients age, duration of diagnosis, and difficulty remembering medication to be the significant predictors of medication noncompliance. Consistent with the study of Boima and colleagues, we also found the elderly (old) to be less compliant than the young. This pattern observed in noncompliance has also been documented in studies carried out in Sub-Saharan Africa [11].

Patients whose disease condition had persisted over a longer period of time were found to be 2 times more likely to be noncompliant. This finding is similar to that of Hyre and colleagues who also found that a longer duration of disease conditions may not only compromise patients' compliance but also affect compliance negatively [18]. A plausible reason for this could be the fear patients have initially when they are diagnosed with an ailment. With time, they see it as a norm and are no longer afraid of the complications that could arise with their default. Also after taking medications for a long time, patients get worn-out and seek for a somewhat permanent cure, the most likely option being resorting to herbal medications which promise a pull-up of the underlying disease cause. In the descriptive analysis we found that majority of the patients did not have difficulty remembering their medication instructions, in the regression analysis; however, we found that patients who did not have difficulty remembering their medication instruction were however 6 times more likely to be noncompliant. A possible explanation to this observation could be due to the fact that once patients understand and have become familiar with their intake routine they could choose to alter it, especially when they begin experiencing some side effects.

5. Limitations

Our study was limited to patients receiving health care at the St. Patrick's Hospital and did not include patients who attended other health centers in the municipality though they might have met the inclusion criteria. This limitation notwithstanding, we anticipate that since the hospital serves as a primary health facility in the municipal, it records majority of the OPD cases and as a result we may have been able to capture most of the patients with chronic conditions. Additionally, engaging in direct observation of clients and pill counting could have made the study findings more robust; however, due to the laboriousness of this methodology it could not be adopted. Despite these limitations, the findings of our study are encouraged.

6. Conclusion

Noncompliance to medication regimen among chronic disease patients is an important issue for public health consideration. This is evidenced by the results of this study which recorded an overall noncompliance level of 55.5%. The factors identified as contributing to medication noncompliance in this study were age, duration of disease condition, and difficulty in remembering medication instructions. To reduce the incidence of medication noncompliance among chronic disease patients, we first recommend that programmes be drawn in the various clinics for the purpose of health education and counselling of the patients during their waiting times with emphasis on the importance of their medications and the consequences of nonadherence. Emphasis must also be placed on the detrimental effects of mixing orthodox medications with herbal preparations. Opportunity should be created at the clinics during the waiting times for patient-to-patient interaction to share their experiences and challenges so that they could encourage themselves through the difficulties of their therapies. Doctor-to-patient relationship must also be improved so patients can freely discuss issues relating to their therapy. The government of Ghana, through the Ministry of Health, could be sought to extend the NHIS to cover more of the medications used by chronic disease patients. This would reduce the financial burden of patients on life-long therapies.

Abbreviations

CHPS: Community-Based Health Planning and Services
GDHS: Ghana Demographic Health Survey
GHS: Ghana Health Service
NHIS: National Health Insurance Scheme.

Ethical Approval

Ethical approval was obtained from the Ethical Review Committee of the KATH through the School of Medical Sciences, KNUST, Kumasi. Permission for the research was granted from the Administration of St. Patrick's Hospital as well as the head of the special clinic of the hospital.

Disclosure

The study was not supported by any external source of funding nor was compensation or monetary benefit given to participants who took part in the study.

Authors' Contributions

Bright Addo and Sally Sencherey conceived the design of the study. Sally Sencherey collected the data; Bright Addo and Michael N. K. Babayara analysed the data. Bright Addo and Sally Sencherey did the literature review and drafted the manuscript. Michael N. K. Babayara reviewed and edited the draft manuscript. All authors revised, read, and approved the final draft for submission.

Acknowledgments

The authors are grateful to all the study participants (patients) who voluntarily consented to participate in the data collection exercise. They also acknowledge the dedicated and hardworking research assistants who assisted during data collection. Lastly, they thank Mr. Emmanuel Kwaku Nakua for his technical input during the conduct of the study.

References

[1] WHO, "Preventing chronic diseases: a vital investment," *World Health Organisation*, 2005, http://www.who.int/chp/chronic_disease_report/en/.

[2] WHO, "Global status report on noncommunicable diseases," *World Health*, p. 176, 2014.

[3] J. Addo, C. Agyemang, and L. Smeeth, "A review of population-based studies on hypertension in Ghana," in *Ghana Medical Journal*, vol. 46, 2012, http://www.ncbi.nlm.nih.gov/pmc/articles/PMC3645150/pdf/GMJ462S-0004.pdf.

[4] A. G. Amoah, S. K. Owusu, and S. Adjei, "Diabetes in Ghana: a community based prevalence study in Greater Accra," *Diabetes Research and Clinical Practice*, vol. 56, no. 3, pp. 197–205, 2002.

[5] WHO, "Diet, nutrition and the prevention of chronic diseases," *World Health Organization Technical Report Series*, p. 916, 2003, http://eutils.ncbi.nlm.nih.gov/entrez/eutils/elink.fcgi?dbfrom=pubmed&id=12768890&retmode=ref&cmd=prlinks%5Cnpapers3://publication/uuid/734F6B31-260B-4545-A8E4-57F7D35DDEB8.

[6] J. G. Laryea, "Factors influencing adherence to oral antihypertensive medication amongst patients attending the Korle-Bu Teaching Hospital, 2013".

[7] M. Nosé, C. Barbui, R. Gray, and M. Tansella, "Clinical interventions for treatment non-adherence in psychosis: Meta-analysis," *The British Journal of Psychiatry*, vol. 183, pp. 197–206, 2003.

[8] N. C. Talam, P. Gatongi, J. Rotich, and S. Kimaiyo, "Factors affecting antiretroviral drug adherence among HIV/AIDS adult patients attending HIV/AIDS clinic at Moi Teaching and Referral Hospital, Eldoret, Kenya," *East African Journal of Public Health*, vol. 5, no. 2, pp. 74–78, 2008.

[9] H. S. Jin, A. R. An, H. C. Choi et al., "Physical activity level of Korean adults with chronic diseases: The Korean National Health and Nutritional Examination Survey, 2010-2012," *Korean Journal of Family Medicine*, vol. 36, no. 6, pp. 266–272, 2015.

[10] S. P. Bruce, F. Acheampong, and I. Kretchy, "WHO. Global status report on noncommunicable diseases 2014," *Pharm Pract (Granada)*, vol. 13, no. 1, p. 176, 2015.

[11] V. Boima, A. D. Ademola, A. O. Odusola et al., "Factors Associated with Medication Nonadherence among Hypertensives in Ghana and Nigeria," *International Journal of Hypertension*, vol. 2015, Article ID 205716, 2015.

[12] A. Bardel, "31 – Factors Associated With Adherence to Drug Therapy, 2015".

[13] Ghana Statistical Service, "2010 Population and Housing Census: National Analytical Report, 2013," http://www.waikato.ac.nz/__data/assets/pdf_file/0007/180592/Norway-2001-en.pdf.

[14] T. Abula and A. Worku, "Compliance to chronic diseases," *Ethiopian Journal of Health Development*, vol. 15, no. 3, pp. 185–192, 2001.

[15] K. O. Buabeng, L. Matowe, and J. Plange-Rhule, "Unaffordable drug prices: the major cause of non-compliance with hypertension medication in Ghana," *Journal of Pharmacy & Pharmaceutical Sciences*, vol. 7, no. 3, pp. 350–352, 2004.

[16] N. K. Joan, E. Owino, and P. N. Agatha, "Non adherence to diabetes treatment at mulago hospital in Uganda—Prevalence and associated factors," *African Health Sciences*, vol. 8, no. 2, pp. 67–73, 2008.

[17] F. I. Abdulazeez, M. Omole, and S. L. Ojulari, "Medication adherence amongst diabetic patients in a tertiary healthcare institution in central Nigeria," *Tropical Journal of Pharmaceutical Research*, vol. 13, no. 6, pp. 997–1001, 2014.

[18] A. D. Hyre, P. Muntner, A. Menke, P. Raggi, and J. He, "Trends in ATP-III-Defined high blood cholesterol prevalence, awareness, treatment and Control Among U.S. Adults," *Annals of Epidemiology*, vol. 17, no. 7, pp. 548–555, 2007.

24

Achievements of Diabetes Goals and Their Determinants in Type 2 Diabetic Patients Attending Outpatient Diabetic Clinic in Northern Ethiopia

Ezra Belay,[1] Abel Abera,[1] Aman Mehari,[1] Gidey Gebremeskel,[1] Asrat Endrias,[1] and Kedir Endris[2]

[1] *Department of Medical Biochemistry, College of Health Sciences, Mekelle University, 1871 Mekelle, Ethiopia*
[2] *Department of Nursing, College of Health Sciences, Mekelle University, 1871 Mekelle, Ethiopia*

Correspondence should be addressed to Ezra Belay; aga.bely@gmail.com

Academic Editor: Katarzyna Zorena

Background. The aim of this study was to assess target diabetic goal achievements and to explore variables associated with them. *Methods.* A cross-sectional study was conducted between December 2015 and April 2016 on 188 type 2 diabetic patients attending Ayder Referral Hospital's outpatient diabetic clinic. Glycemic control was assessed using fasting plasma glucose values and total cholesterol and triglyceride were used to evaluate lipid profiles. Bivariate and multivariate logistic regression analyses were done to identify factors associated with poor glycemic control, hypertension, and dyslipidemia. *Result.* Mean duration of diabetes was 6.5 years. Combined glycemic, lipid, and blood pressure targets were achieved only in 8.5% of the participants. More males achieved combined targets than females. Separately, while above two-thirds of the patients had poor glycemic control (67%), more than half of the participants have had poor lipid (58.5%) and blood pressure (52.1%) control. A significant portion of the patients (68.1%) had also comorbidities other than hyperglycemia. In bivariate and multivariate analyses, longer duration of diabetes disease (AOR: 3.4; $P = 0.013$) and marked month to month fasting plasma glucose (FPG) variability as measured by large standard deviation (AOR: 2.5; $P = 0.023$) were significantly associated with overall poor mean FPG results. Female sex was also significantly associated with dyslipidemia (AOR: 1.9; $P = 0.049$). *Conclusion.* The study showed that achievements of combined diabetic goals are generally poor.

1. Introduction

More than 422 million (8.5%) adult people were living with diabetes at the end of 2014. Tens of millions suffer disabling and life-threatening complications of diabetes such as heart attack, stroke, kidney failure, blindness, and amputation [1, 2]. The proportion of premature deaths due to diabetes is higher in developing countries than in developed countries and the prevalence is rising most rapidly in these least developed countries [2]. According to 2014 International Diabetes Federation (IDF) report, more than 22 million diabetic people (about 7.1%) were living in Africa [3]. Diabetes is becoming a growing health problem along with other noncommunicable diseases in Ethiopia. Cross-sectional studies estimated the prevalence of diabetes to be as high as 7% and 5% of deaths are due to diabetes mellitus [4, 5].

Optimal control of plasma glucose, lipid profile, and blood pressure is central to the management of diabetes mellitus. These are the key factors in reducing morbidity and death from the disease. Several large studies have proven that achieving these diabetic goals averts or considerably delays life-threatening complications of diabetes, enabling people with diabetes to live longer and healthier lives [6, 7]. Despite the strong consensus that excellent management of diabetes prevents both macrovascular and microvascular outcomes in type 1 and type 2 diabetes mellitus, universal studies indicated that majority of diabetic patients did not attain their target diabetic goals [8, 9]. This is even more challenging in developing countries due to a limited access to adequate health services, poor education level, reduced access to medical education, and a lack of standard laboratory tests such as HbA1c for assessing metabolic controls. Moreover, besides the fact that low socioeconomic status is associated with higher prevalence of diabetes and a greater risk for diabetes complications, there are likely many specific elements of low economic status which predispose diabetic patients in resource-limited setting to poor diabetes control [10–12]. The aim of this study was to assess the extent of diabetic goal achievements and failures and their determinants in patients with diabetes in Northern Ethiopia where data are scarce.

2. Methods and Subjects

A cross-sectional study was conducted in type 2 diabetic patients attending outpatient diabetic clinic of Ayder Referral Hospital, Mekelle University, between December 2015 and April 2016 to evaluate the extent of diabetic target achievements and factors associated with them. All type 2 diabetic patients who were attending the outpatient diabetic clinic during the data collection period were included in the study provided that they met all of the following inclusion criteria: visited the diabetic clinic during the data collection period, had been diagnosed with diabetes at least six months earlier, had regular follow-up at diabetic clinic of Ayder Referral Hospital for at least 6 months prior to data collection, and agreed to sign consent form. During their regular follow-up, study participants were recruited into the study by trained data collectors. Patients were allowed to participate only once during the six-month period. Patients whose follow-up was not regular (those who missed three or more follow-ups within six months), patients with less than six-month follow-up, and newly diagnosed diabetic patients (less than six-month duration) were excluded from the study.

2.1. Data Collection. Data on sociodemographic variables (age, sex, income level, education, residency, and marital status), lifestyle variables (dietary variables, alcohol consumption, smoking, and physical activities), and self-monitoring and management practices were collected by trained diabetic nurses using face-to-face interviews and structured questionnaires. After face-to-face interview, information on anthropometric measurements, blood pressure, duration of diabetes, diabetic medications, coexisting comorbidities and other medications, lipid profiles, and current and previous five-month records of fasting plasma glucose (FPG) was collected through clinical laboratory investigation and review of patients' medical records.

2.2. Ethical Approval. Ethical clearance and approval for undertaking this study were obtained from Research and Community Service Council (RCSC) of Mekelle University, College of Health Sciences, before starting the actual data collection. Subsequent permission was obtained from the authorities of Ayder Referral Hospital, including medical director and the head of diabetic clinic. After explaining the aim and objectives of the study, verbal and written informed consent was obtained from each participant.

2.3. Measurements and Operational Definitions. We evaluated achievements of diabetes goal by assessing glycemic control, lipid profile, and blood pressure targets. We used mean and single FPG measurements for glycemic control and total cholesterol and triglyceride test for lipid profile assessments. Glycemic control was classified as good or poor based on the criteria of the American Diabetes Association (ADA) (good: FPG < 130 mg/dL; poor: FPG ≥ 130 mg/dL) [13].

Lipid profiles, blood pressure, and body mass index values were also categorized as normal and high based on criteria of ADA and US National Cholesterol Education Program. Accordingly, hypercholesterolemia was considered when total cholesterol level is ≥200 mg/dl and hypertriglyceridemia refers to a level ≥ 150 mg/dl. Dyslipidemia was defined as the presence of one or both of these abnormalities in serum. Hypertension was defined as systolic blood pressure ≥ 140 mmHg and/or diastolic blood pressure ≥ 90 mmHg or use of antihypertensive medications [13, 14].

Month to month variability of FPG was also assessed using mean, standard deviation (SD), and coefficient of variation (CV) [15]. Mean and standard deviations were calculated for each patient from six-month FPG data. Glycemic variability (GV) was then determined by dividing standard deviation to mean. GV was calculated only when more than three measurements were performed in the last six months including the final measurement done during data collection period. Wide GV was considered when CV of FPG was greater than 25% [15]. Similarly, ideal target for SD was considered when SD multiplied by three was less than mean [16]. We also calculated the approximate HbA1c from mean plasma glucose values using the following formula: mean plasma glucose (MPG) (mg/dl) = (35.6 ∗ HbA1c) − 77.3 [17].

2.4. Laboratory Analysis. Fasting serum value of FPG, total cholesterol, and triglyceride were determined according to their measurement principles and guidelines using Hitachi 902 Autoanalyzer (Roche Diagnostics, Germany). For total cholesterol determination, cholesterol esters in serum are hydrolyzed by cholesterol esterase in the reagent. The free cholesterol is then oxidized by cholesterol oxidase to the corresponding ketone liberating hydrogen peroxide, which is then converted to water and oxygen by the enzyme peroxidase. Para-aminophenazone (4-aminophenazone) takes up the oxygen and together with phenol forms a pink-colored quinoneimine dye and the absorbance was measured at 515 nm wavelength. Triglycerides were measured enzymatically in serum using a series of coupled reactions in which triglycerides were hydrolyzed to produce glycerol. Glycerol is then oxidized using glycerol oxidase, and H_2O_2, one of the reaction products, is measured quantitatively in a peroxidase-catalyzed reaction that produces a color. The color intensity is proportional to triglyceride concentration present in the sample. Absorbance is measured at 500 nm.

2.5. Data/Statistical Analysis. All data were entered into Epi Info software (version 7.1) and analyzed using Statistical Package for the Social Sciences (SPSS) software (version 20.0). First, data were cleaned, edited, and checked for completeness before analysis.

Chi-square test was used to measure the significant differences among different proportions. Binary logistic regression analysis was carried out to identify factors associated with poor glycemic control, hypertension, and dyslipidemia with their 95% confidence interval. At the same time, we performed covariate analysis between continuous variables. A P value of <0.05 was considered as a statistically significant level. All variables with a P value < 0.3 were considered for multivariate logistic regression to determine independent factors predicting poor diabetic control. Model fit to the data (validity and reliability) was assessed by the likelihood ratio χ^2 test and Hosmer-Lemeshow goodness-of-fit test.

3. Result

3.1. Sociodemographic Characteristics of Study's Patients. From the total 188 participants, 104 (58.9%) were males. The median age of the study population was 54 years, ranging from 18 to 80 years. 34% of the study participants were illiterate and 17% were rural residents. Less than one-fifth (16.5%) of the participants have had regular physical exercises and 66% had food selection for their diabetes management. From participants with dietary restriction, 23.4% avoided sugar, salt, and fatty foods, while the rest used vegetables (13.8%), barley (8%), and teff (8%). Majority of the participants visited the diabetic clinic only 3-4 times in the last six months. Only 11.2% patients had their own glucometer for self-monitoring practices (Table 1). Table 1 summarizes the detailed sociodemographic and lifestyle features of the study's participants.

3.2. Clinical Characteristics. Mean duration of diabetes since diagnosis was 6.5 years. A larger proportion of patients (55.3%) were taking oral hypoglycemic agents followed by insulin (37.8). In addition to diabetic treatments, about 40% of the patients were taking other medications. Based on self-report and clinical record review, comorbidities other than hyperglycemia were described in 68.1% of the patients. Peripheral vascular disease (46.8%), hypertension (44.7%), gastrointestinal problems (42.2%), renal diseases (22.3%), retinopathy (18.6%), and heart problems (5.9%) were among the reported comorbidities. Except hypertension, female proportions were higher in all comorbidities (Figure 1).

Based on coefficient of variation of FPG, 93 (49.5%) had marked month to month glycemic variations (CV: FPG ≥ 25) and 61 (32.44%) failed to achieve target SD for FPG (SD $*$ $3 <$ mean). Only 35 (18.6%) patients had HbA1c test record during the last six months. From these, 26/35 had HbA1c value $\geq 7\%$ (poor control). The detailed clinical characteristics of the study's patients are indicated in Table 1.

3.3. Achievements of Diabetic Goals. Based on FPG measurements, 136 (72.3%) had poor glycemic control. After calculating HbA1c values from the corresponding mean FPG values, 110 (58.5%) had HbA1c value ≥ 7 (poor control), while 52.2% of patients were hypertensive and 58.5% had dyslipidemia and either hypercholesterolemia or triglyceridemia or both. Combined glycemic, lipid, and blood pressure targets were achieved only in 8.5% of the participants. While majorities (41.5%) achieved only one of these three goals, 22.3% did not achieve all the three targets. More proportion of males achieved combined targets than females (Table 2).

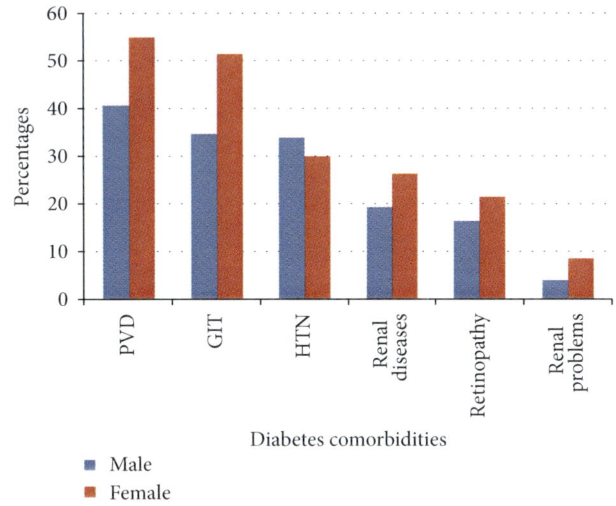

FIGURE 1: Prevalence of diabetes comorbidities among diabetic patients attending outpatient diabetic clinic of Ayder Referral Hospital. PVD: peripheral vascular diseases; GIT: gastrointestinal problem; HTN: hypertension.

3.4. Factors Associated with Poor Diabetic Goals Achievements. Large standard deviation marked FPG variability and longer duration of diabetes were predictors of overall mean glycemic control. Patients with longer duration of diabetes were less likely to achieve overall mean glycemic targets. Similarly, patients with large month to month FPG variability and large standard deviation were more like to have high average FPG. All variables with P value less than 0.3 in binary logistic regression analysis were included in multivariate logistic regression analysis after checking for confounders. In multivariate analysis, these variables retained their significant association (Table 3). Higher body mass index (BMI ≥ 25) and presence of comorbidities other than hyperglycemia were variables that showed statistically significant association with hypertension. Female gender was also significantly associated with dyslipidemia (Table 3).

4. Discussion

This study revealed that only 8.5% of the study population achieved the combined glycemic, lipid, and blood pressure targets and 22.3% of the patients achieved none of these targets. While more than two-thirds of the patients had poor glycemic control, above half of the participants have had poor lipid and blood pressure control. A significant portion of the patients (68.1%) had also comorbidities other than hyperglycemia. Our result is lower as compared to the previous study in Israel, which found 13% of combined target achievements [18]. However, they used low-density lipoprotein cholesterol (LDL-cholesterol) for lipid profile and HbA1c for glycemic control as well as a lower cutoff point for blood pressure assessment, which is different from us. In line with our finding, similar rate of poor glycemic control was reported from Tanzania (69.7%) [19]. However, we found slightly higher prevalence of poor glycemic control based on mean FPG (72.3%) and lower results according to HbA1c

Table 1: Proportion of type 2 diabetic patients with poor glycemic control according to the sociodemographic, lifestyle, and clinical characteristics, attending Ayder Referral Hospital.

Patient characteristics	Total number ($N = 188$), n (%)	Mean glycemia ≥ 130 mg/dL ($N = 136$), n (%)	P value	Current glycemia ≥ 130 mg/dL $N = 126$, n (%)	P value
Age, mean + SD	49.9 + 16.9		0.36	49.9 + 16.9	0.68
≤30 years	5 (2.6)	3 (2.2)		1 (0.07)	
31–45 years	43 (22.9)	33 (24.3)	0.7	29 (23.0)	0.04
46–60 years	88 (46.8)	61 (44.9)		65 (51.6)	
>60 years	52 (27.7)	39 (28.7)		31 (24.6)	
Sex: male, n (%)	104 (58.9)	71 (52.2)	0.17	64 (50.8)	0.08
Education, n (%)					
Illiterate	64 (34.0)	49 (36.0)		47 (37.3)	
Primary education	38 (20.2)	28 (20.5)	0.28	22 (17.5)	0.09
Secondary and above	86 (45.7)	59 (43.3)		57 (45.2)	
Marital status, n (%),					
Single	36 (19.1)	27 (19.6)	0.51	24 (19.1)	0.85
Married	152 (80.8)	109 (80.4)		102 (80.9)	
Residency, n (%)					
Rural	32 (17.0)	26 (19.1)	0.25	23 (18.3)	0.6
Urban	156 (82.9)	110 (80.9)		103 (81.7)	
Income (ETB), n (%)					
None	34 (18.1%)	21 (15.4)		20 (14.7)	
<1000	50 (26.6)	37 (27.2)	0.9	36 (28.6)	0.26
1000–2500	56 (29.8)	44 (32.4)		42 (33.3)	
>2500	48 (25.5)	34 (25.0)		28 (22.2)	
Lifestyles, yes, n (%)					
Smoking	2 (15)	2 (1.5)	NA	2 (1.5)	
Alcohol intake	11 (5.9)	7 (5.1)	0.5	6 (4.8)	
Physical activity	31 (16.5)	21 (15.4)	0.47	17 (13.5)	0.11
Dietary restriction	124 (66.0)	86 (63.2)	0.31	79 (62.7)	0.28
Self-monitoring practices, yes, n (%)	21 (11.1)	15 (11.0)	0.64	12 (9.5)	0.84
Number of visits in 6 months					
3-4 times	106 (56.4)	75 (55.1)	0.58	76 (60.3)	0.12
5-6 times	82 (43.6)	61 (44.9)		50 (39.7)	
Duration of diabetes in years, mean + SD	6.5 + 6.8	-	**0.014**	6.5 + 6.8	0.21
<5 years	94 (50.0)	62 (45.6)		60 (47.6)	
5–10 years	50 (26.6)	39 (28.7)	**0.007**	36 (28.6)	0.14
>10 years	44 (23.4)	35 (25.7)		30 (23.8)	
Glycemic variability ≥ 25	93 (49.5)	77 (56.6)	**0.002**	62 (49.2)	0.91
Large SD (SD ∗ 3 > mean)	61 (32.44)	51 (37.5)	**0.02**	39 (31.0)	0.53
Diabetes drugs, n (%)					
OHA	104 (55.3)	73 (53.7)		68 (54.0)	
Insulin only	71 (37.8)	54 (39.7)	0.67	46 (36.5)	0.14
Combination therapy	13 (6.9)	9 (6.6)		12 (9.5)	
Use of other drugs, yes, n (%)	76 (40.4)	55 (40.4)	0.99	53 (42.1)	0.51
Presence of comorbidities, yes, n (%)	128 (68.1)	93 (68.4)	0.88	85 (67.5)	0.79
BMI ≥ 25	63 (33.5)	41 (30.1)	0.06	39 (31.0)	0.23
Dyslipidemia	110 (58.5)	85 (62.5)	0.10	80 (63.5)	**0.04**
Hypertension	98 (52.1)	70 (51.5)	0.59	65 (51.6)	0.7

SD: standard deviation; ETB: Ethiopian Birr; OHA; oral hypoglycemic agent, BMI: body mass index. P values were calculated using chi-square test.

TABLE 2: Achievements of diabetic goal in patients attending Ayder Referral Hospital, Northern Ethiopia.

Characteristics	Total number (%)	Female	Male	P value
FPG				
Normal (FPG < 130)	62 (33.0)	22 (26.2)	40 (38.5)	0.075
Poor control (FPG ≥ 130)	126 (67.0)	62 (73.8)	64 (61.5)	
Mean FPG				
Normal (FPG < 130)	52 (27.7)	19 (22.6)	33 (31.7)	0.17
Poor control (FPG ≥ 130)	136 (72.3)	65 (77.4)	71 (68.3)	
HbA1c (calculated)				
<7%	78 (41.5)	32 (38.1)	46 (44.2)	0.40
≥7%	110 (58.5)	52 (61.9)	58 (55.8)	
Hypertension				
No	84 (44.7)	43 (51.2)	41 (39.4)	0.093
Yes	98 (52.1)	38 (45.2)	60 (57.7)	
Dyslipidemia				
No	71 (37.8)	25 (29.8)	46 (44.2)	0.028
Yes	110 (58.5)	57 (67.9)	53 (51.0)	
Combined diabetic goal achievements*				
All three goals achieved	16 (8.5)	6 (7.1)	10 (9.6)	0.43
Two goals achieved	52 (27.7)	19 (22.6)	33 (31.7)	
Only one goal achieved	78 (41.5)	39 (46.4)	39 (37.5)	
None of the goals achieved	42 (22.3)	20 (23.8)	22 (21.2)	

FPG: fasting plasma glucose; HbA1c: glycated hemoglobin. *P* values were calculated using binary logistic regression analysis. *Combined diabetic goal: combination of glycemic, lipid, and blood pressure targets.

calculated from mean FPG (58.5%). But we should not use the calculated HbA1c, since approximation results will mislead to wrong inferences. Several other studies described prevalence of poor glycemic control using HbA1c test results. Regardless of these parametric differences, relatively higher rate of poor glycemic control was reported from Malaysia (76%) [20], Saudi Arabia (73%) [21], and South Africa (74.6%) [22], while roughly similar results were found in Jordan (65.1%) [23] and Kuwait (66.7%) [24]. Lower prevalence rate of poor glycemic control was also reported in studies from Pakistan (46.7%) [25] and Spain (50.6%) [26]. Nevertheless, these countries, except Spain, are known for their highest prevalence of diabetes in the world.

In this study, we used FPG test as a tool for assessing glycemic control status. Despite the fact that assessment of FPG is insufficient to obtain optimal glycemic control [27–29] and to achieve long-term diabetic targets, markers such as HbA1c and postprandial plasma glucose tests are not available in the study area. On the other hand, lack of these tests could prevent patients and physicians from taking the necessary actions on time to improve and sustain glycemic control for long time. In fact, in this study, the proportion of patients with high mean FPG value was higher than the proportion of patients with high single FPG measurements (72.3% versus 67.0%). This may partly explain the high rate of poor diabetic goals achievements and high incidences of diabetes comorbidities in the study area.

For blood pressure targets, we found comparable results with studies from Israel (51%) [18] and South Africa (49.6%) [22] and lower than study reports from Brazil (63.2%) [30]. Most of the previous studies used LDL-cholesterol as a tool for assessing lipid profile targets. But because of inaccessibility of the LDL-cholesterol test, we used total cholesterol and triglycerides tests to assess lipid profile targets despite the fact that LDL-cholesterol is more associated with pathogenesis of cardiovascular diseases risks in type 2 diabetic patients.

In bivariate and multivariate analyses, longer duration of diabetes disease (AOR: 3.4) and wide month to month FPG variability as measured by large CV of FPG and large SD (AOR: 2.5) were significantly associated with overall poor mean FPG results. None of these variables were associated with single FPG values. Association of marked FPG variability (CV ≥ 25) with poor mean FPG control, but not with single FPG value, indicates that FPG variability mainly affects the overall long-term results. This can be interpreted as follows: diabetic patients who failed to narrow their month to month FPG variability and maintain its stability are less likely to achieve their long-term control. This may be in turn the reflection of low treatment adherence, low self-management practices, or irregular food intakes.

In accordance with our result, Assunção et al. and Juarez et al. also found significant association between longer duration of diabetes and poor glycemic control [30, 31]. This association may be due to the decreases in β-cell function and insulin secretion as the disease progresses over time.

Similarly, in bivariate analysis, patients with higher BMI (BMI ≥ 25), taking drugs other than antidiabetics, and having coexisting morbidities were more likely to be hypertensive and failed to achieve blood pressure targets. Female diabetic patients and patients with high FPG were also at high risk of

TABLE 3: Bivariate and multivariate analysis for factors associated with wide mean glycemia, hypertension, and dyslipidemia in type 2 diabetic patients attending Ayder Referral Hospital, Northern Ethiopia ($N = 188$).

Characteristics	COR (95% CI)	*P* value	AOR (95% CI)	*P* value
Variables associated with mean glycemia				
Duration of diabetes				
<5 years	Reference			
5–10 years	2.6 (1.13–5.93)	0.025	2.6 (1.12–6.01)	0.027
>10 years	3.5 (1.34–9.06)	0.011	3.4 (1.3–9.0)	0.013
Target SD				
SD * 3 < mean				
SD * 3 > mean	2.5 (1.16–5.5)	0.019	2.5 (1.13–5.5)	0.023
FPG variability				
CV < 25				
CV ≥ 25	2.9 (1.5–5.8)	0.002	R*	R*
Yes	2.0 (1.04–3.7)	0.038		
Variables associated with hypertension				
BMI				
BMI < 25	Reference			
BMI ≥ 25	3.0 (1.54–5.69)	0.001	2.03 (0.88–4.71)	0.098
Presence of other comorbidities				
No	Reference			0.081
Yes	2.9 (1.53–5.76)	0.001	2.114 (0.91–4.9)	
Variables associated with dyslipidemia				
Sex				
Male	Reference			
Female	2.0 (1.071–3.66)	0.029	1.9 (1.002–3.48)	0.049
FPG				
FPG > 130	Reference			0.065
FPG ≥ 130	1.95 (1.04–3.67)	0.038	1.8 (0.96–3.46)	

COR: crude odd ratio; AOR: adjusted odd ratio; CI: confidence interval; SD: standard deviation; CV: coefficient of variation; BMI: body mass index; FPG: fasting plasma glucose. R* indicates that FPG variability was removed from multiple logistic regression analysis because of significant correlation with target SD.

developing dyslipidemia ($P < 0.05$). The association of high BMI with hypertension and female gender and high FPG with dyslipidemia is consistent with the pathogenesis and risk of these diseases. However, the association between presence of coexisting morbidities and hypertension is hard to explain, since frequencies were generated from the data collected by combination of self-report and review of clinical records.

According to clinical record review and self-reports, 68.1% of the study participants have had comorbidities other than hyperglycemia in which peripheral vascular diseases, gastrointestinal problems, hypertension, and renal diseases were most common. Particularly, the high rate of gastrointestinal problem is something uncommon and needs further investigation. Strong evidences demonstrated that poor glycemic control is associated with the development of diabetes complication and other cardiovascular effects [32–34]. However, diabetic patients with multiple disorders could also be challenged by the coexisting comorbidities to sustain their glycemic control and to attain target values.

As a limitation, this study was based on six months' retrospective data analysis and used only routine diagnostic tests available. Another prospective study with inclusion of other diagnostic markers such as postprandial plasma glucose, low-density lipoprotein, and HbA1c is required to fully investigate the prognostic value of glycemic variability and factors affecting it in resource-poor settings.

In conclusion, the results of this study showed that achievements of combined diabetic goals are very poor (only 8.5%). In order to improve combined diabetic goal attainment, patients should be advised to minimize month to month FPG variation and maintain consistent glycemic control.

Abbreviations

ADA: American Diabetes Association
BMI: Body mass index
CV: Coefficient of variation
FPG: Fasting plasma glucose
GV: Glycemic variability
HbA1c: Glycosylated hemoglobin
IDF: International Diabetes Federation
SD: Standard deviation
RCSC: Research and Community Service Council.

References

[1] International diabetes Federation, "Global Diabetes Plan, IDF, 2011–2021".

[2] World Health Organization, "Global report on diabetes," WHO, 2016, http://www.who.int/diabetes/global-report/en/.

[3] International Diabetic Federation, "International diabetic federation, 2014 report," 2014, http://www.idf.org/publications/annual-report.

[4] L. D. Nshisso, A. Reese, B. Gelaye, S. Lemmab, Y. Berhane, and M. A. Williams, "Prevalence of hypertension and diabetes among Ethiopian adults," *Diabetes & Metabolic Syndrome: Clinical Research & Reviews*, vol. 6, no. 1, pp. 36–41, 2012.

[5] A. Misganaw, D. H. Mariam, and T. Araya, "The double mortality burden among adults in Addis Ababa, Ethiopia, 2006–2009," *Preventing Chronic Disease*, vol. 9, no. 4, Article ID 110142, 2012.

[6] American Diabetes Association (ADA), "Standards of medical care in Diabetes," *Diabetes Care*, vol. 37, pp. S14–S80, 2014.

[7] S. J. Beaton, S. S. Nag, M. J. Gunter, J. M. Gleeson, S. S. Sajjan, and C. M. Alexander, "Adequacy of glycemic, lipid, and blood pressure management for patients with diabetes in a managed care setting," *Diabetes Care*, vol. 27, no. 3, pp. 694–698, 2004.

[8] A. Ceriello, S. Colagiuri, J. Gerich, and J. Tuomilehto, "Guideline for management of postmeal glucose," *Nutrition, Metabolism & Cardiovascular Diseases*, vol. 18, no. 4, pp. S17–S33, 2008.

[9] L. Monnier and C. Colette, "Target for glycemic control: concentrating on glucose," *Diabetes Care*, vol. 32, no. 2, pp. S199–S204, 2009.

[10] E. Agardh, P. Allebeck, J. Hallqvist, T. Moradi, and A. Sidorchuk, "Type 2 diabetes incidence and socio-economic position: a systematic review and meta-analysis," *International Journal of Epidemiology*, vol. 40, no. 3, pp. 804–818, 2011.

[11] J. M. Robbins, V. Vaccarino, H. Zhang, and S. V. Kasl, "Socioeconomic status and type 2 diabetes in African American and non-Hispanic White women and men: evidence from the Third National Health and Nutrition Examination Survey," *American Journal of Public Health*, vol. 91, no. 1, pp. 76–83, 2001.

[12] H. K. Seligman, J. Tschann, E. A. Jacobs, A. Fernandez, and A. López, "Food insecurity and glycemic control among low-income patients with type 2 diabetes," *Diabetes Care*, vol. 35, no. 2, pp. 233–238, 2012.

[13] American Diabetes Association, "Standards of medical care in diabetes," *Diabetes Care*, vol. 37, no. 1, pp. S112–S117, 2013.

[14] National Cholesterol Education Program, "ATP III: third report of the expert panel on detection, evaluation, and treatment of high blood cholesterol in adults (adult treatment panel III, or ATP III), Final report," NIH N 02-5215:2002, 2002.

[15] C.-C. Lin, C.-P. Yang, C.-I. Li et al., "Visit-to-visit variability of fasting plasma glucose as predictor of ischemic stroke: competing risk analysis in a national cohort of Taiwan Diabetes Study," *BMC Medicine*, vol. 12, article 165, 2014.

[16] I. B. Hirsch, "Glycemic variability: it's not just about A1C anymore!," *Diabetes Technology & Therapeutics*, vol. 7, no. 5, pp. 780–783, 2005.

[17] C. L. Rohlfing, H. M. Wiedmeyer, R. R. Little, J. D. England, A. Tennill, and D. E. Goldstein, "Defining the relationship between plasma glucose and HbA1c: analysis of glucose profiles and HbA1c in the diabetes control and complications trial," *Diabetes Care*, vol. 25, no. 2, pp. 275–278, 2002.

[18] A. Elis, L. Rosenmann, G. Chodick, A. D. Heymann, E. Kokia, and V. Shalev, "The association between glycemic, lipids and blood pressure control among Israeli diabetic patients," *QJM: An International Journal of Medicine*, vol. 101, no. 4, pp. 275–280, 2008.

[19] A. R. Kamuhabwa and E. Charles, "Predictors of poor glycemic control in type 2 diabetic patients attending public hospitals in Dar es Salaam," *Journal of Drug, Healthcare and Patient Safety*, vol. 6, pp. 155–165, 2014.

[20] M. A. Almutairi, S. Said, and H. Zainuddin, "Predictors of poor glycemic control among type two diabetic patients," *American Journal of Medicine and Medical Science*, vol. 3, no. 2, pp. 17–21, 2013.

[21] S. M. Sadjjadi, S. Ardehali, B. Noman-Pour, V. Kumar, and A. Izadpanah, "Diagnosis of cystic echinococcosis: ultrasound imaging or countercurrent immunoelectrophoresis?" *Eastern Mediterranean Health Journal*, vol. 7, no. 4-5, pp. 671–678, 2001.

[22] Y. Pinchevsky, V. Shukla, N. Butkow, FJ. Raal, and T. Chirwa, "The achievement of glycaemic, blood pressure and LDL cholesterol targets in patients with type 2 diabetes attending a South African tertiary hospital outpatient clinic," *Journal of Endocrinology, Metabolism and Diabetes of South Africa*, vol. 20, no. 2, pp. 81–86, 2015.

[23] M. Khattab, Y. S. Khader, A. Al-Khawaldeh, and K. Ajlouni, "Factors associated with poor glycemic control among patients with Type 2 diabetes," *Journal of Diabetes and its Complications*, vol. 24, no. 2, pp. 84–89, 2010.

[24] F. A. Al-Sultan and N. Al-Zanki, "Clinical epidemiology of type 2 diabetes mellitus in Kuwait," *Kuwait Medical Journal*, vol. 37, no. 2, pp. 98–104, 2005.

[25] S. S. Habib and M. Aslam, "Risk factors, knowledge and health status in diabetic patients," *Saudi Medical Journal*, vol. 24, no. 11, pp. 1219–1224, 2003.

[26] D. Orozco-Beltrán, V. F. Gil-Guillen, F. Quirce et al., "Control of diabetes and cardiovascular risk factors in patients with type 2 diabetes in primary care. The gap between guidelines and reality in Spain," *International Journal of Clinical Practice*, vol. 61, no. 6, pp. 909–915, 2007.

[27] M. Hanefeld, "Post-prandial hyperglycaemia and vascular disease," *International Journal of Clinical Practice*, vol. 112, pp. 13–18, 2000.

[28] L. Rajmohan, V. Mohan, and T. R. Ramanujam, "Postprandial hyperglycaemia—the real challenge in diabetes," *The Journal of the Association of Physicians of India*, vol. 49, pp. 357–360, 2001.

[29] S. Haffner, "The importance of postprandial hyperglycaemia in development of cardiovascular disease in people with diabetes," *International Journal of Clinical Practice*, vol. 123, pp. 24–26, 2001.

[30] M. C. F. Assunção, I. S. Santos, and N. C. J. Valle, "Blood glucose control in diabetes patients seen in primary health care centers," *Revista de Saúde Pública*, vol. 39, no. 2, pp. 183–190, 2005.

[31] D. T. Juarez, T. Sentell, S. Tokumaru, R. Goo, J. W. Davis, and M. M. Mau, "Factors associated with poor glycemic control or wide glycemic variability among diabetes patients in Hawaii, 2006–2009," *Preventing Chronic Disease*, vol. 9, no. 9, Article ID 120065, 2012.

[32] Diabetes Control and Complications Trial (DCCT) Research Group, "The effect of intensive treatment of diabetes on the development and progression of long-term complications in insulin-dependent diabetes mellitus," *The New England Journal of Medicine*, vol. 329, no. 14, pp. 977–986, 1993.

[33] Diabetes Control and Complications Trial (DCCT) Research Group, "The relationship of glycemic exposure (HbA1c) to the risk of development and progression of retinopathy in the diabetes control and complications trial," *Diabetes*, vol. 44, no. 8, pp. 968–983, 1995.

[34] C. Stettler, S. Allemann, P. Jüni et al., "Glycemic control and macrovascular disease in types 1 and 2 diabetes mellitus: meta-analysis of randomized trials," *American Heart Journal*, vol. 152, no. 1, pp. 27–38, 2006.

A Comparison of the Prevalence of the Metabolic Syndrome among Sri Lankan Patients with Type 2 Diabetes Mellitus Using WHO, NCEP-ATP III, and IDF Definitions

H. M. M. Herath,[1] N. P. Weerasinghe,[2] T. P. Weerarathna,[1] and A. Amarathunga[3]

[1] *Department of Medicine, Faculty of Medicine, University of Ruhuna and University Unit, Teaching Hospital, Karapitiya, Galle, Sri Lanka*
[2] *Department of Microbiology, Faculty of Medicine, University of Ruhuna, Galle, Sri Lanka*
[3] *Department of Medicine, Faculty of Medicine, University of Ruhuna, Galle, Sri Lanka*

Correspondence should be addressed to H. M. M. Herath; herathtp@gmail.com

Academic Editor: Tadeusz Robak

Background. Presence of metabolic syndrome (MetS) in patients with type 2 diabetes mellitus (type 2 DM) increases the risk of cardiovascular morbidity and mortality. Therefore, recognition of MetS in type 2 DM is important in initiating the appropriate preventive and therapeutic measures. The commonly used definitions have similarities and discrepancies. Aims of this study was to investigate the prevalence of MetS among patients with type 2DM using all three well known (WHO, IDF, and NCEP-ATP III) definitions and to identify the concordance and the difference of these three definitions. *Methods.* This cross-sectional study included patients with type 2 DM who were followed up at the regional diabetes centre in Galle, Sri Lanka. A total of 2913 type 2 DM patients were recruited by convenient sampling method, and their clinical and biochemical data were collected. *Results.* The mean age (SD) of the sample was 49.9 (10.2) years and the mean duration of diabetes was 5.04 (5.71). Prevalence of MetS was highest by WHO (70%) followed by IDF (44%) and NCEP-ATP III (29%) definitions. The prevalence was significantly higher in women according to all three definitions, and the difference was most marked with NCEP-ATP III and IDF definitions. Around 25% were identified as having MetS by all three definitions whereas around 45% were recognized with MetS by two definitions. While concordances between WHO with IDF (0.37, $p < 0.001$) and NCEP-ATP III (0.24, $p < 0.001$) criteria were poor, they were average (0.53, $p < 0.001$) between NCEP-ATP III and IDF criteria. *Conclusions.* The prevalence of MetS among patients with type 2 DM can significantly be varied based on the definition used and the three definitions of MetS recognized different set of individuals. The highest prevalence of MetS was observed with WHO (70.6%) whereas lowest was observed with NCEP-ATP III definition.

1. Introduction

Type 2 diabetes mellitus (type 2 DM) has become a global epidemic with significant disability, premature death, and enormous medical costs [1]. Total number of people with diabetes is projected to double between 2000 and 2030 with a significantly greater rise in Asia [2, 3]. Among Asian regions, South Asia is developing as the epicentre of this escalating epidemic [4]. South Asians with diabetes have higher risk of developing cardiovascular events (CVD) [3]. This is partly due to the presence of peculiar body phenotype known as South Asian phenotype [5, 6]. It is characterized by increased waist circumference, increased waist hip ratio, excessive body fat mass, increased plasma insulin levels and insulin resistance, and an atherogenic dyslipidaemia, with low levels of HDL cholesterol and increased triglyceride levels [6]. Constellation of such various interrelated cardio metabolic risk factors is referred to as metabolic syndrome (MetS) [7]. There is strong evidence that presence of MetS increased the risk of cardiovascular mortality and morbidity [7, 8]. In addition MetS is also associated with other disorders such as thrombotic and inflammatory conditions, fatty liver disease, and reproductive disorders [1].

Although there is general agreement of the core components of the MetS such as insulin resistance/glucose intolerance, elevated blood pressure, obesity and dyslipidaemia, the diagnostic criteria put forward by various professional bodies differ based on the mandatory inclusion criteria [7]. The first formal definition of the MetS was put forward by the World Health Organization (WHO) in 1998 followed by National Cholesterol Education Program-Adult Treatment Panel III (NCEP:ATP III) and European Group for the Study of Insulin Resistance (EGIR) [7, 9]. The NCEP-ATPIII definition differs from both the WHO and the EGIR definitions as it does not recognize presence of "insulin resistance" as an mandatory criterion [10]. Differences in the diagnostic criteria of MetS led to difficulties in identifying MetS and comparing them between studies. As a solution for these controversies, International Diabetes Federation (IDF) in 2004 proposed new diagnostic criteria for MetS. The IDF diagnostic criteria included central obesity as an essential condition to make the diagnosis of the MetS [11].

Prevalence of MetS ranges from <10% to as high as 84%, depending on factors such as the population studied, ethnicity, geographical region, urban or rural environment, gender, and the definition of MetS used [12, 13]. Overall, it is estimated that 25% of the world's adult population have MetS according to IDF definition [12]. Factors such as higher socioeconomic status, physical inactivity, smoking, family history of diabetes, obesity, and sedentary lifestyle all influence the prevalence of the MetS [12]. There is accumulating evidence that MetS is more common among South Asians compared to the Caucasians [3, 14]. Previous surveys had shown that the prevalence of MetS was 34.8% in Pakistan and 25.3% in India [15]. In Sri Lanka, age-adjusted prevalence of MetS in general population was found to be 24.3% in all adults (males: 18.4%, female: 28.3%) [16].

MetS in patients with type 2 DM increases the risk of cardiovascular mortality and morbidity [17]. Thus, evaluating the MetS in individuals with type 2 DM is of importance for prevention of cardiovascular disease. It is even more important among South Asians with type 2 DM, considering their higher risk of having cardiovascular diseases. However, the prevalence of MetS among diabetes population in Sri Lanka and other South Asians countries is not sufficiently studied. Furthermore, there is no specific diagnostic criteria for MetS in patients with type 2 DM and the validity and performance of the commonly used definitions among individuals with type 2 DM is also not adequately explored. The main aim of this study was to determine the prevalence of MetS among patients with type 2DM using all three well known (WHO, IDF, and NCEP-ATP III) definitions and assess the influence of factors such as gender, glycemic control, and duration of diabetes, on the prevalence of MetS. In addition, performance of above three definitions and their concordance was also assessed.

2. Materials and Methods

This cross-sectional study included patients with type 2 DM who were followed up at the regional diabetes centre in Galle, Southern Sri Lanka, and this study was part of a large study on "cardiovascular risk assessment in patients with diabetes in Sri Lanka." As described elsewhere [18], all previously diagnosed diabetes patients who are being followed up at the diabetes clinic, during the study period (January 2012 to July 2013), were eligible to participate in the study. Subjects were chosen by convenience sampling method for screening for cardio metabolic risk factors on an assigned day, with an average of 30 cases per week.

2.1. Inclusion Criteria. Individuals with ages ≥ 20 years and clinically determined type 2 DM were qualified to participate in the study.

2.2. Exclusion Criteria. Participants aged < 20 years, pregnant, and lactating mothers were excluded from the study. Also patients with other chronic illness including rheumatoid arthritis, severe osteoarthritis, symptomatic heart failure, type 1 DM, myocardial infarction within last 6 months, acromegaly, clinically apparent hypothyroidism, hypogonadism, chronic obstructive airway disease, nephrotic syndrome and chronic kidney disease (stage 3 or more), and chronic liver disease were also excluded. In addition, patients with malignancies and extreme body habitus (BMI >40), those on prolong steroid use, and those who were on active drug treatment for obesity were excluded from the study.

2.3. Data Collection, Anthropometric Measurements, Clinical Examination, and Laboratory Tests. A pretested interviewer-administered questionnaire was used to obtain demographic and medical information such as age, sex, ethnicity, social background, duration of diabetes, and family history of dyslipidaemia, and diabetes among first degree relatives. Anthropometric measurements including waist circumference (cm), weight (Kg), and height (m) were then measured. Waist circumference (WC) was recorded by placing a nonstretchable fibre-glass measuring tape around the waist midway between the last rib and iliac crest with the subject in the standing position. All anthropometric measurements were performed by trained nurses adhering to the WHO guidelines, using calibrated equipment. Blood pressure was measured using an electronic instrument (Omron Corporation, Tokyo, Japan), as the mean of two readings taken five minutes apart. BMI was calculated as weight (kg)/height^2 (m^2).

All chemical analyses were performed in the laboratory attached to the Regional Diabetic Centre mentioned above and same method of biochemical analysis was used throughout the study period. Overnight fasting venous blood samples were collected to measure HDL-C and LDL-C, serum TG, and glucose. Cholesterol esterase oxidase peroxidase-aminopyrine method was used to assess serum cholesterol and for measurement of serum TG glycerol phosphate oxidase peroxidase-aminopyrine method was used. For HDL cholesterol, direct method poly-ethylene-glycol-pretreated enzymes were used.

2.4. Ethical Approval. Ethical clearance for the present study was obtained under the study on "cardiovascular risk assessment in patients with type 2 diabetes in Sri Lanka," from the Institutional Ethics Committee of the Faculty of Medicine, University of Ruhuna. Written informed consent was obtained from all study subjects in the local language.

TABLE 1: Baseline characteristics of study sample.

Category	Total		Male		Female		P
	Mean	SD	Mean	SD	Mean	SD	
Age	49.91	10.77	48.4	10.1	52.8	11.3	.030
Duration in years	5.04	5.71	4.8	5.8	5.4	5.6	.004
Waist circumference	90.32	10.58	90.4	10.0	89.9	11.2	.171
BMI	24.48	4.21	24.2	4.0	24.9	4.7	.060
SBP	124.30	17.40	122.5	17.4	127.5	18.2	.000
HbA1c	7.38	0.96	7.3	1.3	7.3	1.1	.464
TC	200.23	40.05	196.1	47.0	201.1	41.9	.005
LDL	125.35	36.55	122.5	39.5	126.5	37.3	.009
TG	117.15	51.20	118.6	55.9	110.3	44.6	.000
HDL	50.17	8.80	48.6	10.4	51.4	9.9	.000

2.5. Definition of the MetS. The metabolic syndrome (MetS) was defined according to the three well known (WHO, IDF, and NCEP-ATP III) definitions [7, 10].

2.6. IDF Definition. According to the IDF definition, ethnicity specific cut-off value for central obesity should be present as an essential criterion together with two of the following four components to diagnose MetS: raised triglycerides ≥ 150 mg/dL (1.7 mmol/L) or specific treatment for this lipid abnormality; reduced HDL cholesterol < 40 mg/dL (1.03 mmol/L) in males, < 50 mg/dL (1.29 mmol/L) in females or specific treatment for this lipid abnormality; raised blood pressure (BP): systolic BP ≥ 130 or diastolic BP ≥ 85 mm Hg or treatment of previously diagnosed hypertension and; raised fasting plasma glucose (FPG) ≥ 100 mg/dL (5.6 mmol/L), or previously diagnosed type 2 diabetes. The cut-off values of WC ≥90 cm in men or ≥80 cm in women recommended for South Asians for central obesity were used in this study [19].

2.7. NCEP-ATP III Definition. According to NCEP- ATP III definition, an individual can be diagnosed with MetS when any of the three following components are present: WC (>102 cm for males and >88 cm for females); plasma triglycerides (≥ 150 mg/dl); HDL cholesterol (< 40 mg/dl for males and < 50 mg/dl for females); blood pressure (≥ 130/85 mm Hg), and fasting plasma glucose (≥110 mg/dl).

2.8. WHO Definition. According to the WHO definition [9], MetS can be diagnosed in the presence of impaired glucose tolerance, diabetes mellitus, or insulin resistance as an essential criterion together with two or more of the following components: elevated arterial blood pressure ≥140/90 mmHg: raised triglyceride (≥150 mg/dl) or low HDL cholesterol, (<35 mg/dl for males and <39 mg/dl for females): central obesity (waist-to-hip ratio WHR: >0.90 for males and >0.85 for females), and/or BMI (>30 kg/m2): microalbuminuria (urinary albumin excretion rate ≥20 min or albumin: creatinine ratio ≥30 mg/g).

2.9. Statistical Analysis. All numerical data were expressed as means and standard deviations and categorical data were expressed as frequencies and proportions. Statistical significance was assumed at a p value of < 0.05. The significance of the differences between means and proportions (%) was tested using Student's t-test, the chi-square test or ANOVA. Univariate logistic regression analysis was used to identify the associations between individual components and the MetS according to the three definitions. Kappa (κ) statistics was used for finding the agreement between the three definitions. All the data were analyzed using SPSS 17.0.

3. Results

The baseline characteristics of the study population are summarized in Tables 1 and 2. There were 2913 type 2 DM patients, and nearly 65% of them were males. The mean age (standard deviation: SD) was 49.9 (10.2) years and females were significantly older than males ($p = 0.03$). The mean BMI (SD) was 24.5 (4.3) and 37% and 57% had global and visceral obesity, respectively.

Females had significantly higher duration of diabetes, blood pressure, total cholesterol, and LDL cholesterol. The mean values of various anthropometric, clinical, and biochemical variables measured are summarized in Tables 1 and 2 according to the gender.

Table 3 shows the prevalence of MetS according to the three definitions, IDF, NCEP-ATP III, and WHO. Prevalence of MetS was highest by the modified WHO definition (70%) followed by IDF (44%) and NCEP-ATP III (29%) definitions. While nearly 25% (715/2913) were identified to have MetS by all three definitions, around 45% (1311/2913) were found to have MetS by two definitions (Figure 1).

Almost all subjects recognized as having MetS by NCEP-ATP III were also identified as having MetS by one of the other two definitions. However, close to 40% (763/2055) of MetS recognized by WHO were found to have no MetS by the other two definitions. Females had higher prevalence of MetS than male according to all three definitions, and the difference was most obvious with NCEP-ATP III and IDF definitions (Table 3).

Table 4 shows the association between individual components and metabolic syndrome. According to WHO definition, presence of hypertension was associated with the highest

TABLE 2: Baseline characteristics according to the gender.

		Male (n)	%	Female(n)	%
Age groups	20-40	548	28.5	183	28.6
	41-60	1159	60.3	641	60.4
	>60	210	10.9	172	10.9
BMI categories	<18.4	44	2.2	26	2.3
	18.5-22.9	649	33.8	316	32.5
	23-24.9	547	28.5	211	27.3
	>25	677	35.3	443	37.5
Duration of diabetes	Newly diagnosed	654	34.1	255	34.1
	<5 years	500	26.0	245	26.1
	5-10 years	362	18.8	262	18.9
	>10 years	401	23.6	234	21.0
Waist circumference	Normal	828	1.5	125	43.2
	High	1089	87.5	871	56.8
Micro-albuminuria	Present	876	45.6	440	44.1
	Absent	1041	54.4	556	55.9
Total		1917	100	996	100

TABLE 3: Prevalence of metabolic syndrome according to the three different criteria and gender.

		Total (n)	%	Male (n)	%	Female (n)	%
IDF	No MetS	1638	56.2	1279	68	339	34
	MetS	1275	43.8	603	32	658	66
WHO	No MetS	858	29.4	618	33	230	23
	MetS	2055	70.6	1264	67	767	77
ATP 111	No MetS	2070	71.1	1594	85	456	45
	MetS	843	28.9	288	15	541	55

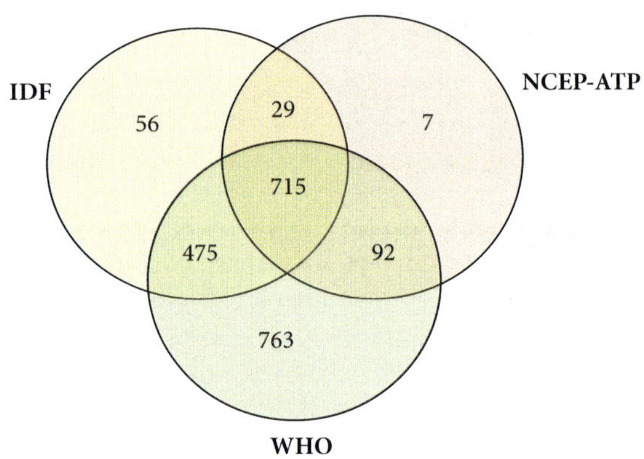

FIGURE 1: Venn diagram of metabolic syndrome according to the three different criteria.

odd of having MetS, whereas with IDF and NCEP-ATP III, low HDL was associated with the highest odds of having MetS.

As shown in Table 5, individuals with MetS according to IDF criteria had significantly higher systolic ($p < 0.05$) and diastolic blood pressure ($p < 0.05$), BMI ($p < 0.05$), and waist circumference ($p < 0.05$) compared to those with MetS based on WHO criteria. Similar observation was seen with NCEP-ATP 111 criteria as well; however, there was no significant difference of BMI and waist circumference between two groups. Individuals with MetS based on NCEP-ATP III criteria also had significantly higher BMI ($p < 0.05$), and waist circumference ($p < 0.05$), higher systolic ($p < 0.05$) and diastolic blood pressure ($p < 0.05$), and lower HDL cholesterol compared to those with MetS based on WHO. Age, duration of diabetes, and glycaemic control as indicated by HbA1c did not differ in individuals identified by the three criteria.

The agreement between the three criteria was assessed by the kappa index. The agreement between IDF with WHO and NCEP-ATP III criteria was 0.37 ($p < 0.001$) and 0.53 ($p < 0.001$), respectively, whereas the agreement between NCEP-ATP III and WHO criteria was 0.24 ($p < 0.001$).

4. Discussion

Even though diabetes itself increases future cardiovascular risk, recognizing MetS among patients with diabetes is vital. Accumulating research showed that the prevalence of cardiovascular diseases was significantly higher in diabetic subjects with MetS compared to those without MetS [17, 20].

TABLE 4: Association between individual components and metabolic syndrome according to the three definitions.

Variables	IDF OR (95% CI)	WHO OR (95% CI)	NCEP-ATP III OR (95% CI)
High WC	2.85 (2.68- 3.03)		7.84 (6.54-9.23)
Low HDL	7.83 (6.19- 9.89)		12.81 (9.32-15.76)
TG>150	3.83 (3.11- 4.70)		5.26 (4.34-6.47)
HT	7.63 (6.45- 9.01)	12.46 (9.07-16.04)	7.31 (6.16-8.16)
High WHR or BMI		14.51 (13.46-16.74)	
Micro-albuminuria		6.92 (5.62- 8.56)	
TG>150 or HDL<35 M, <39 F		6.19 (5.89-7.88)	

TABLE 5: General characteristics of the subjects with metabolic syndrome according to the three definitions.

Variables	IDF		WHO		NCEP-ATP III	
	Mean	SD	Mean	SD	Mean	SD
Duration of diabetes in years	5.5	5.90	5.1	5.74	5.1	5.44
Age in years	47.6	78.63	46.1	62.29	47.3	68.81
Waist circumference (cm)	94.4∗	7.59	93.0#	8.89	94.4	10.09
Body mass index (kg/m^2)	25.8∗	3.94	25.2#	4.16	26.0	4.64
Systolic blood pressure (mmHg)	131.4∗†	17.00	128.4#	17.00	133.6	16.76
Diastolic blood pressure (mmHg)	80.8∗†	9.63	79.7#	9.17	81.8	9.41
HbA_{1C} (%)	7.3	1.06	7.3	0.99	7.3	1.16
Total cholesterol (mg/dL)	201.6	42.05	200.3	40.19	201.6	42.43
LDL cholesterol (mg/dL	124.6	39.16	123.8	36.81	123.9	38.92
HDL cholesterol (mg/dL)	49.0∗†	9.49	49.9#	8.97	48.1	9.98

∗ P< 0.05 compared to WHO criteria.
† $p < 0.05$ compared to NCEP-ATP III criteria.
# $p < 0.05$ compared to NCEP-ATP III criteria.

Different definitions of MetS have been laid down by many different professional bodies; however, the commonly used definitions are WHO, NCEP-ATP III III, and the IDF [21, 22]. These three definitions agree on main components of MetS but differ in the cut-off values and the methods of combining the individual components. Furthermore, all three definitions were primarily used in nondiabetic individuals and, therefore, it is unclear which definition would be most suitable to recognize MetS in diabetic subjects. Overall, the prevalence of the MetS among diabetic subjects has not been adequately studied and the few available studies either had a comparatively small sample size or used only one or two definitions to assess MetS [23–26]. This is the first study to assess the prevalence of MetS among a large cohort of Sri Lankan adults with diabetes.

The most interesting finding in our study is that the prevalence of MetS varied from 28% to 70% depending on the definition used. The overall prevalence of MetS in our study was 28.9%, 43.8%, and 70.6% using NCEP-ATP III, IDF, and WHO criteria, respectively. Previous studies comparing the performance of different definitions of MetS also have shown a varied prevalence of MetS based on the definitions used [27–29]. James Osei-Yeboah et al. reported contrasting performance of the definitions with prevalence of MetS ranging from 43.83% with NCEP-ATP III, 63.58% with WHO, to 69.14% with IDF criteria [29]. In another study in India, prevalence of MetS was estimated to be 57.7% with IDF, 45.9% with NCEP-ATP III, and 28% with WHO criteria [28]. Daya Ram Pokharel et al. reported higher and contrasting prevalence of MetS among Nepalese type 2 diabetic patients (73.9% with NCEP-ATP III, 66.8% with IDF, and 69.9% with WHO) [30]. A large study involving over 4000 diabetic patients in Germany revealed comparatively lower prevalence of MetS with WHO (26.1%) and higher prevalence of MetS with IDF (82.6%) [27]. A study among diabetes patients in Cameroon revealed a comparatively higher prevalence of the MetS with IDF (71.7%) than with NCEP-ATP III (60.4%) [31]. Based on the finding of our study as well as many other studies, it is clear that the different definitions of MetS give rise to different prevalence.

The prevalence of MetS in our study was higher with the WHO definition (70.6%) than with the two other definitions; the difference undoubtedly could be attributed to the study population having diabetes and the presence of microalbuminuria as a component of MetS. In our study, the overall prevalence of microalbuminuria was as high as 45% and it may explain the higher prevalence of WHO-defined MetS. The unexpectedly high prevalence of MetS with WHO definition in our study contrasts with that reported elsewhere [27, 28]. It should be noted however that, in some of these studies, microalbuminuria was not included for analysis even though it is a part of the definition [22, 29]. However, when we look at individual components of MetS and their association with the prevalence of MetS, WHO-defined obesity (raised waist hip ratio, high BMI) appears to account for much of the higher prevalence of WHO-defined MetS in our study. The odds for the MetS in individuals with raised WHR and/or BMI were 14 times higher than the individuals with normal WHR or BMI, and this highlights the fact that raised WHR or BMI as an important predictor of MetS. Predictive ability of central obesity on the prevalence of MetS is less with other two definitions (NCEP-ATP III and IDF) and low HDL appears to be a better predictor of NCEP-ATP III and IDF defined MetS [27, 32].

Of the participants, only around 25% were recognized as having MetS simultaneously by all three definitions, suggesting that the three definitions identify a diverse group of people. Particularly this is true with WHO definition, with roughly 40% (763/2055) being classified as having MetS when other two failed to do so. In contrast, nearly all MetS recognized by the NCEP-ATP III definition were identified as having MetS by one of the other two definitions. In our study, the concordance of individuals with MetS based on IDF criteria with that of WHO and NCEP-ATP III was 0.37 and 0.53, respectively, whereas it was 0.24 between NCEP-ATP III and WHO. In contrast, previous studies revealed comparatively higher concordance between the three definitions, particularly in nondiabetic individuals. A study conducted by Deepa et al. in India had shown that the IDF had a higher agreement (0.58) with WHO definition and similar agreement with NCEP-ATP III (0.58) [22] in compared to our study. Cardiovascular Health Study (CHS) showed almost 80% concordances between NCEP-ATP III and WHO definitions [33]. Thus, the concordance between commonly used definitions of MetS seems to vary depending on factors such as ethnicity (with different cut-off values for central obesity) and presence of diabetes. It is interesting to note that despite all three criteria share most of the components, they were modest in recognizing individuals as having MetS in this study. Another noteworthy finding of our study is that the prevalence of MetS was higher among females as compared to males. Many previous studies described the similar finding of having higher prevalence of MetS in females [27, 28]. Higher prevalence of MetS in females may be due to the higher HDL cut-off and lower waist circumference cut-off values in females as compared to males. Hence, more females than males can be recognized as having central obesity or low HDL.

Identification of MetS among individuals with diabetes is important as it increase the future cardiovascular event. Bonora et al. reported fivefold increase in cardiovascular risk among individuals with type 2 diabetes having MetS compared no MetS [34]. Therefore, it is vital to recognize MetS and manage other risk factors of MetS aggressively. Our study and many other previous studies across the globe have revealed the fact that the MetS continues to be present in majority despite treatment for diabetes and other cardiovascular risk factors. This highlights the continued need for an aggressive risk factor management in individuals with diabetes [35].

As far as we are aware, our study is the first sufficiently large study to examine the prevalence of MetS in diabetic population in Sri Lanka. In addition, other strengths of the present study include its large sample size with close to 3000 individuals with diabetes and being the first ever Sri Lankan study to examine the performance of all commonly used definitions. However, there are few noteworthy limitations of our study. First, cross-sectional design of our study limits the inference of causal relationship between metabolic syndrome and cardiovascular events. Hence, performance of three definitions of MetS in our study is limited to the prevalence of MetS. Second, this study is a single centre study; therefore, generalization of our findings to the whole diabetic population in Sri Lanka may not be feasible.

In conclusion, our study demonstrates that the prevalence of metabolic syndrome among diabetic patients can significantly be varied based on the definition used. The highest prevalence of MetS was observed with WHO (70.6%) whereas lowest was observed with NCEP-ATP III definition. Raised waist circumference is an important predictor of MetS defined by all three definitions.

Abbreviations

CVD:	Cardiovascular disease
MetS:	Metabolic syndrome
NCEP:ATP III:	National Cholesterol Education Program-Adult Treatment Panel III
WHO:	World Health organization
IDF:	International Diabetes Federation
DM:	Diabetes mellitus
WHR:	waist-to-hip ratio
WC:	waist circumference.

Ethical Approval

This study was approved by ethical review committee of the Faculty of Medicine, University of Ruhuna, Galle.

Authors' Contributions

H. M. M. Herath designed this research and guided the other authors (N. P. Weerasinghe, A. Amarathunga) in data collection. Analysis and interpretation of data and literature review were done by H. M. M. Herath, N. P. Weerasinghe, T. P. Weerarathna, and A. Amarathunga. H. M. M. Herath and N. P. Weerasinghe involved in writing up the manuscript and all authors read and approved the final manuscript.

Acknowledgments

The authors would like to acknowledge the staff attached in the diabetes centre and cooperative hospital, Galle, for their assistance during this study.

References

[1] S. O'Neill and L. O'Driscoll, "Metabolic syndrome: a closer look at the growing epidemic and its associated pathologies," *Obesity Reviews*, vol. 16, no. 1, pp. 1–12, 2015.

[2] American Diabetes Association, "Diagnosis and classification of diabetes mellitus," *Diabetes Care*, vol. 36, supplement 1, pp. S67–S74, 2013.

[3] A. Nazir, R. Papita, V. P. Anbalagan, R. M. Anjana, M. Deepa, and V. Mohan, "Prevalence of diabetes in Asian Indians based on glycated hemoglobin and fasting and 2-H post-load (75-g) plasma glucose (CURES-120)," *Diabetes Technology & Therapeutics*, vol. 14, no. 8, pp. 665–668, 2012.

[4] A. Ghaffar, K. S. Reddy, and M. Singhi, "Burden of non-communicable diseases in South Asia," *British Medical Journal*, vol. 328, no. 7443, pp. 807–810, 2004.

[5] A. Shah and A. M. Kanaya, "Diabetes and associated complications in the South Asian population," *Current Cardiology Reports*, vol. 16, no. 5, pp. 476-476, 2014.

[6] R. Unnikrishnan, R. M. Anjana, and V. Mohan, "Diabetes in South Asians: is the phenotype different?" *Diabetes*, vol. 63, no. 1, pp. 53–55, 2014.

[7] M. A. Cornier, D. Dabelea, T. L. Hernandez et al., "The metabolic syndrome," *Endocrine Reviews*, vol. 29, no. 7, pp. 777–822, 2008.

[8] P. A. Sarafidis and P. M. Nilsson, "The metabolic syndrome: a glance at its history," *Journal of Hypertension*, vol. 24, no. 4, pp. 621–626, 2006.

[9] K. G. M. M. Alberti and P. Z. Zimmet, "Definition, diagnosis and classification of diabetes mellitus and its complications. Part 1: diagnosis and classification of diabetes mellitus. Provisional report of a WHO consultation," *Diabetic Medicine*, vol. 15, no. 7, pp. 539–553, 1998.

[10] E. Kassi, P. Pervanidou, G. Kaltsas, and G. Chrousos, "Metabolic syndrome: definitions and controversies," *BMC Medicine*, vol. 9, article 48, 2011.

[11] K. G. M. M. Alberti, P. Zimmet, and J. Shaw, "Metabolic syndrome—a new world-wide definition. A consensus statement from the International Diabetes Federation," *Diabetic Medicine*, vol. 23, no. 5, pp. 469–480, 2006.

[12] G. D. Kolovou, K. K. Anagnostopoulou, K. D. Salpea, and D. P. Mikhailidis, "The prevalence of metabolic syndrome in various populations," *The American Journal of the Medical Sciences*, vol. 333, no. 6, pp. 362–371, 2007.

[13] S. Desroches and B. Lamarche, "The evolving definitions and increasing prevalence of the metabolic syndrome," *Applied Physiology, Nutrition, and Metabolism*, vol. 32, no. 1, pp. 23–32, 2007.

[14] U. P. Gujral, R. Pradeepa, M. B. Weber, K. M. V. Narayan, and V. Mohan, "Type 2 diabetes in South Asians: Similarities and differences with white Caucasian and other populations," *Annals of the New York Academy of Sciences*, vol. 1281, no. 1, pp. 51–63, 2013.

[15] A. Misra and L. Khurana, "The metabolic syndrome in South Asians: epidemiology, determinants, and prevention," *Metabolic Syndrome and Related Disorders*, vol. 7, no. 6, pp. 497–514, 2009.

[16] P. Katulanda, P. Ranasinghe, R. Jayawardana, R. Sheriff, and D. R. Matthews, "Metabolic syndrome among Sri Lankan adults: prevalence, patterns and correlates," *Diabetology & Metabolic Syndrome*, vol. 4, no. 1, article 24, 2012.

[17] B. Isomaa, P. Almgren, T. Tuomi et al., "Cardiovascular morbidity and mortality associated with the metabolic syndrome," *Diabetes Care*, vol. 24, no. 4, pp. 683–689, 2001.

[18] H. M. Herath, T. P. Weerarathna, and N. P. Weerasinghe, "Prevalence and pattern of Dyslipidaemia among patients with newly diagnosed type 2 diabetes mellitus in Southern Sri Lanka; a cross sectional study," *Galle Medical Journal*, vol. 21, no. 2, p. 13, 2016.

[19] A. V. Chobanian, G. L. Bakris, and H. R. Black, "Seventh report of the Joint National Committee on prevention, detection, evaluation, and treatment of high blood pressure," *Hypertension*, vol. 42, no. 6, pp. 1206–1252, 2003.

[20] F. Alsaraj, J. H. McDermott, T. Cawood et al., "Prevalence of the metabolic syndrome in patients with diabetes mellitus," *Irish Journal of Medical Science*, vol. 178, no. 3, pp. 309–313, 2009.

[21] P. Ranasinghe, Y. Mathangasinghe, R. Jayawardena, A. P. Hills, and A. Misra, "Prevalence and trends of metabolic syndrome among adults in the Asia-pacific region: A systematic review," *BMC Public Health*, vol. 17, no. 1, article no. 101, 2017.

[22] M. Deepa, S. Farooq, M. Datta, R. Deepa, and V. Mohan, "Prevalence of metabolic syndrome using WHO, ATPIII and IDF definitions in Asian Indians: The Chennai Urban Rural Epidemiology Study (CURES-34)," *Diabetes/Metabolism Research and Reviews*, vol. 23, no. 2, pp. 127–134, 2007.

[23] C. I. Okafor, "The metabolic syndrome in Africa: current trends," *Indian Journal of Endocrinology and Metabolism*, vol. 16, no. 1, pp. 56–66, 2012.

[24] J. C. G. Lira Neto, M. D. A. Xavier, J. W. P. Borges, M. F. M. D. Araújo, M. M. C. Damasceno, and R. W. J. F. D. Freitas, "Prevalence of Metabolic Syndrome in individuals with Type 2 Diabetes Mellitus," *Revista Brasileira de Enfermagem*, vol. 70, no. 2, pp. 265–270, 2017.

[25] C. M. Alexander, P. B. Landsman, S. M. Teutsch, and S. M. Haffner, "NCEP-defined metabolic syndrome, diabetes, and prevalence of coronary heart disease among NHANES III participants age 50 years and older," *Diabetes*, vol. 52, no. 5, pp. 1210–1214, 2003.

[26] V. Mogre, Z. S. Salifu, and R. Abedandi, "Prevalence, components and associated demographic and lifestyle factors of the metabolic syndrome in type 2 diabetes mellitus," *Journal of Diabetes and Metabolic Disorders*, vol. 13, no. 1, article no. 80, 2014.

[27] C. Koehler, P. Ott, I. Benke, and M. Hanefeld, "Comparison of the prevalence of the metabolic syndrome by WHO, AHA/NHLBI, and IDF definitions in a German population with type 2 diabetes: The Diabetes in Germany (DIG) study," *Hormone and Metabolic Research*, vol. 39, no. 9, pp. 632–635, 2007.

[28] D. Yadav, S. Mahajan, S. K. Subramanian, P. S. Bisen, C. H. Chung, and G. B. Prasad, "Prevalence of metabolic syndrome in type 2 diabetes mellitus using NCEP-ATPIII, IDF and WHO definition and its agreement in Gwalior Chambal region of Central India," *Global Journal of Health Science*, vol. 5, no. 6, pp. 142–155, 2013.

[29] J. Osei-Yeboah, W. K. B. A. Owiredu, G. K. Norgbe et al., "The Prevalence of Metabolic Syndrome and Its Components among People with Type 2 Diabetes in the Ho Municipality, Ghana: A Cross-Sectional Study," *International Journal of Chronic Diseases*, vol. 2017, Article ID 8765804, 8 pages, 2017.

[30] D. R. Pokharel, D. Khadka, M. Sigdel et al., "Prevalence of metabolic syndrome in Nepalese type 2 diabetic patients according

to WHO, NCEP ATP III, IDF and Harmonized criteria," *Journal of Diabetes and Metabolic Disorders*, vol. 13, no. 1, p. 104, 2014.

[31] A. P. Kengne, S. N. Limen, E. Sobngwi, C. F. T. Djouogo, and C. Nouedoui, "Metabolic syndrome in type 2 diabetes: comparative prevalence according to two sets of diagnostic criteria in sub-Saharan Africans," *Diabetology & Metabolic Syndrome*, vol. 4, article 22, 2012.

[32] R. J. Adams, S. Appleton, D. H. Wilson et al., "Population comparison of two clinical approaches to the metabolic syndrome: Implications of the new International Diabetes Federation consensus definition," *Diabetes Care*, vol. 28, no. 11, pp. 2777–2779, 2005.

[33] A. Scuteri, S. S. Najjar, C. H. Morrell, and E. G. Lakatta, "The metabolic syndrome in older individuals: Prevalence and prediction of cardiovascular events: The cardiovascular health study," *Diabetes Care*, vol. 28, no. 4, pp. 882–887, 2005.

[34] E. Bonora, S. Kiechl, J. Willeit et al., "Prevalence of insulin resistance in metabolic disorders: the Bruneck study," *Diabetes*, vol. 47, no. 10, pp. 1643–1649, 1998.

[35] P. Gæde, P. Vedel, N. Larsen, G. V. H. Jensen, H.-H. Parving, and O. Pedersen, "Multifactorial intervention and cardiovascular disease in patients with type 2 diabetes," *The New England Journal of Medicine*, vol. 348, no. 5, pp. 383–393, 2003.

Effectiveness of a Pharmacist-Led Cardiovascular Risk Reduction Clinic in Rural Perry County, Alabama

Pilar Z. Murphy,[1] Charles Sands,[1] and Frances Ford[2]

[1] *Department of Pharmacy Practice, Samford University McWhorter School of Pharmacy, 800 Lakeshore Drive, Birmingham, AL 35229, USA*
[2] *Sowing Seeds of Hope, 1748 S. Washington Street, Marion, AL 36756, USA*

Correspondence should be addressed to Pilar Z. Murphy; pmurphy@samford.edu

Academic Editor: Jens Klotsche

Background. The Cardiovascular Risk Reduction Clinic (CRRC) in Perry County, Alabama, provides free pharmacist-led services. Clinic goals include improving health outcomes and reducing cardiovascular risk factors. *Objective.* To investigate the effectiveness of the CRRC in rural Perry County, Alabama. The reduction of the modifiable cardiovascular risk factors, blood pressure and body mass index, was evaluated to measure a decrease from baseline to last clinic date. *Methods.* This retrospective chart review identified 130 patients with at least two blood pressure and BMI measurements from baseline to June 30, 2010. The patients' paper files were used to collect baseline data and most recent measurements, which were recorded on a data collection sheet. *Results.* There was a statistically significant reduction in systolic blood pressure of 4.08 mmHg, 3.25 mmHg reduction in diastolic blood pressure, and 0.42 kg/m^2 reduction in mean BMI. At their last visit prior to June 30, 2010, 59% of hypertensive patients and 35% of diabetic patients were meeting their blood pressure goals. *Conclusion.* Pharmacist-led management of patients with cardiovascular risk factors significantly reduced blood pressure and allowed more patients to meet their hypertension treatment goals. Despite being modest, reductions in blood pressure and BMI help reduce overall cardiovascular risks.

1. Introduction

Perry County, Alabama, is geographically located approximately 75 miles southwest of Birmingham. It is a rural community of about 10,373 residents, with a majority African American population (68%) [1]. The county is plagued with disproportionately higher rates of hypertension, diabetes, and premature mortality, paralleling the trends of extreme poverty and a stagnated economy [1]. In 2010, Perry County was the worst ranked county for health outcomes in the state of Alabama with a ranking of 67 out of 67. By 2013, Perry County had improved in these rankings to 64 out of 67 [1]. According to the most recent chronic disease burden document published by the Alabama Department of Public Health, the public health area including Perry County has hypertension prevalence of 47% [2]. Hypertension is quantitatively the major risk factor for premature cardiovascular disease and is the most common and most important risk factor for stroke [3–5]. Perry County also has one of the highest stroke death rates in America. While the stroke death rate has decreased nationally and in Perry County, reductions in stroke mortality rates in Perry County continue to lag behind the national averages [6, 7]. Perry County also has increased rates of diabetes (20%) and overweight and obesity (78%) [2]. These percentages are much higher than the Alabama prevalence rates of 27.2% for hypertension, 12.2% for diabetes, and 68.1% for overweight and obesity [2]. Overweight and obesity are defined as "abnormal or excessive fat accumulation that may impair health" and are associated with higher rates of hypertension, diabetes, and cardiovascular disease [3, 4].

In 2004, the Cardiovascular Risk Reduction Clinic (CRRC) was established in Perry County as a collaboration between the nonprofit organization Sowing Seeds of Hope, the Perry County Health Department, and Samford University's McWhorter School of Pharmacy. The CRRC provides free pharmacist-led services at the Perry County Health Department. Population surveys indicate that only 52% of adults in the United States with hypertension actually achieve blood pressure target levels [8]. Involvement of pharmacists in hypertension management has been shown to improve blood pressure control [9]. The goals of the clinic include improving health outcomes for hypertension, diabetes, and obesity and the reduction of cardiovascular risk factors for those utilizing the pharmacist-led clinical services.

Patients are encouraged to attend the weekly clinic where they receive free health screenings and medication therapy management. Medication therapy management (MTM) focuses on the assessment and evaluation of the patient's complete medication therapy regimen to optimize and improve therapeutic outcomes for patients [10]. Patients are counseled on cardiovascular disease risk factors and prevention along with proper medication use, drug indications, and medication compliance. When necessary, patients are referred to their primary care physicians for follow-up. Physicians are contacted with recommendations regarding medication changes and needed laboratory tests following an evidence-based approach and clinical guideline recommendations and algorithms. Although the clinic has been in existence since 2004, no data has been published to determine whether CRRC efforts have reduced cardiovascular risk factors.

2. Objective

The purpose of this study is to investigate the effectiveness of the pharmacist-led CRRC in rural Perry County, Alabama. More specifically, this retrospective chart review looked at the impact of the CRRC on reducing modifiable cardiovascular risk factors in patients utilizing the clinical services provided. Uncontrolled hypertension and obesity are two of the modifiable risk factors related to cardiovascular disease [12–14] and are addressed with all patients utilizing CRRC services. We evaluated whether patients utilizing the clinic had improved blood pressure and lower body mass indexes since it has been noted that the prevalence of obesity is higher in rural communities [11, 15–18].

3. Methods

3.1. Clinic Description. The Cardiovascular Risk Reduction Clinic (CRRC), located in the Perry County Health Department, provides free health screenings, disease state management services, and patient counseling to residents of Perry County, Alabama. The CRRC is staffed by a board certified ambulatory care pharmacy specialist, senior pharmacy students completing Advanced Pharmacy Practice Experience (APPE) rotations, licensed registered nurses, and premedical students. While most patients are self-referred, they can be referred to the pharmacist-led clinic by their primary care provider for education and medication management. Data is unavailable to determine the number of patients who have been referred to the clinic but chose not to use the services. Typical patients include elderly patients needing assistance with medication organization and uninsured patients who are in need of help acquiring their prescription medications, therefore presenting with adherence issues.

During the initial visit, a complete medical history is obtained from the patient, a medication list is compiled, and patients receive a health screening including measuring weight, body mass index (BMI), blood glucose, and blood pressure. Patients are also interviewed about their dietary and exercise habits and receive ongoing counseling about proper diet and exercise to help manage their chronic disease states. Participants are provided with assistive materials such as caloric restriction meal plans, information on adopting the Dietary Approaches to Stop Hypertension (DASH) lifestyle eating plan, Healthy Plate for a Healthy Weight placemats with portion control counseling, and information on reducing sodium/salt intake. They are also encouraged to work with CRRC providers to develop measurable and realistic weight loss and exercise goals, along with developing reminders for taking medications, and provided assistance with obtaining medications through patient assistance programs or discounted medications at specific pharmacies to improve access to medications and adherence. During each follow-up visit, the providers assess the patient's medication adherence, weight loss, dietary and exercise habits, and disease state control according to the latest guidelines. If additional information is needed, patients' primary care providers are contacted to access laboratory results and to request information about prescribed medications. Medication recommendations are also forwarded to the primary care providers if CRRC staff believes there is a need to adjust, change, or add an additional medication to optimize therapy for patients not reaching their Joint National Committee on Prevention, Detection, Evaluation, and Treatment of High Blood Pressure (JNC-7) or American Diabetes Association (ADA) blood pressure or blood glucose goals.

3.2. Patient Population. A chart review of 253 patients who had an encounter with a pharmacist or pharmacy student in the Perry County Cardiovascular Risk Reduction Clinic was performed by reviewing the paper charts of every individual patient who had been seen in the clinic and had a clinic file. Files were evaluated to identify patients who had at least two clinic visits (a necessity to assess any change from baseline in blood pressure, body mass index, blood glucose, or A1c). Baseline data measurements were collected for the earliest encounter on file. Most recent data measurements for comparison were collected for the latest encounter on record prior to June 30, 2010. The patient's most recent visit must have been at least one month after their initial visit to be included in the study. We decided on an interval between the first and the last visit of at least one month based on guideline recommendations to reevaluate blood pressure within one month when modifying or changing antihypertensive therapies. Baseline demographic data included sex, age, weight, body mass index, blood pressure, blood glucose, and A1c if available. Charts were reviewed for medical history, diagnosis of hypertension including systolic and diastolic blood pressure measurements, diagnosis of diabetes, body mass index (BMI), and weight status (underweight, normal weight, overweight, or obesity). Patients were considered to have hypertension or diabetes if it was self-reported, if it was documented in the medical chart, or if there was current use of antihypertensive or antihyperglycemic medications. Patients were considered to be at a healthy weight, to be

TABLE 1: Classification of overweight and obesity by BMI*.

Classification	BMI (kg/m^2)	Obesity class
Underweight	<18.5	
Normal	18.5–24.9	
Overweight	25.0–29.9	
Obesity	30.0–34.9	I
	35.0–39.9	II
Extreme obesity	40.0+	III

*Adapted from the World Health Organization [11].
Body mass index (BMI) is a simple index of weight for height that is commonly used to classify underweight, overweight, and obesity in adults. It is defined as the weight in kilograms divided by the square of the height in meters (kg/m^2).

overweight, or to be obese based on their BMI measurements related to their height and weight. BMI classifications can be found in Table 1.

All patients included in the study were at least 19 years of age or older and had been seen in the CRRC at least twice during the study period to compare their baseline data to their blood pressure, BMI, and weight. There were 130 patients identified who met this criterion. Patients were excluded from the study if they were under 19 years of age, if they only had one clinic visit, or if their subsequent clinic visit was less than one month after their initial visit. Patients were also excluded if they began utilizing the clinic services after June 30, 2010. Demographic data including race, gender, age, and diagnosis of hypertension or diabetes was gathered on all included patients.

3.3. Statistical Analyses. During the time period of the study, every patient chart was reviewed for possible inclusion. All patients meeting the abovementioned criteria were included in the study and a patient list was formulated. Patient information was recorded on data collection sheets (Appendix). The data collection sheet allowed for the assignment of an arbitrary patient number to be used instead of patient names. Each patient received a unique number used specifically for this study. The list of patient names and corresponding numbers was kept separate from the data collection sheets in a locked file cabinet used to store patient files. The primary investigator and senior pharmacy students trained on how to collect the needed information from patient charts were the only ones extracting data for the review. All charts were reviewed on the premises of the CRRC within the Perry County Health Department and were kept confidential in file cabinets currently used to house clinic documents.

We used statistical software SPSS (version 19 for Windows, SPSS Inc.) for data analyses. Clinical value changes from baseline to the last recorded follow-up were analyzed using a matched pair t-test. The paired samples were assessed for normal distribution by employing the 2-tailed t-tests. Statistical significance was recognized as a p value less than or equal to 0.05. This study underwent review and received approval from the Samford University Institutional Review Board (IRB).

TABLE 2: Characteristics of the patients in this study ($n = 130$).

Characteristics	Number	Percentage
Race		
African American	116	89
White	14	11
Sex		
Female	90	69
Male	40	31
Age		
Average (min., max.)	61 (19, 92)	NA
Reported disease states		
Hypertension	80	62
Diabetes	3	2
Hypertension & diabetes	46	35
Other/none	1	<1

4. Results

Patient characteristics of the study population are depicted in Table 2. A total of 130 matched enrollees met all inclusion and exclusion criteria. The study population was 69% female, 89% African American, 62% with hypertension, and 35% with both hypertension and diabetes. The average age of the population was 61 years old.

Outcomes data were collected from the charts of all patients who met the inclusion criteria. The matched pair t-test was used to measure significant differences in systolic blood pressure and the diastolic blood pressure of the study population during pre- and postintervention periods. The t-test assumes that the data is distributed symmetrically. In order to check the violation of the above assumption, we conducted a Wilcoxon Rank Sum test which requires no parametric assumption and showed that the data was distributed symmetrically. At baseline, patients had higher mean systolic/diastolic blood pressure (Figure 1). At the end of the study period, patient groups were successful in reducing systolic/diastolic blood pressure to below 137.49/78.28 mmHg ($p < 0.05$). Mean reduction in systolic blood pressure at the end of the study period was significantly lower from baseline [4.08 (95% confidence interval [CI]: 0.96, 7.19)]. Also, at the end of the study period, the mean diastolic blood pressure significantly changed from baseline [3.25 (95% confidence interval [CI]: 1.31, 5.19)]. There was also a significant reduction in the mean of BMI during the study period. BMI decreased by 0.42 kg/m^2 ($p < 0.05$) (Figure 2).

5. Discussion

We found that the pharmacist-enabled services in the CRRC in Perry County made a significant difference in the blood pressure control of patients. We used the Seventh Report of the Joint National Committee on Prevention, Detection, Evaluation, and Treatment of High Blood Pressure (JNC-7) guidelines to determine whether patients were meeting their blood pressure goals [19]. The JNC-7 guidelines set a hypertension goal for most hypertensive patients at less than

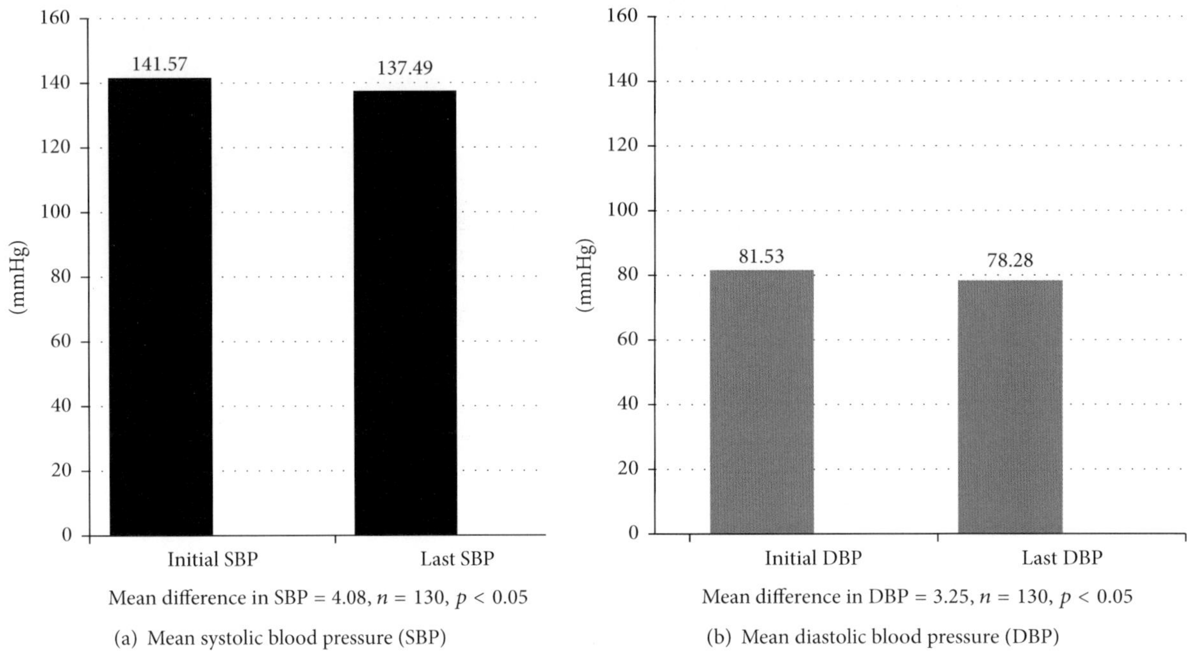

FIGURE 1: Mean differences for systolic blood and diastolic blood pressure.

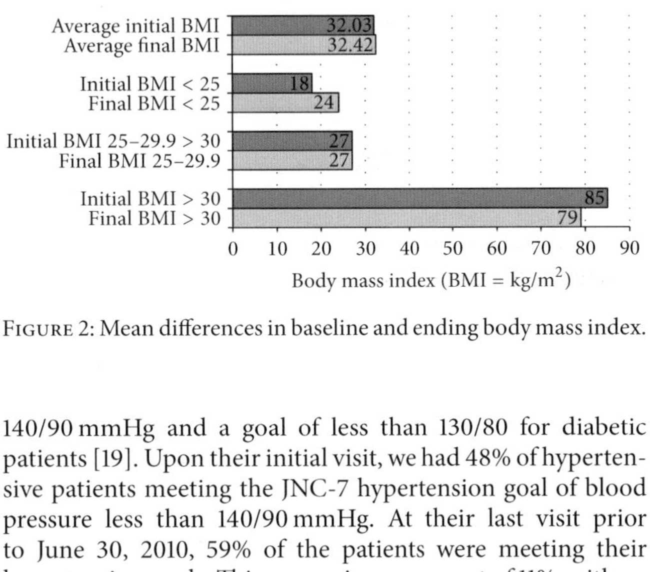

FIGURE 2: Mean differences in baseline and ending body mass index.

140/90 mmHg and a goal of less than 130/80 for diabetic patients [19]. Upon their initial visit, we had 48% of hypertensive patients meeting the JNC-7 hypertension goal of blood pressure less than 140/90 mmHg. At their last visit prior to June 30, 2010, 59% of the patients were meeting their hypertension goals. This was an improvement of 11%, with an additional 11 patients meeting their goal. Upon their initial visit, 29% of our diabetic patients were meeting their JNC-7 goal of blood pressure of less than 130/80 mmHg. At their last visit, 35% of diabetic patients were meeting their blood pressure goal.

We did see small decreases in both systolic and diastolic blood pressure, showing that clinic efforts are making a difference in blood pressure control. There was a statistically significant drop in SBP of 4.08 mmHg and diastolic blood pressure decreased by an average of 3.25 mmHg. The reduction in SBP moved some patients from being above the 140 mmHg goal to being below it at their last clinic visit. While the average BMI remained constant among patients using the CRRC, six patients moved from the obese category to the overweight category, and six patients moved from the overweight to the normal category. This weight reduction, while being modest, is an improvement in risk since obesity is a modifiable risk factor associated with cardiovascular disease, hypertension, myocardial infarction, and stroke.

During each clinic visit, patient parameters were measured along with the provision of education related to reduction of cardiovascular risk factors, meal planning, weight management, and counseling on medication compliance and utilization. When necessary, patient's providers were contacted with recommendations on changing or augmenting therapy based on the clinical guidelines if patients are not meeting the goal. All of these factors probably have played a role in improving the outcomes of patients using the CRRC.

Centers for Disease Control and Prevention (CDC) statistics show that the stroke death rate in Perry County declined by 37.4% between 1991 and 2010 from 190 to 153 per 100,000 people [7]. While we do not take full credit for this decrease in stroke mortality among patients in Perry County, we do believe that our efforts have had an impact due to increased awareness, patients being educated on the need to seek treatment early, and learning the warning signs of heart attack and stroke. Pharmacy faculty and students provide medication therapy management services to patients utilizing the clinic by making medication review charts and counseling on medication adherence and proper usage, along with providing coaching for lifestyle changes to improve cardiovascular health. Students employ a wallet card provided by the Alabama Department of Public Health which lists the classification of blood pressure, warning signs of a stroke, and the ABCs of heart disease that can be used to talk to patients about aspirin use and smoking cessation. Our model does not propose to be the substitution of physicians

Effectiveness of Pharmacist-Enabled Hypertension and Diabetes Clinics in Perry County

Data collection sheet

Record #_________

Gender ☐ Male ☐ Female

Race ☐ African American ☐ Caucasian

☐ Hispanic ☐ Other __________________

Disease state(s) present? ☐ Hypertension ☐ Diabetes

	Date of 1st visit (mm/dd/yyyy)	Last visit (must be prior to July 1, 2010) (mm/dd/yyyy)	Number of recorded clinic visits		
Weight (lbs)					
Blood pressure					
BMI					
BMI classification (healthy, overweight, obese)					
BG					
A1C (if available)					

FIGURE 3

in the care of patients with chronic disease states, but rather a division of labor to aid in disease state management and medication therapy management. Our results suggest that pharmacist-enabled clinics do reduce both systolic and diastolic blood pressure among patients and help patients reach their predetermined blood pressure goals. We consider that this clinic model such as ours is a realistic and cost-effective way to provide clinical services to underserved patients, especially those in rural areas.

While many Americans gain weight each year, participants in the CCRC are controlling and maintaining their weight. While only six participants moved from the obese category to the overweight category, the same number of patients moved from being overweight to being in the healthy/normal weight category according to their BMI. Acquiring a normal weight significantly reduces cardiovascular risk factors.

There were limitations to our study. First, there were inconsistencies in documentation in the patient charts. More than 200 charts were reviewed, but, due to documentation errors, omitted information, and incomplete SOAP notes, many patients had to be omitted from the study. Patients were also excluded because they had only one office visit. This loss to follow-up was most concerning to investigators as patients often came to the initial office visit due to symptoms of uncontrolled hypertension or diabetes. These patients may have been referred to their primary care physicians or the emergency room for follow-up but did not return to our clinic for disease state management. Second, there was a lack of a control group for comparison. The lack of a control group prevented us from being able to determine whether clinic efforts were fully responsible for the decreases in blood pressure and weight. Third, we had limited comparison data parameters. We originally wanted to determine whether we had made a difference in diabetes control among patients; however, there was not enough blood glucose data to compare among diabetic patients. Ideally, hemoglobin A1c is a clinical marker used in guidelines and its measurements would be compared to give a more definitive evaluation of blood sugar control.

6. Conclusion

The residents of rural Perry County, Alabama, are working to close the gap in cardiovascular health disparities by taking charge of their health and utilizing the CRRC at the Perry County Health Department. The CRRC aims to increase awareness about disease states among patients and to teach patients how to control their risk factors along with taking charge of their comorbid disease state. In summary, the Perry County CRRC model may be an innovative model that is effective in screening patients with hypertension and narrowing the health disparity gap among patients in a rural area. Questions remain as to whether this model is replicable in other areas and whether further improvement in blood pressure control has been realized in patients beyond the study period. The study has also shown the need for more consistent documentation, periodic measurements for hemoglobin A1c and lipids, and an electronic medical record for clinic staff.

Appendix

See Figure 3.

Competing Interests

The authors declare that they have no competing interests.

References

[1] Robert Wood Johnson Foundation and the University of Wisconsin Population Health Institute, 2013 County Health Rankings, 2013, http://www.countyhealthrankings.org/app/#/alabama/2013/perry/county/outcomes/overall/snapshot/by-rank.

[2] Alabama Department of Public Health, *The Risk of Heart Disease and Stroke in Alabama: Burden Document Finding the Path to Cardiovascular Health 2010*, 2010, http://www.adph.org/cvh/assets/2010_HeartDiseaseStroke_Alabama_Burden.pdf.

[3] S. M. Grundy, H. B. Brewer Jr., J. I. Cleeman, S. C. Smith Jr., and C. Lenfant, "Definition of metabolic syndrome: report of the National Heart, Lung, and Blood Institute/American Heart Association conference on scientific issues related to definition," *Circulation*, vol. 109, no. 3, pp. 433–438, 2004.

[4] L. E. Fields, V. L. Burt, J. A. Cutler, J. Hughes, E. J. Roccella, and P. Sorlie, "The burden of adult hypertension in the United States 1999 to 2000: a rising tide," *Hypertension*, vol. 44, no. 4, pp. 398–404, 2004.

[5] C. M. M. Lawes, S. V. Hoorn, and A. Rodgers, "Global burden of blood-pressure-related disease, 2001," *The Lancet*, vol. 371, no. 9623, pp. 1513–1518, 2008.

[6] Alabama Department of Public Health, Center for Health Statistics, Division of Statistical Analysis, *County Health Profiles Alabama 2006*, Alabama Department of Public Health, Montgomery, Ala, USA, 2007.

[7] Centers for Disease Control and Prevention, *Heart Disease and Stroke Maps*, CDC, 2015, http://nccd.cdc.gov/DHDSPAtlas/reports.aspx?geographyType=county&themeSubClassId=3&filterIds=4,3,2,7,10,9&filterOptions=1,1,1,1,1,1#.

[8] T. Nwankwo, S. S. Yoon, V. Burt, and Q. Gu, *Hypertension Among Adults in the US: National Health and Nutrition Examination Survey, 2011-2012. NCHS Data Brief, No. 133*, National Center for Health Statistics, Centers for Disease Control and Prevention, US Dept of Health and Human Services, Hyattsville, Md, USA, 2013.

[9] V. Santschi, A. Chiolero, B. Burnand, A. L. Colosimo, and G. Paradis, "Impact of pharmacist care in the management of cardiovascular disease risk factors: a systematic review and meta-analysis of randomized trials," *Archives of Internal Medicine*, vol. 171, pp. 1441–1453, 2011.

[10] American Pharmacists Association and the National Association of Chain Drug Stores Foundation Medication Therapy Management in Pharmacy Practice Core Elements of an MTM Service Model Version 2.0 March 2008, http://www.pharmacist.com/sites/default/files/files/core_elements_of_an_mtm_practice.pdf.

[11] M. C. Kegler, C. Escoffery, I. Alcantara, D. Ballard, and K. Glanz, "A qualitative examination of home and neighborhood environments for obesity prevention in rural adults," *International Journal of Behavioral Nutrition and Physical Activity*, vol. 5, pp. 65–74, 2009.

[12] S. Yusuf, S. Hawken, S. Ounpuu et al., "Effect of potentially modifiable risk factors associated with myocardial infarction in 52 countries (the INTERHEART study): case-control study," *The Lancet*, vol. 364, pp. 937–952, 2004.

[13] G. Mancia, R. Fagard, K. Narkiewicz et al., "2013 ESH/ESC Guidelines for the management of arterial hypertension: the task force for the management of arterial hypertension of the European Society of Hypertension (ESH) and of the European Society of Cardiology (ESC)," *Journal of Hypertension*, vol. 31, no. 7, pp. 1281–1357, 2013.

[14] S. C. Fagan and D. C. Hess, "Stroke," in *Pharmacotherapy: A Pathophysiologic Approach*, J. T. Dipiro, R. L. Talbert, G. C. Yee, G. R. Matzke, B. G. Wells, and L. M. Posey, Eds., p. 353, McGraw-Hill, New York, NY, USA, 8th edition, 2011.

[15] L. M. Vadheim, K. A. Brewer, D. R. Kassner et al., "Effectiveness of a lifestyle intervention program among persons at high risk for cardiovascular disease and diabetes in a rural community," *The Journal of Rural Health*, vol. 26, no. 3, pp. 266–272, 2010.

[16] P. D. Patterson, C. G. Moore, J. C. Probst, and J. A. Shinogle, "Obesity and physical inactivity in rural America," *The Journal of Rural Health*, vol. 20, no. 2, pp. 151–159, 2004.

[17] C. J. Aguero, M. N. Luftiyya, and Y. Patel, *Are There Disparities in Diabetes Care? A Comparison of Care Received by US Rural and Urban Adults with Diabetes*, North American Primary Care Research Group, Leawood, Kan, USA, 2008.

[18] M. W. Murimi and T. Harpel, "Practicing preventive health: the underlying culture among low-income rural populations," *The Journal of Rural Health*, vol. 26, no. 3, pp. 273–282, 2010.

[19] A. V. Chobanian, G. L. Bakris, H. R. Black et al., "The Seventh Report of the Joint National Committee on Prevention, Detection, Evaluation, and Treatment of High Blood Pressure: the JNC 7 report," *The Journal of the American Medical Association*, vol. 289, no. 19, pp. 2560–2571, 2003.

27

Screening for Nephropathy in Diabetes Mellitus: Is Micral-Test Valid among All Diabetics?

Koubaa Afifa,[1] Sriha Belguith Asma,[2] Harzallah Nabil,[3] Bellaleh Ahlem,[4] Sahtout Mounira,[5] Younes Kawthar,[1] Triki Sonia,[6] Hellara Ilhem,[6] Neffati Fadoua,[6] Najjar Fadhel,[6] and Soltani Mohamed[2]

[1] *Stah Jabeur Primary Health Center, Monastir Health Group, 5000 Monastir, Tunisia*
[2] *Department of Preventive Medicine and Epidemiology, Faculty of Medicine, Monastir, Tunisia*
[3] *Primary Health Center, Monastir Health Group, Monastir, Tunisia*
[4] *Department of Pathology, Monastir, Tunisia*
[5] *C2 Primary Health Center, Monastir Health Group, Monastir, Tunisia*
[6] *Biochemistry Laboratory, Faculty of Pharmacy, Monastir, Tunisia*

Correspondence should be addressed to Sriha Belguith Asma; belguith_asma@yahoo.fr

Academic Editor: Jens Klotsche

Background. Using Micral-test (MT) for screening microalbuminuria (MA) among type 2 diabetics (T2D) is helpful. We aimed at determining prevalence of MA and at describing the MT validity. *Methods.* We studied 182 T2D followed up in family medicine. Two 24-hour urinary quantitative assays of MA had been used as a gold standard. *Results.* Prevalence of MA was 23%, CI 95%: 16.9–29.1. MT validity was 77% for sensitivity, 88% for negative predictive value, and 0.2 for Kappa coefficient ($p = 0.001$). Among subjects having a blood pressure ≥130/80 mmHg, having a CHT/HDL ratio ≥ 3, being a T2D for more than 5 years, and being women, negative predictive values were, respectively, 91%, 89%, 95%, and 91%. The area under the ROC curve was 0.81 in men ($p = 0.008$) and 0.80 when diabetes duration exceeds 5 years ($p = 0.001$). The MA value at 100% Sp for MT was 35 mg/L. *Conclusion.* The use of MT in primary healthcare for yearly screening for MA in T2D must be accentuated especially when diabetes duration exceeds 5 years or when associated with other cardiovascular risks.

1. Introduction

Screening and management of early stage of diabetes are insured by the family practitioner, while Tunisian diabetics with complications are managed by specialists. Diabetic nephropathy (DN) is the commonest cause of end-stage renal disease (ESRD) [1]. Screening for microalbuminuria (MA) is required in primary healthcare centers to prevent the progression of this serious complication [2–5]. The prevalence of DN is increasing along with the diabetes prevalence [6]. It should be detected and treated by the family doctor, at the stage of MA which is potentially reversible and associated with an increased risk of cardiovascular morbidity and mortality [7, 8]. The determination of MA by the semiquantitative method, Micral-test (MT), is a rapid screening tool. It is the easiest method, using urinary strips and a spot urine specimen. It is simple and inexpensive [9, 10]. The aim of this study was to assess the validity of MT criteria to detect DN among subgroups of diabetics and therefore to establish prevalence of MIA in diabetics managed in primary healthcare centers.

2. Methods

2.1. Design. This is a cross-sectional study, conducted from January 2013 to December 2014, to screen diabetic patients for elevated urinary albumin excretion with Micral-test in general practice.

2.2. Patients. We have included type 2 diabetics (T2D) without known complications followed up in two primary healthcare centers based in Monastir ("Stah Jabeur" and "C2").

Patients with fever, transitory diabetes decompensation, urinary infection, hematuria, or DN managed by a specialist were excluded from the study.

2.3. Study Area. Monastir is a coastal city located in the central eastern part of Tunisia. It includes 7 primary healthcare centers. Over than 20,000 inhabitants are followed up in "Stah Jabeur" and "C2" centers. Those centers were chosen because they manage diabetics at early stage.

2.4. Methods. The participants benefited from screening using the MT, done at the primary healthcare center. For the gold standard, two quantitative assays of MA on the urine of 24 hours were performed at one-month interval, at the Biochemistry Laboratory of the University Hospital of Monastir. MA was considered pathological if urinary albumin concentration (UAC) was between 30 and 300 mg in the urine of 24 hours. A third quantitative assay was performed in case of discordance. The MT is a semiquantitative strip test done on a urine sample in order to determinate MA. A comparative color scale is used to assess the results of MT: at a concentration of 0 mg/L of microalbumin in the urine, the strip remains white; it turns to light pink at 20 mg/L, to dark pink at 50 mg/L, and finally to very dark pink at more than 100 mg/L. A therapeutic education session was conducted on the test's day in primary healthcare center to improve patients' participation to MT and quantitative assays. Answerable nurse received information about this study.

2.5. Parameters. The participants also benefited from multiple blood tests. The studied parameters were sociodemographic data (age, gender), information about diabetes (diabetes duration, fasting blood glucose levels, glycated hemoglobin (HbA1C)), and risk factors associated with T2D (blood pressure, total cholesterol, and HDL cholesterol (HDL-C)). Total cholesterol to HDL-C ratio was calculated; the patient was considered as being at low risk of overload if this ratio was less than 3, at intermediate risk between 3 and 4.4, and at high risk if more than 4.5 [11]. Controlled glycemia is defined as the ADA [12]. Renal function was assessed by the measurement of glomerular filtration rate (GFR) calculated using the MDRD formula (modification of diet and renal disease). Some variables influence AUC, as was found in the literature. So we have analyzed validity criteria of MT according to demographic variables, blood pressure, CH/HDL-C ratio, and T2D duration.

2.6. Statistical Analysis. Statistical data were performed on SPSS 17.0 computer software. Sensitivity and specificity were calculated to determine the diagnostic properties of MT in predicting a UAC greater than or equal to 30 mg/24 hours. To determine the confidence intervals for sensitivity and specificity, we used the guidelines of Gardner and Altman. The coefficient Kappa (κ) was used to assess the concordance between the MT and the quantitative measurement of MIA. A value of $p < 0.05$ was considered as the cut-off of significance. The cut-off point for 100% specificity and the equilibrium point between sensibility and specificity were determined. We assessed, according to the subgroups, diagnostic sensitivity, specificity, positive and negative predictive values, Kappa coefficient, positive likelihood ratio, and negative likelihood ratio. The ROC curves of MT in diurnal random urine specimen for screening of MA according to the subgroups were plotted.

3. Results

3.1. Description of the Study's Population. We have included 182 T2D among whom 122 were followed up in the primary healthcare center "Stah Jabeur" and 60 in "C2" center. The mean age of the patients was 61.4 years (SD: 11.9). Females represented 69.2% of the studied population (sex ratio = 0.44) and 62% had hypertension. The mean duration of diabetes was 8.1 years (SD: 6.4). Fasting blood glucose levels value was <7 mmol/L in 31% of the cases and the HbA1C <7% in 30% of T2D. Blood pressure was ≥130/80 mmHg in 66% of the studied population and 49% of the patients were obese. Mild renal impairment was present in 47.6% of diabetics. The prevalence of MA was 23%; CI 95% = 16.9–29.1.

3.2. Variability of Micral-Test Validity. The MT had 77% sensitivity, CI 95%: 65.5–88.9, 46% specificity, and a negative predictive value (NPV) of 88%. The positive likelihood ratio was 1.4 and the negative likelihood ratio was 0.5. The validity of MT was better in women (NPV = 91%; $\kappa = 0.3$; $p = 0.008$), subjects having a blood pressure ≥130/80 mmHg (NPV = 91%; $\kappa = 0.24$; $p = 0.005$) or a total CHT/HDL ratio ≥3 (NPV = 89%; $\kappa = 0.36$; $p = 0.01$), and patients who have had T2D for more than 5 years (NPV = 95%; $\kappa = 0.38$; $p = 0.001$) (Table 1). The cut-off point for 100% specificity was 35 mg/L for all studied subgroups. The equilibrium point between sensitivity and specificity was 10 mg/L (Table 2). The area under the ROC curves was 0.72: CI 95% = 0.581–0.863 ($p = 0.001$) for the entire study population. It was 0.81 in men ($p = 0.008$) and 0.80 when diabetes duration exceeds 5 years ($p = 0.001$) (Figure 1).

4. Discussion

The highlight of this study is that it was conducted in first-line therapy for diabetes in early stage. It allowed us to determine the accuracy of the MT in the detection of MA among diabetics subgroups and to estimate MA prevalence. This subject was little discussed in the Tunisian studies contrary to world literature [9, 10, 13–17].

Our diabetic population was characterized by a female majority, as described in the literature [18, 19]. Different distributions were found though [20, 21]. The mean age (61.4 years) and the mean duration of diabetes (8.1 years (SD: 6.4)) were similar to those reported by other authors [13, 22]. We found that 30% of diabetics had a good glycemic control, and this result matches those observed in other Arab countries (Morocco, Kuwait, and Emirates) [13, 23, 24]. The glycemic control was better in China [25]. The review of literature shows a great variability in the prevalence of MA in T2D (Table 3); this prevalence ranged from 11.5 to 58.2% [13, 26].

TABLE 1: Assessment of validity of Micral-test according to subgroups of diabetics.

Cut-off value: 20 mg/L	Sensibility (%)	Specificity (%)	Kappa	p	NPV	PLR	NLR
Entire population	77.2 *CI 95%* [65.5–88.9]	46.3 *CI 95%* [32.4–60.2]	0.2	0.001	88.4	27.8	
Gender:							
(i) Male	66.6%	46.6%	0.103	0.008	77.7%	1.2	0.74
(ii) Female	77%	66%	**0.323**	0.006	**90.6%**	**2.26**	0.34
BP ≥ 130/80 mmHg	81%	54.1%	0.236	0.005	**90.7%**	1.76	0.35
CHT/C-HDL ratio ≥ 3	83.3%	60.1%	**0.363**	0.011	89.4%	2.07	**0.28**
T2D duration > 5 years	91%	60.6%	**0.378**	0.001	**95.2%**	**2.27**	**0.15**

NPV: negative predictive value.
PLR: positive likelihood ratio.
NLR: negative likelihood ratio.

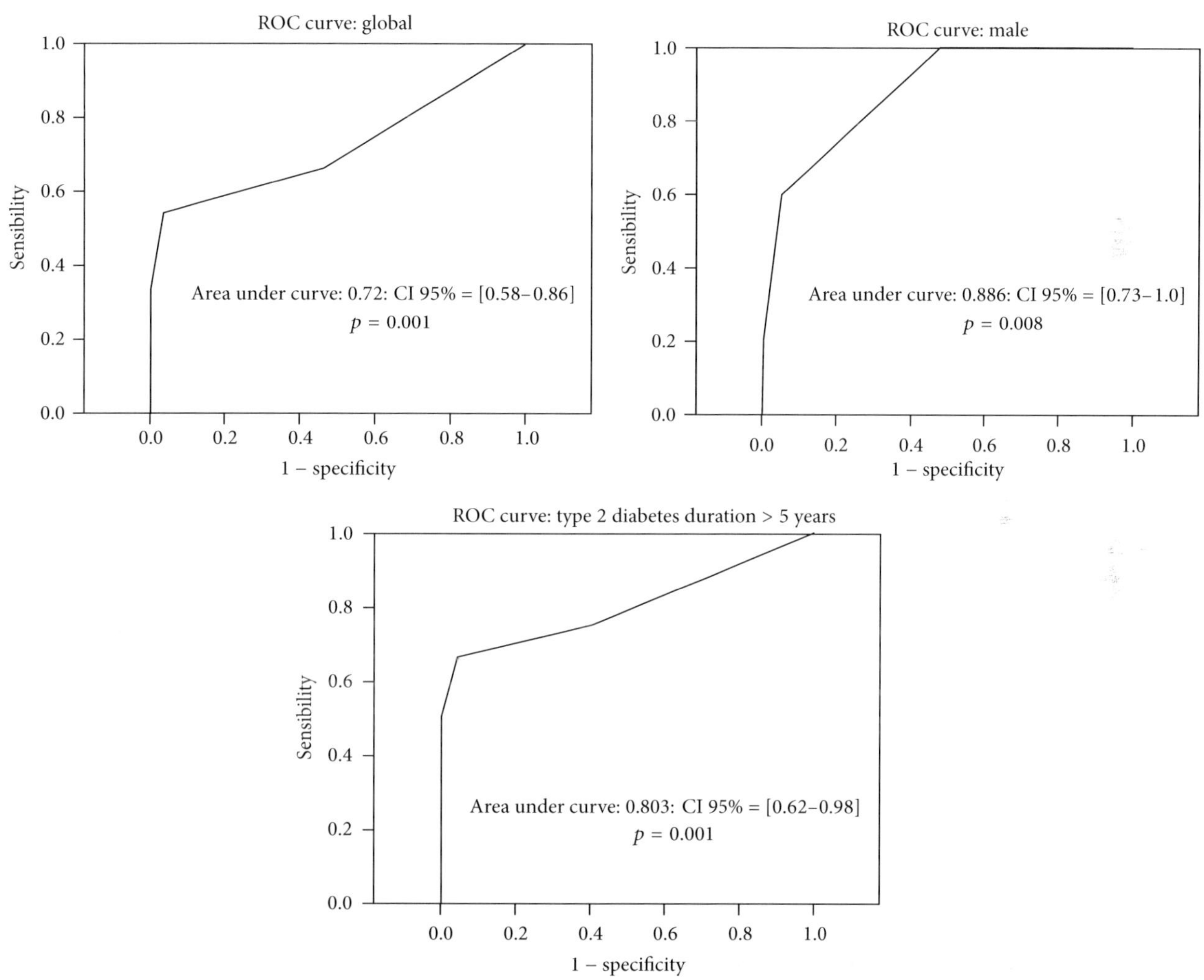

FIGURE 1: The area under the ROC curve of Micral-test (mg/L) in microalbuminuria screening.

This variation can be mainly attributed to the genetic and the ethnic dissimilarities between the studied groups [27] and to the difference in the classifications system. Among the studied population, 36 patients had MA (23%). This finding is comparable to those obtained in the United Kingdom Prospective Diabetes Study (UKPDS) [28] and in Adler et al.'s study [28] and Arfa et al.'s work [29] done in Tunisian specialized departments. MA's prevalence was lower in an Argentinean study [25] and greater in Canadian and Moroccan studies [13, 30, 31]. Several methods were used for the detection of the MA. The quantitative methods include the determination of the urinary albumin concentration (UAC)

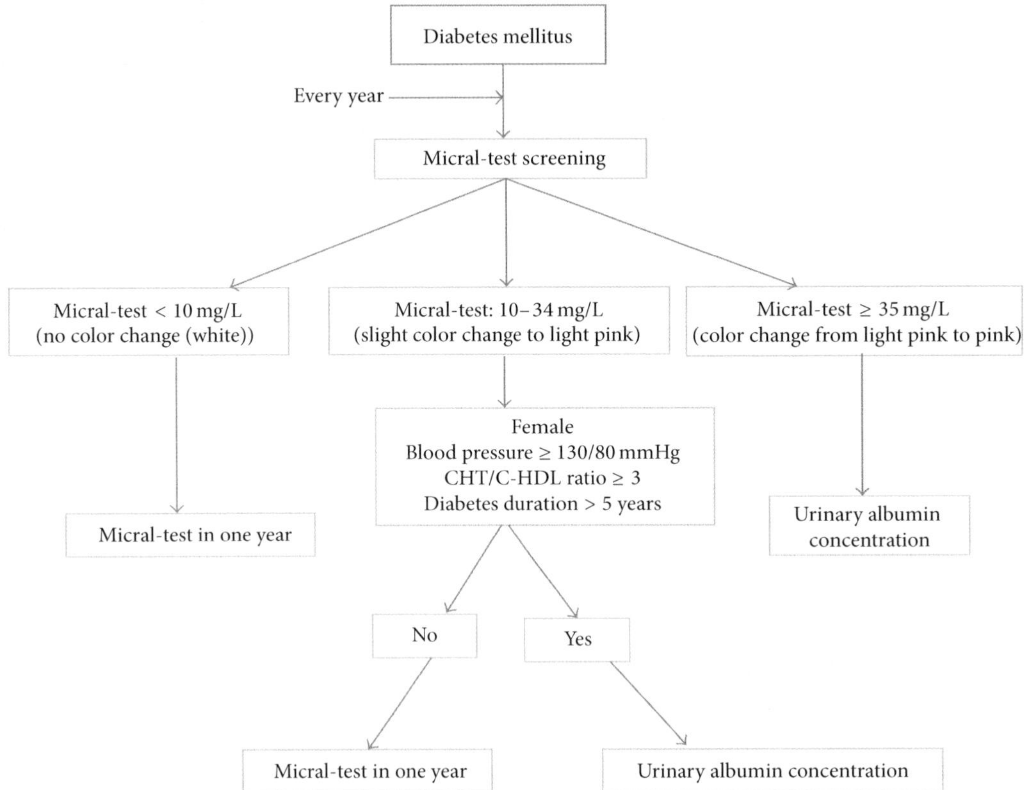

FIGURE 2: Algorithm for screening nephropathy in diabetes mellitus with Micral-test.

TABLE 2: Sensitivity and specificity among subgroups depending on the chosen point.

	Cut-off point for 100% specificity for MT	Equilibrium point between sensibility and specificity
Entire population	*35 mg/L*	*10 mg/L*
Sensitivity	54.2%	66.7%
Specificity	100%	53.6%
Gender: male	35 mg/L	10 mg/L
Sensitivity	60%	**100%**
Specificity	100%	52.4%
BP ≥ 130/80 mmHg	35 mg/L	10 mg/L
Sensitivity	52.4%	66.7%
Specificity	100%	53.6%
CHT/C-HDL ratio ≥ 3	35 mg/L	10 mg/L
Sensitivity	58.3%	58.3%
Specificity	100%	57.5%
T2D duration >5 years	35 mg/L	10 mg/L
Sensitivity	**66.7%**	75%
Specificity	100%	60%

and the urinary albumin-to-creatinine ratio (UACR) in a first morning urine sample, 24 h urine collection, or timed urine collection. These two methods are performed in the laboratory by radioimmunoassay, radial immunodiffusion, enzyme immunoassay (ELISA), or immunoturbidimetric means. Among semiquantitative methods, the MT has been the most used screening tool for the detection of MA in many countries [32]. This test involves the immunochromatographic principle. Initially, the labeled antibody is combined with the sample albumin. Then, during the migration, excess conjugate is retained by the immobilized human albumin. Finally, the complex spread by migration on the strip to a revelation area. A more or less intense pink color appears in the play area based on the initial concentration of albumin [33, 34]. In different studies (Table 4), the MT precision varied from 67 to 96.7% and the specificity ranged from 46 to 96% [9, 32, 33, 35–39]. Table 5 shows a comparison between Micral-test and Multistix® commonly used for detection of DN in Tunisia. Our results are similar to Incerti's findings [36] for the same cut-off (20 mg/L). The MT validity was better in men ($p = 0.008$), subjects having a BP ≥130/80 mmHg ($p = 0.005$) or a cholesterol/C-HDL ratio ≥3 ($p = 0.011$), and patients who have had T2D for more than 5 years ($p = 0.001$). The point for 100% specificity (0% false positives) was 35 mg/L among all subgroups. The equilibrium point between sensibility and specificity was 10 mg/L; it was between 26 and 32 mg/L in Incerti et al.'s study [36]. Several studies have shown that the MT is commonly used worldwide, that it is a good screening tool for MA [32, 33, 36, 37, 39], and that positive results should be confirmed and quantified by a reference assay [33, 36]. Few authors have discussed the limitation of the diagnosis value of MT due to the rate of false positive [40], high costs, and the possibility of false negative

TABLE 3: Microalbuminuria's prevalence in the literature.

Study	Number of patients	MA measurement method	MA's prevalence (%)
Our study	182	24-hour urinary UAC: 30–300 mg/d	23%
Kuwait, 2008 [23]	440	Micral-test	14.2%
Argentina, 2011 [26]	88	24-hour urinary UAC: 30–300 mg/d	46.2%
Albania, 2013 [43]	222	Matinal urine UACR: 30–300 mg/g	38.6%
Italy, 1996 [41]	1574	Night urine UAC: 20–200 μg/min	32.1%
Tunisia, 2014 [44]	120	—	27.5%
Tunisia, 2008 [29]	141	24-hour urinary UAC: 30–300 mg/d	25.5%
Morocco, 2009 [13]	728	24-hour urinary UAC: 30–300 mg/d	11.5%

UAC: urinary albumin concentration.
UACR: urinary albumin creatinine ratio.

TABLE 4: Micral-test's validity in literature.

Study	Number of patients	Sensibility (%)	Specificity (%)	NPV (%)	Area under curve
Our study	**182**	**77**	**46**	**88**	**0.72**
De Grauw et al. [35]	401	67	93		0.84
Incerti et al. [36]	278	90	46		0.84
Mogensen et al. [37]	2228	96.7	71		—
Parikh et al. [38]	444	88	80		—
Sarafidis et al. [39]	165	70	83		—
Cortés-Sanabria et al. [9]	71	83	96	88	0.91
Larijani et al. [32]	200	93	87	92	
Le Floch et al. [33]	302	79	81	95	—
Mogensen et al. [37]	530	78	77		

NPV: negative predictive value.

TABLE 5: Comparison of commonly used dipsticks for the detection of albuminuria.

	Micral-test	Multistix 10 SG, Bayer [45]
Type	Semiquantities	Qualitative
Level of detection	20 mg/L	200 mg/L
Level of 100% specificity	35 mg/L	—
Negative predictive value	88% (20 mg/L)	73.7% (200 mg/L)
Time for reading	1 mn	1 mn
Cost	++	+
Efficacy of treatment (IEC) at screening	+++	±

results [32, 34]. Taking into consideration accuracy and cost, the measurement of the UAC in a random urine specimen, having 15 mg/L as the cut-off point for diagnosis, or the UACR on first morning micturition was considered by other authors as the best choice for MA screening patients with diabetes [36, 41]. Several advantages of MT have been described such as the economic benefit [42], the rapidity of the test (total time of 3 minutes), and its validity and reliability as a screening method for albuminuria on a single urine sample. It does not require 24-hour urine collection, feasible on a morning urine sample and especially adequate in the elderly [9, 32, 33]. We propose the algorithm (Figure 2) for screening ND.

5. Conclusion

Detecting MA in diabetic patients leads the family doctor to speed up the adaptation of the therapeutic goals in order to have the finest metabolic control, an improvement of health-related behaviors, and an optimal treatment of the associated risk factors. Screening for MA has to be improved in primary healthcare centers. The use of reliable, cheap, and easily semiquantitative methods such as the MT seems to be a promising strategy to achieve that purpose.

Competing Interests

The authors declare that they have no competing interests.

Acknowledgments

The authors thank the nurse staff of the healthcare centers Stah Jabeur and C2 in Monastir, where this study was conducted, for their invaluable contribution in implementing the study. Their special thanks extend to Dr. Jebara Hassen, Headmaster of the Regional Department of the Basic Healthcare in Monastir, for his help to supply the Micral-test. This work was financially supported by research committees in Monastir University.

References

[1] A. T. Reutens, L. Prentice, and R. Atkins, "The epidemiology of diabetic kidney disease," in *The Epidemiology of Diabetes Mellitus*, pp. 499–518, John Wiley & Sons, 2nd edition, 2008.

[2] H. Préneuf, "Néphropathies diabétiques," *EMC—Nephrologie*, vol. 1, no. 1, pp. 1–16, 2011.

[3] T. Ninomiya, V. Perkovic, B. E. De Galan et al., "Albuminuria and kidney function independently predict cardiovascular and renal outcomes in diabetes," *Journal of the American Society of Nephrology*, vol. 20, no. 8, pp. 1813–1821, 2009.

[4] L. H. Opie and H.-H. Parving, "Diabetic nephropathy: can renoprotection be extrapolated to cardiovascular protection?" *Circulation*, vol. 106, no. 6, pp. 643–645, 2002.

[5] N. S. Anavekar and M. A. Pfeffer, "Cardiovascular risk in chronic kidney disease," *Kidney International*, vol. 92, pp. S11–S15, 2004.

[6] P. C. W. Van Dijk, K. J. Jager, B. Stengel, C. Grönhagen-Riska, T. G. Feest, and J. D. Briggs, "Renal replacement therapy for diabetic end-stage renal disease: data from 10 registries in Europe (1991–2000)," *Kidney International*, vol. 67, no. 4, pp. 1489–1499, 2005.

[7] G. Pylypchuk and E. Beaubien, "Diabetic nephropathy. Prevention and early referral," *Canadian Family Physician*, vol. 46, pp. 636–642, 2000.

[8] E. Ritz, "Diabetic nephropathy," *Saudi Journal of Kidney Diseases and Transplantation*, vol. 17, no. 4, pp. 481–490, 2006.

[9] L. Cortés-Sanabria, H. R. Martínez-Ramírez, J. L. Hernández, E. Rojas-Campos, J. L. Canales-Muñoz, and A. M. Cueto-Manzano, "Utility of the Dipstick Micraltest II in the screening of microalbuminuria of diabetes mellitus type 2 and essential hypertension," *Revista de Investigación Clínica*, vol. 58, p. 190, 2006.

[10] A. Szymanowicz, E. Blanc-Bernard, C. Roche, M. J. Neyron, M. Perrin, and K. Nourdine, "Evaluation du micral test en vue du dépistage de la microalbuminurie en biologie délocalisée," *Immuno-Analyse et Biologie Spécialisée*, vol. 23, pp. 109–115, 2008.

[11] P. Giannuzi and D. A. Wood, "Guidelines on primary prevention of cardiovascular disease," *European Journal of Cardiovascular Prevention and Rehabilitation*, vol. 14, pp. S1–S113, 2007.

[12] American Diabetes Association, "Standards of medical care in diabetes—2013," *Diabetes Care*, vol. 36, supplement 1, pp. S11–S66, 2012.

[13] T. Bouattar, S. Ahid, S. Benasila et al., "The factors for progression of the diabetic nephropathy: management and evolution," *Nephrologie et Therapeutique*, vol. 5, no. 3, pp. 181–187, 2009.

[14] M. Marre, A. Girault, and D. Vasmant, "Prévalence de la microalbuminurie chez les diabétiques de type 2 français suivis par leur médecin généraliste," *Diabète et Métabolisme*, vol. 21, pp. 34–40, 1995.

[15] P. Sabouret, T. Denolle, M. Krempf, S. Om, and M. Laville, "Enquête microalb: dépistage de la microalbuminurie chez l'hypertendu diabétique de type 2 par le médecin généraliste en France métropolitaine," *Archives des Maladies du Coeur et des Vaisseaux*, vol. 99, pp. 712–717, 2006.

[16] A. Guerin, O. Savary, and S. Del Puppo, "Enquête mira: épidémiologie de la microalbuminurie et des comorbidités associées chez le diabétique de type 2," *Archives des Maladies du Coeur et des Vaisseaux*, vol. 98, pp. 783–787, 2005.

[17] L. Bendriss, A. Lebbaq, H. Jallal, S. Mrani, and A. Khatouri, "Intérêt de la microalbuminurie au sein du syndrome métabolique dans la prédiction des évènements cardiovasculaires. Étude prospective à propos de 78 cas," *Annales de Cardiologie et d'Angéiologie*, vol. 61, no. 1, pp. 15–19, 2012.

[18] A. Al-Adsani, "Risk factors associated with albuminuria in Kuwaiti adults with type 2 diabetes," *Saudi Journal of Kidney Diseases and Transplantation*, vol. 23, no. 4, pp. 860–865, 2012.

[19] U. Krairittichai, S. Potisat, A. Jongsareejit, and C. Sattaputh, "Prevalence and risk factors of diabetic nephropathy among Thai patients with type 2 diabetes mellitus," *Journal of the Medical Association of Thailand*, vol. 94, pp. S1–S5, 2011.

[20] K. D. Prasad and P. Rajaseker, "Study of microalbuminuria as a cardiovascular risk factor in type 2 diabetes mellitus," *Asian Journal of Pharmaceutical and Clinical Research*, vol. 5, pp. 42–43, 2012.

[21] F. A. Rahamtalla, "Prevalence of microalbuminuria among sudanese type 2 diabetic patients at elmusbah center at ombadda—omdurman," *IOSR Journal of Pharmacy*, vol. 2, no. 5, pp. 51–55, 2012.

[22] H.-H. Parving, J. B. Lewis, M. Ravid, G. Remuzzi, and L. G. Hunsicker, "Prevalence and risk factors for microalbuminuria in a referred cohort of type II diabetic patients: a global perspective," *Kidney International*, vol. 69, no. 11, pp. 2057–2063, 2006.

[23] M. Shebl and M. Atteia, "High prevalence of MicroAlbuminuria (MA) in type 2 diabetic patients," *Health Care*, vol. 21, pp. 221–232, 2008.

[24] F. Al-Maskari, M. El-Sadig, and E. Obineche, "Prevalence and determinants of microalbuminuria among diabetic patients in the United Arab Emirates," *BMC Nephrology*, vol. 9, article 1, 2008.

[25] W. Jia, X. Gao, C. Pang et al., "Prevalence and risk factors of albuminuria and chronic kidney disease in Chinese population with type 2 diabetes and impaired glucose regulation: Shanghai diabetic complications study (SHDCS)," *Nephrology Dialysis Transplantation*, vol. 24, no. 12, pp. 3724–3731, 2009.

[26] P. Sánchez Azcona and N. B. Quaglia, "A higher prevalence of microalbuminuria in women in a diabetes management program at a public hospital in the south of Santa Fe province," *Revista Argentina de Endocrinologia y Metabolismo*, vol. 48, no. 3, pp. 158–163, 2011.

[27] S. Maeda, N. Osawa, T. Hayashi, S. Tsukada, M. Kobayashi, and R. Kikkawa, "Genetic variations associated with diabetic nephropathy and type II diabetes in a Japanese population," *Kidney International*, vol. 72, no. 106, pp. S43–S48, 2007.

[28] A. I. Adler, R. J. Stevens, S. E. Manley, R. W. Bilous, C. A. Cull, and R. R. Holman, "Development and progression of nephropathy in type 2 diabetes: the United Kingdom Prospective Diabetes Study (UKPDS 64)," *Kidney International*, vol. 63, no. 1, pp. 225–232, 2003.

[29] I. Arfa, A. Abid, S. Nouira et al., "Lack of association between the angiotensin-converting enzyme gene (I/D) polymorphism and diabetic nephropathy in Tunisian type 2 diabetic patients," *Journal of the Renin-Angiotensin-Aldosterone System*, vol. 9, no. 1, pp. 32–36, 2008.

[30] J. M. Zacharias, T. K. Young, N. D. Riediger, J. Roulette, and S. G. Bruce, "Prevalence, risk factors and awareness of albuminuria on a Canadian First Nation: a community-based screening study," *BMC Public Health*, vol. 12, article 290, 2012.

[31] P. Gæde, H. Lund-Andersen, H.-H. Parving, and O. Pedersen, "Effect of a multifactorial intervention on mortality in type 2 diabetes," *The New England Journal of Medicine*, vol. 358, no. 6, pp. 580–591, 2008.

[32] B. Larijani, P. Hemati, A. Javadi, M. Mahmoudi, and A. Shafaee, "Screening for Microalbuminuria in the early detection of diabetic nephropathy: a cheap and simple method," *Acta Medica Iranica*, vol. 40, pp. 1–2, 2002.

[33] J. P. Le Floch, M. Marre, M. Rodier, and P. H. Passa, "Interest of clinitek® microalbumin in screening for microalbuminuria: results of a multicentre study in 302 diabetic patients," *Diabetes and Metabolism*, vol. 27, no. 1, pp. 36–39, 2001.

[34] P. McFarlane and B. Culleton, "La néphropathie chronique en présence de diabète," *Canadian Journal of Diabetes*, vol. 32, pp. S139–S147, 2008.

[35] W. J. C. De Grauw, E. H. Van de Lisdonk, H. J. M. Van den Hoogen et al., "Screening for microalbuminuria in type 2 diabetic patients: the evaluation of a dipstick test in general practice," *Diabetic Medicine*, vol. 12, no. 8, pp. 657–663, 1995.

[36] J. Incerti, T. Zelmanovitz, J. L. Camargo, J. L. Gross, and M. J. de Azevedo, "Evaluation of tests for microalbuminuria screening in patients with diabetes," *Nephrology Dialysis Transplantation*, vol. 20, no. 11, pp. 2402–2407, 2005.

[37] C. E. Mogensen, G. C. Viberti, E. Peheim et al., "Multicenter evaluation of the Micral-Test II test strip, an immunologic rapid test for the detection of microalbuminuria," *Diabetes Care*, vol. 20, no. 11, pp. 1642–1646, 1997.

[38] C. R. Parikh, M. J. Fischer, R. Estacio, and R. W. Schrier, "Rapid microalbuminuria screening in type 2 diabetes mellitus: simplified approach with Micral test strips and specific gravity," *Nephrology Dialysis Transplantation*, vol. 19, pp. 1881–1885, 2004.

[39] P. A. Sarafidis, J. Riehle, Z. Bogojevic, E. Basta, A. Chugh, and G. L. Bakris, "A comparative evaluation of various methods for microalbuminuria screening," *American Journal of Nephrology*, vol. 28, no. 2, pp. 324–329, 2008.

[40] D. J. Webb, D. J. Newman, N. Chaturvedi, and J. H. Fuller, "The use of the Micral-Test strip to identify the presence of microalbuminuria in people with insulin dependent diabetes mellitus (IDDM) participating in the EUCLID study," *Diabetes Research and Clinical Practice*, vol. 31, pp. 93–102, 1996.

[41] G. Bruno, P. Cavallo-Perin, G. Bargero et al., "Prevalence and risk factors for micro-and macroalbuminuria in an Italian population-based cohort of NIDDM subjects," *Diabetes Care*, vol. 19, no. 1, pp. 43–47, 1996.

[42] D. Jacobs, W. DeMott, H. Grady, R. Horvat, D. Huestis, and B. Kasten, *Laboratory Test Handbook*, Lexi-Comp, Cleveland, Ohio, USA, 1996.

[43] N. Pasko, F. Toti, E. Zekollari, A. Strakosha, V. Kacori, and N. Thereska, "Prevalence of microalbuminuria in type 2 diabetes patients in Tirana, a preliminary multicenter study," *Journal of Diabetes Mellitus*, vol. 3, no. 3, pp. 145–149, 2013.

[44] H. Ben Ahmed, K. Bouzid, M. Hassine et al., "Prévalence des facteurs de risque cardiovasculaire non conventionnels chez les sujets diabétiques tunisiens," *La Presse Médicale*, vol. 43, no. 1, pp. e9–e16, 2014.

[45] C. Garcia, L. Bordier, P. Burnat et al., "Urinary dipsticks must not be used to detect diabetes-induced incipient nephropathy," *La Presse Médicale*, vol. 35, no. 7-8, pp. 1117–1121, 2006.

28

Prevalence of Anemia, Overweight/Obesity, and Undiagnosed Hypertension and Diabetes among Residents of Selected Communities in Ghana

Alex Kojo Anderson

Department of Foods and Nutrition, University of Georgia, Athens, GA 30602, USA

Correspondence should be addressed to Alex Kojo Anderson; fianko@uga.edu

Academic Editor: Srinivas Kondalsamy-Chennakesavan

The increasing numbers of lifestyle related chronic diseases in developing countries call for awareness, early detection, and effective management. The objective of this paper is to report the prevalence of undiagnosed hypertension, diabetes, overweight/obesity, and anemia among residents of selected communities in Ghana. The data comes from a community screening conducted in Ghana as part of the University of Georgia Summer Service Learning Program. Descriptive statistics were used to summarize the data while chi-square and independent t-test compared groups. A total of 976 participants (37.9% males and 62.1% females), 18 years and older, were screened. Mean age was 46.25 ± 17.14 years, BMI was 25.44 ± 5.26 kgm^{-2}, and hemoglobin was 12.04 ± 2.22 g/dL. 3.1% and 12.6% reported existing diagnosis for diabetes and hypertension, respectively. Almost half (47.8%) were overweight/obese; 27.0% were hypertensive while 34.0% had diabetes. Also, 28.8% males compared to 37.8% females had diabetes ($P = 0.015$), while 28.2% males compared to 26.2% females were hypertensive ($P = 0.635$). There were differences in BMI ($P < 0.0001$), anemia ($P = 0.007$), and undiagnosed diabetes ($P < 0.0001$) and hypertension ($P < 0.0001$) by community (Takoradi versus Cape Coast) where the screening took place. Findings from the screening exercise call for improved public health education with a focus on lifestyle habits and health seeking behaviors among Ghanaians.

1. Introduction

Hypertension (raised blood pressure), one of the major diseases of the 21st century, is reported to affect over 1 billion of the world's population with about three-fourths living in developing countries and almost half (46%) in Africa [1–3]. Hypertension is also a major risk factor for a number of chronic diseases including heart disease, heart attack/failure, stroke, cerebrovascular disease, diabetes mellitus, and renal failure. Unfortunately, because of the asymptomatic nature of hypertension during the early stages of the disease, it has not been a priority for primary healthcare workers, particularly in developing countries with limited resources and poor healthcare infrastructure.

Type 2 diabetes (due to insulin insensitivity and/or poor blood glucose management) currently affects 1 in 11 adults, and a predicted 642 million people are expected to be living with diabetes in the world by the year 2040 [4, 5]. Recent reports suggest that almost 3 of every 4 diabetics reside in low- and middle-income countries, expected to further increase by the year 2030 [6, 7]. Poorly managed diabetes increases the risk of cardiovascular disease, blindness, kidney failure, amputations, and early death. It is projected that the prevalence of diabetes in Africa will increase and surpass those of the other regions of the world by the year 2035 [8–10].

Anemia (low blood hemoglobin concentration) is one of the significant public health problems (hidden hunger) plaguing the world today [11]. Globally, over 1.6 billion people are reported to be anemic [12]. Anemia occurs through the lifecycle but disproportionately affects children and women and individuals from low-income, resource limited areas of the world. Although iron deficiency is the significant cause of anemia, there are other contributing causes of anemia which include parasitic infections, malaria, heavy blood loss as a result of menstruation among females, and other nutrient deficiencies including folate, vitamin B_{12}, riboflavin, and copper. Because of the silent nature of anemia, it often goes undiagnosed and poorly managed, leading to poor cognitive and physical development of children and negative physical performance and work productivity among adults [13].

The prevalence and risk of death from hypertension and diabetes are on the increase in most developing countries as a result of the ongoing nutrition transition and poor health infrastructure in these countries [8, 14–23]. The impact of the nutrition transition on the dietary habit is the resulting change from traditionally less processed foods to Western food habits and lifestyles which include the consumption of foods high in calories, sugar, salt, and total fat [24, 25]. These dietary changes have led to increased prevalence of obesity, metabolic syndrome, diabetes, and hypertension in most low- to middle-income countries [26, 27]. This is compounded by poor health seeking behaviors, poor healthcare infrastructure and resource allocation, and inadequate access to preventative health services. Because of the limited healthcare resources, governments of developing countries, including Ghana, tend to focus most of their effort and resources on infectious diseases and not chronic diseases [19, 28]. Another major problem is the lack of awareness and magnitude of these chronic diseases and their early detection and intervention among populations of developing countries, including Ghana [26]. Thus, in this paper we report the prevalence of undiagnosed hypertension and diabetes, overweight/obesity, and anemia among residents of selected communities in Ghana and their public health implications.

2. Methods

2.1. Study Design and Setting. This was a secondary data analysis of data generated from a community nutrition and health screening/education which is part of service learning activities conducted by students from the University of Georgia who participated in a Service Learning Program in Ghana directed by the author. The community nutrition and health screening/education was conducted between June and July 2016. Participants were free living adult community residents who came forward to participate in the screening exercise. The use of the data in this study was approved by the Human Subject Institutional Review Board of the University of Georgia.

The community nutrition and health screening/education exercises occurred in Sekondi-Takoradi, capital city of the Western Region and Cape Coast, capital city of the Central Region of Ghana. The mobile clinics for the nutrition and health screening/education were in two (2) communities (Collins Avenue and Star of the Sea Cathedral) in Takoradi and Apewosika community in Cape Coast.

Sekondi-Takoradi is located at the southeastern part of the Western Region. According to the 2010 Population and Housing Census, the total population of the Sekondi-Takoradi is 559,548 (23.5% of the region's total population). Over 67% of the population are 15 years and older. Over 96% of the population in Sekondi-Takoradi resides in urban areas. Almost 91% of the population in the Metropolis are literate (having some form of formal education) while 90% of the adult population are employed. Health facilities include the regional hospital, 2 district hospitals, and a number of clinics that provide healthcare services to residents of the area and other neighboring communities.

The total population of Cape Coast is 169,894 (constituting about 7.7% of the total population of the Central Region) of which over 120,000 are 15 years and older. Cape Coast is predominantly urban with three-quarters of the population residing in urban areas. Over 90% of the population of Cape Coast is literate compared to 78.2% and 74.1% for the Central Region and Ghana, respectively. Almost 91% of adults are employed. Cape Coast is the home of the regional hospital which also serves as a referral center. It also has a district hospital and a number of clinics that provide healthcare to the population of the Metropolis.

2.2. Data Collection Procedures. Data for this study was generated from adults 18 years and older who voluntarily participated in the University of Georgia Ghana Summer Service Learning from June to July 2016. The data available included community where the screening occurred, age, gender, weight, height, blood hemoglobin, fasting blood glucose, and blood pressure.

2.3. Anthropometric Measurement. Weight and height were measured using calibrated weighing scale and stadiometer following standard protocol [29]. Because these anthropometric measurements were conducted in the open, the requirement for minimum clothing during weight measurement was not possible. Weight was measured with participants wearing their regular clothing devoid of other clothing accessories in the case of women and wallets and so forth in the pocket of men. Weight was measured to the nearest 0.1 kg. Height was measured to the nearest 0.1 cm without shoes, cap, or headgear. Weight and height measurements were used to estimate body mass index (BMI = weight in kg ÷ [height in meters]^2). BMI was further classified as underweight (BMI < 18.5 kgm^{-2}), normal weight (BMI = 18.5–24.9 kgm^{-2}), overweight (BMI = 25.0–29.9 kgm^{-2}), and obese (BMI > 30.0 kgm^{-2}).

2.4. Hemoglobin. Blood hemoglobin level was measured using HemoCue Hb201$^+$. To measure blood hemoglobin level, the patient's forefinger was prepared by wiping the tip with alcohol to sterilize the area and then allowed to dry. The sterilized area was then pricked with a lancet and a drop of blood collected into a microcuvette. The microcuvette filled with the blood was then inserted into the HemoCue Hb201$^+$ for the hemoglobin measurement. The measured hemoglobin was classified as normal (Hb > 13 g/dL for men and Hb > 12 g/dL for women), mild anemia (Hb: 11.0–12.9 g/dL for men versus Hb: 11.0–11.9 g/dL for women), moderate anemia (Hb: 8.0–10.9 g/dL), and severe anemia (Hb < 8 g/dL).

2.5. Fasting Blood Glucose. Blood glucose concentration was measured using HemoCue Glucose 201$^+$. For blood glucose measurement, the patient forefinger was prepared as described for hemoglobin measurement above. A drop of blood was collected from a finger prick into a microcuvette and inserted into the HemoCue Glucose 201$^+$ for blood glucose measurement. The measured blood glucose was later classified as normal (FBG < 100 mg/dL), prediabetes (FBG: 100–125 mg/dL), and diabetes (FBG > 126 mg/dL) [30].

2.6. Blood Pressure. Blood pressure was measured at least 10 minutes from the patient's arrival at the mobile screening clinic. Participants were seated and made comfortable with one arm resting on a table. The BP was measured using an automated (digital) sphygmomanometer. The cuff was inflated by turning on the sphygmomanometer for the blood pressure measurement. The measured blood pressure was classified as normal (systolic: less than 120 mmHg; diastolic: less than 80 mmHg), prehypertension (systolic: 120–139 mmHg; diastolic: 80–90 mmHg), and hypertension (systolic: ≥140 mmHg; diastolic ≥ 90 mmHg).

2.7. Statistical Analysis. The statistical package IBM SPSS Statistics 23 for Windows (IBM SPSS Inc., Armonk, NY, USA) was used for data entry and analysis. Descriptive statistics were used to summarize the data and results reported as percentages (frequencies) and means (± standard deviation). Student's unpaired, two-sided t-test was used to compare means between Takoradi and Cape Coast. Pearson Chi-squared test (Fisher's exact test) was used to compare the independent variables (place of resident, age, and gender) and outcome variables (indicators of anemia, obesity, diabetes, and hypertension). All P values were two-sided, and criterion for statistical significance was set at $P < 0.05$.

3. Results

A total of 976 adults (597 from Takoradi and 379 from Cape Coast) participated in the screening with data for the study. The average age was 46.25 ± 17.14 (range: 18–100) years and was similar in the two Metropolises. Majority of the participants were over 40 years old. Participants were fairly distributed by gender ($P = 0.437$) in the two cities with over 60% being females (Table 1). For individuals who participated in the screening exercise, 12.6% (13.7% in Takoradi versus 10.8% in Cape Coast) and 3.1% (3.7% in Takoradi versus 2.1% in Cape Coast) reported known (existing) diagnosis for hypertension and diabetes, respectively.

3.1. Participant Hemoglobin. The mean hemoglobin level was 12.04 ± 2.22 g/dL (range: 2.00–17.80). There were differences in hemoglobin levels by gender and screening community. The mean blood hemoglobin concentration was significantly lower among females compared to males (11.43 ± 2.17 g/dL versus 13.03 ± 2.17 g/dL, $P < 0.0001$) and Takoradi compared to Cape Coast (11.85 ± 2.38 g/dL versus 12.34 ± 1.92 g/dL, $P = 0.001$), although these were within the normal range. Overall, 47.0% of the participant had mild to severe anemia. About a third of males (30.5%) and a little over half (52.2%) of females had mild to severe anemia according to their blood hemoglobin concentration (Figure 1). Prevalence of anemia was significantly ($P = 0.007$) higher among participants from Takoradi compared to their counterparts from Cape Coast (Table 1).

3.2. Participant Weight. Overall, almost half (47.8%) of the participants were either overweight or obese (BMI > 25 kgm^{-2}). The average BMI was 26.06 ± 5.32 kgm^{-2} versus 24.45 ± 5.01 kgm^{-2} for participants in Takoradi and Cape Coast, respectively ($P < 0.0001$). 18.4% of the participants were obese. Whereas 53.7% of participants from Takoradi were either overweight or obese, only 38.4% of those from Cape Coast were overweight or obese ($P < 0.0001$). The prevalence of overweight/obesity was higher among female participants compared to male participants ($P < 0.0001$) (Figure 1).

3.3. Blood Pressure. Generally, measured systolic and diastolic blood pressures were higher for participants from Takoradi compared to those from Cape Coast. The measured blood pressure shows that majority of the participants were either prehypertensive or hypertensive. The overall prevalence of hypertension was 27.0%. Of those with hypertensive blood pressure, only 12.6% (123/976) had prior diagnosis for hypertension. The prevalence of hypertension detected from the screening exercise was significantly ($P < 0.0001$) higher among participants from Takoradi (30.4%) compared to their counterparts from Cape Coast (21.8%). There was overall significant ($P = 0.002$) difference in hypertension by participant gender, with males having slightly higher prevalence compared to females (Figure 1). Similar trends were observed in Takoradi and Cape Coast (data not shown).

3.4. Fasting Blood Glucose. Majority of the participants had fasting blood sugar levels classified as either prediabetes or diabetes. The measured fasting blood glucose showed 39.2% prevalence for diabetes of which 3.1% (30/976) reported known diabetes diagnosis. Almost 40% of participants from Takoradi were diabetics compared to 24.6% from Cape Coast based on their measured fasting blood sugar ($P < 0.0001$) (Table 1). Most (39.8%) of the participants from Cape Coast compared to 28.4% from Takoradi had measured fasting blood sugar level in the normal range. There was statistical difference in fasting blood sugar level by participant gender with 37.1% of females compared to 28.8% of males who were diabetics ($P = 0.015$) (Figure 1).

4. Discussion

Ghana, as is the case of many low- and middle-income countries, is dealing with the triple burden of malnutrition (undernutrition, micronutrient deficiencies, and increasing prevalence of overweight/obesity and related chronic diseases) because of changes in their food systems due to their degree of economic development and adopting Western food culture [31]. The situation poses a threat to the healthcare infrastructure and productivity and creates a financial burden for these countries. There is therefore a need to bring attention to awareness and early intervention to mitigate the human resource and economic burden of these countries. In this study, we examined the problem of undiagnosed hypertension and diabetes, overweight/obesity, and anemia among residents of Takoradi and Cape Coast, Ghana. We observed high prevalence of undiagnosed hypertension and diabetes, overweight/obesity, and anemia among residents who participated in the screening exercise.

Table 1: Characteristics of participants.

	Takoradi Mean ± SD	Cape Coast Mean ± SD	P value
Age (years)	46.45 ± 16.69	45.92 ± 17.86	0.637
BMI (kgm^{-2})	26.06 ± 5.32	24.45 ± 5.01	<0.0001
Systolic blood pressure (mmHg)	136.89 ± 24.80	134.27 ± 25.53	0.114
Diastolic blood pressure (mmHg)	86.98 ± 14.62	81.81 ± 14.04	<0.0001
Fasting blood glucose (mg/dL)	123.46 ± 43.41	112.86 ± 38.37	<0.0001
Hemoglobin (g/dL)	11.85 ± 2.38	12.34 ± 1.92	0.001
	n (%)	n (%)	
Age (years)			
<25	61 (10.2)	45 (11.9)	
25–40	177 (29.6)	120 (31.7)	0.661
41–60	222 (37.2)	136 (35.9)	
>60	137 (22.9)	78 (20.6)	
Sex			
Male	228 (38.2)	142 (37.5)	0.437
Female	369 (61.8)	237 (62.5)	
Weight status			
Underweight	21 (3.5)	25 (6.6)	
Normal weight	255 (42.8)	208 (55.0)	<0.0001
Overweight	196 (32.9)	90 (23.8)	
Obese	124 (20.8)	55 (14.6)	
Measured blood pressure			
Normal	204 (34.2)	184 (48.5)	
Prehypertensive	211 (35.4)	113 (29.8)	<0.0001
Hypertensive	181 (30.4)	82 (21.6)	
Fasting blood glucose			
Normal	169 (28.4)	149 (39.8)	
Prediabetes	189 (31.8)	133 (35.6)	<0.0001
Diabetes	237 (39.8)	92 (24.6)	
Hemoglobin			
Normal	305 (51.1)	211 (56.1)	
Mild anemia	150 (25.1)	100 (26.6)	0.007
Moderate anemia	98 (16.4)	56 (14.9)	
Severe anemia	44 (7.4)	9 (2.4)	

The findings of the present study show overall prevalence of undiagnosed hypertension and diabetes to be 53.2% (77.3% in Takoradi and 0.0% in Cape Coast) and 90.9% (90.5% in Takoradi and 91.3% in Cape Coast), respectively. Our finding is consistent with findings from a study by Amoah and colleagues conducted in Accra, Ghana, where they reported prevalence of undiagnosed diabetes [32]. However, the prevalence of undiagnosed diabetes among participants in the current study from Takoradi and Cape Coast is higher than reported by Amoah and colleagues [32]. This suggests a lack of awareness or knowledge of symptoms and general education of these diseases among residents of Takoradi and Cape Coast. This is a major public health problem as previous studies have shown that awareness and early detection leads to effective management of hypertension and diabetes [33–36]. This observation paints a bleak health picture for both Takoradi and Cape Coast as this stands to affect the work productivity and quality of life of the adult population of these areas, which will eventually have a negative impact on their economic growth as these adults constitute the workforce. This situation also has the potential of posing a great challenge to the healthcare infrastructure and increasing healthcare costs for the government of Ghana and the individuals involved as well as their respective families.

The prevalence of overweight and obesity was disproportionately higher among participants from Takoradi compared to those from Cape Coast ($P < 0.0001$). Over half of participants from Takoradi compared to about a third from Cape Coast were either overweight or obese. This is higher than previously reported among the adult population in Ghana and other developing countries [37]. For example, a recent systematic review and analysis conducted by Ofori-Asenso and colleagues of 43 studies conducted across the 10 regions of Ghana reported that about 43% of the adult

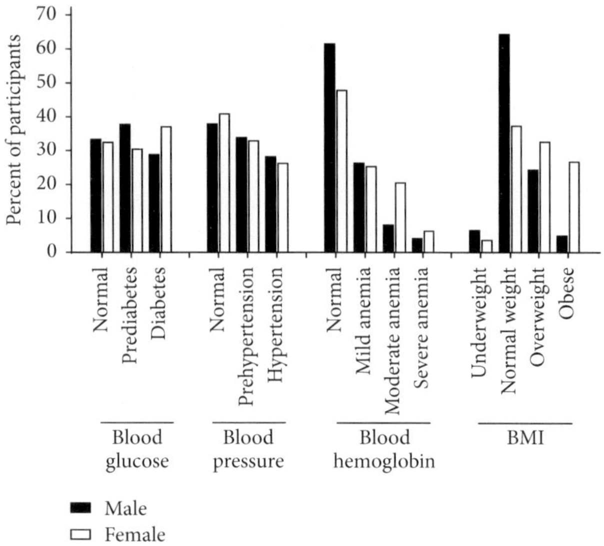

FIGURE 1: Prevalence of undiagnosed diabetes and hypertension, anemia, and obesity.

population are either overweight or obese. Women generally had a higher prevalence of overweight/obesity compared to men [37]. This differential and high prevalence rate of overweight/obesity by gender as was observed in the current study has been attributed to cultural perception of body size. In most African countries including Ghana, being overweight or obese is associated with good health, wellbeing, and high social class [20, 23, 38–43]. Prevailing knowledge of the strong association between obesity and chronic diseases including hypertension and diabetes paints a gloomy picture of the health of Ghanaian adults should this continue [44–46]. There is therefore a need for culturally appropriate interventions that target healthy weight management among Ghanaian adults, especially women, so they understand the health risks associated with overweight and obesity and that being overweight or obese is not necessarily an indication of good health status and wellbeing.

The prevalence of anemia observed among participants in this study was similar to that reported in a number of systematic reviews of global level data [11, 12, 47]. This observation is a significant public health problem as anemia has direct effect on one's performance and productivity. In the current study we could not ascertain the cause of the high anemia prevalence due to our inability to obtain information on potential causes and general lifestyle of the participants. The high anemia prevalence could be due to a number of factors including genetic make-up (such as sickle cell trait and thalassemia), dietary habits (micronutrient deficiencies), infections such as hookworm and schistosomiasis, and disease states such as malaria or inflammation [48]. Other evidences suggest increased risk for anemia among patients with diabetes [49]. This is evidential in the current study with high prevalence of undiagnosed diabetes and anemia.

This study comes with a number of limitations which should inform the interpretation of the findings. First, this is a secondary data analysis, and the data used came from a community screening exercise, thus the likelihood of selection bias. Second, we did not have data to examine the predictors of anemia, overweight/obesity, hypertension, and diabetes. Third, the screening exercise took place within communities in Takoradi and Cape Coast; therefore, our findings may not be representative of respective regions limiting the generalizability of the findings; thus results should be interpreted with caution. However, the study had a large sample size, which is a strength, and also highlights the lack of awareness of hypertension, diabetes, overweight/obesity, and anemia in communities in Ghana to inform public health interventions.

5. Conclusions

The situation of high prevalence of obesity, anemia, and undiagnosed hypertension and diabetes has significant public health implications for health planners of a country such as Ghana which has limited health infrastructure with a heavy burden of undernutrition and infectious diseases among its population. There is therefore an urgent need for health policies focused on primary prevention and early detection of these chronic disease conditions within the Ghanaian population. The ongoing nutrition and epidemiologic transition and urbanization in Ghana have affected the traditional food culture and general lifestyle. The situation poses a serious threat to the wellbeing, quality of life, and productivity of Ghana's workforce if immediate steps are not taken to reverse these rising trends.

Ethical Approval

The proposal for this paper was reviewed and approved by the Human Subjects Institutional Review Board of the University of Georgia.

Disclosure

Because the study only used data generated from a community health and nutrition screening exercise, waiver was given for documenting participant consent.

Authors' Contributions

Alex Kojo Anderson conceived the idea, sought IRB approval, conducted the data analysis, and wrote the manuscript.

Acknowledgments

First and foremost, the author would like to thank all University of Georgia students who participated in the 2016 Ghana Summer Service Learning Program who worked diligently to screen residents of selected communities in Ghana. The author also wants to thank Evan S. Johnson for entering and cleaning the data for analysis and, lastly, the residents of Takoradi and Cape Coast in Ghana who participated in the screening exercise that generated the data for this paper.

References

[1] WHO, *The world health report 2002: reducing risks, promoting healthy life*, World Health Organization, Geneva, Switzerland, 2002.

[2] WHO, *WHO Global Report. Preventing chronic disease a vital investment*, World Health Organization, Geneva, Switzerland, 2005.

[3] WHO, *A global brief on HYPERTENSION. Silent killer, global public health crisis*, World Health Organization, Geneva, Switzerland, 2013.

[4] International Diabetes Federation (IDF), Primary Care Diabetes Europe (PCDE), and World Heart Federation (WHF), *The Berlin Declaration: a Collective Ambition for Policy Change to Drive Early Action in Type 2 Diabetes*, International Diabetes Federation, Berlin, Germany, 2016.

[5] *IDF Diabetes Atlas*, International Diabetes Federation (IDF), 2015.

[6] R. Sicree, J. Shaw, and P. Zimme, "Diabetes and Impaired Glucose Tolerance," in *proceedings of the International Diabetes Federation*, Geneva, Switzerland, 2010.

[7] C. Murray and A. D. Lopez, *Global Burden of Disease: A Comprehensive Assessment of Mortality and Disability from Diseases, Injuries and Risk Factors in 1990 and Projected to 2020*, Harvard School of Public Health, Cambridge, MA, USA, 1996.

[8] L. Guariguata, D. Whiting, I. Hambleton, J. Beagley, U. Linnenkamp, and J. Shaw, "Global estimates of diabetes prevalence for 2013 and projections for 2035," *Diabetes Research and Clinical Practice*, vol. 103, no. 2, pp. 137–149, 2014.

[9] J. E. Shaw, R. A. Sicree, and P. Z. Zimmet, "Global estimates of the prevalence of diabetes for 2010 and 2030," *Diabetes Research and Clinical Practice*, vol. 87, no. 1, pp. 4–14, 2010.

[10] J. Mattei, V. Malik, N. M. Wedick et al., "Reducing the global burden of type 2 diabetes by improving the quality of staple foods: The Global Nutrition and Epidemiologic Transition Initiative," *Globalization and Health*, vol. 11, no. 1, article no. 23, 2015.

[11] E. McLean, M. Cogswell, I. Egli, D. Wojdyla, and B. De Benoist, "Worldwide prevalence of anaemia, WHO Vitamin and Mineral Nutrition Information System, 1993–2005," *Public Health Nutrition*, vol. 12, no. 4, pp. 444–454, 2009.

[12] N. J. Kassebaum et al., "A systematic analysis of global anemia burden from 1990 ti 2010," *Blood*, vol. 23, pp. 615–624, 2014.

[13] WHO, "Iron deficiency anaemia: assessment, prevention, and control," in *A guide for Programme Managers*, World Health Organization, Geneva, Switherland, 2001.

[14] P. M. Kearney, M. Whelton, K. Reynolds, P. Muntner, P. K. Whelton, and J. He, "Global burden of hypertension: analysis of worldwide data," *The Lancet*, vol. 365, no. 9455, pp. 217–223, 2005.

[15] R. Funetes et al., "Hypertension in developing economies: a review of population-based studies carried out from 1980-1998," *Journal of Hypertension*, vol. 18, pp. 521–529, 2000.

[16] R. Edwards, N. Unwin, F. Mugusi et al., "Hypertension prevalence and care in an urban and rural area of Tanzania," *Journal of Hypertension*, vol. 18, no. 2, pp. 145–152, 2000.

[17] J. Tran, M. Mirzaei, and S. Leeder, "Hypertension: its prevalence and population-attributable fraction for mortality from stroke in the Middle East and North Africa," *Circulation*, vol. 122, article e155, 2010.

[18] D. Yach, C. Hawkes, C. L. Gould, and K. J. Hofman, "The global burden of chronic diseases: overcoming impediments to prevention and control," *The Journal of the American Medical Association*, vol. 291, no. 21, pp. 2616–2622, 2004.

[19] V. Perkovic, R. Huxley, Y. Wu, D. Prabhakaran, and S. MacMahon, "The burden of blood pressure-related disease: a neglected priority for global health," *Hypertension*, vol. 50, no. 6, pp. 991–997, 2007.

[20] A. M. Prentice, "The emerging epidemic of obesity in developing countries," *International Journal of Epidemiology*, vol. 35, no. 1, pp. 93–99, 2006.

[21] WHO, "Global Strategy on Diet, Physical Activity & Health," in *Obesity and Overweight*, World Health Organization, Geneva, Switherland, 2003.

[22] B. M. Popkin and P. Gordon-Larsen, "The nutrition transition: Worldwide obesity dynamics and their determinants," *International Journal of Obesity*, vol. 28, pp. S2–S9, 2004.

[23] L. McLaren, "Socioeconomic status and obesity," *Epidemiologic Reviews*, vol. 29, no. 1, pp. 29–48, 2007.

[24] J. Schmidhuber and P. Shetty, "The nutrition transition to 2030: why developing countries are likely to bear the major burden," in *Proceedings of the 97th Seminar of European Association of Agricultural Economists*, vol. 2, pp. 150–166, Food and Agriculture Organization (FAO), Reading, UK, 2005.

[25] B. M. Popkin, L. S. Adair, and S. W. Ng, "Global nutrition transition and the pandemic of obesity in developing countries," *Nutrition Reviews*, vol. 70, no. 1, pp. 3–21, 2012.

[26] M. M. Ibrahim and A. Damasceno, "Hypertension in developing countries," *The Lancet*, vol. 380, no. 9841, pp. 611–619, 2012.

[27] G. Danaei, M. M. Finucane, J. K. Lin et al., "National, regional, and global trends in systolic blood pressure since 1980: systematic analysis of health examination surveys and epidemiological studies with 786 country-years and 5·4 million participants," *The Lancet*, vol. 377, no. 9765, pp. 568–577, 2011.

[28] O. Adeyi, O. Smith, and S. Robles, *Public Policy and the Challenge of Chronic Noncommunicable Diseases*, World Bank, Washington, DC, USA, 2007.

[29] R. S. Gibson, *Principles of Nutritional Assessment*, Oxford University Press, Oxford, UK, 2005.

[30] Centers for Disease Control and Prevention, "Current trends CDC criteria for anemia in children and childbearing-aged women," *Morbidity and Mortuligy Weekly Report (MMWR)*, vol. 38, no. 22, pp. 400–404, 1989.

[31] B. M. Popkin, "Global nutrition dynamics: the world is shifting rapidly toward a diet linked with noncommunicable diseases," *The American Journal of Clinical Nutrition*, vol. 84, no. 2, pp. 289–298, 2006.

[32] A. G. Amoah, S. K. Owusu, and S. Adjei, "Diabetes in Ghana: a community based prevalence study in Greater Accra," *Diabetes Research and Clinical Practice*, vol. 56, no. 3, pp. 197–205, 2002.

[33] M. M. Ibrahim, H. Rizk, L. J. Appel et al., "Hypertension prevalence, awareness, treatment, and control in Egypt: Results from the Egyptian National Hypertension Project (NHP)," *Hypertension*, vol. 26, no. 6 I, pp. 886–890, 1995.

[34] C. Agyemang, M. A. Bruijnzeels, and E. Owusu-Dabo, "Factors associated with hypertension awareness, treatment, and control in Ghana, West Africa," *Journal of Human Hypertension*, vol. 20, no. 1, pp. 67–71, 2006.

[35] K. Wolf-Maier, R. S. Cooper, H. Kramer et al., "Hypertension treatment and control in five european countries, Canada, and the United States," *Hypertension*, vol. 43, no. 1, pp. 10–17, 2004.

[36] P. Primatesta and N. R. Poulter, "Improvement in hypertension management in England: results from the Health Survey for

England 2003," *Journal of Hypertension*, vol. 24, no. 6, pp. 1187–1192, 2006.

[37] R. Ofori-Asenso, A. A. Agyeman, A. Laar, and D. Boateng, "Overweight and obesity epidemic in Ghana - A systematic review and meta-analysis," *BMC Public Health*, vol. 16, no. 1, article no. 1239, 2016.

[38] P. Bovet, A. G. Ross, J.-P. Gervasoni et al., "Distribution of blood pressure, body mass index and smoking habits in the urban population of Dar es Salaam, Tanzania, and associations with socioeconomic status," *International Journal of Epidemiology*, vol. 31, no. 1, pp. 240–247, 2002.

[39] P. Craig, V. Halavatau, E. Comino, and I. Caterson, "Perception of body size in the Tongan community: Differences from and similarities to an Australian sample," *International Journal of Obesity*, vol. 23, no. 12, pp. 1288–1294, 1999.

[40] N. J. Pollock, "Cultural elaborations of obesity-fattening practices in pacific societies," *Asia Pacific Journal of Clinical Nutrition*, vol. 4, pp. 357–360, 1995.

[41] M. Holdsworth, A. Gartner, E. Landais, B. Maire, and F. Delpeuch, "Perceptions of healthy and desirable body size in urban Senegalese women," *International Journal of Obesity*, vol. 28, no. 12, pp. 1561–1568, 2004.

[42] T. Puoane, J. M. Fourie, M. Shapiro, L. Rosling, N. C. Tshaka, and A. Oelofse, "'Big is beautiful' - An exploration with urban black community health workers in a South African township," *South African Journal of Clinical Nutrition*, vol. 18, no. 1, pp. 6–15, 2005.

[43] M. Rguibi and R. Belahsen, "Body size preferences and sociocultural influences on attitudes towards obesity among Moroccan Sahraoui women," *Body Image*, vol. 3, no. 4, pp. 395–400, 2006.

[44] G. A. Colditz, W. C. Willett, A. Rotnitzky, and J. E. Manson, "Weight gain as a risk factor for clinical diabetes mellitus in women," *Annals of Internal Medicine*, vol. 122, no. 7, pp. 481–486, 1995.

[45] E. S. Ford, D. F. Williamson, and S. Liu, "Weight change and diabetes incidence: findings from a national cohort of US adults," *American Journal of Epidemiology*, vol. 146, no. 3, pp. 214–222, 1997.

[46] R. Scranton, H. D. Sesso, M. J. Stampfer, J. W. Levenson, J. E. Buring, and J. M. Gaziano, "Predictors of 14-year changes in the total cholesterol to high-density lipoprotein cholesterol ratio in men," *American Heart Journal*, vol. 147, no. 6, pp. 1033–1038, 2004.

[47] G. A. Stevens, M. M. Finucane, L. M. De-Regil et al., "Global, regional, and national trends in haemoglobin concentration and prevalence of total and severe anaemia in children and pregnant and non-pregnant women for 1995–2011: a systematic analysis of population-representative data," *The Lancet Global Health*, vol. 1, no. 1, pp. E16–E25, 2013.

[48] World Health Organization, *Assessing the iron status of populations*, World Health Organization, Geneva, Switherland, 2007.

[49] D. R. Bosman, A. S. Winkler, J. T. Marsden, I. C. Macdougall, and P. J. Watkins, "Anemia with erythropoietin deficiency occurs early in diabetic nephropathy," *Diabetes Care*, vol. 24, no. 3, pp. 495–499, 2001.

29

Musculoskeletal Disorders and Perceived Work Demands among Female Nurses at a Tertiary Care Hospital in India

Apexa S. Raithatha and Daxa G. Mishra

KM Patel Institute of Physiotherapy, Shree Krishna Hospital, Gokal Nagar, Karamsad, Gujarat 388325, India

Correspondence should be addressed to Apexa S. Raithatha; apexa.raithatha@gmail.com

Academic Editor: Mario Cardiel

Introduction. Musculoskeletal disorders (MSD) are common among nurses and can affect patient outcomes. There is a dearth of literature on MSD among Indian nurses. The study objective was to measure prevalence of MSD and their association with perceived work demands and sociodemographic variables among female nurses at a tertiary care hospital in rural India. *Methods*. A cross-sectional study was undertaken in 2013 through interviewer administered questionnaires which comprised three parts: sociodemographic data, modified Nordic questionnaire, and perceived physical and psychological work demands. *Results*. 296 nurses with a mean age of 30.4 years participated. Prevalence of any MSD in the last seven days was 60.5% with low back pain being the most common and elbow pain the least common. Occurrence of any MSD was associated with age, number of children, working hours at home, BMI, and total work experience. High perceived physical demands score was associated with lower back (OR: 3.06) and knee pain (OR: 7.73). *Conclusion*. Prevalence of MSD was high and occurrence of lower back and knee MSD was associated with perceived physical demands. This information should be used as a benchmark and guiding tool for designing work place interventions to improve working conditions and health of nurses.

1. Introduction

"Musculoskeletal disorders" (MSD) include a wide range of inflammatory and degenerative conditions affecting the muscles, tendons, ligaments, joints, peripheral nerves, and supporting blood vessels [1]. Work related MSD by definition are a subset of musculoskeletal disorders that arise from occupational exposures [2]. They are common among health care workers. The nursing population, that constitutes about 33% of the hospital workforce accounts for 60% of these MSD [3]. The job requirements of nursing personnel associated with providing medications to patients, maintaining hygiene of patients, looking after the dietary needs, and so forth predispose them to a very high risk for development of MSD.

The most commonly reported biomechanical risk factors for MSD include excessive repetition, awkward postures, and heavy lifting [4]. Nurses often conduct patient handling by bending their waist and maintaining an uncomfortable posture towards the opposite side of the bed or chair, increasing the risk of back pain [5]. Shift work may be a demanding situation because it raises problems for restoring work and no work activities. Shift schedules that involve night duties also disturb circadian rhythm and put different workload demands and reduce adequate communication and participation in preventive activities than the other work schedules [6]. MSD have a significant impact on the quality of life [1]. They contribute to lost work time or absenteeism and reduced work participation and quality of work output, resulting in a considerable economic burden on the individual, the organization, and the society as a whole [3, 5].

Several authors have reported the prevalence of MSD among nurses in the developed populations worldwide [3, 7–9]. However, data on prevalence of MSD are limited in India. The overburdened health care system of India due to the lack of adequate and skilled medical and paramedical personnel puts additional demands on its human resources. Moreover majority of the nursing staff in India are females who have added responsibilities of looking after their families which increases the physical and psychological burden further.

In such a scenario, the Indian nurses appear to be at a higher risk of development of MSD as compared to their western counterparts. In order to gain an understanding about the prevalence of MSD and its associated risk factors, this study was undertaken at a rural tertiary care hospital in India. The findings of the study can be utilised to plan and evaluate work place interventions to reduce the burden of MSD among nurses.

2. Materials and Methods

A cross-sectional descriptive study was undertaken at a tertiary care hospital located in the Anand district of the Gujarat state located in the western part of India. Ethical clearance was obtained from the institutional Human Research Ethics Committee. The inclusion criteria were female nurses working at the hospital for at least one year. Nurses reporting as having congenital deformities, traumatic conditions, neurological conditions, and gynaecological conditions were excluded from the study. The data was collected by administering a structured, coded, and pretested questionnaire on a one-to-one basis in local language. The questionnaire consisted of mainly three divisions, namely, demographic data, Nordic questionnaire, and perceived physical and psychological demand items. The Nordic questionnaire has been validated to screen musculoskeletal disorders in different populations [10, 11]. Additional questions on frequency of MSD were added to Nordic's questionnaire to obtain better information regarding musculoskeletal problems. For the purpose of analysis the outcome variable for presence of MSD was calculated on the basis of frequencies. All those having a frequency of "often" or "almost daily" were considered as having high frequency MSD. Self-perception of their work conditions was measured by using a structured and coded questionnaire based on the study by [8] and the Job Content Questionnaire (JCQ) [12]. Physical and psychological demand scores were calculated based on responses to different questions. For physical items, responses were dichotomised (1 and 2 versus 3 and 4) and then summed up to produce a total score which ranged from 0 to 12. Thereafter the scores were classified into three categories, as low (0 to 3), medium (3 to 9), and high (10 to 12). Items for perceived psychological demands were also dichotomised and summed up to produce a total score which ranged from 0 to 8. The scores were then categorised as low (0 to 5) and high (6 to 8) [8].

Data entry was done using Microsoft Excel 2007 and data analysis was done with the SPSS version 15.0. Means, 95% Confidence Intervals (CI), frequencies, and percentages were used for descriptive analysis. Cronbach's alpha was calculated to measure internal consistency of various items for the physical demand score and psychological demand score. For univariate analysis, the normality of numerical variables was tested using the Kolmogorov-Smirnov test. To test the association between numerical independent variables and occurrence of MSD, Mann-Whitney U test was applied as the variables were not normally distributed [13]. Chi-square (χ^2) test was used for testing associations between categorical variables. Association of MSD with individual items of perceived physical and psychological demands was measured using Multiple Binary Logistic Regression analysis.

Table 1: Descriptive analysis: sociodemographic and work related information.

Variable	Value
Mean age (95% CI)	30.44 (29.46–31.42)
Mean number of family members (95% CI)	5.13 (4.88–5.39)
Mean number of children (95% CI)	0.65 (0.55–0.75)
Family type (percent)	
Nuclear family	187 (63.2%)
Joint family	109 (36.8%)
Marital status (percent)	
Unmarried	133 (44.9%)
Married	162 (54.7%)
Others	1 (0.4%)
Appointment of housemaid at home (percent)	
Yes	60 (20.3%)
No	236 (79.7%)
Mean duration of domestic work in hours (95% CI)	3.81 (3.6–4.03)
Clinical posting (percent)	
OPD	19 (6.4%)
Ward	119 (40.2%)
OT	32 (10.8%)
ICU	110 (37.2%)
Emergency care unit	16 (5.4%)
Type of shifts	
Rotatory	248 (83.8%)
Fixed	48 (16.2%)
Mean years of work experience (95% CI)	7.96 (7.10–8.81)

(OPD: outpatient department, OT: operation theater, and ICU: intensive care unit).

3. Results

There were a total of 320 nurses eligible for the study out of which 296 participated in the study (response rate: 92.5%). Table 1 describes the sociodemographic and work profile of the participants. Mean age was 30.44 years (95% CI: 29.46–31.42) with majority of the participants in the age group of 20–25 years (44.9%). Mean duration of work done by nurses at home was 3.81 hours per day. 248 (83.8%) nurses were having shifting duties and total duration of work in a week was 48 hours for each of them. The mean duration of total work experience was 7.96 years and that at the current hospital was 7 years. Among the participants, majority (89.5%) were staff nurses. The mean BMI was 21.58 kg/m^2 (95% CI: 21.14–22.02) and 19.3% and 16.2% were underweight and obese, respectively.

TABLE 2: Prevalence of different types of MSD over the last 12 months and last 7 days and with high frequency.

MSD	Prevalence (last 12 month)[a]	Prevalence (last 7 days)[b]	Prevalence with high frequency*
Any MSD	264 (89.2%)	179 (60.5%)	176 (59.5%)
Neck	102 (34.5%)	48 (16.2%)	36 (12.2%)
Shoulder	62 (20.9%)	26 (8.8%)	22 (7.5%)
Elbow	4 (1.4%)	2 (0.7%)	1 (0.3%)
Wrist/hands	55 (18.6%)	24 (8.1%)	15 (5.1%)
Upper back	86 (29.1%)	46 (15.5%)	35 (12.0%)
Lower back	206 (69.6%)	120 (40.5%)	108 (37.0%)
Thighs/hips	14 (4.7%)	10 (3.4%)	9 (3.1%)
Knees	78 (26.4%)	35 (11.8%)	37 (12.7%)
Ankle/foot	80 (27.0%)	38 (12.8%)	34 (11.6%)

Note: [a]occurrence of MSD in the last 12 months.
[b]Occurrence of MSD in the last 7 days.
*Prevalence with high frequency: if the participant responded as having the MSD "often" or "almost daily", it was considered as high frequency.
MSD: musculoskeletal disorders.

TABLE 3: Association of MSD with various sociodemographic variables (univariate analysis).

Variable	Any MSD		p value
	Yes	No	
Mean age (95% CI)	31.76	28.63	**0.01**[a]
Family type			
Nuclear family	110 (59.8%)	77 (40.2%)	0.842[b]
Joint family	64 (59.3%)	45 (40.7%)	
Number of family members			
≤5 members	120 (58.8%)	88 (40.2%)	0.739[b]
>5 members	53 (60.9%)	35 (30.1%)	
Mean number of children (95% CI)	0.8333	0.3814	**<0.001**[a]
Duration of working hours at home	4.1322	3.3602	**0.001**[a]
Appointment of housemaid at home			
Yes	45 (75.00%)	15 (25.00%)	**0.006**[b]
No	129 (55.6%)	107 (44.4%)	
Marital status			
Unmarried	62 (47.3%)	71 (52.7%)	**<0.001**[b]
Married	111 (69.4%)	51 (30.6%)	

[a]Mann-Whitney U test.
[b]Pearson Chi-square test.
A p value of <0.05 was considered as significant and it has been made bold wherever it was found significant.

The prevalence of different MSD is shown in Table 2. Prevalence of any MSD in the last 12 months and past 7 days was 89.2% and 60.5%, respectively. Low back pain was the most commonly reported MSD whereas elbow pain was the least commonly reported. Table 3 shows association of any MSD with important sociodemographic variables tested through univariate analysis. The mean age of the participants, mean number of children at home, mean duration of working hours at home, mean duration of work experience at the current hospital, and mean duration of total work experience were significantly higher in those having any MSD as compared to those not having any MSD. Moreover the prevalence of any MSD was higher in those having a housemaid at home and married nurses as compared to those not having a housemaid and those who were unmarried, respectively. The difference in the prevalence of MSD across different categories of the nursing staff position, posting in different areas, and the type of duty shifts was not significant.

Table 4 shows association of various items related to physical demands at work and psychological demands at work with the occurrence of any MSD tested through Multiple Binary Logistic Regression. Among all the items, the physical demand perception "in my job, I am working for long periods with my body in awkward positions" was significantly associated with the occurrence of any MSD. Cronbach's alpha for the physical and psychological work demands items was found to be 0.833 and 0.762, respectively. Thereafter a logistic regression analysis (Table 5) was done with the total physical demands score, total psychological demands score, age, BMI, work experience, number of children < 5 years of age, duration of work at home, and having a housemaid as independent variables and occurrence of different MSD as the dependent variable. It was found that a high score for perceived physical demands was significantly associated with the occurrence of MSD in the lower back and knee regions, presence of housemaid at home with MSD in neck and lower back, and presence of children with upper and lower back regions.

4. Discussion

This was a cross-sectional study carried out at a tertiary care hospital in Gujarat, India, to find the prevalence of musculoskeletal disorders and its association with self-perceived work demands and other sociodemographic and work related variables among the female nursing staff.

The prevalence of MSD in any body part was 89.2% in the last 12 months and 60.5% in the past 7 days and 59.5% of the nurses reported occurrence of MSD with high frequency, that is, MSD occurring "often" or "almost daily." The prevalence of MSD in the last 12 months in the lower back region (69.6%) was the highest followed by the same in the neck (34.5%), upper back (29.1%), ankle/feet (27.0%), and knee (26.4%) regions in the last 12-month period. This finding is consistent with the findings obtained from several other studies [3, 7, 9, 14, 15]. The prevalence of MSD in the elbow region was the least. Similar finding was also obtained in the study conducted by [7] and in a study conducted in rural Japan nurses [16]. The mean age of the participants with MSD in any body part was higher than that of those without MSD and the difference was statistically significant. Similar findings were also observed in the study undertaken on Nigerian nurses by Tinubu et al. [3]. It is a well-known fact that as the age increases, functional capacity of an individual decreases resulting in a higher incidence of MSD [17].

TABLE 4: Association of occurrence of any MSD with perceived physical and psychological demands at work, Multiple Logistic Regression analysis.

Perceived physical and psychological demand items	OR for any MSD (95% CI)
Perceived physical demand items	
My job requires lots of physical efforts	1.383 (0.744–2.573)
My job requires rapid and continuous physical activity	1.215 (0.613–2.407)
In my job, I am often moving/lifting very heavy loads	0.746 (0.414–1.342)
In my job, I am working for long periods with my head or arms in awkward positions	0.731 (0.359–1.489)
In my job, I am working for long periods with my body in awkward positions	**2.723 (1.336–5.549)**
Lift or lower patients/objects to/from floor	0.817 (0.438–1.523)
Lift or lower objects to/from shoulder height	1.820 (0.912–3.629)
Work while bent or twisted at waist	1.575 (0.908–2.731)
Push/pull heavy objects or people	1.427 (0.740–2.752)
Stand in one place/static position (>30 minutes)	0.648 (0.366–1.148)
Perform repetitive motions with hands/wrists	1.023 (0.574–1.823)
Apply pressure with hands/fingers (e.g., to prevent bleeding)	1.274 (0.711–2.282)
Perceived psychological demand items	
My job requires working very hard	0.952 (0.480–1.889)
My job requires working very fast	1.113 (0.443–2.798)
My job requires an excessive amount of work	1.275 (0.670–2.427)
My job requires long periods of intense concentration on the task	1.736 (0.859–3.508)
My job requires enough time to get the job done	1.095 (0.639–1.875)
My job is free from conflicting demands that others make	0.928 (0.515–1.673)
My job requires waiting on work from other people or departments	1.288 (0.727–2.281)
My job has tasks that are often interrupted before they can be completed	1.155 (0.654–2.039)

TABLE 5: Association of different MSD with total physical demands score, total psychological demands score, and selected sociodemographic and work related variables (Multiple Logistic Regression analysis with each MSD).

Independent variables	Neck	Upper back	Lower back	Knee	Ankle
Age	1.088 (0.945–1.252)	0.829 (0.668–1.028)	0.946 (0.846–1.058)	1.073 (0.945–1.218)	0.996 (0.859–1.156)
BMI	0.927 (0.826–1.040)	0.981 (0.876–1.098)	0.981 (0.907–1.060)	1.065 (0.957–1.184)	0.996 (0.892–1.112)
Work experience	0.968 (0.818–1.145)	1.184 (0.943–1.488)	1.034 (0.911–1.174)	0.985 (0.848–1.144)	1.025 (0.865–1.214)
Number of children under 5 years of age	2.002 (0.747–5.362)	**3.604 (1.387–9.363)**	**2.202 (1.044–4.646)**	0.967 (0.322–2.904)	1.028 (0.360–2.935)
Duration of work at home	1.049 (0.840–1.310)	0.870 (0.681–1.110)	**1.228 (1.046–1.440)**	1.107 (0.882–1.388)	1.129 (0.899–1.418)
Having a housemaid at home	**2.935 (1.306–6.596)**	1.378 (0.579–3.277)	**2.723 (1.470–5.045)**	0.371 (0.120–1.148)	1.159 (0.480–2.800)
Physical demands					
Low	1	1	1	1	1
Medium	0.841 (0.254–2.790)	1.117 (0.304–4.103)	1.987 (0.846–4.668)	1.980 (0.577–6.793)	1.062 (0.892–1.792)
High	2.255 (0.530–9.586)	1.839 (0.382–8.856)	**3.061 (1.005–9.325)**	**7.726 (1.716–34.785)**	1.890 (0.901–2.100)
Psychological demands	1.873 (0.828–4.238)	1.106 (0.506–2.417)	0.994 (0.579–1.706)	0.757 (0.332–1.722)	0.870 (0.398–1.900)

The mean number of children ($p < 0.001$) and mean number of domestic work hours' duration ($p = 0.001$) were higher in the group having any MSD as compared to those not having any MSD which could be because of the fact that the greater amount of workload and responsibility at home leads to higher prevalence of MSD. Marital status was significantly associated ($p < 0.001$) with any MSD, which could be due to the fact that, in Indian culture, after marriage the responsibility increases and so does the domestic work, thus increasing the physical demands of work. Those having a housemaid were having a higher prevalence of any MSD as compared to those not having the housemaid. Similar findings were obtained for the prevalence of low back pain. The duration of domestic work was also associated with increased odds of MSD over lower back region which reflects the effect of higher domestic work demands on the occurrence of MSD over lower back region. It has been known that the double work burden or the simultaneous engagement in two different types of tasks, namely, paid job and household work, increases psychological and physical demands from an individual resulting in an increased risk of MSD [18]. On doing further analysis it was found that as the frequency of the back pain increased the proportion of nurses having a housemaid increased sequentially. It reflects that the higher frequency of lower back pain might be leading to appointment of a house maid for doing routine household work. It can be explained by the concept of reverse causality [19].

A significant difference was not found in the prevalence of any MSD in those having rotating or fixed duty shifts. It could be due to the fact that the shift duties are worked out in such a way that no one is required to do more than two consecutive shifts (i.e., morning, evening, and night) and the shifts are arranged in forward manner (i.e., morning, evening, and night) which is known to reduce side effects like fatigue. This is a well-known strategy to reduce the burden of rotating duties [20]. The mean work experience in years was significantly higher in those having MSD in any body part as compared to those not having the same. Similar findings were also seen in the study by Tinubu et al. [3]. As worker's seniority and job experience increase they tend to have fixed shift, so fixed shift is associated with increased years of employment and increased age which was also seen in our study [21]. It was found that the odds of development of any MSD were significantly higher (2.723 (95% CI: 1.336–5.549)) among those who perceived that they had to work for long periods with the body in awkward positions. This finding was further supported by other studies as well [8, 22, 23].

The findings of the study should be generalised with caution. The variability of the workload and ergonomics knowledge of the study respondents in different areas of the hospital may influence homogeneity. In a cross-sectional study survivor effects will typically decrease the observed associations between symptomatic disorders and physically demanding jobs [24]. Since the analysis was limited to currently working nurses, we may have excluded nurses who had left jobs due to MSD or other health conditions during the study time. The MSD reported here may be work related or due to other factors and it is very difficult to distinguish the two [25]. Furthermore, the cross-sectional design prevented us from drawing conclusions on the temporal order of relationships. Further studies may be undertaken with posture analysis systems to get an in-depth understanding of the issues. Detailed ergonomic evaluation of the work place should be done to thorough observations and other techniques to get important clues related to the problem.

5. Conclusions

The study reported a high prevalence of MSD and occurrence of lower back and knee MSD was associated with perceived physical demands among nurses in a rural based tertiary care medical college hospital. The findings of such a study can be utilised in the development of a work place intervention addressing the risk factors and preventive measures for the MSD identified. The findings can serve as a benchmark for evaluation of the effect of the intervention.

Competing Interests

The authors declare that they have no competing interests.

Acknowledgments

The authors thank Ms. Archana Gupta, nursing in-charge, Shree Krishna Hospital, Karamsad, for supporting the study, and Dr. R Harihara Prakash, Principal, KM Patel Institute of Physiotherapy, for providing valuable inputs in conducting the study.

References

[1] L. Punnett and D. H. Wegman, "Work-related musculoskeletal disorders: the epidemiologic evidence and the debate," *Journal of Electromyography and Kinesiology*, vol. 14, no. 1, pp. 13–23, 2004.

[2] M. S. Forde, L. Punnett, and D. H. Wegman, "Pathomechanisms of work-related musculoskeletal disorders: conceptual issues," *Ergonomics*, vol. 45, no. 9, pp. 619–630, 2002.

[3] B. M. S. Tinubu, C. E. Mbada, A. L. Oyeyemi, and A. A. Fabunmi, "Work-related musculoskeletal disorders among nurses in Ibadan, South-West Nigeria: a cross-sectional survey," *BMC Musculoskeletal Disorders*, vol. 11, article 12, 2010.

[4] B. R. Da Costa and E. R. Vieira, "Risk factors for work-related musculoskeletal disorders: a systematic review of recent longitudinal studies," *American Journal of Industrial Medicine*, vol. 53, no. 3, pp. 285–323, 2010.

[5] K. J. June and S.-H. Cho, "Low back pain and work-related factors among nurses in intensive care units," *Journal of Clinical Nursing*, vol. 20, no. 3-4, pp. 479–487, 2011.

[6] D. Camerino, M. Sandri, S. Sartori, P. M. Conway, P. Campanini, and G. Costa, "Shiftwork, work-family conflict among Italian nurses, and prevention efficacy," *Chronobiology International*, vol. 27, no. 5, pp. 1105–1123, 2010.

[7] A. Choobineh, M. Movahed, S. H. Tabatabaie, and M. Kumashiro, "Perceived demands and musculoskeletal disorders in operating room nurses of Shiraz city hospitals," *Industrial Health*, vol. 48, no. 1, pp. 74–84, 2010.

[8] A. M. Trinkoff, J. A. Lipscomb, J. Geiger-Brown, C. L. Storr, and B. A. Brady, "Perceived physical demands and reported musculoskeletal problems in registered nurses," *American Journal of Preventive Medicine*, vol. 24, no. 3, pp. 270–275, 2003.

[9] S. Ando, Y. Ono, M. Shimaoka et al., "Associations of self estimated workloads with musculoskeletal symptoms among hospital nurses," *Occupational and Environmental Medicine*, vol. 57, no. 3, pp. 211–216, 2000.

[10] A. Descatha, Y. Roquelaure, J. F. Chastang et al., "Validity of Nordic-style questionnaires in the surveillance of upper-limb work-related musculoskeletal disorders," *Scandinavian Journal of Work, Environment and Health*, vol. 33, no. 1, pp. 58–65, 2007.

[11] A. P. Dawson, E. J. Steele, P. W. Hodges, and S. Stewart, "Development and test-retest reliability of an extended version of the Nordic Musculoskeletal Questionnaire (NMQ-E): a screening instrument for musculoskeletal pain," *The Journal of Pain*, vol. 10, no. 5, pp. 517–526, 2009.

[12] R. Karasek, C. Brisson, N. Kawakami, I. Houtman, P. Bongers, and B. Amick, "The Job Content Questionnaire (JCQ): an instrument for internationally comparative assessments of psychosocial job characteristics," *Journal of Occupational Health Psychology*, vol. 3, no. 4, pp. 322–355, 1998.

[13] M. P. Fay and M. A. Proschan, "Wilcoxon-Mann-Whitney or *t*-test? On assumptions for hypothesis tests and multiple interpretations of decision rules," *Statistics Surveys*, vol. 4, pp. 1–39, 2010.

[14] D. R. Smith, J.-W. Choi, M. Ki, J.-Y. Kim, and Z. Yamagata, "Musculoskeletal disorders among staff in South Korea's largest nursing home," *Environmental Health and Preventive Medicine*, vol. 8, no. 1, pp. 23–28, 2003.

[15] A. Lorusso, S. Bruno, and N. L'Abbate, "A review of low back pain and musculoskeletal disorders among Italian nursing personnel," *Industrial Health*, vol. 45, no. 5, pp. 637–644, 2007.

[16] D. R. Smith, N. Kondo, E. Tanaka, H. Tanaka, K. Hirasawa, and Z. Yamagata, "Musculoskeletal disorders among hospital nurses in rural Japan," *Rural and Remote Health*, vol. 3, no. 3, article 241, 2003.

[17] T. W. Olanre Okunribido, "Ageing and work-related musculoskeletal disorders. A review of the recent literature," Report RR799, Health and Safety Laboratory, 2010, http://www.hse.gov.uk/research/rrpdf/rr799.pdf.

[18] L. F. Portela, L. Rotenberg, and W. Waissmann, "Health, sleep and lack of time: relations to domestic and paid work in nurses," *Revista de Saúde Pública*, vol. 39, no. 5, pp. 802–808, 2005.

[19] G. S. Marquis, J.-P. Habicht, C. F. Lanata, R. E. Black, and K. M. Rasmussen, "Association of breastfeeding and stunting in Peruvian toddlers: an example of reverse causality," *International Journal of Epidemiology*, vol. 26, no. 2, pp. 349–356, 1997.

[20] P. Knauth and S. Hornberger, "Preventive and compensatory measures for shift workers," *Occupational Medicine*, vol. 53, no. 2, pp. 109–116, 2003.

[21] C. C. Caruso and T. R. Waters, "A review of work schedule issues and musculoskeletal disorders with an emphasis on the healthcare sector," *Industrial Health*, vol. 46, no. 6, pp. 523–534, 2008.

[22] J. Smedley, P. Egger, C. Cooper, and D. Coggon, "Manual handling activities and risk of low back pain in nurses," *Occupational and Environmental Medicine*, vol. 52, no. 3, pp. 160–163, 1995.

[23] E. C. Alexopoulos, A. Burdorf, and A. Kalokerinou, "A comparative analysis on musculoskeletal disorders between Greek and Dutch nursing personnel," *International Archives of Occupational and Environmental Health*, vol. 79, no. 1, pp. 82–88, 2006.

[24] H. M. Arrighi and I. Hertz-Picciotto, "The evolving concept of the healthy worker survivor effect," *Epidemiology*, vol. 5, no. 2, pp. 189–196, 1994.

[25] B. O. A. Adegoke, A. K. Akodu, and A. L. Oyeyemi, "Work-related musculoskeletal disorders among Nigerian physiotherapists," *BMC Musculoskeletal Disorders*, vol. 9, article 112, 2008.

30

Tenofovir-Based Highly Active Antiretroviral Therapy Is Associated with Superior CD4 T Cells Repopulation Compared to Zidovudine-Based HAART in HIV 1 Infected Adults

Vitus Sambo Badii,[1] Kwame Ohene Buabeng,[2] Thomas Agyarko Poku,[3] Arnold Donkor Forkuo,[1] Bright Boafo Boamah,[1] Stephen Mensah Arhin,[1] and Daniel Edem Kpewou[4]

[1] *Department of Pharmacology, Faculty of Pharmacy and Pharmaceutical Sciences, Kwame Nkrumah University of Sciences and Technology, Kumasi, Ghana*
[2] *Department of Pharmacy Practice, Faculty of Pharmacy and Pharmaceutical Sciences, Kwame Nkrumah University of Sciences and Technology, Kumasi, Ghana*
[3] *Suntreso Government Hospital, Kumasi, Ghana*
[4] *Department of Biochemistry and Biotechnology, College of Science, Kwame Nkrumah University of Sciences and Technology, Kumasi, Ghana*

Correspondence should be addressed to Kwame Ohene Buabeng; kchiefb@yahoo.co.uk

Academic Editor: Tadeusz Robak

Tenofovir-based highly active antiretroviral therapy (HAART) is one of the preferred first-line therapies in the management of HIV 1 infection. Ghana has since 2014 adopted this recommendation; however there is paucity of scientific data that reflects the safety and efficacy of the tenofovir-based therapy compared to zidovudine in the Ghanaian health system. This study sought to assess the comparative immune reconstitution potential between tenofovir and zidovudine-based HAART regimens, which includes lamivudine and efavirenz in combination therapy. It also aimed to investigate the adverse drug reactions/events (ADREs) associated with pharmacotherapy with these agents in a total of 106 HAART naïve HIV patients. The study included 80 patients in the tenofovir cohort while 26 patients were on the zidovudine regimen. The occurrence of HIV comorbidities profile was assessed at diagnosis and throughout the study period. The baseline CD4 T cells count of the participants was also assessed at diagnosis and repeated at a median period of five months (range 4–6 months), after commencing treatment with either tenofovir- or zidovudine-based HAART. After five months of the HAART, the tenofovir cohort recorded higher CD4 T cell count change from baseline compared to the zidovudine cohort ($p < 0.0001$). The patients on the tenofovir-based HAART and female sex however appeared to be associated with more multiple ADREs.

1. Introduction

The main physiological derangement in HIV infection is an uncontrolled CD4 T cells decline [1–3]. Studies suggest CD4 T cell death via cytolysis, chronic immune activation [3–5], cytotoxic T cells response, and gp120-envelop induced immune reactions [6–8] to partly account for the overall decline. Furthermore, the failure of thymus T cell hemostatic function due to HIV-induced thymopathy and infection of hematopoietic progenitor cells helps to establish this progressive CD4 T cell decline in chronic HIV infection [3, 6]. As a result, people living with HIV/AIDS (PLWHA) often present with low CD4 T cell count which permits dormant human flora and other potential pathogens to revert to overt forms causing opportunistic infections and rare cancers such as Kaposi sarcoma [3, 9, 10].

The advent of Highly Active Antiretroviral therapy (HAART) has revolutionized the management of PLWHA over the past decades [10, 11]. It inhibits viral replication and suppresses HIV RNA with resultant regression in HIV associated immune activation and CD4 cell death [4, 12, 13]. The success of any HAART combination to cause CD4 T cell repopulation is premised on choosing a regimen that is efficacious, tolerable, and safe in PLWHA [3, 14]. The rate of CD4 T cell repopulation is believed to vary with different HAART combinations and is also affected by both human (age, gender, baseline and CD4 and CD8 count) and viral (baseline viral load) factors [3, 10, 11, 15–17]. The world health organization (WHO) guidelines and Ghana in its 2014 ART guidelines have recommended tenofovir, lamivudine/emtricitabine, and efavirenz combination as the most preferred first line for management of HIV 1 over the most available zidovudine-based and other first-line combinations [18–20]. Both Spaulding et al. and Gallant et al. suggest a superior immune reconstitution and adverse drug reactions/events (ADREs) profile with tenofovir-based regimen relative to zidovudine regimen based on studies conducted in developed countries [3, 12, 21]. However, Joshi et al. and other related studies have shown there exist inter- and intrapopulation difference in response to HAART along with other host and viral factors [3, 6, 10, 14, 15, 21–23]. Since the introduction of tenofovir-based regimen in Ghana in 2014, there has been little or no scientific data that reflect the local scientific reality as a developing country and must be addressed and put into perspective.

This study therefore sought to evaluate and compare the efficacy (immune reconstitution propensity) and safety (adverse drug reactions/events, ADREs) of tenofovir, lamivudine, and efavirenz regimen (tenofovir cohort) to zidovudine, lamivudine, and efavirenz regimen (zidovudine cohort) and further assess how human related factors affect efficacy and safety of these HAART regimens in PLWHA.

2. Study Design and Targeted Population

This was a prospective observational study involving only participants who enrolled on a naïve tenofovir, lamivudine, and efavirenz regimen known as tenofovir cohort and those on zidovudine, lamivudine, and efavirenz also known as zidovudine cohort at Komfo Anokye Teaching Hospital (KATH) in 2016. The above-mentioned HAART regimens are the commonly used and readily available first-line therapeutic options for the management of HIV 1 infections at KATH and in Ghana, with tenofovir regimen believed to have a favorable dosing schedule and more tolerable effects than the zidovudine regimen. The only difference between the two cohorts was either the use of tenofovir or zidovudine in the respective cohorts, with all other variables being constant. Also the sampling technique used for selection of patients for participation in the study was systematic random sampling and thus did not interfere with the choice of treatment. The selection of HAART regimen was thus the sole responsibility of the clinician in charge of the adult HIV clinic at the study site, guided by patients' comorbidities, tolerability, and acceptance. A total of 106 patients were recruited for the study estimated from the annual HIV/AIDS cases at KATH. A total of 80 participants were in the tenofovir cohort while 26 were in zidovudine cohort.

2.1. Inclusion and Exclusion Criteria. Included in the study were adults aged 18 years and above and newly diagnosed of HIV 1 in 2016. In addition, only those with no past exposure to HAART known as HAART naïve were considered for the study. Furthermore and more importantly, to be considered for the study, one must have been on any two of the commonly prescribed regimens, namely, tenofovir with lamivudine and efavirenz (tenofovir cohort) or zidovudine with lamivudine and efavirenz. Only those with baseline CD4 T cells with or without viral load determined before the initiation of a naive HAART were considered. Those with HIV 2 infection or both HIV1 and HIV 2 were excluded from the study. These were necessary to limit confounding factors and provide similar conditions for a plausible comparison.

2.2. Data Collection. Each patient who consented for inclusion in the study was given a unique identification number and allocated a designated location in the data collection notebook in an ordered fashion. Data on demographics and vital signs (age, sex, disclosure, weight, height, lifestyle, herbal medicine use, and blood pressure) were obtained from patients' folders and laboratory reports. Patients were made to undertake CD4 T cell absolute count, viral load, and full blood count before the initiation of naïve HAART. Patients were followed up to assess the occurrence of adverse drug reactions/events especially during the first five weeks after HAART initiation. Study subjects were made to repeat CD4 T cells absolute count using flow cytometer (BD FACS caliber) per manufacturer's protocol (normal reference range 400–1400 cells/μL) at a median period of five months (range 4–6 months) after HAART initiation at the serology unit of the Komfo Anokye Teaching Hospital.

2.3. Statistical Analysis. STATA version 12 was used for data analysis. Normality test was carried out on all continuous variables and presented as either mean ± standard deviation or median with range values for normally and nonnormally distributed data, respectively. The within-group variations of the paired differences between CD4 T cell count before and after five months of treatment were compared using Wilcoxon Signed Ranks Test in each cohort and overall effect. The Mann–Whitney U test was used to test for differences in CD4 T cell absolute count change across the treatments cohorts and human factors. A multivariate regression analysis was performed to assess predictors of CD4 T cell change after HAART. All categorical variables are presented as frequencies and/or proportions.

2.4. Ethical Considerations. Approval was sought from the management of the Komfo Anokye Teaching Hospital. This was to ensure that the hospital has prior knowledge of the research and to affirm if the facility is equipped enough to enable the proper execution of the research work. Ethical Clearance with reference number CHRPE/AP/499/16 was granted by the Committee on Human Research, Publications and Ethics of the Kwame Nkrumah University of Science and

Table 1: Demographic and baseline characteristics of the study participants at diagnosis.

Variable	Observations	Mean age	Std. Dev.	Min	Max
Females	69 (65.1%)	39.09	11.8	20	78
Males	37 (34.9%)	42.30	11.0	22	72
Total	106	42.63	11.4	20	78
Distribution of participants across treatment groups before and during follow-up					
Treatment group	Initial distribution			Follow-up distribution	
TLE (tenofovir cohort)	80 (75.5%)			68 (76.4%)	
ZLE (zidovudine cohort)	26 (24.5%)			21 (23.6%)	
Total	106 (100%)			89 (100%)	
Comorbidities				Number of participants	
Tuberculosis				21	
Hepatitis B				7	
Hepatitis C				1	
Kaposi sarcoma				4	
Cerebral toxoplasmosis				1	
Total comorbidities				34	
Stage of HIV (CD4 count/cells/μL)	Number of participants			Percentage Freq. (%)	
Stage I ($\geq$500)	11			10.4	
Stage II (200–499)	35			33.0	
Stage III (0–199)	60			56.6	
Total number	106			100	

The table shows the baseline characteristics of study participants before and during the initiation of therapy. It shows their age distribution across gender at diagnosis and the comorbidity profile of participants determined before and during treatment with HAART. The stage of HIV was determined at baseline depicting the degree of progression to AIDS using the CD4 T cells count.

Technology, KNUST, and Komfo Anokye Teaching Hospital (KATH) to ensure the research protocol does not breach research ethics involving human subjects. Finally, during recruitment of study subjects, a written informed consent was obtained from the study participants freely, after the purpose of the study has been explained to them, and they or their immediate relations have been assured of client confidentiality and anonymity of data.

3. Results

3.1. Demographics and Comorbidities. As shown in Table 1, a total of 106 HAART naive HIV patients were enrolled with 89 successfully followed up out of which 68 (76.4%) were in the tenofovir cohort while 21 (23.6%) were in the zidovudine cohort. In this study, there were 65.1% (69) females and 34.9% (37) males. The participants were found to have a mean age of 42.6 $\pm$ 11.4. However, females were relatively younger with a mean age of 39.1 $\pm$ 11.6 compared to males with mean age of 42 $\pm$ 11 with both sexes showing considerable age variability. HIV is known to exist with several comorbidities and, in this study, 34 (32%) had comorbidities. The most prevalent comorbidity was tuberculosis with 21 (19.8%) subjects contracting the disease and this was followed by hepatitis B virus infection, where 7 participants were seropositive to HbsAg. Also in this study, and in accordance with WHO clinical staging of HIV/AIDS at baseline, about 57% of participants had progressed to stage III (CD4 count < 200 cells/μL) with 33% at stage II (200–499 cells/mL).

3.2. Immune Reconstitution across Treatment Groups. Out of 106 participants recruited into the study, 17 were lost to follow-up while 89 were successfully followed up for a median period of five months (20th week). From Table 2, after 5 months of initiating a naïve HAART, there was a significantly higher median CD4 T cells count in all subjects 327 (45–972) compared to 142.5 (0–556) cells/μL at baseline ($p < 0.0001$). Also, within each treatment group, there was significant increase in posttreatment CD4 T cells count from baseline after 5 months of treatment. The extent of CD4 count change between baseline and posttreatment was assessed between the two cohorts. Tenofovir regimen (TLE) recorded a significantly ($p < 0.0001$) higher median CD4 cell increase of 214 (0–795) cells/μL compared to zidovudine regimen (ZLE) which recorded a median increase of 109.5 (21–275) cells/μL. Furthermore, the univariate Mann–Whitney tests to determine the CD4 count change between those with and without individual comorbidities and young and older adults were unexpectedly found not to be significantly associated with any difference in CD4 count change after HAART as observed. Interestingly, females were found to have higher median CD4 T cell change 217 (7–516) cells/μL compared to males 149.5 (21–401) cells/μL. However in a multivariate analysis gender and likewise other variables were found not to be associated with CD4 T cell change. Thus the significant change in the CD4 T count recorded among the study participants prior to TLE/ZLE administration within 5 months was independent of age, gender, comorbidities (TB and hepatitis B infections), and baseline CD4 and CD8 cell

TABLE 2: Comparison of CD4 T cells count change between treatment groups and how other variables affect CD4 T cells reconstitution following the initiation of HAART.

Comparison between baseline CD4 count and outcome after median of 5 months after HAART				
Group	Pretreatment cells/μL	Posttreatment cells/μL		p value
Overall	142.5 (0–556)	327 (45–972)		**<0.0001**
ZLE	104 (0–509)	200 (45–889)		**<0.0001**
TLE	150 (3–556)	337 (69–972)		**<0.0001**
Determination of the effect HIV co-morbidities, gender, and increasing age on with CD4 T cell reconstitution				
Parameter				p value
	Gender			
	Male	Female		
	149.7 (21–401)	217 (7–516)		**0.0094**
	Age group (years)			
	20 to 40	>40		
	364.5 (45–972)	352.1 (76–697)		0.3184
	TB status			
CD4+ count change after 5 months of TLE/ZLE treatment	No	Yes		
	190.1 (0–500)	211.9 (21–578)		0.5717
	Hepatitis B status			
	No	Yes		
	172 (0–578)	215.6 (52–319)		0.3059
	Treatment group			
	ZLE	TLE		
	109.5 (21–275)	214 (0–795)		**<0.0001**
Multivariate model to predict the influencing variables on CD4 change after HAART F (8, 78) = 1.03, Prob > F = 0.4176, R^2 = 0.0959, adjusted R^2 = 0.0032				
CD4 change	Coefficient	Standard error	t	p value
Gender	−89.999	47.207	−1.91	0.060
Age	−0.313	1.758	−0.18	0.859
Hepatitis B	73.777	87.532	0.84	0.402
Tuberculosis	61.796	54.536	1.13	0.261
Baseline CD4	0.066	0.1292	0.52	0.607
Baseline Hb	15.814	11.682	1.35	0.180
Baseline CD8	−0.0123	0.015	−0.82	0.412
Herbs use	−46.145	42.435	−1.09	0.280

From the table, data is presented as median with range values. TLE: tenofovir, lamivudine, and efavirenz and ZLE: zidovudine, lamivudine, and efavirenz. p is significant at 0.05. Mann–Whitney test was used to compare the median CD4 cells count increase between the tenofovir treatment group (TLE) and the zidovudine treatment group (ZLE) and likewise the effect age, gender, and comorbidities at univariate level. The last part of the table is a multivariate regression analysis to identify variables that may predict CD4 T cells count change. t is the test-statistic, and $p > t$ is the probability of predictive value of each variable on CD4 T cells count significant at 0.05. R^2 measures the degree of correlation between variables with CD4 T cells count change.

counts. Contrary to that, the observed CD4+ count change among the study participants varied significantly across the treatment groups.

3.3. Safety Assessment of HAART (TLE/ZLE) on Study Participants. In this study during follow-up, one participant each on TLE and ZLE died with the one from ZLE cohort said to have had Kaposi sarcoma. Two participants on TLE change from efavirenz to nevirapine due to intolerable CNS effects (psychosis) while one patient on ZLE was switched to TLE due to unfavorable dosing schedule and side effects. In terms of serious ADRE, one participant with Kaposi sarcoma in tenofovir cohort experienced tenofovir induced nephropathy and two experience intolerable psychosis. Figure 1 shows the distribution of adverse drug reaction/events (ADREs) occurrences within the ZLE and TLE treatments groups. In all, 11.4% participants on ZLE treatment experienced ADR compared to 36.3% in the TLE treatment group. Moreover, out of the proportion of participants who reported side effects in each treatment arm, 33.3% of the ZLE treatment group compared to 48.3 percent of the TLE treatment group recorded multiple ADREs. Figure 1 shows 32% males and 28% females experienced ADREs. However females are more likely to experience multiple ADREs as 60% of females who experienced ADREs compared to 25% of males who experienced ADREs had multiple events.

TABLE 3: Classification/distribution of ADREs in the treatment groups and gender.

ADREs description	Overall	Treatment groups		Gender	
		TLE	ZLE	Male	Female
Cutaneous	14 (31.1%)	11 (78.6%)	3 (21.4%)	4 (28.6%)	10 (71.4%)
GIT effects	10 (22.2%)	10 (100%)	0 (0%)	3 (21.4%)	7 (78.6%)
CNS effects	15 (33.3%)	14 (93.3%)	1 (6.7%)	5 (33.3%)	10 (66.7%)
Mitochondrial toxicity	6 (13.3%)	6 (100%)	0 (0%)	1 (16.7%)	5 (83.3%)
Total	45 (100%)				
*Serious ADREs observed	3	3	0	0	3

The table shows the distribution of the specific ADREs experienced at each level of comparison under four broad classification.

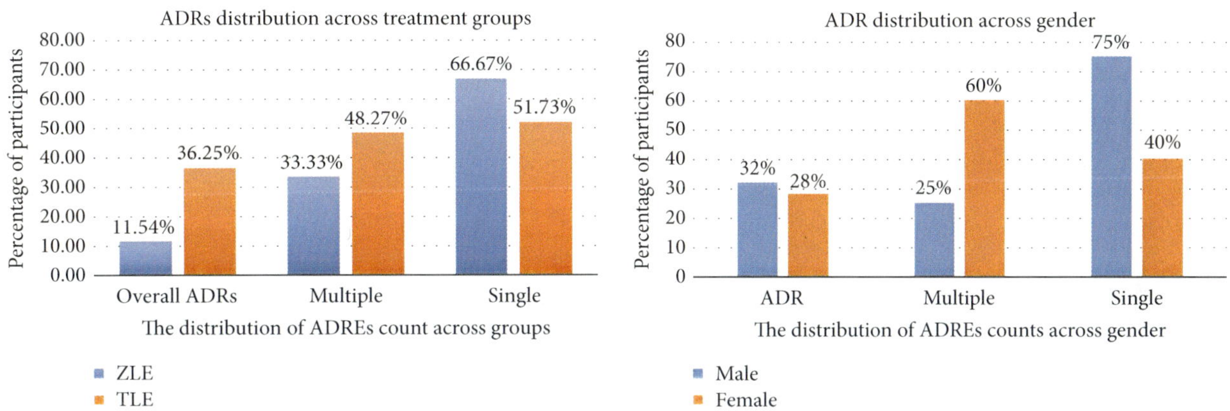

FIGURE 1: The figure shows the distribution of adverse drug reactions/events (ADREs) across comparison groups. The figure shows how treatment type and gender affect the occurrence of adverse drug reactions/events (ADREs) among participants. ADR refers to the proportion of participants who experienced adverse drug reactions/events in each comparison group. Single: the proportion of persons who had only one ADRE out of the number of persons with ADREs in each group. Multiple: the proportion of persons who had two or more ADREs out of the number of persons with ADREs in each group.

From Table 3, the most prevalent ADREs category was CNS effects with diverse manifestations accounting for about 33% (dizziness accounted for 12% while other CNS ADREs like nightmare, insomnia, psychosis, and excessive sleep accounted for about 21% of all reported cases). The most prevalent reported single ADRE was skin rash as 20% of reported ADREs were rash with overall cutaneous ADREs accounting for 31.1% of all ADREs. GIT effects were all attributable to tenofovir therapy with about 77% experienced by females.

4. Discussion

Many studies support the assertion that HAART enhances immune recovery which partly is reflected as an increase in absolute CD4 T cell count [3, 11]. However this property is believed to be affected by the type of HAART combination and other factors [3, 10, 14, 21]. In this study, participants were initiated on a naïve HAART comprised of lamivudine and efavirenz in combination with either tenofovir or zidovudine. Their propensity to repopulate CD4 T cell and ADREs experienced in PLWHA were subsequently assessed. Close to 56% of the study participants were in stage III which suggests late diagnosis of HIV in these participants. Overall, participants exhibited a significant ($p < 0.0001$) increase in median CD4 T cell absolute count after five months of being on HAART compared to baseline CD4 T cell absolute count before HAART initiation. This study finding agrees with many studies that HAART enhances immune recovery [3, 10, 15, 19].

The extent of CD4 cells change five months to HAART between the two cohorts when assessed. Tenofovir treatment arm yielded a significantly ($p < 0.0001$) higher median increase in CD4 T cell absolute count of 214 (0–795) cells/μl compared to zidovudine treatment arm of 109.5 (21–275) cells/μl five months after HAART. The finding is consistent with a systematic review by Gallant et al. which purported tenofovir-based HAART to elicit superior immune recovery rate than zidovudine-based HAART but an equipotent in virologic suppression [12, 21, 24, 25] while another study found tenofovir to be noninferior to zidovudine in both immune recovery and virologic suppression [12, 21]. From other studies, the ability of any HAART regimen to effect CD4 cell repopulation is premised on enhancing thymic functionality for improve thymopoiesis [3, 15, 25]. Additionally, their ability to reverse HIV-induced chronic immune activation enhancing positive selection of naïve CD4 T cells in the thymus gland is widely acknowledged [4]. Immune reconstitution as a property of HAART has also been associated with the reduction in the cytotoxic effect of *naf*, *vpr*, and *tat* viral proteins on CD4 T cells through the activation of NF-kappa β and TNF-α [2]. The observed immune recovery in this study may be due to reduction in chronic immune activation, cytolysis, cytotoxic viral proteins, and an increase in thymic function though there is not much data on these parameters for analysis to support this claim [2, 7, 15, 26]. However the observed higher CD4 T cells absolute count increase in the tenofovir cohort compared to zidovudine cohort may be attributable to the postulated zidovudine induced stasis of CD4 T cells expansion. Zidovudine seems to enhance cytotoxic lymphocytes activity leading to infected CD4 T cells death via cytolysis. It also impedes antigen and lectin-induced T cells proliferation and mitosis causing an impaired T cells expansion [17].

The significant change in the CD4+ count recorded among the study participants prior to TLE/ZLE administration was found to be independent of age and HIV comorbidities (TB and hepatitis B infections). In a univariate analysis, gender was associated with CD4 count change as females recorded a significantly ($p = 0.0094$) elevated median CD4 count 217 (7–516) compared to males 149.7 (21–401) cells/μL. However in a multivariate analysis, the association was not statistically significant. This was unexpected as it finds no association between any of the variables evaluated. With regard to age, children and younger adults generally have lager thymic volume reserve at baseline than the elderly and are expected to have superior immune recovery [15, 27]. However this study excluded children and adolescence but only considered young and old adults. Also, more than half of the study participants were in stage III and are normally known to have reduced baseline thymic reserve due to long standing HIV infection [15]. These could account for the fact that there is no significant difference in immune reconstitution between the older and young adults and even across sex.

Despite the enormous gains since the advent of HAART, adverse drug reactions/events continue to be a major setback to the success of most HAART pharmacotherapies. In most instances, noncompliance and treatment discontinuation are due largely to the development of HAART related ADREs in PLWHA [28–33]. An Indian study estimated over 90% PLWHA starting a naïve HAART reacted adversely while a Cameroon-based study reported about 20% of such ADRs [32, 34]. The Lartey et al. study conducted in Ghana revealed ADR prevalence of 9.4% among HAART users with diarrhea and anemia being the commonest [30].

Altogether, ADREs were reported in about a third of the study participants. Those in the tenofovir cohort somehow appeared to have experienced more of the ADRs and multiple adverse events compared to the zidovudine cohort. The unexpected higher incidence of ADREs associated with tenofovir compared to zidovudine can be explained as follows. First, there was high incidence of cutaneous ADREs manifesting as skin rash, itching, and others of varying degrees and this may be attributed to synergistic cutaneous adverse effects of tenofovir and efavirenz as more than two-thirds of the cutaneous ADREs experienced in this study (78%) were in the tenofovir group. Likewise, the most common ADREs category was CNS side effects with over 93% CNS effects experienced by those in the tenofovir cohort. This also reveals a possible potentiated interaction of tenofovir and efavirenz resulting in synergized CNS adverse effects of the tenofovir regimen. Efavirenz and its metabolite 8-hydroxyefavirenz are known to reach higher concentrations in the CSF and likewise tenofovir increasing the risk of neurotoxicity and disturbance of brain bioenergetics from an inconclusive brain mitochondrial polymerase-γ activity inhibition and activation of inducible nitric oxide synthetase [15, 28–30, 32, 35]. Only one patient had tenofovir induced nephropathy (TIN) as serious ADR. This TIN is due to the selective mitochondrial toxicity of tenofovir on the renal tubules due to inhibition of MtDNA polymerase-γ resulting in acute tubular necrosis [31]. One patient in the tenofovir also reported serious psychiatric disorders resulting in subsequent change to nevirapine. Gender related difference in side effects exists with females estimated to possess higher likelihood of experiencing adverse events to HAART though some found no or contradicting results [14, 23]. There was no significant difference between males and females in this study; however, females appeared to experience more multiple ADRs than males. In all, the unexpected higher ADREs associated with tenofovir compared to zidovudine may be due population variation and synergistic ADREs (cutaneous and neuropsychiatric effects) associated with tenofovir and efavirenz. Also the higher number of participants in the tenofovir cohort and female gender compared to the zidovudine and male gender, respectively, may have also influenced the proportions of ADREs as observed [15, 28–30, 32, 35].

Despite the evidence generated in this study, data on the HIV RNA load, a primary biomarker, could not be obtained for all of the study patients during the follow-up phase in the study, due to breakdown of Cobas Ampliprep HIV 1 analyzer at the facility. If this were done the evidence generated in this study could have been more robust. This study could not also obtain follow-up data for LFT, FBC, and RFT on about two-thirds of the study participants due to financial constraints and hence results on these parameters could not be assessed for more definitive evaluation of safety of the HAART pharmacotherapy. Again the number of participants involved in the study was relatively small ($n = 106$), and this could be attributed to the difficulty the investigators had in getting naïve HAART patients to enroll at the beginning of the study. The individuals who participated in this study however are a reflection of the annual estimate of HAART naïve HIV cases that visited the hospital and the attrition rate is also found to be below the 20% margin [36]. Finally about 17 patients were lost to follow-up and thus could not be traced for assessment. This was believed to be the result of movement of the patients or their relations out of catchment area of the hospital or might have travelled to live in other locations outside the catchment area of the hospital. All these notwithstanding, the evidence generated is interesting and can be described as a true reflection of the safety and efficacy of the various HAART regimen for HIV/AIDs case management and care at the study site.

5. Recommendation for Further Research

We therefore recommend a study with a much more robust design such as a multicenter noninferiority trial or a national cohort study to compare the efficacy and safety of tenofovir-based HARRT regimens and zidovudine-based HAART regimens in Ghana. Also we recommend an evaluation of the comparative effect of tenofovir-based and Zidovudine-based HAART regimens on markers of thymic functionality and immune activation in people living with HIV/AIDS.

6. Conclusion

The tenofovir-based cohort had a superior immune reconstitution potential compared to zidovudine-based cohort. Patients on the zidovudine regimen also improved significantly with regard to CD4 T cell repopulation. The immune reconstitution potentials of both HAART pharmacotherapy were independent of age, gender, baseline CD4 and CD8 T cells count, herbal medicine use, and HIV related comorbidities. Patients on the tenofovir-based regimen and females reported to have had more ADREs compared to those on zidovudine-based regimen. Although the tenofovir treatment arm in this study showed a superior immunological recovery, its use must be closely monitored to address the occurrence of ADREs to improve compliance.

Acknowledgments

The authors acknowledge the staff of chest clinic and serology and virology laboratory units of Komfo Anokye Teaching Hospital for their cooperation and support during this research work. To GETFUND, the authors appreciate the support giving to them in the conduct of this research. To lecturers and colleagues of the Department of Pharmacology, KNUST, the authors really appreciate your intellectual contribution that has aided the compilation of this manuscript.

References

[1] G. Doitsh and W. C. Greene, "Dissecting how CD4 T cells are lost during HIV infection," *Cell Host Microbiology*, vol. 19, no. 3, pp. 280–291, 2016.

[2] M. Lenassi, G. Cagney, M. Liao et al., "HIV Nef is secreted in exosomes and triggers apoptosis in bystander CD4$^+$ T cells," *Traffic*, vol. 11, no. 1, pp. 110–122, 2010.

[3] P. Corbeau and J. Reynes, "Immune reconstitution under antiretroviral therapy: the new challenge in HIV-1 infection," *Blood*, vol. 117, no. 21, pp. 5582–5590, 2011.

[4] M. Paiardini and M. Müller-Trutwin, "HIV-associated chronic immune activation," *Immunological Reviews*, vol. 254, no. 1, pp. 78–101, 2013.

[5] M. Paiardini and M. Müller-Trutwin, "HIV-associated chronic immune activation," *NIH Public Access*, vol. 254, no. 1, pp. 78–101, 2013.

[6] A. Joshi, M. Sedano, B. Beauchamp et al., "HIV-1 Env glycoprotein phenotype along with immune activation determines CD4 T cell loss in HIV patients," *The Journal of Immunology*, vol. 196, no. 4, pp. 1768–1779, 2016.

[7] G. Ferrari, B. F. Haynes, S. Koenig, J. L. Nordstrom, D. M. Margolis, and G. D. Tomaras, "Envelope-specific antibodies and antibody-derived molecules for treating and curing HIV infection," *Nature Reviews Drug Discovery*, vol. 15, no. 12, pp. 823–834, 2016.

[8] E. Scully and G. Alter, "NK Cells in HIV Disease," *Current HIV/AIDS Reports*, vol. 13, no. 2, pp. 85–94, 2016.

[9] V. C. Marconi, G. A. Grandits, A. C. Weintrob et al., "Outcomes of highly active antiretroviral therapy in the context of universal access to healthcare: The U.S. Military HIV Natural History Study," *AIDS Research and Therapy*, vol. 7, article no. 14, 2010.

[10] C. J. Smith, C. A. Sabin, M. S. Youle et al., "Factors influencing increases in CD4 cell counts of HIV-positive persons receiving long-term highly active antiretroviral therapy," *The Journal of Infectious Diseases*, vol. 190, no. 10, pp. 1860–1868, 2004.

[11] R. Verheggen, "Immune restoration in patients with HIV infection: HAART and beyond," *Journal of the Association of Nurses in AIDS Care*, vol. 14, no. 6, pp. 76–82, 2003.

[12] J. E. Gallant, E. Dejesus, J. R. Arribas et al., "Tenofovir DF, emtricitabine, and efavirenz vs. zidovudine, lamivudine, and efavirenz for HIV," *The New England Journal of Medicine*, vol. 354, no. 3, pp. 251–260, 2006.

[13] R. Ofori-Asenso and A. A. Agyeman, "Hepatitis B in Ghana: A systematic review & meta-analysis of prevalence studies (1995-2015)," *BMC Infectious Diseases*, vol. 16, no. 1, article no. 130, 2016.

[14] M. Floridia, M. Giuliano, L. Palmisano, and S. Vella, "Gender differences in the treatment of HIV infection," *Pharmacological Research*, vol. 58, no. 3-4, pp. 173–182, 2008.

[15] E. Ruiz-Mateos, A. Rubio, A. Vallejo et al., "Thymic volume is associated independently with the magnitude of short- and long-term repopulation of CD4+ T cells in HIV-infected adults after highly active antiretroviral therapy (HAART)," *Clinical & Experimental Immunology*, vol. 136, no. 3, pp. 501–506, 2004.

[16] V. C. Marconi, G. Grandits, J. F. Okulicz et al., "Cumulative viral load and virologic decay patterns after antiretroviral therapy in HIV-infected subjects influence CD4 recovery and AIDS," *PLoS ONE*, vol. 6, no. 5, Article ID e17956, 2011.

[17] S. Francke, C. G. Orosz, J. Hsu, and L. E. Mathes, "Immunomodulatory effect of zidovudine (ZDV) on cytotoxic T lymphocytes previously exposed to ZDV," *Antimicrobial Agents and Chemotherapy*, vol. 46, no. 9, pp. 2865–2871, 2002.

[18] Ghana Anti-retroviral Therapy guideline, 2014.

[19] World Health Organization (WHO), *Consolidated Guidelines on the Use of Antiretroviral Drugs for Treating and Preventing HIV Infection, 2013*, World Health, Geneva, Switzerland, 2013, http://apps.who.int/iris/bitstream/10665/85321/1/9789241505727_eng.pdf.

[20] World Health Organization W. H., *Treat all people living with HIV, offer antiretrovirals as additional prevention choice for people at "substantial" risk*, World Health Organization, 2015.

[21] A. Spaulding, G. W. Rutherford, and N. Siegfried, "Tenofovir or zidovudine in three-drug combination therapy with one nucleoside reverse transcriptase inhibitor and one non-nucleoside reverse transcriptase inhibitor for initial treatment of HIV infection in antiretroviral-naïve individuals.," *Cochrane Database of Systematic Reviews (Online)*, no. 10, p. CD008740, 2010.

[22] J. L. Castilho, V. V. Melekhin, and T. R. Sterling, "Sex differences in HIV outcomes in the highly active antiretroviral therapy era: A systematic review," *AIDS Research and Human Retroviruses*, vol. 30, no. 5, pp. 446–456, 2014.

[23] E. Nicastri, C. Angeletti, L. Palmisano et al., "Gender differences in clinical progression of HIV-1-infected individuals during long-term highly active antiretroviral therapy," *AIDS*, vol. 19, no. 6, pp. 577–583, 2005.

[24] R. Landman, S. Koulla-Shiro, P. S. Sow et al., "Evaluation of four tenofovir-containing regimens as first-line treatments in Cameroon and Senegal: The ANRS 12115 DAYANA trial," *Antiviral Therapy*, vol. 19, no. 1, pp. 51–59, 2014.

[25] B. H. Chi, A. Mwango, M. J. Giganti et al., "Comparative outcomes of tenofovir-based and zidovudine-based antiretroviral therapy regimens in Lusaka, Zambia," *Journal of Acquired Immune Deficiency Syndromes*, vol. 58, no. 5, pp. 475–481, 2011.

[26] D. L. Pitrak, R. M. Novak, R. Estes et al., "Short communication: Apoptosis pathways in HIV-1-infected patients before and after highly active antiretroviral therapy: Relevance to immune recovery," *AIDS Research and Human Retroviruses*, vol. 31, no. 2, pp. 208–216, 2015.

[27] P. Subramaniam and P. Usha, "Aging and immune function: molecular mechanisms to interventions," *Antioxidants and Redox Signaling*, vol. 14, no. 8, 2011.

[28] M. Nagpal, V. Tayal, S. Kumar, and U. Gupta, "Adverse drug reactions to antiretroviral therapy in AIDS patients at a tertiary care hospital in India: A prospective observational study," *Indian Journal of Medical Sciences*, vol. 64, no. 6, pp. 245–252, 2010.

[29] A. Jena, R. K. Sachdeva, A. Sharma, and A. Wanchu, "Adverse drug reactions to nonnucleoside reverse transcriptase inhibitor-based antiretroviral regimen: A 24-week prospective study," *Journal of the International Association of Physicians in AIDS Care*, vol. 8, no. 5, pp. 318–322, 2009.

[30] M. Lartey, A. Asante-Quashie, A. Essel, E. Kenu, V. Ganu, and A. Neequaye, "Adverse drug reactions to antiretroviral therapy during the early art period at a tertiary hospital in Ghana," *The Pan African Medical Journal*, vol. 18, no. 25, 2014.

[31] A. Maagaard and D. Kvale, "Mitochondrial toxicity in HIV-infected patients both off and on antiretroviral treatment: A continuum or distinct underlying mechanisms?" *Journal of Antimicrobial Chemotherapy*, vol. 64, no. 5, Article ID dkp316, pp. 901–909, 2009.

[32] H. Namme Luma, M.-S. Doualla, S.-P. Choukem et al., "Adverse drug reactions of Highly Active Antiretroviral Therapy (HAART) in HIV infected patients at the General Hospital, Douala, Cameroon: a cross sectional study," *The Pan African Medical Journal*, vol. 12, no. 87, 2012.

[33] B. Kayaaslan and R. Guner, "Adverse effects of oral antiviral therapy in chronic hepatitis B," *World Journal of Hepatology*, vol. 9, no. 5, pp. 227–241, 2017.

[34] V. Tayal, U. Gupta, M. Nagpal, and S. Kumar, "Adverse drug reactions to antiretroviral therapy in AIDS patients at a tertiary care hospital in India: A prospective observational study," *Indian Journal of Medical Sciences*, vol. 64, no. 6, pp. 245–252, 2010.

[35] N. Apostolova, H. A. Funes, A. Blas-Garcia, M. J. Galindo, A. Alvarez, and J. V. Esplugues, "Efavirenz and the CNS: What we already know and questions that need to be answered," *Journal of Antimicrobial Chemotherapy*, vol. 70, no. 10, Article ID dkv183, pp. 2693–2708, 2015.

[36] M. S. Fewtrell, K. Kennedy, A. Singhal et al., "How much loss to follow-up is acceptable in long-term randomised trials and prospective studies?" *Archives of Disease in Childhood*, vol. 93, no. 6, pp. 458–461, 2008.

31

Diabetes Mellitus as Hub for Tuberculosis Infection: A Snapshot

Rahul Pal, Moiz A. Ansari, Saif Hameed, and Zeeshan Fatima

Amity Institute of Biotechnology, Amity University Haryana, Gurgaon, Manesar 122413, India

Correspondence should be addressed to Saif Hameed; saifhameed@yahoo.co.in and Zeeshan Fatima; drzeeshanfatima@gmail.com

Academic Editor: Katarzyna Zorena

Tuberculosis (TB) still remains the thorn in the flesh of efficient therapeutics affecting one-third of global population annually. There are several factors that enhance the susceptibility to TB infections including malnutrition, smoking, and immunocompromised conditions such as AIDS. In the recent years, growing body of evidence has gained considerable prominence which suggests that Diabetes Mellitus (DM) is individual risk factor leading to complicated TB infections. In this article the authors have attempted to summarize the link of type 2 DM with TB, the mechanistic action of how DM sensitizes for developing the active TB infection from the latent infection, and problems faced during treatment followed by possible preventive measures. We have tried to give account of the alterations that occurred in DM making a person more prone to develop TB.

1. Introduction

Tuberculosis (TB) continues to be a considerable worldwide health issue, provoking millions of new cases and one-third deaths annually. Around 2 billion of the population of the world are considered to be infected with latent TB and out of which approximate 5–10% grows in to active TB [1, 2]. Previously it was thought that TB emerges only in low economic countries but in recent years it is spreading its tentacles to high income countries as well. This shift in the scenario is mainly because of predisposing factors like malnutrition, smoking, and immunocompromised conditions such as AIDS [3–6]. Among various challenging conditions Diabetes Mellitus (DM) is emerging out to be one of the leading factors after HIV/AIDS [7–9]. Epidemiological reports have proved a strong link between DM and TB [10]. DM is a condition developed due to either the pancreas not producing enough insulin (type 1) or the cells of the body not responding enough to the insulin produced (type 2). Type 1 DM was previously referred to as "Insulin-Dependent Diabetes Mellitus" (IDDM) or "juvenile diabetes." Type 2 DM begins with insulin resistance, a condition in which cells fail to respond to insulin properly and as the disease progresses a lack of insulin may also develop. This form was previously referred to as "Non-Insulin-Dependent Diabetes Mellitus" (NIDDM) or "adult-onset diabetes." Type 2 DM is more prevalent than type 1 DM and occurs in 90% of the cases. The pervasiveness of DM growing worldwide is predicted to attain an approximate total of 300 million people by 2025. It is believed that DM patients are thrice more susceptible to develop TB as compared to normal individuals without DM. Thus addressing the problem of DM in achieving the long term goal of curing TB is also needed. Various case studies revealed unsuccessful TB treatment outcome in DM-TB patients (Figure 1) as compared to only TB patients [11–13]. Considering the impact of DM on development and treatment of TB, this article on a common platform focuses on the link of type 2 DM with TB, the mechanistic action of how DM sensitizes for developing the active TB infection from the latent infection, and problems faced during treatment followed by possible preventive measures.

2. Predisposing Factors Endorsing TB Infection in DM

2.1. Latent to Active Transition. TB is an airborne disease that is transferred from one person to another either through aerosol formation or through contaminated air within the population. However based on the PPD test results survey, usually, only 30% of the population gets successfully infected when coming in contact with MTB. In remaining 70% of

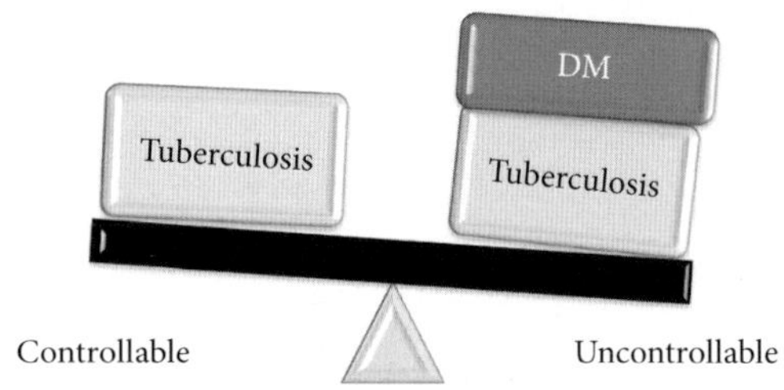

FIGURE 1: Twin burden of TB infection and DM: TB infections are controllable in comparison to diabetics suffering from TB infection.

the population the boosted level of immunity prevents the onset of MTB infection and prolongs the latent condition. Under this condition most MTB are distorted and the few viable ones are transferred to the latent state because of their hampered metabolism. TB and DM both interact with each other on various levels, one making worse situation for the other [14]. Under diabetic conditions the possibility of death with TB enhances and moreover if it is cured, the chances of reappearance of this infection are high under diabetic condition (Figure 2). Literature also shows that people suffering from DM stay infected more than people who do not have DM. Additionally, the level of blood sugar is elevated temporarily beyond normal in TB; this condition is termed as "impaired glucose tolerance," which makes a chance for developing DM, and this condition is also called "prediabetes," a state of hyperglycemia [15–17].

2.2. Immunocompromised. To attain the minimal level of defense against MTB, body develops the immunologic responses in the form of first-line defense through innate immunity where eradication occurs through phagocytosis. However, because of the increased burden of MTB the innate immunity further develops the adaptive immunity leading to the activation of localized T-helper 1 (Th1) along with several cytokines (TNF-α, IL-1β, and IL-12), lymphocytes, monocytes, natural killer T cells, and B lymphocytes that form granulomas and kill almost all MTB preventing the growth of those that remain viable. However in the diabetic conditions the immunologic responses weaken making the individual immunocompromised (Figure 3). In recent in vitro study on diabetic cells the reduced level of MTB phagocytosis was observed in the diabetic monocytes probably due to alteration in diabetic monocytes and C3 component of complement system mainly responsible for MTB phagocytosis [18]. Further, the study on 2-week infected mice with DM leads to reduced uptake of MTB through macrophages which clearly depict the delayed or loss of innate immunity to MTB in diabetic condition and these delays make DM patients at high risk of TB [18]. Moreover, not only innate but adaptive immunity is also affected in the DM more than the normal condition. In many studies the altered level of several cytokines such as IFN-γ, IL-12, IL-2, and TNF-α was observed in DM-TB conditions.

2.3. Drug-Drug Interaction. Anti-TB drug rifampicin is a strong hepatic enzyme-inducer. It boosts the metabolism of various oral hypoglycemic factors, primarily sulphonylureas and biguanides, and also decreases their level in plasma leading to hyperglycemia in diabetic patients. In nondiabetics, it increases the intestinal absorption of glucose and may mimic the symptoms of diabetes [19]. Additionally, some of the anti-TB drugs (particularly rifampicin) make the situation sometime worsen to control DM. This kind of problem arises when anti-TB and DM medication, that is, ATT drug rifampicin, interact with each other. Some concept has been emerged that DM medicines can reduce the impact of anti-TB drug [20, 21]. INH, unlike Rif, inhibits the metabolism of oral hypoglycaemic factors which increases the plasma levels of these drugs. INH mainly interacts with sulphonylureas and leads to diminish control of medicines on DM by antagonizing the effect [22]. It also impairs the release of insulin and causes hyperglycemia even in nondiabetics.

3. Consequences of DM on Clinical Characteristics of TB

3.1. Age. Data available till now proves that DM-TB patients are of older age than those who do not suffer from DM; the reason may be because DM type 2 persists more in old age people [23].

3.2. Gender. It is still controversial that DM-TB is gender specific or not; however, some reports show it is indeed gender specific and persists more in men than women [24, 25].

3.3. Symptoms. Symptoms of DM and TB are weight loss and fatigue which are common for both diseases [21]. However, some literature states that body weight of DM-TB patient is usually more than the TB patients not affected by diabetes [12, 23].

3.4. Pulmonary/Extrapulmonary. Involvement of extrapulmonary cases has been reported to be less common among diabetic TB patients than in nondiabetics and found more in pulmonary cases [23].

3.5. Hemoglobin Level. HbA1C is an abbreviation of hemoglobin A1c that binds to glucose which is also known as glycohemoglobin. In DM-TB patients HbA1C is found to be higher than in patients with DM without TB infection; however few reports suggest that there is no such difference in DM-TB with or without TB [12, 26].

3.6. Diagnosis. Similarly some conflicts have been also reported regarding the negative and positive sputum smears in DM-TB [12]. Some reports suggest DM as an independent risk factor for numerous acid fast bacilli on the sputum smear examination [25] and others showed no association between DM and patients [27]. Conflict in these clinical characteristics might be due to the availability of limited studies on status of DM-TB twin burden (Table 1).

4. DM Enhances Susceptibility to TB Infection

As already discussed, DM is a global epidemic disease affecting both the developed and developing countries. Due to

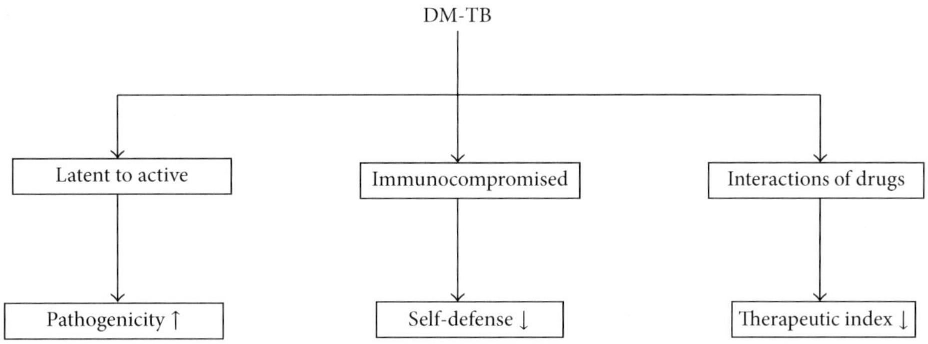

FIGURE 2: Predisposing factors endorsing TB in DM: DM leads to frequent development of latent to active TB having enhanced pathogenicity; compromised immunity causing loss in self-defense and the interaction of anti-TB drug with antidiabetic drugs causing decreased therapeutic index.

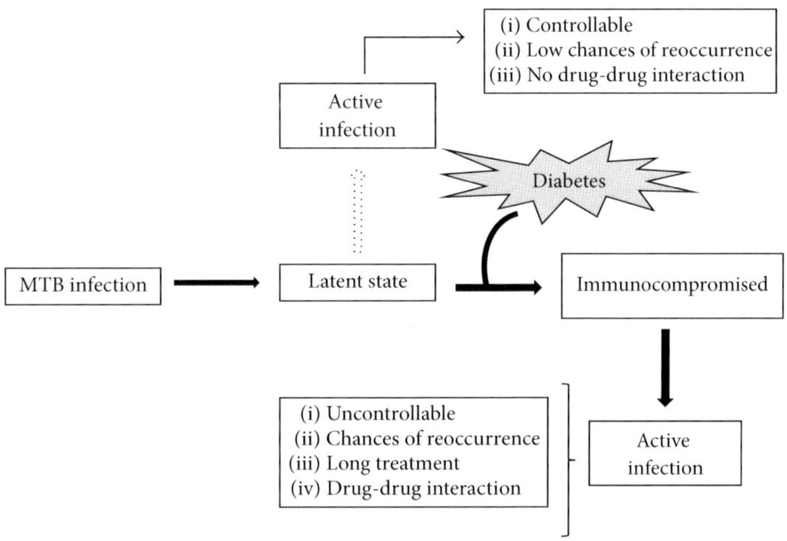

FIGURE 3: Implications of DM on TB: MTB resides as latent condition which could develop to active TB (shown by dotted arrow) but still is curable. Under diabetic condition immunocompromised state develops making condition prone to develop active TB (shown by bold arrows) which becomes incurable.

the immunosuppressed conditions developed in diabetic condition, it makes the individual become more susceptible to MTB infection and to several other diseases linked with immunocompromised condition leading to treatment failure and death. The immense rate of TB with increasing DM has been studied extensively but the complete mechanistic rationale for how DM is making TB more susceptible is still comparatively less understood. The immune response upon the invasion of MTB in the host is well studied through various workers.

Inflammatory responses in the host against MTB begin with the first-line defense through nonspecific mechanistic action of macrophages such as phagocytosis and cytokines production (Figure 4). On recognizing the MTB epitope on macrophages, Th1 cytokines like IFN-γ and IL-2 are produced by specific CD4$^+$ lymphocytes [28]. The functioning of macrophages is enhanced by IFN-γ killing or suppressing the replication of phagosome residing organism [29]. IFN-γ arouses the TNF and VitD$_3$ production that suppresses the growth of MTB in human macrophages through ROS generation, nitrogen intermediate, and alteration in intracellular iron level [30]. IL2 functions by promoting the proliferation of activated lymphocytes. It is seen that if any mutation in IFN-γ, IL-12 production, and IL-12 receptor happens that leads to inactivation or nonfunctioning of these cytokines it results in enhanced susceptibility to MTB. If IFN-γ in particular has become inactive or nonfunctional particularly in DM then MTB attack is more rigorous (Figure 4) [31]. Several T-lymphocytes are involved in the inflammatory response against MTB such as CD-1 restricted T cells, CD4$^+$ T cells, CD8$^+$ T cells, and γ/δ. Among all, CD4$^+$ T cells and CD8$^+$ T cells play a critical role in immune response against MTB [32, 33]. It has been shown that, in comparison to healthy individuals, the patients with mild, moderate, or advanced pulmonary disease were having enhanced levels of IFN-γ, IL-2, IL-4, and IL-10. Further it was observed that IFN-γ and IL-2 were higher in mild and moderate patients compared with the patients suffering from advanced disease. However,

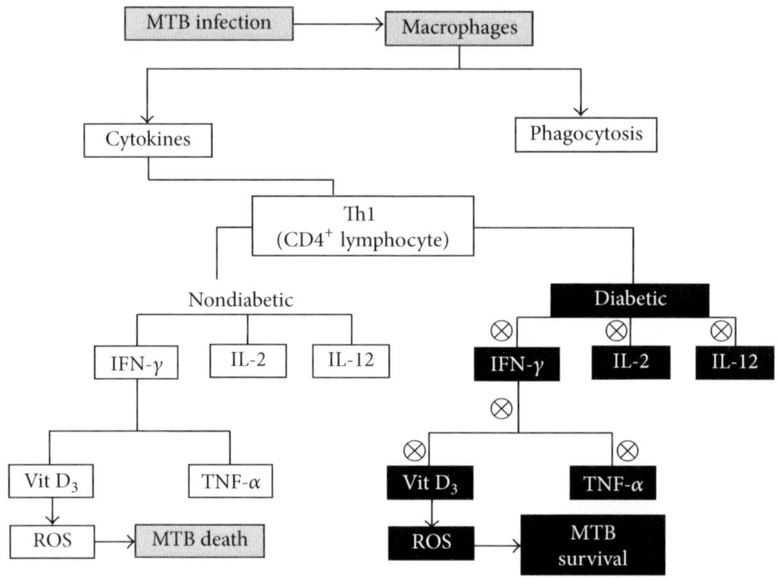

Figure 4: Mechanisms involved in enhancing TB infection during DM: during MTB infection the host innate immunity activates macrophages which causes phagocytosis and activates cytokines. Under nondiabetic condition cytokines become activated leading to ROS generation subsequently killing MTB. Under diabetic condition due to immunocompromised state the alteration in cytokine release leads to the survival of MTB due to suppressed ROS generation.

Table 1: Showing differences in clinical characteristics between TB and DM-TB.

Characteristics	TB	DM-TB
Age	Not defined and persisting at any age	Usually persisting in adults and in old age
Gender	Men or women	Persisting more in men
Symptoms	Higher body weight loss, less fatigue, low breathlessness, less hemoptysis, more fever, more expectoration	Lesser body weight loss, more fatigue, higher breathlessness, more hemoptysis, less fever, lower expectoration
Pulmonary/ extrapulmonary	Both pulmonary and extrapulmonary involvement	Only pulmonary and few extrapulmonary involvement
Hemoglobin level	Anemia	HbA1C is higher
Diagnosis	Can be diagnosed	Difficulty in diagnosis

the patients with moderate and advanced pulmonary disease were having enhanced levels of cytokines IL4 and IL-10 in contrast to mild disease patients [34]. Apart from IFN-γ and IL-2, the in vitro studies of relation with the signaling pattern of these cytokines with some other cytokines which are assumed to be involved in the pathogenesis of MTB were also studied, such as TGF-β and IL-1β [35].

The immune responses in DM cases showed that alterations in humoral innate immune responses are mediated through change in cytokine levels (Figure 4). Deeper studies reflected the declination in the functioning of DM affected macrophages and polymorphonuclear cells through affected chemotaxis, phagocytosis, and killing efficiency [36]. Evidences show the alteration in TNF-α and IL-6 level without any stimuli in DM type 1 and DM type 2, respectively. However, under similar condition IL-8 concentration was altered in both DM type 1 and DM type 2 [37, 38]. In the presence of stimuli, such as LPS, the IL-1 secretion of PBMC was found to be downregulated in both type 1 and 2 diabetic PBMC but no difference was found in the level of TNF-α [39]. Literatures also suggest that IL-1 and IL-6 production were found to be lowered after LPS stimulation in monocytes of DM type 1 when compared with DM type 2 and control patients, but again no difference was found in TNF-α level. Moreover no effect of glucose or insulin stimulation was observed on either of these cytokines which substantially points out that defective LPS may be the important property of diabetic cells [40].

Although the immunologic responses in TB and DM conditions are extensively studied, the responses against MTB in diabetic condition are still not completely understood. However in recent study it was shown that the intracellular level of cytokines, such as IFN-γ, IL-2, TNF-α, and IL-17, is found to be diminished in the patients with DM or pre-DM. Further it was seen that this diminished level of cytokines is associated with proinflammatory cytokines such as IL-1β and IL-18 which were also found to be diminished; however no links were found with the diminished level of type 2 cytokines. Moreover, patient suffering from DM was found to have inhibited level of MTB antigen specific cytokines (type 1 and type 17) [41]. Elevation in resistin level, a protein produced by immune cells in humans, diminishes the activation of mycobacterium-induced inflammasome through suppressing ROS production in leukocytes [42]. In some studies Vitamin D is proposed as an adjuvant for MTB treatment.

It was seen that the expression of TLR-2/1 receptor and CYP27B1-hydroxylase enzyme increases upon stimulation and catalyzes the conversion of Vitamin D from its active form to induce antimicrobial peptide cathelicidin finally leading to the MTB execution. Further investigation reported the expression level of CYP27B1-hydroxylase enzyme, VDR, and antimicrobial peptides gene and compared the DM type 2 and TB patients with healthy control. They found that DM type 2 individuals were having lower VDR and antimicrobial peptides expression, however when MDM isolated from DM type 2 patients having low VDR expression upon Vitamin D supplementation were efficiently inhibiting the MTB functioning [43]. GSH level was downregulated in DM type 2 individuals through hyperactivation of transforming growth factor-β (TGF-β), a cytokine responsible for lowering the GCLC expression. This suggests that the lower level of GSH in DM type 2 individuals makes MTB more susceptible. In DM individuals, level of cytokines such as IL-6 and IL-17 was also found to be increased leading to the enhanced free radicals formation which confirms the degraded level of GSH in DM type 2 individuals. However, it was observed that the increment in the GSH level advances the action against MTB infections. Moreover, cytokines accountable for MTB infection at cellular level, such as TNF-α, IL-1β, IL-2, IFN-γ, and IL-12, were found to be altered in DM type 2 individuals; interestingly the augmented level of some immunosuppressive cytokines such as IL-10 was also found in the same individual [44]. Even short chain fatty acid could also be responsible for the enhanced susceptibility of MTB where the effect of butyrate on different immunologic condition of cytokines in PBMC of diabetic individuals was studied. It was found that the MTB induced proinflammatory cytokine responses were decreased by butyrate treatment in DM individuals; however IL-10 concentration was increased [45]. These links of immunologic condition with DM and MTB suggest that the DM provokes the MTB by providing a conducive environment for its pathogenesis.

5. Preventive Measures to Combat DM-TB

Controlling the level of glucose probably minimizes the chances of developing TB among DM people; however sufficient research is still to be conducted which might give awareness whether it is minimizing the TB risk or saving people from death. Gliptins, a new agent for the treatment of type 2 DM also known as DPP-4 inhibitors (inhibitors of dipeptidyl peptidase 4), control the glucagon release and stimulate the release of insulin which lowers the blood glucose level [45]. Therefore, the dose of insulin should be modified while prescribing these drugs to patients [46]. Furthermore, till now how to standardize the control of glucose level in people who are suffering from both TB and DM is not clear. It has been recommended to perform tuberculin skin test (TST) in all the diabetic patients by the American Thoracic Society with purified protein derivative (PPD). If the skin becomes firm reddish bump and is found to be more than 10 mm, then it is suggested to take precautionary treatment with isoniazid (INH) for 6 to 12 months; however, some investigators have challenged the authenticity of this recommendation. Consequently, the persistence of TB infection in DM is high and the sensitiveness of TST may be low [26]. Few studies have explained the benefit of TB prophylaxis in DM patients. The first one was done in Germany in the 1950s where they evaluated the recurrence rate of TB and found it to be lower in DM patients where the treatment has been completed with INH [47]. Second study was done in Russia in the 1960s, where administration of INH analogue in DM patient decreases the occurrence of TB 2-3-fold [48]. Both studies were controversial because of lack of sufficient data regarding interventions [49]. Therefore, only through a randomized controlled trial can the true effectiveness be properly addressed. To attain success in TB-DM disease consequently it needs a cooperate response from each level of the health system, that is, from the administration of public policies to the management of health disease control programs. Policies maker may take steps for establishing new policies and new global health services. Agenda can be focused on combating against this serious threat before it causes more damage to human health as well as economy. Research community synergistically with clinicians and policy makers is required to work in tandem to bring forth some potential measure for the management of the twin burden of TB-DM.

6. Conclusion

Patients suffering from DM are more prone to develop TB as it compromises treatment of TB in diabetic patients. Moreover, DM is associated with enhanced risk of multiple outcomes of not only treatment failure but relapse and death during TB treatment. Therefore, extensive studies on TB management with DM are required. Considering the increasing disease burden of DM, particularly in highly prevalent TB areas, TB control programs will need to expand their efforts and focus on treatment of patients with DM and TB.

Abbreviations

TB:	Tuberculosis
DM:	Diabetes Mellitus
AIDS:	Acquired immune deficiency syndrome
HIV:	Human immunodeficiency virus
MTB:	*Mycobacterium tuberculosis*
PPD:	Purified protein derivative
Anti-TB:	Antituberculosis
ATT:	Antituberculosis therapy
INH:	Isoniazid
Rif:	Rifampicin
TST:	Tuberculin skin test
IFN-γ:	Interferon-gamma
IL-2:	Interleukin-2
TNF:	Tumor necrosis factor
VitD3:	Vitamin D3
TGF-β:	Transforming growth factor-β
LPS:	Lipopolysaccharide
PBMC:	Peripheral blood mononuclear cells
ROS:	Reactive oxygen species
VDR:	Vitamin D receptor

MDM: Monocytes derived from macrophages
GSH: Glutathione
GCLC: Glutamine-cysteine ligase.

Competing Interests

The authors declare that they have no competing interests.

Authors' Contributions

Rahul Pal and Moiz A. Ansari contributed equally to this work.

References

[1] World Tuberculosis Day: WHO enjoins all to end TB by 2030, report 2016.

[2] World Health Organization: Tuberculosis country profiles, 2010.

[3] P. Narasimhan, J. Wood, C. R. MacIntyre, and D. Mathai, "Risk factors for tuberculosis," *Pulmonary Medicine*, vol. 2013, Article ID 828939, 11 pages, 2013.

[4] R. R. Pathak, B. K. Mishra, P. K. Moonan et al., "Can intensified tuberculosis case finding efforts at nutrition rehabilitation centers lead to pediatric case detection in Bihar, India?" *Journal of Tuberculosis Research*, vol. 4, no. 1, pp. 46–54, 2016.

[5] K. B. Gupta, R. Gupta, A. Atreja, M. Verma, and S. Vishvkarma, "Tuberculosis and nutrition," *Lung India*, vol. 26, no. 1, pp. 9–16, 2009.

[6] S. H. Jee, J. E. Golub, J. Jo, I. S. Park, H. Ohrr, and J. M. Samet, "Smoking and risk of tuberculosis incidence, mortality, and recurrence in South Korean men and women," *American Journal of Epidemiology*, vol. 170, no. 12, pp. 1478–1485, 2009.

[7] Q. M. Trinh, H. L. Nguyen, V. N. Nguyen, T. V. A. Nguyen, V. Sintchenko, and B. J. Marais, "Tuberculosis and HIV co-infection-focus on the Asia-Pacific region," *International Journal of Infectious Diseases*, vol. 32, pp. 170–178, 2015.

[8] C. R. Diedrich, J. O'Hern, and R. J. Wilkinson, "HIV-1 and the *Mycobacterium tuberculosis* granuloma: a systematic review and meta-analysis," *Tuberculosis*, vol. 98, pp. 62–76, 2016.

[9] L. M. A. J. Muller, K. J. Gorter, E. Hak et al., "Increased risk of common infections in patients with type 1 and type 2 diabetes mellitus," *Clinical Infectious Diseases*, vol. 41, no. 3, pp. 281–288, 2005.

[10] A. O'Garra, P. S. Redford, F. W. McNab, C. I. Bloom, R. J. Wilkinson, and M. P. R. Berry, "The immune response in tuberculosis," *Annual Review of Immunology*, vol. 31, pp. 475–527, 2013.

[11] M. J. Magee, R. R. Kempker, M. Kipiani et al., "Diabetes mellitus is associated with cavities, smear grade, and multidrug-resistant tuberculosis in Georgia," *International Journal of Tuberculosis and Lung Disease*, vol. 19, no. 6, pp. 685–692, 2015.

[12] B. Alisjahbana, E. Sahiratmadja, E. J. Nelwan et al., "The effect of type 2 diabetes mellitus on the presentation and treatment response of pulmonary tuberculosis," *Clinical Infectious Diseases*, vol. 45, no. 4, pp. 428–435, 2007.

[13] M. A. Baker, A. D. Harries, C. Y. Jeon et al., "The impact of diabetes on tuberculosis treatment outcomes: a systematic review," *BMC Medicine*, vol. 9, article 81, 2011.

[14] J.-T. Chang, H.-Y. Dou, C.-L. Yen et al., "Effect of type 2 diabetes mellitus on the clinical severity and treatment outcome in patients with pulmonary tuberculosis: a potential role in the emergence of multidrug-resistance," *Journal of the Formosan Medical Association*, vol. 110, no. 6, pp. 372–381, 2011.

[15] B. I. Restrepo and L. S. Schlesinger, "Host-pathogen interactions in tuberculosis patients with type 2 diabetes mellitus," *Tuberculosis*, vol. 93, pp. S10–S14, 2013.

[16] M. M. Singh, S. K. Biswas, S. Ashok, K. R. Ashok, and P. P. Singh, "Impaired glucose tolerance in active pulmonary tuberculosis," *Indian Journal of Tuberculosis*, vol. 31, no. 3, pp. 118–121, 1984.

[17] F. Jawad, A. S. Shera, R. Memon, and G. Ansari, "Glucose intolerance in pulmonary tuberculosis," *The Journal of the Pakistan Medical Association*, vol. 45, no. 9, pp. 237–238, 1995.

[18] K. E. Dooley and R. E. Chaisson, "Tuberculosis and diabetes mellitus: convergence of two epidemics," *The Lancet Infectious Diseases*, vol. 9, no. 12, pp. 737–746, 2009.

[19] H. M. J. Nijland, R. Ruslami, J. E. Stalenhoef et al., "Exposure to rifampicin is strongly reduced in patients with tuberculosis and type 2 diabetes," *Clinical Infectious Diseases*, vol. 43, no. 7, pp. 848–854, 2006.

[20] T. F. Blaschkc and M. H. Skinner, "The clinical pharmucokmcticsof rifabutin," *Clinical Infectious Disease*, vol. 22, supplement, p. 515, 1996.

[21] A. Guptan and A. Shah, "Tuberculosis and diabetes: an appraisal," *Indian Journal of Tuberculosis*, vol. 47, no. 3, pp. 2–8, 2000.

[22] G. Mandcll and M. A. LSande, "Drugs used in the chemotherapy of tuberculosis and leprosy," in *Goodman and Oilman's-The Pharmacological Basis of Therapeutics*, A. G. Oilman, L. S. Goodman, and A. Gilman, Eds., p. 1200, Macmillan, London, UK, 6th edition, 1980.

[23] R. Ruslami, R. E. Aarnoutse, B. Alisjahbana, A. J. A. M. Van Der Ven, and R. Van Crevel, "Implications of the global increase of diabetes for tuberculosis control and patient care," *Tropical Medicine and International Health*, vol. 15, no. 11, pp. 1289–1299, 2010.

[24] A. Jabbar, S. F. Hussain, and A. A. Khan, "Clinical characteristics of pulmonary tuberculosis in adult Pakistani patients with co-existing diabetes mellitus," *Eastern Mediterranean Health Journal*, vol. 12, no. 5, pp. 522–527, 2006.

[25] R. Singla, N. Khan, N. Al-Sharif, M. O. Ai-Sayegh, M. A. Shaikh, and M. M. Osman, "Influence of diabetes on manifestations and treatment outcome of pulmonary TB patients," *International Journal of Tuberculosis and Lung Disease*, vol. 10, no. 1, pp. 74–79, 2006.

[26] E. A. Webb, A. C. Hesseling, H. S. Schaaf et al., "High prevalence of Mycobacterium tuberculosis infection and disease in children and adolescents with type 1 diabetes mellitus," *International Journal of Tuberculosis and Lung Disease*, vol. 13, no. 7, pp. 868–874, 2009.

[27] F. Bacakoglu, Ö. K. Başoglu, G. Çok, A. Sayiner, and M. Ateş, "Pulmonary tuberculosis in patients with diabetes mellitus," *Respiration*, vol. 68, no. 6, pp. 595–600, 2001.

[28] W. H. Boom, "The role of T-cell subsets in Mycobacterium tuberculosis infection," *Infectious Agents and Disease*, vol. 5, no. 2, pp. 73–81, 1996.

[29] L. Bulat-Kardum, G. E. Etokebe, J. Knezevic et al., "Interferon-γ receptor-1 gene promoter polymorphisms (G-611A; T-56C) and susceptibility to tuberculosis," *Scandinavian Journal of Immunology*, vol. 63, no. 2, pp. 142–150, 2006.

[30] G. A. W. Rook, J. Steele, and L. Fraher, "Vitamin D3, gamma interferon, and control of proliferation of *Mycobacterium tuberculosis* by human monocytes," *Immunology*, vol. 57, no. 1, pp. 159–163, 1986.

[31] F. Altare, E. Jouanguy, S. Lamhamedi, R. Döffinger, A. Fischer, and J.-L. Casanova, "Mendelian susceptibility to mycobacterial infection in man," *Current Opinion in Immunology*, vol. 10, no. 4, pp. 413–417, 1998.

[32] S. Baumann, A. N. Eddine, and S. H. E. Kaufmann, "Progress in tuberculosis vaccine development," *Current Opinion in Immunology*, vol. 18, no. 4, pp. 438–448, 2006.

[33] T. H. M. Ottenhoff, F. A. W. Verreck, M. A. Hoeve, and E. van de Vosse, "Control of human host immunity to mycobacteria," *Tuberculosis*, vol. 85, no. 1-2, pp. 53–64, 2005.

[34] D. Dlugovitzky, A. Torres-Morales, L. Rateni et al., "Circulating profile of Th1 and Th2 cytokines in tuberculosis patients with different degrees of pulmonary involvement," *FEMS Immunology and Medical Microbiology*, vol. 18, no. 3, pp. 203–207, 1997.

[35] D. Dlugovitzky, M. L. Bay, L. Rateni et al., "In vitro synthesis of interferon-γ, interleukin-4, transforming growth factor-β, and interleukin 1-β by peripheral blood mononuclear cells from tuberculosis patients. Relationship with the severity of pulmonary involvement," *Scandinavian Journal of Immunology*, vol. 49, pp. 210–217, 1999.

[36] S. E. Geerlings and A. I. M. Hoepelman, "Immune dysfunction in patients with diabetes mellitus (DM)," *FEMS Immunology and Medical Microbiology*, vol. 26, no. 3-4, pp. 259–265, 1999.

[37] D. Zozulinska, A. Majchrzak, M. Sobieska, K. Wiktorowicz, and B. Wierusz-Wysocka, "Serum interleukin-8 level is increased in diabetic patients," *Diabetologia*, vol. 42, no. 1, pp. 117–118, 1999.

[38] J. Mysliwska, K. Zorena, A. Bakowska, A. Skuratowicz-Kubica, and A. Mysliwski, "Significance of tumor necrosis factor-α in patients with long-standing type-1 diabetes mellitus," *Hormone and Metabolic Research*, vol. 30, pp. 158–161, 1998.

[39] Y. Ohno, N. Aoki, and A. Nishimura, "In vitro production of interleukin-1, interleukin-6, and tumor necrosis factor-α in insulin-dependent diabetes mellitus," *Journal of Clinical Endocrinology and Metabolism*, vol. 77, no. 4, pp. 1072–1077, 1993.

[40] H. W. L. Ziegler-Heitbrock, A. Wedel, W. Schraut et al., "Tolerance to lipopolysaccharide involves mobilization of nuclear factor κB with predominance of p50 homodimers," *Journal of Biological Chemistry*, vol. 269, no. 25, pp. 17001–17004, 1994.

[41] P. Kumari and L. S. Meena, "Factors affecting susceptibility to *Mycobacterium tuberculosis*: a close view of immunological defence mechanism," *Applied Biochemistry and Biotechnology*, vol. 174, no. 8, pp. 2663–2673, 2014.

[42] W.-C. Chao, C.-L. Yen, Y.-H. Wu et al., "Increased resistin may suppress reactive oxygen species production and inflammasome activation in type 2 diabetic patients with pulmonary tuberculosis infection," *Microbes and Infection*, vol. 17, no. 3, pp. 195–204, 2015.

[43] N. Lopez-Lopez, I. Gonzalez-Curiel, J. Castañeda-Delgado et al., "Vitamin D supplementation promotes macrophages' antimycobacterial activity in type 2 diabetes mellitus patients with low vitamin D receptor expression," *Microbes and Infection*, vol. 16, no. 9, pp. 755–761, 2014.

[44] M. Lagman, J. Ly, T. Saing et al., "Investigating the causes for decreased levels of glutathione in individuals with type II diabetes," *PLoS ONE*, vol. 10, no. 3, Article ID e0118436, 2015.

[45] I. Idris and R. Donnelly, "Dipeptidyl peptidase-IV inhibitors: a major new class of oral antidiabetic drug," *Diabetes, Obesity and Metabolism*, vol. 9, no. 2, pp. 153–165, 2007.

[46] E. Lachmandas, C. N. A. M. Van Den Heuvel, M. S. M. A. Damen, M. C. P. Cleophas, M. G. Netea, and R. Van Crevel, "Diabetes mellitus and increased tuberculosis susceptibility: the role of short-chain fatty acids," *Journal of Diabetes Research*, vol. 2016, Article ID 6014631, 15 pages, 2016.

[47] S. Madsbad, "Treatment of type 2 diabetes with incretin-based therapies," *The Lancet*, vol. 373, no. 9662, pp. 438–439, 2009.

[48] R. Pfaffenberg and H. Jahler, "Isoniazid & recurrence of tuberculosis in diabetics," *Zeitschrift für Tuberkulose*, vol. 111, no. 3-4, pp. 167–173, 1958.

[49] A. V. Lesnichii and L. Z. Karpina, "Experience with the chemoprophylaxis of pulmonary tuberculosis in diabetes mellitus patients," *Problemy Tuberkuleza*, vol. 47, no. 12, pp. 1–3, 1969.

32

Lipid Profile in Tuberculosis Patients with and without Human Immunodeficiency Virus Infection

Gebremedhin Gebremicael,[1] Yemane Amare,[2] Feyissa Challa,[1] Atsbeha Gebreegziabxier,[1] Girmay Medhin,[3] Mistire Wolde,[4] and Desta Kassa[1]

[1] *HIV and TB Research Directorate, Ethiopian Public Health Institute (EPHI), Addis Ababa, Ethiopia*
[2] *Institute of Biomedical Science, College of Health Sciences, Mekelle University, Mekele, Ethiopia*
[3] *Aklilu Lemma Institute of Pathobiology, Addis Ababa University, Addis Ababa, Ethiopia*
[4] *Department of Medical Laboratory Sciences, Addis Ababa University, Addis Ababa, Ethiopia*

Correspondence should be addressed to Gebremedhin Gebremicael; kudus12@gmail.com

Academic Editor: Jochen G. Schneider

Background. Understanding whether the preceding low lipid profile leads to active tuberculosis (TB) or active TB leads to low lipid profile is crucial. *Methods.* Lipid profile concentrations were determined from 159 study participants composed of 93 active TB patients [44 HIV coinfected (HIV+TB+) and 49 HIV negative (HIV−TB+)], 41 tuberculin skin test (TST) positive cases [17 HIV coinfected (HIV+TST+) and 24 HIV negative (HIV−TST+)], and 25 healthy controls (HIV−TST−). Cobas Integra 400 Plus was used to determine lipid profiles concentration level. *Results.* The concentrations of total cholesterol (TC), triglyceride (TG), low-density lipoprotein cholesterol (LDL-C), and high-density lipoprotein cholesterol (HDL-C) in HIV−TB+ patients were significantly lower compared to HIV−TST+ and to HIV−TST− individuals. Similarly, the concentrations of the TC, LDL-C, and HDL-C in HIV+TB+ were significantly lower compared to HIV−TB+ patients. After the 6 months of anti-TB treatment (ATT), the concentration levels of TC, LDL-C, and HDL-C in HIV−TB+ patients were higher compared to the baseline concentration levels, while they were not significantly different compared to that of HIV−TST+ concentration. *Conclusion.* The low concentration of lipid profiles in TB patients may be a consequence of the disease and significantly increased in TB patients after treatment.

1. Introduction

Cholesterol regulates hormones in the body and basic cellular metabolism. LDL and HDL transport cholesterol back and forth between tissues and liver [1]. Cholesterol is used to make fluidic of cell membrane structure, participating in the activity of enzymes and in the functions of phagocytosis and cell growth [2, 3]. Accumulation of cholesterol in the blood vessels narrows the blood tube and causes atherosclerosis [4].

Current recommendations for the treatment of noncommunicable diseases are all geared towards reducing the serum cholesterol levels [5]. However, increasing evidence indicates a link between low blood cholesterol levels and a number of human diseases including tuberculosis (TB) [6]. TB has remained a major global health threat for centuries [7]. About 90–95% of immune-competent latent TB infected persons will not develop TB disease in their lives. Nevertheless, when the immune systems become weak, especially those with HIV infection patients, the developing TB diseases are considerably higher [8]. Hypocholesterolemia promotes the development of TB whereas hypercholesterolemia leads to protection against TB with *Mycobacterium tuberculosis* (Mtb) [9].

Cholesterol in the lymphocyte cell membrane is important for their cytotoxic function [10]. Activated lymphocyte subsets including CD4+, CD8+, and T cells recruit macrophages and release molecules, such as interferon and tumour necrosis factor that render them more efficient in killing Mtb [11]. The inability of macrophages to uptake Mtb due to a low cholesterol content of their cell membrane might constitute a key defect in the host defence system against TB [11]. The level and function of lipids profile were negatively affected by pulmonary TB [12]. TB makes malnutrition worse, and malnutrition weakens immunity, thereby increasing the likelihood that latent TB will develop into active disease [13]. But it is not clear whether the preceding low lipid profile leads to an advancement of the disease or active TB leads to low lipid profile. In Ethiopia, there is not enough data on lipid profiles level in TB patients with and without HIV infection, though there is a study done by Tadewos et al. [14] which assessed the prevalence of dyslipidemia among HIV-infected patients on first-line HAART in Southern Ethiopia. Therefore, the aim of this study was to determine any differences in lipid profile between TB patients with and without HIV infection and controls (latent TB and healthy controls) and to determine the level of lipid profiles in response to TB treatment.

2. Methods

2.1. Study Designs and Populations. An observational study was conducted at St. Peter Specialized TB Hospital, Akaki and Kality Health Centers, Addis Ababa, Ethiopia, between April 2007 and January 2011. A total of 159 adults of both sexes ranging between 15 and 65 years of age were enrolled. Study participants were composed of 93 active TB patients with newly diagnosed tuberculosis (never treated) [44 HIV coinfected (HIV+TB+) and 49 HIV negative (HIV−TB+)], 41 latent TB cases [17 HIV coinfected (HIV+TST+) and 24 HIV negative (HIV−TST+)], and 25 healthy controls (HIV−TST−). At recruitment, all study participants were interviewed using a standard questionnaire and demographic data were collected. A control group of 49 (HIV−TST+ and HIV−TST−) subjects without a prior diagnosis of TB was recruited from the group of individuals who works at Ethiopian Public Health Institute (former name Ethiopian Health and Nutrition Research Institute) as daily labourer without any clinical symptoms or signs of illness due to active TB. The blood plasma was separated from each patient's whole blood at HIV national laboratory and then stored in a deep freezer until use. Demographic data were collected at the baseline during recruitment. Exclusion criteria for enrollment were refusal of HIV testing, pregnancy, comorbidity with diabetes mellitus or chronic bronchitis, receiving steroid therapy, receiving TB and/or HAART treatment (at recruitment or previously), and alcohol or drug abuse that could compromise reliability. All active TB cases confirmed at enrollment were treated according to the national guideline [15].

2.2. Diagnostic Assessments. The HIV status of study participants was determined using the Determine HIV-1/2 (Abbott laboratories, Japan) as the screening test, the Capillus HIV-1/2 (Trinity Biotech, Ireland) as the confirmatory test and Uni-Gold HIV-1/2 recombinant (Trinity Biotech, Ireland) as a tie breaker test [15]. The CD4 T cell count was determined by flow cytometry using a FACSCalibur Flow cytometer (Becton Dickinson, San Jose, USA).

Active TB diagnosis was based on both clinical and bacteriological parameters. At least two sputum smears ("spot-early morning") were required to be positive by microscopy for Acid Fast Bacilli (AFB) using the Ziehl-Neelsen staining method and X-ray positive for those participants presenting with a dry cough [15]. A TST test to detect latent TB infection was performed at baseline visits for all participants except active TB patients according to the national guidelines [15]. A 0.1 ml tuberculin solution (RT23, State Serum Institute, Copenhagen) was injected intradermally into the dorsal surface of the forearm: TST positivity was classified as skin induration diameter $\geq$ 5 mm in HIV-infected individuals while being $\geq$10 mm in HIV negative individuals [15].

2.3. Lipid Profiles Testing. TC, TG, HDL-C, and LDL-C were measured using stored plasma samples separated from fasting blood sample collected from a peripheral vein and Cobas Integra 400 Plus clinical chemistry machine (Roche, Switzerland). Two levels of quality control materials (PreciControl CliniChem Multi 1 and 2, Roche 05 117 208 922, 05 117 291 922) were run prior to sample testing and analysis each day to set instrument sensitivity. In addition, the Cobas Integra 400 Plus instrument at the national reference laboratory was enrolled in an external quality assurance program (EQA- One world Accuracy) to maintain good laboratory practice (GLP). The instrument passed the EQA assessment during the study and during the preceding year of EQA panels. A sample of the individuals with a result of TC < 130 mg/dl, TG < 90 mg/dl, LDL-C < 100 mg/dl, and HDL-C < 40 mg/dl were considered as hypolipidemic while individuals with the result of TC $\geq$ 200, TG $\geq$ 150, LDL-C $\geq$ 130 mg/dl, or HDL-C > 40 mg/dl were classified as hyperlipidemic in both groups [5].

2.4. Statistical Analyses. A Kruskal-Wallis test was used to compare medians between more than two clinical groups, while a two-tailed Wilcoxon rank-sum (Mann–Whitney) test was used to compare two unpaired data items or a Wilcoxon signed-rank test for two paired group data items. A Chi^2 test was used to compare proportions of dichotomous variables across the groups. Logistic regression analysis was performed in patients and controls for factors affecting TB. All data analysis was done using STATA version 11.0 (College Station, Texas, USA). P value of 5% was taken as a cutoff to determine statistical significance.

3. Results

3.1. Characteristics of the Study Population at Baseline. A total of 93 TB patients [49 HIV−TB+ and 44 HIV+TB+], 41 latent TB cases [17 HIV+TST+ and 24 HIV−TST+], and 25 HIV−TST− were included in the study. Table 1 shows the demographic, nutritional, and clinical status of the patients and controls. Malnutrition (Body Mass Index (BMI) < 18.5 kg/m2) was not detected in all study groups. There was no statistically significant difference in the median BMI of the study groups (P value > 0.05). The proportion of patients with the CD4-T cell of less than 200 cells/μl had significant difference among the groups (P = 0.003), and HIV+TB+ and HIV−TB+ individuals had been with the higher proportion (Table 1).

TABLE 1: Baseline study population characteristics.

Characteristics	HIV+TB+ ($n = 44$)	HIV−TB+ ($N = 49$)	HIV+TST+ ($N = 17$)	HIV−TST+ ($N = 24$)	HIV−TST− ($N = 25$)	P value
Demographic data						
Median age, years	30.5 ± 16.2	39 ± 13.8	44 ± 12.9	41 ± 13.3	41 ± 12.9	0.0737
Female, n (%)	21 (48)	24 (49)	8 (47)	11 (46)	12 (48)	0.999
Median of BMI, kg/m2 (IQR)	26.5 (24–28)	27 (23.5–28)	27 (23–29)	27 (24.5–29)	28 (26–30)	0.0641
Nutritional status						
Severe malnutrition, n (%)	0 (0)	0 (0)	0 (0)	0 (0)	0 (0)	
Moderate malnutrition, n (%)	0 (0)	0 (0)	0 (0)	0 (0)	0 (0)	
Mild malnutrition, n (%)	0 (0)	0 (0)	0 (0)	0 (0)	0 (0)	
Normal, n (%)	13 (30)	16 (33)	7 (41)	6 (25)	4 (16)	
Overweight, n (%)	31 (70)	33 (67)	10 (59)	18 (75)	21 (84)	
CD4+ T cell count						
Median CD4+ count (IQR)	180 (112–239.5)	234 (146–345)	200 (146–267)	333 (234–478)	345 (234–401)	**0.0001**
Median CD4+ T cell count ≤ 200, n (%)	24 (42)	19 (33)	6 (11)	3 (5)	5 (9)	**0.003**

Data indicate medians ± standard deviations unless stated otherwise. BMI cutoff of <18. Kg/m^2 was used to define underweight. A CD4+ T cell count cutoff of <200 cells/μl was used to define lymphocytopenia, n (%): number of patients (percentage of patients); BMI: Body Mass Index.

3.2. Lipid Profile Status of Active and Latent TB in HIV Negative Study Groups. The concentrations of four lipid profiles (TC, TG, LDL-C, and HDL-C) were significantly lower in HIV−TB+ compared to HIV−TST+ and HIV−TST−. However, there were no statistically significant differences in concentrations of TC, TG, LDL-C, and HDL-C between HIV−TST+ and HIV−TST− (Table 2(a)).

Table 2(b) shows the proportion of hypolipidemia and hyperlipidemia of the patients and controls. The hypolipidemia of TC, TG, LDL-C, and HDL-C was significantly more prevalent in HIV−TB+ than in HIV−TST+ and HIV−TST− ($P < 0.05$). The proportion of hypolipidemia of all four lipid profiles (TC, TG, LDL-C, and HDL-C) was detected in 44% of HIV−TB+ compared to 3% of HIV−TST+ and 0% of HIV−TST− (Table 2(b)). In the bivariate logistic regression analysis, hypolipidemia of TC, TG, LDL-C, and HDL-C was associated with TB (odds ratio: 2.9, 1.75, 1.64, and 1.89, resp., $P < 0.007$). Hypolipidemia of TC, TG, LDL-C, and HDL-C was not associated with latent TB; this finding could be due to the low numbers of patients with this hypolipidemia.

3.3. The Effect of HIV on the Concentration of Lipid Profile in Active TB and Latent TB Study Participants. The concentrations of the three lipid profiles (TC, LDL-C, and HDL-C) were significantly lower in HIV+TB+ patients compared to HIV−TB+ patients. Moreover, the concentrations of these three lipid profiles were lower in HIV+TST+ patients compared to HIV−TST+ patients (Table 3). There was no significant difference on the concentration level of TG between HIV+TB+ and HIV−TB+ patients and between HIV+TST+ and HIV−TST+ patients (Table 3). The proportion of hypolipidemia of all four lipid profiles (TC, TG, LDL-C, and HDL-C) was detected in 40% of HIV+TB+ patients (Table 2(b)).

3.4. Anti-TB Treatment (ATT) Response on Lipid Profile Concentration in HIV−TB+ Patients. In this study, we assessed also the effect of ATT treatment on the level lipid profiles. Thus, the concentrations of TC, TG, LDL-C, and HDL-C in HIV−TB+ patients were measured at six months (M6) of ATT and compared to the baseline value (M0) of the same patients (HIV−TB+) and with that of apparently healthy control (HIV−TST+ and HIV−TST− groups).

The concentrations of TC, LDL-C, and HDL-C were significantly higher in HIV−TB+ patients at the end of ATT compared to HIV−TB+ patients at baseline, while the concentration of TG was not different between before and after ATT of HIV−TB+ patients (Table 4).

Although baseline concentrations of the lipids were lower in HIV−TB+ individuals compared to HIV−TST+ and HIV−TST− (Table 2(a)); the concentration of all the lipids (TC, TG, LDL-C, and HDL-C) after ATT in HIV−TB+ had no significant difference compared to that of HIV−TST+ groups, while the concentration of all the lipids (TC, TG, LDL-C and HDL-C) remained lower in the HIV−TB+ patients compared to HIV−TST− ($P < 0.05$ for all comparisons). Moreover, the CD4+ T cell count was significantly higher in HIV−TB+ after ATT compared to HIV−TB+ patients at baseline and normalized to the CD4+ T cell count of HIV−TST+ and/or HIV−TST+ at baseline (Table 4).

4. Discussion

This study was conducted to assess any difference in concentration of lipid profiles (TC, TG, LDL-C, and HDL-C) between TB patients with and without HIV infection and latent TB or healthy control individuals and to determine the level of lipid profiles in response to TB treatment.

TABLE 2

(a) Baseline lipid profile levels (mg/dl) among HIV negative study groups (month 0)

Lipid name	HIV−TB+ (n = 49)	HIV−TST+ (n = 24)	HIV−TST− (n = 25)	P value: HIV−TB+ versus HIV−TST+ P value	HIV−TB+ versus HIV−TST− P value	HIV−TST+ versus HIV−TST− P value
TC	108 (87–130)	149 (140.5–162)	158 (150–192)	**<0.001**	**<0.001**	0.119
TG	75 (66–84)	83.5 (73–110.5)	119 (82–119)	**0.027**	**<0.001**	0.180
LDL	59.3 (46.9–73.2)	73.35 (63.8–87.2)	80.4 (73.5–105.1)	**0.001**	**<0.001**	0.072
HDL	26.5 (21.1–31.8)	42.4 (37.05–49.3)	44.7 (37.4–54.6)	**<0.001**	**<0.001**	0.276

Median (interquartile range) micronutrient level values are shown at baseline and significant differences between study groups were determined using Kruskal-Wallis H and Wilcoxon Mann–Whitney test.

(b) The proportional of the abnormality of lipid profile level among study groups at baseline

Lipid name	HIV+TB+ (n = 44)	HIV−TB+ (n = 49)	HIV+TST+ (n = 17)	HIV−TST+ (n = 24)	HIV−TST− (n = 25)	P value using Pearson Chi^2
TC < 130 mg/dl, N (%)	38 (86)	36 (73)	11 (65)	2 (8)	4 (4)	**<0.001**
TC ≥ 200 mg/dl, N (%)	0 (0)	0 (0)	0 (0)	1 (4)	6 (24)	**<0.001**
TG < 90 mg/dl, N (%)	30 (68)	40 (82)	13 (76)	14 (58)	8 (32)	**0.001**
TG ≥ 150 mg/dl, N (%)	0 (0)	0 (0)	0 (0)	2 (8)	2 (8)	0.056
LDL < 100 mg/dl, N (%)	43 (98)	46 (94)	15 (88)	19 (79)	17 (68)	**0.002**
LDL ≥ 130 mg/dl, N (%)	0 (0)	1 (2)	0 (0)	1 (4)	1 (4)	0.652
HDL < 40 mg/dl, N (%)	43 (98)	43 (88)	13 (76)	10 (42)	9 (36)	**<0.001**
HDL > 40 mg/dl, N (%)	1 (2)	6 (12)	4 (24)	14 (58)	16 (64)	**0.000**
TC < 130 & TG < 90 & LDL < 100 & HDL < 40	25 (40)	28 (44)	8 (13)	2 (3)	0 (0)	

TABLE 3: Lipid profile levels (mg/dl) of active TB and latent TB coinfected with HIV compared to without HIV infection.

Lipid name	HIV+TB+ (n = 40)	HIV−TB+ (n = 20)	$^*P$ value	HIV+TST+ (n = 20)	HIV−TST+ (n = 20)	$^‡P$ value
TC	88 (71.5–112)	108 (87–130)	**0.012**	106 (83–140)	149 (140.5–162)	**<0.001**
TG	76 (68–94)	75 (66–84)	0.200	80 (67–89)	83.5 (73–110.5)	0.315
LDL-C	42 (32.45– 63.1)	59.3 (46.9–73.2)	**0.008**	54.2 (41–70.2)	73.35 (63.8–87.2)	**0.004**
HDL-C	17.65 (12.35–22.65)	26.5 (21.1–31.8)	**<0.001**	25.3 (18.1–37.6)	42.4 (37.05– 49.3)	**<0.001**

Median (interquartile range) of lipid profile level values at baseline is shown. Comparison among the groups was determined using Wilcoxon Mann–Whitney test; $^*P$ value for the comparison between active TB groups with and without HIV; $^‡P$ value for the comparison between latent TB groups with and without HIV.

TABLE 4: ATT response on lipid profile concentration in HIV−TB+ patients after treatment.

Lipid profile name	HIV−TB+ at M0	HIV−TB+ at M6	HIV−TST+	HIV−TST−	HIV−TB+ (M6) versus HIV−TB+ (M0) *P* value	HIV−TB+ (M6) versus HIV−TST+ (M0) *P* value	HIV+TB+ (M6) versus HIV−TST− (M0) *P* value
TC	108 (87–130)	137 (122–166)	149 (140.5–162)	158 (150–192)	**0.0000**	0.8638	**0.0047**
TG	75 (66–84)	76 (65–87)	83.5 (73–110.5)	119 (82–119)	0.4212	0.1046	**0.0007**
LDL-C	59.3 (46.9–73.2)	71.2 (56.8–92.4)	73.35 (63.8–87.2)	80.4 (73.5–105.1)	**0.0120**	0.7253	**0.0110**
HDL-C	26.5 (21.1–31.8)	35.9 (32.4–45.1)	42.4 (37.05–49.3)	44.7 (37.4–54.6)	**0.0000**	0.9466	**0.0027**
CD4+	234 (146–345)	345 (234–566)	333 (234–478)	345 (234–401)	**0.0063**	0.4321	0.3865

Median (interquartile range) of lipid profile concentration and CD4+ T-cell count values are shown. Significant differences between HIV−TB+ patients at M0 and M6 were determined using Wilcoxon signed-rank test. Significant differences between HIV−TB+ patients at M6 and HIV−TST+ or HIV−TST− at M0 were determined using Wilcoxon Mann–Whitney test.

At the baseline, our result shows the concentration of lipid profiles (TC, TG, LDL-C, and HDL-C) in HIV negative active TB patients was lower compared to both HIV negative latent TB and healthy controls, while those lipid parameters in latent TB groups were not significantly different from healthy groups.

Low TC, LDL-C, and HDL-C concentrations observed in Ethiopian active TB patients were in line with the studies conducted in Turkey [12], Egypt [16], and Benin [17]. In addition, low cholesterol concentration was observed in the homeless TB patients compared to nonhomeless TB patients and healthy men elsewhere [18]. The low concentration of lipid profiles in patients with pulmonary tuberculosis is correlated with disease severity and improper functioning of the immune system [6, 19]. Our findings showed that 73, 82, 94, and ≈88% of TB patients had low TC, TG, LDL, and HDL-C concentration levels, respectively, at the baseline compared to 4, 32, 68, and 36% of healthy controls. This alerts physicians to encourage regular lipid profile testing. Even though researchers recommend TC, HDL, and LDL concentration levels as biomarkers for pulmonary tuberculosis [20], these parameters are not yet used in Ethiopia. Therefore, our findings suggest the need to test lipid profiles in TB patients at the baseline for better patient management and treatment outcomes. Further research is also warranted to investigate the factors contributed to the lower lipid profile in TB patients as well as investigate the effect of the lower lipid profile in disease severity in TB patients.

We also showed low concentration of TC, LDL-C, and HDL-C in HIV+TB+ patients compared with HIV−TB+ and HIV+TST+ patients compared to HIV−TST+ groups. A study conducted in Nigeria shows the significantly reduced level of HDL-C and TC in HIV positive patients compared with HIV negative controls [21]. This is similar to our result which is lower concentration of HDL-C and TC in HIV+TB+ and HIV+TST+ compared to HIV−TB+ and HIV−TST+, respectively, which might be related to the main feature of AIDS, that is, depletion of CD4+ T cells and inhibiting other immune systems [22]. Active TB and TB-HIV coinfection pose an additional metabolic, physical, and nutritional burden, resulting in further increase in energy expenditure, malabsorption, and micronutrient deficiency [13]. In fact, the combination of malnutrition leading to decreased "supplementation" of lipid and reduction of immune parameters might be representing a pathogenic loop of TB. The Mtb activates invaded macrophages resulting in free radical burst. High serum levels of the free radicals and high concentration of lipid peroxidation products are characteristics of patients with advanced tuberculosis [17, 23, 24]. The peroxidation could cause reduced concentration of serum lipids and tissue inflammation [25]. The previous study demonstrated that the CD4+ T cell and/or FoxP3 gene expression had been correlation with both TC and LDL-C [26]. The increasing of lipid profiles was also stimulation of immune system to increase the white blood cell [27]. Another previous study confirmed that hypercholesterolemia induced an accumulation of regulatory T lymphocytes in the atherosclerotic aorta and spleens in mice, but the expression of functional selectin ligands was decreased [28].

We assessed also the level of lipids in response to ATT. We showed that the concentration level of TC, TG, LDL-C, and HDL-C was significantly increased in ATT treated TB patients at 6 months compared to baseline. The concentration of those lipid parameters in TB patients at the end of ATT treatment was similar compared to concentrations in latent TB infection, while still being significantly lower compared to healthy controls

The finding that TB patients with ATT significantly increased the lipid profile concentration compared to baseline is consistent with the previous findings [17, 28], while the concentration of the lipid profile level in TB patients at the end of ATT treatment was not normalized to the level of healthy controls. The increment of lipid profile concentration after taking ATT treatment in TB patients might be due to the nutritional status and immune function improing [29] and the cleaning of circulating of bacilli in the blood [30]. Our results also showed an increase in lipid concentration levels in ATT treated TB patients which might be related to increasing in CD4 cells from baseline to 6 months' follow-up.

Our findings should be interpreted within the context of the study and its limitations. We used a five-year stored plasma sample which had little effect (≈2% decrement for TC, TG, and HDL-C) of 7 years' stored plasma samples studied in United States of America [31, 32]. We did not collect individual-level dietary history and cannot comment on the role of dietary intake. We do not have data on regional body composition or blood pressure, so we were unable to assess the risk of metabolic syndrome or coronary heart disease or develop predictors for the same in this population; furthermore, we were unable to compare lipid levels with other well-known markers of inflammation (C-reactive protein (CRP) and albumin concentrations) because there is no data from the prospective study. Our follow-up end point at 6 months may not have been enough to assess long-term changes in lipids. The limited sample size may affect the adequate statistic power to test the study hypothesis.

In conclusion, according to our finding, we found that patients with pulmonary TB have low lipid profiles (TC, TG, LDL-C, and HDL-C) that indicate TB diseases might be a risk factor for low lipid profiles at diagnosis time point. These low lipid profiles appear to be correctable to normal levels of HIV−TST+ (but not HIV−TST−) after anti-TB treatment. Further research is needed with larger number of patients with individual-level dietary history and longer follow-up periods in order to provide additional support to this finding.

Ethical Approval

The study obtained ethical clearance from the Scientific and Ethics Research Office (Ref. EHNRI 6.13/01), the Ethiopian Public Health Research Institute, and Addis Ababa University, Department of Medical Laboratory Sciences Ethics Review Committee (Ref. A. A. U/23-5/2014).

Authors' Contributions

Gebremedhin Gebremicael and Yemane Amare were lead authors in planning, implementation of the study, data analysis, writing of the draft, and final version of the manuscript; Feyissa Challa and Atsbeha Gebreegziabxier participated in laboratory tests; Girmay Medhin, Mistire Wolde, and Desta Kassa were involved during data analysis and in writing during the draft interim and final version of the manuscript. All authors have seen and approved the final manuscript.

Acknowledgments

The authors thank all patients who participated in this study, all study nurses involved, and Simret Tesfaye for the data management.

References

[1] J.-Y. Chien, J.-S. Jerng, C.-J. Yu, and P.-C. Yang, "Low serum level of high-density lipoprotein cholesterol is a poor prognostic factor for severe sepsis," *Critical Care Medicine*, vol. 33, no. 8, pp. 1688–1693, 2005.

[2] E. C. Jury, F. Flores-Borja, and P. S. Kabouridis, "Lipid rafts in T cell signalling and disease," *Seminars in Cell & Developmental Biology*, vol. 18, no. 5, pp. 608–615, 2007.

[3] G. van Meer, D. R. Voelker, and G. W. Feigenson, "Membrane lipids: where they are and how they behave," *Nature Reviews Molecular Cell Biology*, vol. 9, no. 2, pp. 112–124, 2008.

[4] J.-X. Song, J.-Y. Ren, and H. Chen, "Primary and secondary hypocholesterolemia," *Beijing Da Xue Xue Bao*, vol. 42, no. 5, pp. 612–615, 2010.

[5] Expert Panel on Detection, Evaluation, and Treatment of High Blood Cholesterol in Adults, "Executive summary of the third report of the National Cholesterol Education Program (NCEP) expert panel on detection, evaluation, and treatment of high blood cholesterol in adults (adult treatment panel III)," *Journal of the American Medical Association*, vol. 285, no. 19, pp. 2486–2497, 2001.

[6] C. Pérez-Guzmán, M. H. Vargas, C. Salas-Mártir et al., "Lipid profile in household contacts of patients with pulmonary tuberculosis," *Revista Médica Del Instituto Mexicano Del Seguro Social*, vol. 46, no. 3, pp. 247-52, 2008.

[7] M. Vitoria, R. Granich, C. F. Gilks et al., "The global fight against HIV/AIDS, tuberculosis, and malaria: current status and future perspectives," *American Journal of Clinical Pathology*, vol. 131, no. 6, pp. 844–848, 2009.

[8] TB Elimination: The Difference between Latent TB Infection and TB Disease, 2011, https://www.cdc.gov/tb/publications/factsheets/general/ltbiandactivetb.pdf.

[9] R. F. Wilson, J. F. Barletta, and J. G. Tyburski, "Hypocholesterolemia in sepsis and critically ill or injured patients," *Critical Care*, vol. 7, no. 6, pp. 413-414, 2003.

[10] M. P. Dabrowski, W. E. Peel, and A. E. R. Thomson, "Plasma membrane cholesterol regulates human lymphocyte cytotoxic function," *European Journal of Immunology*, vol. 10, no. 11, pp. 821–827, 1980.

[11] D. Kaul, P. K. Anand, and I. Verma, "Cholesterol-sensor initiates M. tuberculosis entry into human macrophages," *Molecular and Cellular Biochemistry*, vol. 258, no. 1-2, pp. 219–222, 2004.

[12] O. Deniz, S. Gumus, H. Yaman et al., "Serum total cholesterol, HDL-C and LDL-C concentrations significantly correlate with the radiological extent of disease and the degree of smear positivity in patients with pulmonary tuberculosis," *Clinical Biochemistry*, vol. 40, no. 3-4, pp. 162–166, 2007.

[13] Development United States Agency for International (UNAIDs), *Nutrition and Tuberculosis: A Review of the Literature and Considerations for TB Control Programs*, 2010.

[14] A. Tadewos, Z. Addis, H. Ambachew, and S. Banerjee, "Prevalence of dyslipidemia among HIV-infected patients using first-line highly active antiretroviral therapy in Southern Ethiopia: a cross-sectional comparative group study," *AIDS Research and Therapy*, vol. 9, article no. 31, 2012.

[15] WHO, *Tuberculosis, Leprosy and TB/HIV Prevention and Control Programme Manual*, 4th edition, 2008.

[16] M. M. Metwally and H. A. Raheem, "Lipid profile in tuberculous patients: A preliminary report," *Life Science Journal*, vol. 9, no. 1, pp. 719–722, 2012.

[17] D. C. Akpovi, L. H. S. Gbaguidi, E. Anago et al., "Tuberculosis treatment raises total cholesterol level and restores high density lipoprotein cholesterol (HDLC) in patients with pulmonary tuberculosis," *African Journal of Biotechnology*, vol. 12, no. 41, 2013.

[18] K. Yamanaka, S. Sakai, F. Nomura, T. Akashi, and T. Usui, "A nutritional investigation of homeless patients with tuberculosis," *Kekkaku*, vol. 76, no. 4, pp. 363–370, 2001.

[19] Y. Wondimeneh, D. Muluye, and Y. Belyhun, "Prevalence of Pulmonary tuberculosis and immunological profile of HIV co-infected patients in Northwest Ethiopia," *BMC Research Notes*, vol. 5, article 331, 2012.

[20] O. Y.-C. Lee, I. D. Bull, E. Molnár et al., "Integrated strategies for the use of lipid biomarkers in the diagnosis of ancient mycobacterial disease," in *Proceedings of the 12th Annual Conference of the British Association for Biological Anthropology and Osteoarchaeology*, pp. 63–69, 2012.

[21] O. O. Adewole, S. Eze, Y. Betiku et al., "Lipid profile in HIV/AIDS patients in Nigeria," *African Health Sciences*, vol. 10, no. 2, pp. 144–149, 2010.

[22] A. Pawlowski, M. Jansson, M. Sköld, M. E. Rottenberg, and G. Källenius, "Tuberculosis and HIV co-infection," *PLoS Pathogens*, vol. 8, no. 2, Article ID e1002464, 2012.

[23] V. Wagh, S. Rajopadhye, S. Mukherjee, A. Urhekar, and D. Modi, "Assessment of oxidative stress in serum of pulmonary tuberculosis patients," *International Journal of Research in Medical Sciences*, vol. 4, no. 8, pp. 3328–3332, 2016.

[24] S. O. Oyedeji, N. R. Oguntuase, A. Esan, A. A. Adesina, and O. T. Oke, "Oxidative Stress and Lipid Profile Status in Pulmonary Tuberculosis Patients in South Western Nigeria," *Greener Journal of Medical Sciences*, vol. 3, no. 6, pp. 228–232, 2013.

[25] B. M. Rothschild, L. D. Martin, G. Lev et al., "Mycobacterium tuberculosis complex DNA from an extinct bison dated 17,000 years before the present," *Clinical Infectious Diseases*, vol. 33, no. 3, pp. 305–311, 2001.

[26] L. Guasti, A. M. Maresca, L. Schembri et al., "Relationship between regulatory T cells subsets and lipid profile in dyslipidemic patients: A longitudinal study during atorvastatin treatment," *BMC Cardiovascular Disorders*, vol. 16, no. 1, article no. 26, 2016.

[27] B. A. Rashid, "Relation ship between increased WBC with increased lipid profile in blood," *Diyala Journal of Medicine*, vol. 5, no. 2, pp. 83–90, 2013.

[28] O. A. Iyamu, J. E. Ugheoke, M. O. Ozor et al., "The effect of nutritional lipid supplementation on serum lipid levels and effectiveness of antitubercular chemotherapy," *American Journal of Biomedical Research*, vol. 2, no. 2, pp. 36–41, 2014.

[29] W. M. El-Sadr, C. M. Mullin, A. Carr et al., "Effects of HIV disease on lipid, glucose and insulin levels: results from a large antiretroviral-naïve cohort," *HIV Medicine*, vol. 6, no. 2, pp. 114–121, 2005.

[30] J. M. Cliff, J. S. Lee, N. Constantinou et al., "Distinct phases of blood gene expression pattern through tuberculosis treatment reflect modulation of the humoral immune response," *The Journal of Infectious Diseases*, vol. 207, no. 1, pp. 18–29, 2013.

[31] Y. M. Stokes, C. E. Salmond, L. M. Carpenter, and T. J. Welby, "Stability of total cholesterol, high-density-lipoprotein cholesterol, and triglycerides in frozen sera," *Clinical Chemistry*, vol. 32, no. 6, pp. 995–999, 1986.

[32] S. Cuhadar, M. Koseoglu, A. Atay, and A. Dirican, "The effect of storage time and freeze-thaw cycles on the stability of serum samples," *Biochemia Medica*, vol. 23, no. 1, pp. 70–77, 2013.

33

The Prevalence of Metabolic Syndrome and Its Components among People with Type 2 Diabetes in the Ho Municipality, Ghana

James Osei-Yeboah,[1] William K. B. A. Owiredu,[2,3] Gameli Kwame Norgbe,[4] Sylvester Yao Lokpo,[1] Jones Gyamfi,[1] Emmanuel Alote Allotey,[1] Romeo Asumbasiya Aduko,[1] Mark Noagbe,[5] and Florence A. Attah[6]

[1]*Department of Medical Laboratory Sciences, School of Allied Health Sciences, University of Health and Allied Sciences, Ho, Ghana*
[2]*Department of Molecular Medicine, School of Medical Sciences, Kwame Nkrumah University of Science and Technology, Kumasi, Ghana*
[3]*Department of Clinical Biochemistry, Diagnostic Directorate, Komfo Anokye Teaching Hospital, Kumasi, Ghana*
[4]*School of Allied Health Sciences, University of Health and Allied Sciences, Ho, Ghana*
[5]*Laboratory Department, Ho Municipal Hospital, Ghana Health Service, Ho, Volta Region, Ghana*
[6]*Diabetic Clinic, Ho Municipal Hospital, Ghana Health Service, Ho, Volta Region, Ghana*

Correspondence should be addressed to James Osei-Yeboah; joyeboah@uhas.edu.gh

Academic Editor: Jochen G. Schneider

The cooccurrence of diabetes mellitus and metabolic syndrome potentiates the cardiovascular risk associated with each of the conditions; therefore characterizing metabolic syndrome among people with type 2 diabetes is beneficial for the purpose of cardiovascular disease prevention. This study aims at evaluating the prevalence of metabolic syndrome and its components among 162 patients with type 2 diabetes attending the diabetic clinic of the Ho Municipal Hospital, Ghana. Data obtained included anthropometric indices, blood pressure, serum lipids, glucose, and sociodemographics and clinical information. The overall prevalence of metabolic syndrome among the study population was 43.83%, 63.58%, and 69.14% using the NCEP-ATP III, the WHO, and the IDF criteria, respectively. The most predominant component among the study population was high blood pressure using the NCEP-ATP III (108 (66.67%)) and WHO (102 (62.96)) criteria and abdominal obesity (112 (69.14%)) for IDF criteria. High blood pressure was the most prevalent component among the males while abdominal obesity was the principal component among the females. In this population with type 2 diabetes, high prevalence of metabolic syndrome exists. Gender vulnerability to metabolic syndrome and multiple cluster components were skewed towards the female subpopulation with type 2 diabetes.

1. Introduction

There is a growing interest in a cluster of synergistically interacting cardiovascular risk factors called metabolic syndrome (MetS) [1]. The syndrome has also been described as Insulin Resistance Syndrome, Deadly Quartet, and Syndrome X [2, 3]. The main components associated with the metabolic syndrome include raised blood pressure, dyslipidaemia (raised triglycerides and lowered high density lipoprotein cholesterol), raised fasting glucose, and central/abdominal obesity [1, 4].

Metabolic syndrome is an extremely important parallel risk contributor to heart disease [5]. Isomaa et al. [6] reported a threefold increased risk of coronary heart disease and stroke, as well as markedly increased cardiovascular mortality among subjects with metabolic syndrome. There is a surge in prevalence of many of the attributable components of MetS, causing a worldwide pandemic with implication for both clinical and public health [7]. The available evidence indicates that in most countries, 20% to 30% of the adult population can be characterized as having MetS [7–9].

In Ghana, various studies among various subpopulations have reported different prevalence rates based on different definitive criteria. Among them, Gyakobo et al. [3] reported a prevalence of 35.9% using the International Diabetes Federation (IDF) criteria and 15.0% using the National Cholesterol Education Program Adult Treatment Panel III (NCEP-ATP III) in a rural community. Kow Nanse Arthur et al. [10] reported a prevalence of 14.4%, 25.6%, 29.2%, and 30.4% using the World Health Organization (WHO) criteria, the NCEP-ATP III criteria, the IDF criteria, and the Harmonised Metabolic Syndrome (H_MS) criteria, respectively, among adult females.

Diabetes mellitus is a group of metabolic diseases that is associated with disturbance in the body's metabolism and energy utilization from carbohydrates, lipids, and proteins [11, 12]. Patients with diabetes are prone to complications driven by both modifiable and nonmodifiable risk factors [13]. A strong association between MetS and incident diabetes exists [14]. The cooccurrence of diabetes mellitus and MetS potentiates the cardiovascular risk associated with each condition [15]. Some investigators favour keeping the risk factors separated for purposes of clinical management, whereas others believe that identifying individuals with an aggregation of risk factors provides additional useful information to guide clinical management [4, 16]. Thus characterizing MetS among patients with diabetes is beneficial for multiple risk reduction including lifestyle factors with the ultimate purpose of preventing cardiovascular disease [4, 16].

Among the Ghanaian population with diabetes, predominantly high prevalence of MetS (24–78.8%) has been reported at different locations, with different definitive criteria [1, 13, 17–19]. Due to the influence of genetic and lifestyle factors in the development of MetS, the prevalence and principal components of the syndrome vary among populations [20]. There is a dearth of information in the Ghanaian literature on metabolic syndrome among people with type 2 diabetes within the regional jurisdiction of the current work (Volta region). Using three definitive criteria (NCEP-API III, WHO, and IDF), this study is aimed at evaluating the prevalence of metabolic syndrome (MetS) and its component among people living with type 2 diabetes in the Ho Municipality.

2. Materials and Methods

2.1. Sampling. A hospital-based cross-sectional study was conducted between February 2016 and April 2016. One hundred and sixty-two (162) previously diagnosed patients with type 2 diabetes attending diabetic management clinic at the Ho Municipal Hospital in the Volta Region, Ghana, were conveniently and purposively recruited for this study. The study populations were of consent age (25–86 years) and were all living in the Ho Municipality.

2.2. Sociodemographic Data Capture (Questionnaire). Self-reported semistructured questionnaire was administered to determine duration of diabetes and treatment status, educational level, occupation, smoking status, alcohol intake, sugar intake, fat intake, and physical activity.

2.3. Haemodynamic Parameter

2.3.1. Blood Pressure (BP) Measurement. After participants had sat quietly for at least ten minutes, their blood pressure (BP) measurements were done using the OMRON digital fully automatic blood pressure monitor (OMRON Healthcare, IntelliSense BP785, HEM-7222). Three measurements were taken using an appropriate sized cuff at one-minute interval on the right arm in a seated position, with the arm supported at heart level and feet flat on the floor [21].

2.3.2. Anthropometric Measurements. Using a dual-purpose weight and height scale, body weight of participants was measured to the nearest 0.1 kg and height to the nearest 0.1 cm, with participants standing erect, back straight, heels together, feet slightly spread without shoes, and in light clothing (Health O meter® Professional Scales, 9500 West 55th St. McCook, IL 60525-7110, USA). Waist circumference (to the nearest centimeter) was measured with a Gulick II spring-loaded measuring tape (Gay Mills, WI) midway between the inferior angle of the ribs and the suprailiac crest. The hip circumference was measured as the maximal circumference over the hip circumference (HC) at the level of the widest diameter around the gluteal protuberance in centimeters. Body mass index (BMI) was calculated by dividing weight (kg) by the square of the height (m^2). The waist-to-hip ratio (WHR) was calculated by dividing the waist circumference (cm) by the hip circumference (cm). Waist-to-height ratio was calculated by dividing the waist circumference (cm) by the height (cm). Other calculated adiposity indices were as follows:

(1) Conicity Index (CI) [22]:

$$\text{CI} = \frac{\text{Waist Circumference (m)}}{\left[0.109 \times \sqrt{\text{Weight (Kg)}/\text{Height (m)}}\right]}. \quad (1)$$

(2) Abdominal Volume Index (AVI) [23]:

$$\text{AVI} = \frac{\left[2\,(\text{Waist C (cm)})^2 + 0.7\,(\text{Waist C (cm)} - \text{Hip C (cm)})^2\right]}{1000}. \quad (2)$$

(3) Body Adiposity Index (BAI) [24]:

$$\text{BAI} = \frac{\text{Hip Circumference (cm)}}{[\text{Height (m)}]^{1.5}} - 18. \quad (3)$$

(4) Visceral Adiposity Index (VAI) [23]:

$$\text{Males: VAI} = \frac{\text{Waist Circumference (m)}}{36.58 + (1.89 \times \text{BMI})} \times \frac{\text{TG}}{1.03} \times \frac{1.31}{\text{HDL-C}}$$

$$\text{Females: VAI} = \frac{\text{Waist Circumference (m)}}{36.58 + (1.89 \times \text{BMI})} \times \frac{\text{TG}}{0.81} \times \frac{1.52}{\text{HDL-C}}. \quad (4)$$

2.4. Metabolic Syndrome Diagnosis Criteria

2.4.1. National Cholesterol Education Program, Adult Treatment Panel III (NCEP-ATP III). According to the National Cholesterol Education Programme, Adult Treatment Panel III (NCEP-ATP III), the criteria for the diagnosis of MetS include individuals with any three or more of the following five components: (1) abdominal obesity (waist circumference > 102 cm for men, or > 88 cm for women), (2) high triglyceride (TG) ≥ 1.7 mmol/L, (3) lowered high density lipoprotein cholesterol (HDL-C): men < 0.9 mmol/L or women < 1.0 mmol/L; (4) high blood pressure (BP) (systolic BP ≥ 130 mmHg or diastolic BP ≥ 85 mmHg or treatment of hypertension); and (5) high fasting glucose ≥ 6.1 mmol/L. However all participants were previously diagnosed patients with type 2 diabetes under management and, therefore, were classified as hyperglycaemic irrespective of the level of fasting blood glucose at the time of sampling [25].

2.4.2. International Diabetes Federation (IDF) Criteria. According to the International Diabetes Federation (IDF), MetS can be diagnosed if central obesity (waist measurement > 90 cm for men or >80 cm for women) is accompanied by any two (2) of the following four (4) factors: (1) TG levels ≥ 1.7 mmol/L, (2) HDL-C < 1.03 mmol/L for men or <1.29 mmol/L for women, (3) high blood pressure (BP) of 130/85 mmHg or greater or treatment of previously diagnosed hypertension, and (4) a fasting blood glucose (FBG) of 5.6 mmol/L or greater or previously diagnosed type 2 diabetes [26].

2.4.3. World Health Organization (WHO) Criteria. World Health Organization criteria also require the presence of diabetes mellitus, impaired glucose tolerance or insulin resistance, and any two of the following: (1) body mass index (BMI) ≥ 30 kg/m^2 and/or waist-to-hip ratio >0.90 (male), >0.85 (female); (2) blood pressure ≥140/≥90 mmHg or on hypertension medication; and (3) triglyceride ≥ 1.7 mmol/L and/or HDL-C < 0.91 mmol/L (male), <1.01 mmol/L (female) [27].

2.5. Laboratory Assays. All serum biochemistry assays were carried out at the Ho Municipal Hospital Laboratory using the Random Access Fully Automated Vitalab Selectra Junior Chemistry autoanalyzer (Vital Scientific, BV Kanaalweg 24, Netherlands). After an overnight fast between 7 am and 10 am, about 5 mL venous blood samples was drawn from the antecubital vein of which four (4) milliliters was dispensed into a Vacutainer® serum separator tube using the closed vacutainer system and one (1) mL into fluoride oxalate tubes. The samples were centrifuged at 2500 rpm for 5 minutes to obtain the serum and plasma used for the assays. Using predetermined methods by the reagent manufacturer (ELITech Clinical Systems, SAS, Zone Indusrrielle-61500 SEES, France), the separated plasma and serum were used for the following assays: fasting blood glucose (FBG), total cholesterol (TC), triglyceride, and high density lipoprotein cholesterol. Very low density lipoprotein cholesterol (VLDL-C) and low density lipoprotein cholesterol (LDL-C) were calculated using the Fredrickson-Friedewald formula

$$\text{LDL-C} = \text{TC} - \text{HDL} - \frac{\text{TG}}{2.2}, \qquad (5)$$

where VLDL-C = TG/2.2.

2.6. Statistical Analysis. Normality of all continuous variables was tested. Continuous parametric variables were expressed as their mean ± standard deviation; continuous nonparametric variables were expressed as median (minimum and maximum), whereas categorical variables were expressed as frequency and proportion. Gender comparisons of parameters were performed using unpaired t-tests, Mann–Whitney U test, Chi square (χ^2) test, or Fisher exact test where appropriate. A $p < 0.05$ was considered as statistically significant for all analyses. IBM Statistical Package for the Social Sciences version 22.00 was used for data analysis (SPSS Inc., Chicago, USA; http://www.spss.com).

3. Results

As shown in Table 1, one hundred and sixty-two (162) participants with a mean age of 56.42 ± 10.64 were recruited into this study. Sixty-one (37.65%) were males and 101 (62.35%) were females with matched average ages of 55.93±11.25 and 56.71± 10.29, respectively. The majority of the study participants were married 119 (73.46%), with a higher proportion of the male participants reported married (56 (91.80%)) compared to their female counterparts (63 (62.38%)). A greater proportion (74.69%) of the study participants had attained at least secondary education at the time of this study. The majority (43.40%) of the study participants worked in the informal sector. Intake of dietary salt, sugar, and fat was generally low among the study population (see Table 1).

In general, the female participants presented with significantly higher anthropometric indices than their male counterparts. The exception, however, was seen with height where the males were averagely taller. Weight and waist-to-hip ratio were found to be comparable among the male and the female participants (see Table 2).

There was no significant gender difference in the levels of haemodynamic parameters measured for this study (SP and DP). Among the biochemical parameters assayed, the atherogenic lipid parameters such as total cholesterol, LDL-cholesterol, as well as triglyceride levels were observed to be significantly higher in the female population compared to the male population. Fasting blood glucose levels were found to be similar between both sexes (see Table 3).

The overall prevalence of metabolic syndrome among the study population was 63.58%, 43.83%, and 69.14% using the World Health Organization (WHO), the National Cholesterol Education Program, Adult Treatment Panel III (NCEP-ATP III), and the International Diabetes Federation (IDF) criteria, respectively. The prevalence was significantly higher among women using the WHO and the IDF criteria. However no statistical difference was observed between genders when the NCEP-ATP III criteria were used (Table 4).

Table 1: Sociodemographic characteristics of the population under study stratified by gender.

Parameter	Total	Male	Female
Total respondents	162 (100)	61 (37.65)	101 (62.35)
Age	56.42 ± 10.64	55.93 ± 11.25	56.71 ± 10.29
Marital status			
Married	119 (73.46)	56 (91.80)	63 (62.38)
Single	43 (26.54)	5 (8.20)	38 (37.62)
Education background			
None	10 (6.17)	1 (1.64)	9 (8.91)
Basic	31 (19.14)	8 (13.11)	23 (22.77)
Secondary	69 (42.59)	21 (34.43)	48 (47.53)
Tertiary	52 (32.10)	31 (50.82)	21 (20.79)
Occupation			
None	49 (30.82)	16 (27.59)	33 (32.67)
Informal	69 (43.40)	20 (34.48)	49 (48.52)
Formal	41 (25.78)	22 (37.93)	19 (18.81)
Salt intake			
None	131 (82.39)	46 (79.31)	85 (84.16)
Moderate	25 (15.72)	9 (15.52)	16 (15.84)
High	3 (1.89)	3 (5.17)	0 (0.00)
Sugar intake			
None	127 (80.89)	42 (72.41)	85 (85.86)
Moderate	4 (2.55)	2 (3.45)	2 (2.02)
High	26 (16.56)	14 (24.14)	12 (12.12)
Fat intake			
None	137 (86.71)	52 (89.65)	85 (85.00)
Moderate	10 (6.33)	2 (3.45)	8 (8.00)
High	11 (6.96)	4 (6.90)	7 (7.00)

Data are presented as frequency with percentage in parenthesis or mean ± standard deviation.

Table 2: Anthropometric parameters of patients with type 2 diabetes seeking care at the Ho Municipal Hospital stratified by gender.

Parameter	Total	Male	Female	p value
Weight (Kg)	73.08 ± 14.26	71.59 ± 13.5	73.98 ± 14.69	0.3040
Height (m)	1.64 ± 0.08	1.69 ± 0.07	1.60 ± 0.08	<0.0001
BMI (Kg/m^2)	27.46 ± 5.88	25.09 ± 4.55	28.89 ± 6.15	<0.0001
WC (cm)	93.52 ± 13.33	89.03 ± 10.01	96.24 ± 14.35	0.0014
HC (cm)	102.67 ± 15.48	98.79 ± 14.85	105.02 ± 15.45	0.0135
WHR	0.92 ± 0.08	0.91 ± 0.09	0.92 ± 0.07	0.5492
WHtR	0.57 ± 0.09	0.53 ± 0.06	0.60 ± 0.1	<0.0001
CI	1.29 ± 0.11	1.26 ± 0.09	1.30 ± 0.11	0.0140
AVI	18.00 ± 5.07	16.28 ± 3.51	19.04 ± 5.58	0.0017
BAI	31.39 ± 8.91	27.15 ± 7.69	33.94 ± 8.64	<0.0001
VAI	1.62 (0.30–7.89)	1.07 (0.30–6.01)	2.01 (0.42–7.89)	0.0231

Data are presented as mean ± standard deviation of the mean or median with minimum and maximum in parenthesis. BMI: body mass index, WC: waist circumference, HC: hip circumference, WHR: waist-to-hip ratio, WHtR: waist-to-height ratio, CI: Conicity Index, AVI: Abdominal Volume Index, BAI: Body Adiposity Index, and VAI: Visceral Adiposity Index.

Among the study population, there was no individual without a metabolic score, irrespective of the definitive criteria used. Also, there was no individual who had three or more metabolic syndrome scores but did not present with metabolic syndrome (see Table 4).

The prevalence of abdominal obesity was 48.15% using the NCEP-ATP III criteria and 69.14% using the IDF criteria. Using the WHO criteria, 30.86% of the study participants were classified as having central obesity. Abdominal/central obesity irrespective of the criteria used was found to be predominant among the female participants (Table 5).

Comorbidity of diabetes with hypertension ranged from 62.96% to 66.67% using the WHO and the IDF/NCEP-ATP III, respectively. No gender variation of diabetes with

TABLE 3: Haemodynamic and biochemical parameters of study population stratified by gender.

Parameter	Total	Male	Female	*p* value
SP	129.42 ± 20.07	129.72 ± 20.17	129.24 ± 20.11	0.8820
DP	79.15 ± 11.37	79.51 ± 11.46	78.93 ± 11.37	0.7550
FBG	7.35 ± 1.93	7.16 ± 2.12	7.47 ± 1.82	0.9870
Total cholesterol	4.90 ± 1.36	4.49 ± 1.17	5.15 ± 1.41	0.0030
Triglyceride	1.11 (0.38–5.30)	0.97 (0.38–4.46)	1.23 (0.42–5.30)	0.0110
HDL	1.25 ± 0.38	1.25 ± 0.44	1.25 ± 0.34	0.9740
LDL	3.02 ± 1.07	2.71 ± 0.99	3.21 ± 1.07	0.0030
VLDL	0.51 (0.17–2.03)	0.44 (0.17–2.03)	0.56 (0.19–1.66)	0.0120

Data is presented as mean ± standard deviation of the mean and median with minimum and maximum in parenthesis. SP: systolic blood pressure, DP: diastolic blood pressure, FBG: fasting blood glucose, HDL: high density lipoprotein, LDL: low density lipoprotein, and VLDL: very low density lipoprotein.

TABLE 4: Prevalence of metabolic syndrome and metabolic score among the population stratified by gender.

Parameters	Total $N = 162$	Male $N = 61$	Female $N = 101$	*p* value
Prevalence of metabolic syndrome				
WHO	103 (63.58)	32 (52.46)	71 (70.30)	0.0285
NCEP-ATP III	71 (43.83)	26 (42.62)	45 (44.55)	0.8708
IDF	112 (69.14)	24 (39.34)	88 (87.13)	<0.0001
Prevalence of clustering of one or more components of metabolic syndrome				
WHO				
1	10 (6.17)	6 (9.84)	4 (3.96)	
2	49 (30.25)	23 (37.70)	26 (25.74)	0.7306
>2 without MetS	0 (0.00)	0 (0.00)	0 (0.00)	
NCEP-ATP III				
1	13 (8.02)	8 (13.12)	5 (4.95)	
2	78 (48.15)	27 (44.26)	51 (50.50)	0.1208
>2 without MetS	0 (0.00)	0 (0.00)	0 (0.00)	
IDF				
1	50 (30.86)	37 (60.66)	13 (12.87)	<0.0001
>2 without MetS	0 (0.00)	0 (0.00)	0 (0.00)	

Data is presented as frequency with corresponding percentage in parenthesis. WHO: World Health Organization, NCEP ATP III: National Cholesterol Education Program, Adult Treatment Panel III, IDF: International Diabetes Federation, and MetS: metabolic syndrome. *p* is significant at 0.05.

hypertension comorbidity was observed. Atherogenic levels of triglyceride were significantly tilted towards the female (see Table 5).

4. Discussion

The prevalence of metabolic syndrome (MetS) is increasing worldwide in both developing and developed countries [28, 29]. In the current study, the overall prevalence of metabolic syndrome observed among the study population was 43.83%, 63.58%, and 69.14% using NCEP-ATP III, WHO, and IDF criteria, respectively. Irrespective of the criteria used, there was no individual who possessed three or more metabolic scores and yet did not have metabolic syndrome. This is in agreement with earlier reports indicating that metabolic syndrome is a common phenomenon among the Ghanaian type 2 diabetes mellitus population. The prevalence of metabolic syndrome among people with type 2 diabetes in the Ghanaian population ranged within 43.3% NCEP-ATP III [19], 43.4% NCEP-ATP III, and 51.8% IDF [18] and 55.9% NCEP-ATP III [1], 58% NCEP-ATP III [13], and 78.8% WHO [18]. Similar reports in other jurisdictions of high prevalence rates of metabolic syndrome (63.6%, 51%, and 56%) have been recorded among people with type 2 diabetes, respectively, in North-Central Nigeria and Saudi Arabia [30–32]. The prevalence of metabolic syndrome was significantly higher in women than in men using the WHO and IDF criteria. The observation compares favourably with that of Titty et al. [1] and Nsiah et al. [13] where femininity accounted for higher metabolic syndrome scores. Similarly, a study in South-Western Nigeria reported a female preponderance to metabolic syndrome in a ratio of 3 : 2 to males among the people living with type 2 diabetes using the WHO criteria [32]. In contrast, observations in Jos, North-Central Nigeria, and the United States of America using the IDF definitive criteria revealed significantly higher occurrence of metabolic syndrome among the male subpopulation with diabetes compared to their female counterparts [30, 33]. The use of

TABLE 5: Prevalence of the various components of metabolic syndrome among the study population stratified by gender.

Parameter	Total	Male	Female	p value
NCEP-ATP III				
Abdominal obesity	78 (48.15)	5 (8.20)	73 (72.28)	<0.0001
Raised TG	27 (16.67)	4 (6.56)	23 (22.77)	0.0083
Reduced HDL	38 (23.46)	15 (24.59)	23 (22.77)	0.8491
High blood pressure	108 (66.67)	39 (63.93)	69 (68.32)	0.6079
WHO				
Central obesity	50 (30.86)	8 (13.11)	42 (41.58)	0.0001
Raised TG	27 (16.67)	4 (6.56)	23 (22.77)	0.0083
Reduced HDL	40 (24.69)	17 (27.87)	23 (22.77)	0.5731
High blood pressure	102 (62.96)	36 (59.02)	66 (65.35)	0.5021
IDF				
Abdominal obesity	112 (69.14)	24 (39.34)	88 (87.13)	<0.0001
Raised TG	27 (16.67)	4 (6.56)	23 (22.77)	0.0083
Reduced HDL	77 (47.53)	24 (39.34)	53 (52.48)	0.1437
High blood pressure	108 (66.67)	39 (63.93)	69 (68.32)	0.6079

Data is presented as frequency with corresponding percentage in parenthesis. TG: triglyceride, HDL: high density lipoprotein, WHO: World Health Organization, NCEP-ATP III: National Cholesterol Education Program, Adult Treatment Panel III, and IDF: International Diabetes Federation. p is significant at 0.05.

different diagnostic criteria for the definition of metabolic syndrome has been shown to account for the inconsistency in gender ratios observed in various populations [30].

The most predominant component of MetS abnormality among the study population was high blood pressure using the NCEP-ATP III (66.67%) and the WHO (62.96) criteria and abdominal obesity (69.14%) using the IDF criteria. Consistent with the findings of this study, Puepet et al. [30], Unadike et al. [34], and Nsiah et al. [13] have reported similar findings. Hypertension is identified as an independent cardiovascular risk factor and, in combination with insulin resistance, will have a synergistic effect which results in a grave risk for severe vascular events [34]. Abdominal/central obesity is associated with high amount of visceral fat, which is metabolically active, producing free fatty acids and inflammatory cytokines that drain directly into the liver via the portal circulation [20, 35]. This could elicit various complex injurious mechanisms leading to atherosclerosis and cardiovascular disease [35, 36].

Compared to previous studies in Ghanaian populations with diabetes, one of the strengths of the current study is the expanded scope of anthropometric parameters to include less commonly used candidate adiposity indices in this setting (Conicity Index, Abdominal Volume Index, Body Adiposity Index, and Visceral Adiposity Index). In general, the female subpopulation presented with significantly higher average anthropometric indices than their male counterparts (Table 2). The leading component of the MetS among the females with diabetes was abdominal/central obesity (Table 5). A previous study has recorded significantly higher measurements of obesity and adiposity among the females with type 2 diabetes compared to their male counterparts [16]. Though the reasons for this occurrence could not be directly inferred from the current study, gender disparities in obesity are influenced by acculturation through complex sociocultural pathways that are known to facilitate female weight gain in developing countries like those found in sub-Saharan Africa [37]. According to Nsiah et al. [13] women in Ghana are less likely to participate in physical exercises and live sedentary lifestyles than men and this may account for the odds of higher obesity and overweight.

Dyslipidaemia has been commonly demonstrated in subjects with metabolic syndrome [38]. The altered lipid levels associated with atherogenic dyslipidaemia are individual and collective risk factors for cardiovascular diseases [39]. Among the biochemical parameters assayed in this study, the atherogenic lipid parameters such as total cholesterol (TC), low density lipoprotein cholesterol (LDL-C), and triglyceride (TG) levels were found to be significantly higher among the female participants compared to their male counterparts (Table 3). This, however, contradicts the report by Gilani et al. [40]. In explaining the gender difference in lipid-lowering treatment outcome among the Chinese population, Zhang et al. [41] reported the biological baseline gender disparities in lipid levels as an attributed factor.

Though the mechanism of dyslipidaemia in persons with glycaemic dysregulation is not fully elucidated, there is compelling evidence implicating insulin resistance [42, 43]. Among the constellation of effects in an insulin resistant state is reduced suppression of lipolysis in adipose tissue, leading to a high free fatty acid influx and increased hepatic very low density lipoprotein (VLDL) secretion, thus causing hypertriglyceridemia and reduced plasma levels of high density lipoprotein (HDL) cholesterol [44].

5. Conclusion

In this population of people living with diabetes, high prevalence of metabolic syndrome exists. Gender vulnerability to metabolic syndrome and multiple cluster components are tilted towards the female subpopulation with diabetes.

Ethical Approval

Ethical approval for the study was granted by the facility authorized committee in a letter (HMH/G-207 [Vol3]). The study was anonymous and nonlinked. Confidentiality of participant's information was assured and no patient was denied the appropriate care for declining to participate in this study.

Competing Interests

The authors have declared that no competing interests exist.

Authors' Contributions

This work was carried out with collaboration between all authors. Authors James Osei-Yeboah, William K. B. A. Owiredu, Gameli Kwame Norgbe, Sylvester Yao Lokpo, Jones Gyamfi, Emmanuel Alote Allotey, Romeo Asumbasiya Aduko, Mark Noagbe, and Florence A. Attah conceptualized and designed the study. Authors James Osei-Yeboah, Sylvester Yao Lokpo, Emmanuel Alote Allotey, Romeo Asumbasiya Aduko, Mark Noagbe, and Florence A. Attah recruited participants and generated the data. Authors James Osei-Yeboah, William K. B. A. Owiredu, Gameli Kwame Norgbe, Sylvester Yao Lokpo, Jones Gyamfi, Emmanuel Alote Allotey, and Romeo Asumbasiya Aduko analyzed the data. Authors James Osei-Yeboah, William K. B. A. Owiredu, Gameli Kwame Norgbe, Sylvester Yao Lokpo, Jones Gyamfi, Emmanuel Alote Allotey, Romeo Asumbasiya Aduko, Mark Noagbe, and Florence A. Attah drafted the manuscript. Authors James Osei-Yeboah, William K. B. A. Owiredu, Gameli Kwame Norgbe, Sylvester Yao Lokpo, Jones Gyamfi, Emmanuel Alote Allotey, Romeo Asumbasiya Aduko, Mark Noagbe, and Florence A. Attah reviewed the manuscript for intellectual content and each author approved the final manuscript.

Acknowledgments

The authors acknowledge the help they received from the diabetic clinic and laboratory scientists at the Ho Municipal Hospital in conducting this study.

References

[1] F.-V. K. Titty, W. K. B. A. Owiredu, and M. T. Agyei-Frempong, "Prevalence of metabolic syndrome and its individual components among diabetic patients in Ghana," *Journal of Biological Sciences*, vol. 8, no. 6, pp. 1057–1061, 2008.

[2] J. Akpalu, A. Akpalu, and F. Ofei, "The metabolic syndrome among patients with cardiovascular disease in Accra, Ghana," *Ghana Medical Journal*, vol. 45, no. 4, pp. 161–166, 2011.

[3] M. Gyakobo, A. G. B. Amoah, D.-A. Martey-Marbell, and R. C. Snow, "Prevalence of the metabolic syndrome in a rural population in Ghana," *BMC Endocrine Disorders*, vol. 12, article no. 25, 2012.

[4] K. G. M. M. Alberti, R. H. Eckel, S. M. Grundy et al., "Harmonizing the metabolic syndrome: a joint interim statement of the international diabetes federation task force on epidemiology and prevention; national heart, lung, and blood institute; American heart association; world heart federation; international atherosclerosis society; and international association for the study of obesity," *Circulation*, vol. 120, no. 16, pp. 1640–1645, 2009.

[5] M. Larkin, ""Metabolic syndrome" targeted in new US cholesterol guidelines," *The Lancet*, vol. 357, no. 9268, p. 1594, 2001.

[6] B. Isomaa, P. Almgren, T. Tuomi et al., "Cardiovascular morbidity and mortality associated with the metabolic syndrome," *Diabetes Care*, vol. 24, no. 4, pp. 683–689, 2001.

[7] S. M. Grundy, "Metabolic syndrome pandemic," *Arteriosclerosis, Thrombosis, and Vascular Biology*, vol. 28, no. 4, pp. 629–636, 2008.

[8] J. V. van Vliet-Ostaptchouk, M.-L. Nuotio, S. N. Slagter et al., "The prevalence of metabolic syndrome and metabolically healthy obesity in Europe: a collaborative analysis of ten large cohort studies," *BMC Endocrine Disorders*, vol. 14, no. 1, article 9, 13 pages, 2014.

[9] B. Xi, D. He, Y. Hu, and D. Zhou, "Prevalence of metabolic syndrome and its influencing factors among the Chinese adults: the China Health and Nutrition Survey in 2009," *Preventive Medicine*, vol. 57, no. 6, pp. 867–871, 2013.

[10] F. Kow Nanse Arthur, M. Adu-Frimpong, J. Osei-Yeboah, F. Obu Mensah, and L. Owusu, "The prevalence of metabolic syndrome and its predominant components among pre-and postmenopausal Ghanaian women," *BMC Research Notes*, vol. 6, no. 1, article no. 446, 2013.

[11] L. Siva, S. Mythili, J. Rani, and P. S. Kumar, "Biochemical and haematological aberrations in type I and type II diabetic patients in South India-a comparative study," *International Journal of Research in Pharmaceutical and Biomedical Sciences*, vol. 3, no. 2, pp. 967–977, 2012.

[12] C. Varım, T. Kaya, A. Nalbant, A. Uçar, and A. Tamer, "Effects of glucose control on hematological indices in patients with diabetes mellitus," *Macedonian Journal of Medical Sciences*, vol. 7, no. 1, pp. 83–88, 2014.

[13] K. Nsiah, V. Shang, K. Boateng, and F. Mensah, "Prevalence of metabolic syndrome in type 2 diabetes mellitus patients," *International Journal of Applied and Basic Medical Research*, vol. 5, no. 2, p. 133, 2015.

[14] J.-A. Shin, J.-H. Lee, S.-Y. Lim et al., "Metabolic syndrome as a predictor of type 2 diabetes, and its clinical interpretations and usefulness," *Journal of Diabetes Investigation*, vol. 4, no. 4, pp. 334–343, 2013.

[15] N. D. Wong, J. C. Nelson, T. Granston et al., "Metabolic syndrome, diabetes, and incidence and progression of coronary calcium: the Multiethnic Study of Atherosclerosis study," *JACC: Cardiovascular Imaging*, vol. 5, no. 4, pp. 358–366, 2012.

[16] A. P. Kengne, S. N. Limen, E. Sobngwi, C. F. T. Djouogo, and C. Nouedoui, "Metabolic syndrome in type 2 diabetes: comparative prevalence according to two sets of diagnostic

criteria in sub-Saharan Africans," *Diabetology and Metabolic Syndrome*, vol. 4, article 22, 2012.

[17] V. Mogre, Z. S. Salifu, and R. Abedandi, "Prevalence, components and associated demographic and lifestyle factors of the metabolic syndrome in type 2 diabetes mellitus," *Journal of Diabetes and Metabolic Disorders*, vol. 13, no. 1, article no. 80, 2014.

[18] N. Amidu, W. K. Owiredu, H. Alidu, C. Sarpong, C. K. Gyasi-Sarpong, and L. Quaye, "Association between metabolic syndrome and sexual dysfunction among men with clinically diagnosed diabetes," *Diabetology and Metabolic Syndrome*, vol. 5, no. 1, article no. 42, 2013.

[19] F.-V. K. Titty, "Glycaemic control, dyslipidaemia and metabolic syndrome among recently diagnosed diabetes mellitus patients in tamale teaching hospital, Ghana," *West African Journal of Medicine*, vol. 29, no. 1, pp. 8–11, 2010.

[20] W. Owiredu, N. Amidu, E. Gockah-Adapoe, and R. Ephraim, "The prevalence of metabolic syndrome among active sportsmen/sportswomen and sedentary workers in the Kumasi metropolis," *Journal of Science and Technology (Ghana)*, vol. 31, no. 1, 2011.

[21] I. K. Owusu, C. Aryee, W. K. Owiredu, J. Osei-Yeboah, E. Owusu-Dabo, and E. F. Laing, "Analysis of atherogenic and anthropometric profiles of normotensive and hypertensive ghanaians in the kumasi metropolis," *British Journal of Medicine and Medical Research*, vol. 7, no. 5, pp. 378–397, 2015.

[22] M. Ruperto, G. Barril, and F. J. Sánchez-Muniz, "Conicity index as a contributor marker of inflammation in haemodialysis patients," *Nutricion Hospitalaria*, vol. 28, no. 5, pp. 1688–1695, 2013.

[23] M. Vuga, "Conceptual review of issues with practical abdominal obesity measures," in *JSM Section on Statistics in Epidemiology*, 2009.

[24] R. Lategan, V. L. Van den Berg, and C. M. Walsh, "Body adiposity indices are associated with hypertension in a black, urban Free State community: original research," *African Primary Health Care and Family Medicine*, vol. 6, no. 1, pp. 1–7, 2014.

[25] C. M. Alexander, P. B. Landsman, S. M. Teutsch, and S. M. Haffner, "NCEP-defined metabolic syndrome, diabetes, and prevalence of coronary heart disease among NHANES III participants age 50 years and older," *Diabetes*, vol. 52, no. 5, pp. 1210–1214, 2003.

[26] E. S. Ford, "Prevalence of the metabolic syndrome defined by the international diabetes federation among adults in the U.S.," *Diabetes Care*, vol. 28, no. 11, pp. 2745–2749, 2005.

[27] K. G. M. M. Alberti, P. Zimmet, and J. Shaw, "Metabolic syndrome—a new world-wide definition. A consensus statement from the International Diabetes Federation," *Diabetic Medicine*, vol. 23, no. 5, pp. 469–480, 2006.

[28] X. Ruan and Y. Guan, "Metabolic syndrome and chronic kidney disease," *Journal of Diabetes*, vol. 1, no. 4, pp. 236–245, 2009.

[29] M. Aguilar, T. Bhuket, S. Torres, B. Liu, and R. J. Wong, "Prevalence of the metabolic syndrome in the United States, 2003–2012," *JAMA*, vol. 313, no. 19, pp. 1973–1974, 2015.

[30] F. Puepet, A. Uloko, I. Akogu, and E. Aniekwensi, "Prevalence of the metabolic syndrome among patients with type 2 diabetes mellitus in urban North-Central Nigeria," *African Journal of Endocrinology and Metabolism*, vol. 8, no. 1, 2009.

[31] D. Akbar, "Metabolic syndrome is common in Saudi type 2 diabetic patients," *Hypertension*, vol. 12, no. 2, pp. 47–49, 2002.

[32] O. Adediran, A. Edo, A. Jimoh, and A. Ohwovoriole, "Prevalence of the metabolic syndrome among Nigerians with type 2 diabetes," *Diabetes International*, vol. 15, no. 1, pp. 13–14, 2007.

[33] E. S. Ford, W. H. Giles, and A. H. Mokdad, "Increasing prevalence of the metabolic syndrome among U.S. adults," *Diabetes Care*, vol. 27, no. 10, pp. 2444–2449, 2004.

[34] B. Unadike, N. Akpan, E. Peters, I. Essien, and O. Essien, "Prevalence of the metabolic syndrome among patients with type 2 diabetes mellitus in Uyo, Nigeria," *African Journal of Endocrinology and Metabolism*, vol. 8, no. 1, 2009.

[35] L. W. Johnson and R. S. Weinstock, "The metabolic syndrome: concepts and controversy," *Mayo Clinic Proceedings*, vol. 81, no. 12, pp. 1615–1620, 2006.

[36] G. T.-C. Ko, C. S. Cockram, C.-C. Chow et al., "High prevalence of metabolic syndrome in Hong Kong Chinese - Comparison of three diagnostic criteria," *Diabetes Research and Clinical Practice*, vol. 69, no. 2, pp. 160–168, 2005.

[37] R. Kanter and B. Caballero, "Global gender disparities in obesity: a review," *Advances in Nutrition*, vol. 3, no. 4, pp. 491–498, 2012.

[38] C. I. Okafor, "The metabolic syndrome in Africa: current trends," *Indian Journal of Endocrinology and Metabolism*, vol. 16, no. 1, pp. 56–66, 2012.

[39] H. N. Ginsberg and P. R. MacCallum, "The obesity, metabolic syndrome, and type 2 diabetes mellitus pandemic: part I. Increased cardiovascular disease risk and the importance of atherogenic dyslipidemia in persons with the metabolic syndrome and type 2 diabetes mellitus," *Journal of the CardioMetabolic Syndrome*, vol. 4, no. 2, pp. 113–119, 2009.

[40] S. Y. Gilani, S. Bibi, N. Ahmed, and S. R. Shah, "Gender differences of dyslipidemia in type 2 diabetics," *Journal of Ayub Medical College, Abbottabad : JAMC*, vol. 22, no. 3, pp. 146–148, 2010.

[41] R. Zhang, L. Zhao, L. Liang, G. Xie, and Y. Wu, "Factors explaining the gender disparity in lipid-lowering treatment goal attainment rate in Chinese patients with statin therapy," *Lipids in Health and Disease*, vol. 11, article no. 59, 2012.

[42] S. J. Robins, A. Lyass, J. P. Zachariah, J. M. Massaro, and R. S. Vasan, "Insulin resistance and the relationship of a dyslipidemia to coronary heart disease: the framingham heart study," *Arteriosclerosis, Thrombosis, and Vascular Biology*, vol. 31, no. 5, pp. 1208–1214, 2011.

[43] J. D. Brunzell and J. E. Hokanson, "Dyslipidemia of central obesity and insulin resistance," *Diabetes Care*, vol. 22, no. 3, pp. C10–C13, 1999.

[44] R. K. Avramoglu, H. Basciano, and K. Adeli, "Lipid and lipoprotein dysregulation in insulin resistant states," *Clinica Chimica Acta*, vol. 368, no. 1-2, pp. 1–19, 2006.

34

Hierarchical Modeling of Patient and Physician Determinants of Blood Pressure Outcomes in Hypertensive Patients with and without Diabetes: Pooled Analysis of Six Observational Valsartan Studies with 15,282 Evaluable Patients

Noha Ashy,[1,2] Thanh-Nga Nguyen,[2,3] Kris Denhaerynck,[4,5,6] Mahdi Gharaibeh,[2] Abdulaziz Alhossan,[2,7] Stefaan Vancayzeele,[8] Heidi Brié,[8] Ann Aerts,[9] Karen MacDonald,[4] and Ivo Abraham[2,4,10,11]

[1] *College of Pharmacy, King Abdulaziz University, P.O. Box 80200, Jeddah 21589, Saudi Arabia*
[2] *Center for Health Outcomes and PharmacoEconomic Research, University of Arizona, 1295 N Martin, Tucson, AZ 85721, USA*
[3] *College of Pharmacy, University of Wyoming, 1000 E University Ave, Laramie, WY 82071, USA*
[4] *Matrix45, 6159 W Sunset Rd, Tucson, AZ, USA*
[5] *Institute of Nursing Science, University of Basel, Bernoullistrasse 29, 4001 Basel, Switzerland*
[6] *Cardiovascular Research Institute Basel, University Hospital Basel, Spitalstrasse 2, 4056 Basel, Switzerland*
[7] *College of Pharmacy, King Saud University, P.O. Box 89885, Riyadh 11692, Saudi Arabia*
[8] *Novartis Pharma, Medialaan 40, 1800 Vilvoorde, Belgium*
[9] *Novartis Foundation, Novartis Campus, Forum 1-3.97, 4002 Basel, Switzerland*
[10] *Department of Pharmacy Practice and Science, College of Pharmacy, University of Arizona, 1295 N Martin, Tucson, AZ 85721, USA*
[11] *Department of Family and Community Medicine, College of Medicine-Tucson, University of Arizona, 1295 N Martin, Tucson, AZ 85721, USA*

Correspondence should be addressed to Ivo Abraham; abraham@pharmacy.arizona.edu

Academic Editor: Jochen G. Schneider

We pooled data from 6 valsartan-related studies including 3,658 diabetic and 11,624 nondiabetic patients to evaluate blood pressure (BP) outcomes after approximately 90 days of second- or later-line valsartan treatment. Hierarchical linear and logistic regressions were applied to identify determinants of BP outcomes. Similar reductions in BP values and similar BP control rates were achieved in both groups after approximately 90 days of therapy. The modeling analyses identified several common and different patient- and physician-related determinants of BP outcomes for both groups, many of which are modifiable or clinically manageable. Through varying in terms of association and influence between the diabetic and nondiabetic groups, patient-related determinants included age, BP at diagnosis of hypertension, risk factors, valsartan regimen, concomitant antihypertensive treatment, and adherence; and physician-related determinants included gender, years in practice, and hypertension management. In summary, in both diabetic and nondiabetic patients, the use of valsartan-centric treatment regimens in second- or later-line antihypertensive treatment is associated with significant reductions in BP level and improvement in BP control. The determinants identified in modeling provide guidance to clinicians in the common and differential management of hypertension in diabetic and nondiabetic patients.

1. Introduction

Hypertension and glucose intolerance are highly associated chronic conditions. Over two-thirds of diabetic patients have elevated blood pressure [1]. Diabetes and hypertension have long been known to be major risk factors for cardiovascular mortality and morbidity [2]. Diabetes increases the risk of cardiovascular disease twofold to threefold, while high blood pressure (BP) is associated with a 72% rise in all-cause mortality risk and a 57% rise of cardiovascular events in diabetic individuals [3, 4].

For long, the recommended systolic blood pressure (SBP) and diastolic blood pressure (DBP) targets were <140 mmHg and <90 mmHg for nondiabetic patients but <130 mmHg and <80 mmHg for diabetic patients. The most recent European [5] and North American [6] guidelines now recommend SBP < 140 mmHg and DBP < 90 mmHg in the general adult population for both diabetic and nondiabetic patients. It is more difficult to achieve blood pressure control in diabetic patients [5], but the revised targets for these patients have resulted in nominally higher BP control rates in this population.

We have conducted seven observational studies on real-world practice patterns and associated outcomes in patients with hypertension treated for approximately 90 days (hereafter "90 days") with valsartan (Novartis, Basel, Switzerland), an angiotensin receptor blocker [7]. All patients were treated by general practitioners (GPs) in Belgium in second- or later-line antihypertensive therapy because prior antihypertensive treatment failed or was not tolerated. Because of similarities in design and data model, in particular the assessment of medication adherence, we pooled six of these studies to yield a data set of 15,282 evaluable patients recruited by 2,832 general practitioners (GPs) (Table 1). Of these patients, 3,658 (23.9%) had a diagnosis of either type 1 or type 2 diabetes mellitus.

Lowering blood pressure and especially achieving blood pressure control are more difficult in diabetic than in nondiabetic patients, as both randomized controlled trials and observational studies have shown [4–6]. There is a continued need to validate the known determinants of these differential outcomes and to identify other determinants, especially in the real-world setting of routine clinical practice. Similarly, there is a need to examine which determinants of outcome are common (and to what extent) among diabetic and nondiabetic patients and where these two cohorts differ (and to what extent) in terms of determinants. By necessity, randomized controlled trials evaluate treatments under conditions of relative homogeneity in patients, settings, clinicians, and treatment protocols. In contrast, studies in the real-world setting assess treatments under conditions of heterogeneity in patients, settings, clinicians, and treatment approaches.

In the comparative analysis reported here, we aimed (1) to evaluate blood pressure values (in mmHg) and blood pressure control rates (in %) observed after 90 days of treatment with a valsartan-centric regimen and (2) to identify patient-related and clinician-related determinants of these blood pressure outcomes using hierarchical linear and logistic regressions. Implicit to the choice for hierarchical models of statistical analysis was the hypothesis, evaluated and confirmed in each of the constituent studies in this pooled analysis; that part of the variance in BP values at the end of the observation period could be attributed to a class effect for the treating physician. Also, our aim was to evaluate similarities and differences in the determinants of blood pressure outcomes between diabetic and nondiabetic patients as strata and therefore we opted for our analysis method rather than evaluating models of determinants and using diabetic status as a cofactor. The studies were conducted before the change in guidelines concerning BP targets from <140 mmHg/90 mmHg for patients in general but <130 mmHg/80 mmHg for diabetic patients. However, we adopted the recent <140 mmHg/<90 mmHg targets as the threshold for BP control.

2. Methods

The methodology common to all of the studies included in this pooled analysis has been described in detail elsewhere [7]. We summarize key aspects here.

2.1. Design, Subjects, and Data. All six studies were prospective, multicenter, pharmacoepidemiological studies of hypertensive patients in the setting of routine "real-world" clinical practice involving hypertensive patients whose GPs prescribed a valsartan formulation, in monotherapy or combination therapy, as second- or later-line antihypertensive therapy because prior treatment failed to achieve the intended therapeutic benefit or was not tolerated. Patients BP was measured when valsartan therapy was initiated and again after approximately 90 days of therapy. The latter visit occurred as physician and patient schedules permitted in routine clinical practice and may not have been exactly 90 days (hereafter referred to as "90 days"). The decision to prescribe valsartan was made by the prescribing physician per best clinical judgment.

Note that the one study excluded from this pooled analysis did not collect data using the Basel Assessment of Adherence Scale and in particular the item asking patients whether they had missed any doses in the preceding four weeks. Consistently, previous analyses have shown adherence to be a significant determinant of blood pressure outcomes and this single item has been shown to be highly predictive of outcomes [8]. Hence, this one study was not included in this pooled analysis.

As the constituent studies were observational in design, all data were recorded as available from routine clinical practice. There were no mandatory tests or other assessments. The common data model for this study has been described extensively elsewhere [7]. In addition to patient-related variables, the data model also included several physician-related variables.

A subject was considered evaluable if SBP and DBP values (mmHg) were available at both baseline and 90 days. Patients were stratified as diabetic or nondiabetic based on whether a diabetes diagnosis was recorded by their treating physician.

We treated diabetic status as a stratification variable and hence distinguished between the strata of diabetic and nondiabetic patients. This was driven by our aim to evaluate not only blood pressure outcomes but also especially the similarities and differences in the determinants of blood pressure outcomes between diabetic and nondiabetic patients as strata. Hence, we did not use diabetic status as a cofactor in an omnibus model and opted for stratified analyses.

2.2. Statistical Analysis. We assumed that the patients recruited by a given GP had the commonality of being treated by the same GP and thus within the knowledge, experience,

TABLE 1: Studies included in pooled analysis.

	PREVIEW	IMPROVE	INSIST	eNOVA	BSCORE	EXCELLENT	Total
Study characteristics							
Year initiated	2004	2004	2006	2006	2008	2008	
Diabetic	627	781	225	253	815	957	3658
Nondiabetic	2424	2818	470	701	2622	2589	11624
Number of physicians	504	684	308	284	354	698	2832
	PREVIEW	IMPROVE	INSIST	eNOVA	BSCORE	EXCELLENT	Weighted average
Patient characteristics							
Age, y, mean (±SD)	63.4 ± 11.9	63.2 ± 12.3	63.6 ± 12.0	64.0 ± 11.4	63.8 ± 12.0	63.8 ± 11.7	63.6 ± 12.0
Male gender (%)	47.7	48.7	48.5	49.0	52.3	53.9	50.5
Valsartan formulation							
80 mg	√	√		√	√		
160 mg	√	√		√	√		
80/12.5 mg HCTZ	√	√		√	√		
160/12.5 mg HCTZ		√		√	√		
160/25 mg HCTZ		√	√		√		
80/5 mg amlodipine						√	
160/5 mg amlodipine						√	
160/10 mg amlodipine						√	

HCTZ: hydrochlorothiazide; SD: standard deviation.

treatment preferences, and practice patterns of this GP. This violates the statistical assumption of independence of observations, which can be corrected by hierarchical (multilevel or mixed-effects) modeling. In this modeling, the variance observed in an outcome variable (in this case, blood pressure outcomes) is partitioned between the treating physicians and the patients being treated. This enables differentiation of the proportion of variance attributable to, in this case, the treating physician as a class effect (expressed in the metric of intraclass correlation coefficient [ICC]) and the residual variance to the patients being treated [9]. Conditional two-level (physician level and patient level) mean effect mixed models analysis was performed to determine mean SBP and DBP, quantify the treatment effect after 90 days, and, using backward manual elimination, identify physician-level and patient- level determinants of BP values in the diabetic and nondiabetic groups. Adjusted logistic regression model with backward manual elimination was used to identify predictors of uncontrolled SBP (≥140 mm Hg), DBP (≥90 mm Hg), and combined SBP/DBP in the diabetic and nondiabetic cohorts. Backward manual elimination was used to identify independent variables included in the logistic regression model while assuring clinical relevance over statistical prioritization. Because of the relative lack of uniformity in goodness-of-fit metrics for hierarchical and logistic regression modeling, we chose not to rely on prespecified metrics for two reasons. First, we chose to evaluate the goodness-of-fit metrics for hierarchical linear and hierarchical logistic modeling. Second, we monitored for the precision of estimates generated in the modeling analyses.

The constituent studies differed to some extent in the potency of the valsartan formulations that were evaluated (Table 1). Hence studies were considered a proxy for the formulation(s) being evaluated and included in the analyses as a potential patient-level determinant. Any study effects retained in the modeling were identified by the study's name (Table 1).

All tests were two-tailed and a P value less than 0.05 was considered as statistically significant. Statistical analyses were performed using SAS v.9.4 (SAS Institute, Cary, NC, USA).

3. Results

3.1. Patients. Of the 15,282 patients in the evaluable sample, 3,658 (23.9%) were diabetic and 11,624 (76.1%) were nondiabetic. Table 2 summarizes patient demographics, cardiovascular risk factors and history, and antihypertensive treatment patterns at baseline (initiation of valsartan treatment) for the nondiabetic and diabetic cohorts. There were no statistically significant differences between both cohorts except for higher proteinuria and diabetic nephropathy rates in the diabetic group.

3.2. BP Values and Control Rates at 90 Days Compared to Baseline. In both the diabetic and nondiabetic groups, SBP and DBP values (mmHg) decreased significantly over the course of treatment (all $P < 0.001$) (Table 3). The nominal differences in recorded SBP and DBP reductions were statistically similar (all P = n.s.). Similarly, SBP, DBP, and combined SBP/DBP control rates improved significantly during the 90-day study period (all $P < 0.001$). The nominal differences in control rates were statistically similar as well (all P = n.s.).

3.3. Linear Modeling of SBP Values. In the diabetic group, from an intercept of 111.02 mmHg, SBP values increased as a

Table 2: Patient characteristics by diabetes status.

	Diabetic	Nondiabetic	*P*
Demographics			
Age, y, (M ± SD)	65.44 ± 10.38	63.10 ± 12.24	n.s.
Male gender (%)	51.18	51.66	n.s.
Cardiovascular risk factors and history			
Smoking (%)	22.03	25.64	n.s.
Claudication (%)	9.44	5.59	n.s.
Adherence (%)	71.29	73.26	n.s.
Total cholesterol, mg/dl, mean (±SD)	205.9 ± 43.3	214.7 ± 39.0	n.s.
Fasting LDL, mg/dl, mean (±SD)	111.3 ± 45.0	119.5 ± 42.3	n.s.
Fasting HDL, mg/dl, mean (±SD)	67.6 ± 34.1	68.4 ± 33.9	n.s.
Microalbuminuria (%)	24.80	4.16	n.s.
Proteinuria (%)	11.95	2.00	<0.010
Renal impairment (creatinine > 1.5 mg/dl) (%)	6.92	2.70	n.s.
Diabetic nephropathy (%)	12.13	0.42	<0.003
Amputation (%)	0.66	0.14	n.s.
Angina (%)	20.05	13.12	n.s.
Transient ischemic attacks (%)	9.44	7.00	n.s.
Peripheral bypass/stent (%)	7.99	5.19	n.s.
Coronary revascularization (%)	12.53	7.68	n.s.
Cerebrovascular accident (ischemic) (%)	6.99	5.10	n.s.
Myocardial infarct (%)	11.27	7.62	n.s.
Left ventricular hypertrophy (%)	19.89	12.40	n.s.
Congestive heart failure (%)	6.70	3.73	n.s.
Cerebrovascular accident (hemorrhagic) (%)	1.15	0.76	n.s.
Antihypertensive treatment patterns			
Valsartan 80 mg (%)	4.93	7.15	n.s.
Valsartan, 160 mg (%)	35.14	40.70	
Valsartan 80/12.5 mg HCTZ (%)	5.77	6.78	
Valsartan 160/12.5 mg HCTZ (%)	16.06	14.89	
Valsartan 160/25 mg HCTZ (%)	11.90	8.20	
Valsartan 80/5 mg amlodipine (%)	2.24	2.69	
Valsartan 160/5 mg amlodipine (%)	15.96	15.38	
Concomitant diuretic (%)	28.70	22.29	n.s.
Concomitant alpha-blocker (%)	4.76	2.06	n.s.
Concomitant beta-blocker (%)	37.07	32.79	n.s.
Concomitant calcium antagonist (%)	48.80	37.01	n.s.
Concomitant ACE inhibitor (%)	6.45	2.48	n.s.

M: mean; SD: standard deviation; n.s.: nonsignificant; ACE: angiotensin-converting enzyme.

Table 3: SBP and DBP at baseline and 90 days by diabetes status.

	Diabetic				Nondiabetic			
	Baseline	90 days	Δ	*P*	Baseline	90 days	Δ	*P*
Blood pressure (mmHg)								
SBP (M ± SD)	155.0 ± 15.2	137.9 ± 12.5	−17.1	<0.001	156.1 ± 15.5	137.2 ± 11.7	−18.9	<0.001
DBP (M ± SD)	90.4 ± 9.7	81.6 ± 7.6	−8.8	<0.001	91.8 ± 9.5	81.9 ± 7.5	−9.9	<0.001
	140/90 mmHg				140/90 mmHg			
Blood pressure control (%)								
SBP	7.8	51.2	43.4	<0.001	7.9	52.5	44.6	<0.001
DBP	34.6	81.2	46.6	<0.001	29.0	80.6	51.6	<0.001
SBP/DBP	6.3	48.0	41.7	<0.001	6.1	48.8	42.6	<0.001

SBP: systolic blood pressure; DBP: diastolic blood pressure; SBP/DBP: combined SBP & DBP; M: mean; SD: standard deviation.

Table 4: Hierarchical linear modeling of SBP and DBP at 90 days by diabetes status.

	Diabetic				Nondiabetic			
	Estimate	SE	*t*	*P*	Estimate	SE	*t*	*P*
SBP								
Intercept	111.02	2.8471	38.99	<0.001	105.79	2.0141	52.53	<0.001
Patient determinants								
Age (per 1 year)					0.0312	0.0112	2.78	0.006
SBP at diagnosis of HT (per 1 mmHg)	0.1097	0.0137	7.99	<0.001	0.1262	0.0089	14.20	<0.001
Renal impairment					−2.0430	0.7882	−2.59	0.010
Cardiovascular disease (MI & coronary)	−1.9713	0.6510	−3.15	0.002	−1.7733	0.4235	−4.19	<0.001
Total cholesterol (per 1 mg/dl)	0.0168	0.0054	3.12	0.002	0.0145	0.0035	4.12	<0.001
Body mass index (per 1 kg/m^2)					0.0407	0.0151	2.69	0.007
Valsartan dose (0/80/160 mg)	1.8257	0.5433	3.36	0.001	1.1446	0.3190	3.59	<0.001
Hydrochlorothiazide (0/12.5/25 mg)	2.3898	0.5253	4.55	<0.001	3.0290	0.3188	9.50	<0.001
Concomitant beta-blocker	1.3436	0.4913	2.73	0.006	0.9209	0.2962	3.11	0.002
Adherence	−2.3483	0.5105	−4.60	<0.001	−2.1193	0.2969	−7.14	<0.001
Study: PREVIEW[¥]	3.3340	0.5693	5.86	<0.001				
Physician determinants								
Years in practice (per 1 year)					0.0794	0.0217	3.67	<0.001
Male gender	2.0623	0.7377	2.80	0.005	1.1902	0.5645	2.11	0.035
HT patients seen in past year (per 1 patient)					−0.0013	0.0006	−2.10	0.036
Intraclass correlation coefficient	0.25				0.23			
DBP								
Intercept	74.14	1.9590	37.85	<0.001	69.26	1.2184	56.84	<0.001
Patient determinants								
Age (per 1 year)	−0.0580	0.01337	−4.33	<0.001	−0.0363	0.0069	−5.23	<0.001
DBP at diagnosis of HT (per 1 mmHg)	0.0964	0.01304	7.40	<0.001	0.1139	0.0084	13.54	<0.001
Cardiovascular disease (MI & coronary)	−0.7409	0.3668	−2.02	0.044				
Total cholesterol (per 1 mg/dl)	0.0075	0.00323	2.33	0.020	0.0091	0.0022	4.17	<0.001
Body mass index (per 1 kg/m^2)					0.0249	0.0097	2.55	0.011
Valsartan dose (0/80/160 mg)	0.9529	0.3214	2.97	0.003	0.3616	0.1969	1.84	0.066
Hydrochlorothiazide (0/12.5/25 mg)	1.2184	0.3194	3.81	<0.001	1.5947	0.2000	7.97	<0.001
Adherence	−1.5461	0.3037	−5.09	<0.001				
Study: IMPROVE[¥]	−1.3811	0.5008	−2.76	0.006				
Study: INSIST[¥]					−2.7437	0.6520	−4.21	<0.001
Study: PREVIEW[¥]	1.0204	0.4858	2.10	0.036				
Physician determinants								
Years in practice (per 1 year)	0.0499	0.01797	2.78	0.006				
Male gender					0.7676	0.3452	2.22	0.026
HT patients seen in past year (per 1 patient)					−0.0009	0.0004	−2.20	0.028
Duration of visit with newly diagnosed patient	−0.0636	0.02561	−2.48	0.013				
Intraclass correlation coefficient	0.24				0.24			

SBP: systolic blood pressure; DBP: diastolic blood pressure; HT: hypertension; MI: myocardial infarct; SE: standard error. [¥]Reference study: EXCELLENT.

function of the SBP recorded at the time of the hypertension diagnosis, total cholesterol levels at start of the study, higher valsartan and hydrochlorothiazide (HCTZ) doses prescribed (including a study effect for the PREVIEW study), and the need for concomitant beta-blocker therapy. At the physician level, being treated by a male GP was associated with higher SBP values (Table 4). In contrast, patient adherence had a mitigating effect on SBP as did, perhaps counter-intuitively, the presence of cardiovascular disease. The ICC for the SBP model in the diabetic cohort was 0.25.

In the nondiabetic group, from an intercept of 105.79 mmHg, SBP values rose as a function of patient age, the SBP recorded at the time the hypertension diagnosis was made, total cholesterol levels, body mass index (BMI), higher valsartan and hydrochlorothiazide (HCTZ) doses prescribed, and the need for concomitant beta-blocker therapy. At the physician level, years in practice and male gender were associated with higher SBP values (Table 4). Patient adherence had a mitigating effect as did, perhaps counter-intuitively, the presence of renal impairment and cardiovascular disease. The ICC for the SBP model in the nondiabetic group was 0.23.

3.4. Linear Modeling of DBP Values. In the diabetic group, from an intercept of 74.14 mmHg, DBP values rose as a function of the DBP recorded at the time of the hypertension diagnosis, total cholesterol levels at start of the study, and higher valsartan and hydrochlorothiazide (HCTZ) doses (including a study effect for the PREVIEW study). At the physician level, years the GP had been in practice were associated with higher DBP readings (Table 4). Alternately, patient age and patient adherence had a mitigating effect on DBP as did, perhaps counter-intuitively, the presence of cardiovascular disease and (per the study effect observed for the IMPROVE study) higher valsartan and HCTZ doses when in single-pill combinations with valsartan. At the physician level, the time typically taken with a newly diagnosed hypertension patient in the first visit also had a mitigating effect on DBP. The ICC for the SP model in the diabetic group was 0.24.

In the nondiabetic group, from an intercept of 69.26 mmHg, DBP values increased as a function of the DBP recorded at the time of hypertension diagnosis, total cholesterol levels, body mass index (BMI), and higher valsartan and hydrochlorothiazide (HCTZ) doses prescribed. At the physician level, male gender was associated with higher DBP values (Table 4). Patient age had a mitigating effect as did the number of hypertensive patients the treating GP had seen in the preceding year. The study effect for the INSIST study indicated the therapeutic benefit of the single-pill combination of 160 mg valsartan and 25 mg HCTZ. The ICC for the SBP model in the nondiabetic cohort was 0.24.

3.5. Logistic Modeling of SBP Control Rates. In the diabetic cohort, the odds of controlled SBP at 90 days decreased as a function of total cholesterol levels and the need for higher valsartan and HCTZ doses (Table 5). The odds of controlled SBP at 90 days in this cohort also decreased if patients were started on low valsartan and/or HCTZ doses (as indicated by the study effect for the PREVIEW study) (Table 5). Perhaps counter-intuitively, the odds of controlled SBP in the diabetic group rose if patients had cardiovascular disease.

In the nondiabetic cohort, the likelihood of controlled SBP at 90 days increased if the patient was adherent and (per the INSIST study effect) was treated with the single-pill combination of 160 mg valsartan and 25 mg HCTZ (Table 5). Impairing the probability of controlled SBP in this group were patient age, the SBP recorded at the time of diagnosis, renal impairment, total cholesterol levels, the need for higher valsartan and HCTZ doses, and, at the physician level, the years the treating GP had been in practice.

3.6. Logistic Modeling of DBP Control Rates. In the diabetic group, the likelihood of controlled DBP at 90 days increased as a function of patient age, patient adherence, and treatment with proportionately more potent valsartan and HCTZ formulations (as indicated by the study effect for the IMPROVE study) (Table 5). The odds of controlled DBP at 90 days decreased as a function of the DBP recorded at the time the hypertension diagnosis was made, total cholesterol levels, and the need for higher HCTZ dose at the start of the study.

In the nondiabetic cohort, the odds of controlled SBP at 90 days increased with age and if the patient was adherent and (per the INSIST study effect) was treated with the single-pill combination of 160 mg valsartan and 25 mg HCTZ and, counter-intuitively, had cardiovascular disease (Table 5). At the physician level, the number of hypertension patients seen in the prior year also increased the odds of controlled DBP at 90 days. Decreasing the likelihood of controlled DBP in this group were the DBP recorded at the time of diagnosis, total cholesterol levels, and the need for higher valsartan and HCTZ doses.

3.7. Logistic Modeling of Combined SBP and DBP Control Rates. In the diabetic group, the odds of having both SBP and DBP controlled at 90 days were a function of patient adherence and the counterintuitive finding of having cardiovascular disease (Table 5). The odds of controlled SBP/DBP at 90 days decreased as a function of the SBP level at the time the hypertension diagnosis was made, total cholesterol levels, and the need for higher valsartan and HCTZ doses at the start of the study (as also indicated by the study effect for the PREVIEW study).

In the nondiabetic cohort, the likelihood of controlled SBP/DBP increased with patient adherence and treatment with potent valsartan and HCTZ formulations (per the INSIST study effect) (Table 5). Lowering the odds of controlled SBP/DBP in this group were the SBP at the time of hypertension diagnosis, total cholesterol levels, the need for higher valsartan and HCTZ doses (as also indicated by the study effect for the PREVIEW study), and, at the physician level, the number of years the GP had been in practice.

4. Discussion

The first principal finding of this pooled analysis comparing 3,658 patients with diabetes and 11,624 patients without diabetes treated with valsartan (second or later line) is that similar reductions in BP values and similar BP control rates can be achieved in both groups. However, the patient- and physician-level determinants of these outcomes differ between these groups. On average, in diabetic patients, SBP was reduced by 17.1 mmHg and DBP by 8.8 mmHg, compared to 18.9 mmHg and 9.9 mmHg in nondiabetic patients. In both groups, at follow-up, eight out of ten patients had controlled DBP, half of the patients had controlled SBP, and slightly less than half had controlled SBP/DBP. Thus, in our analysis, diabetic patients showed similar decreases in blood pressure values and achieved similar blood pressure control rates as nondiabetic patients. These findings are remarkable for diabetic patients because of the known difficulty in lowering BP and achieving BP control in this population.

The second principal finding is that the diabetic and nondiabetic strata have some common but also some unique

Table 5: Logistic regression modeling of controlled 90-day BP by diabetes status (140/90 mmHg).

	Diabetic		Nondiabetic	
	OR (95% CI)	*P*	OR (95% CI)	*P*
SBP control at 90 days				
Patient determinants				
Age (per 1 year)			0.996 (0.992–0.999)	0.022
SBP at diagnosis of HT (per 1 mmHg)	0.986 (0.981–0.991)	<0.001	0.980 (0.977–0.983)	<0.001
Adherence			1.443 (1.301–1.601)	<0.001
Renal impairment			0.696 (0.507–0.954)	0.024
Total cholesterol (per 1 mg/dL)	0.998 (0.981–1.000)	0.033	0.997 (0.996–0.999)	<0.001
Cardiovascular disease (MI & coronary)	1.300 (1.055–1.601)	0.014		
Valsartan dose (0/80/160 mg)	0.754 (0.632–0.900)	0.002	0.814 (0.731–0.907)	<0.001
HCTZ dose (0/12.5/25 mg)	0.770 (0.646–0.918)	0.004	0.672 (0.601–0.751)	<0.001
Study: PREVIEW[¥]	0.568 (0.438–0.737)	<0.001	0.699 (0.590–0.826)	<0.001
Study: INSIST[¥]			1.670 (1.196–2.332)	0.003
Physician determinants				
Years in practice (per 1 year)			0.988 (0.981–0.994)	<0.001
DBP control at 90 days				
Patient determinants				
Age (per 1 year)	1.015 (1.005–1.024)	0.002	1.007 (1.003–1.012)	0.003
DBP at diagnosis of HT (per 1 mmHg)	0.969 (0.956–0.979)	<0.001	0.965 (0.959–0.971)	<0.001
Adherence	1.348 (1.096–1.659)	0.005	1.443 (1.270–1.640)	<0.001
Cardiovascular disease (MI & coronary)			1.238 (1.016–1.510)	0.034
Total cholesterol (per 1 mg/dL)	0.998 (0.995–1.000)	0.020	0.998 (0.997–1.000)	0.0119
Valsartan dose (0/80/160 mg)			0.845 (0.734–0.972)	0.019
HCTZ dose (0/12.5/25 mg)	0.669 (0.541–0.827)	<0.001	0.650 (0.566–0.748)	<0.001
Study: INSIST[¥]			1.941 (1.248–3.019)	0.003
Study: IMPROVE[¥]	1.761 (1.230–2.519)	0.002	1.347 (1.055–1.719)	0.017
Physician determinants				
HT patients seen in past year(per 1 patient)			1.000 (1.000–1.001)	0.0063
SBP/DBP control at 90 days				
Patient determinants				
SBP at diagnosis of HT (per 1 mmHg)	0.986 (0.981–0.991)	<0.001	0.981 (0.978–0.984)	<0.001
Adherence	1.619 (1.367–1.917)	<0.001	1.473 (1.299–1.589)	<0.001
Cardiovascular disease (MI & coronary)	1.310 (1.066–1.609)	0.010		
Total cholesterol (per 1 mg/dL)	0.998 (0.996–0.999)	0.007	0.997 (0.996–0.999)	<0.001
Valsartan dose (0/80/160 mg)	0.726 (0.608–0.867)	<0.001	0.803 (0.720–0.894)	<0.001
HCTZ dose (0/12.5/25 mg)	0.757 (0.635–0.903)	0.002	0.683 (0.611–0.764)	<0.001
Study: INSIST[¥]			1.630 (1.173–2.265)	0.004
Study: PREVIEW[¥]	0.560 (0.431–0.728)	<0.001	0.721 (0.610–0.851)	<0.001
Physician determinants				
Years in practice (per 1 year)			0.988 (0.982–0.995)	<0.001

SBP: systolic blood pressure; DBP: diastolic blood pressure; HT: hypertension; HCTZ: hydrochlorothiazide; CI: confidence interval; OR: odds ratio; MI: myocardial infarct. [¥]Reference study: EXCELLENT.

determinants of blood pressure outcomes. Where the same determinants were observed, the strata often differed in the impact and weight of a given determinant on blood pressure outcomes. Table 6 presents a conceptual summary of the determinants by strata.

Summarizing key results, higher blood pressure at the time of diagnosis, elevated total cholesterol, and higher valsartan and concomitant HCTZ doses were associated with an undesired effect on blood pressure outcomes in both strata of patients. However, generally, these effects were more pronounced in diabetic patients. In contrast, adherence had a desired effect on blood pressure outcomes in both strata but especially among diabetic patients.

There were also some isolated effects, desired and undesired, for diabetic and nondiabetic patients. The need for concomitant beta-blocker therapy was associated with worse

TABLE 6: Summary of determinants retained in hierarchical linear and logistic regression modeling (any occurrence of determinant).

	Diabetic					Nondiabetic				
	BP values		BP control			BP values		BP control		
	SBP	DBP	SBP	DBP	SBP/DBP	SBP	DBP	SBP	DBP	SBP/DBP
Patient determinants										
Demographics										
Age, per 1 year		+		+		−	+	−	+	
Blood pressure										
SBP at diagnosis of HTN, per 1 mm Hg	−		−		−	−		−		−
DBP at diagnosis of HTN, per 1 mm Hg		−		−			−		−	
Risk factors										
Renal impairment						+		−		
Cardiovascular disease (MI & coronary)	+	+	+		+	+			+	
Body mass index, per 1 kg/m^2						−	−			
Total cholesterol, per 1 mg/dL	−	−	−	−	−	−	−	−	−	−
Valsartan dose (0/80/160 mg)	−	−	−		−	−	−	−	−	−
HCTZ dose (0/12.5/25 mg)	−	−	−	−	−	−	−	−	−	−
Adherence	+	+		+	+	+		+	+	+
Concomitant antihypertensive treatment										
β-Blocker	−					−				
Studies										
PREVIEW	−	−	−		−			−		−
IMPROVE		+		+					+	
INSIST							+	+	+	+
Physician determinants										
Year in practice, per 1 year		−				−		−		−
Duration of visit of newly diagnosed HTN patients		+								
HTN patients in past year (per 1 patient)						+	+		+	
Male gender	−					−	−			

BP: blood pressure; DBP: diastolic blood pressure; SBP: systolic blood pressure; HCTZ: hydrochlorothiazide; HTN: hypertension. Negative impact is denoted by a minus (−) sign: increases BP levels and decreases odds of BP control. Positive impact is denoted by a plus (+) sign: decreases BP levels and increases odds of BP control.

BP outcomes. There was also a trend of poorer outcomes among patients whose GP had been in practice longer and, we can presume, may therefore also have been older. In both diabetic and nondiabetic patients, age was associated with better DBP outcomes. In contrast, among nondiabetic patients, age was associated with poorer SBP outcomes. BMI had an undesired effect on blood pressure values in nondiabetic patients.

At the physician level, diabetic patients benefitted from their physicians spending more time with them when they were diagnosed with hypertension. Nondiabetic patients, in contrast, showed better BP outcomes if their GPs had a large volume of hypertensive patients. For both diabetic and nondiabetic patients, there was an association between male physician gender and poorer blood pressure outcomes. This may be tied also to the observed association of poorer outcomes in patients followed by older physicians.

We determined BP control rates using the most recent European [5] and North American [6] criteria of SBP < 140 mmHg and DBP < 90 mmHg. However, if the criteria for diabetics at the time of the conduct of the studies were applied, that is, SBP < 130 mmHg and DBP < 80 mmHg, control rates would have been 17.6% for SBP, 25.5% for DBP, and 9.5% for combined SBP/DBP. This suggests that one-third of diabetic patients had SBP between 130 mmHg and 140 mmHg and over half had DBP between 80 mmHg and 90 mmHg at follow-up (data not reported). The encouraging BP control rates reported here are directly related to the recent change in BP criteria.

At the time of the studies, valsartan was indicated for second- or later-line treatment if prior-line treatment did not achieve the intended therapeutic benefit or was not tolerated. Our analyses yielded a perhaps paradoxical finding: higher doses of valsartan and HCTZ, and perhaps the addition of a beta-blocker, were associated with poorer BP outcomes in both diabetic and nondiabetic patients. Keeping in mind that the studies were in the GP setting, this may reflect that these clinicians were trying to bring this previously uncontrolled BP under control but may not have yet achieved this for many patients during the 90-day observation period. Also, note that being a subject in the IMPROVE (valsartan 80 mg to 160 mg, with or without HCTZ 12.5 mg to 25 mg) and PERSIST (valsartan/HCTZ 160 mg/25 mg) studies was associated with better BP outcomes to which can be added the EXCELLENT study (valsartan/amlodipine 80–160 mg/ 5–10 mg) as this was the reference study. These two trends in the data may reflect the real-world fact that, despite being treated with combination therapies, some patients may still not achieve the desired BP outcomes, while other patients receiving the same or different combination therapies do show beneficial BP outcomes. The issue may not be whether or not combination therapies are indicated. Rather, there may be a need to assess which combinations of agents are effective for which profiles of patients. Future studies, in first instance in diabetic patients, are needed to evaluate which antihypertensive combination therapies will yield for specific patients the greater reductions in BP and larger proportions of patients with controlled BP. This need for additional investigations, especially in diabetic patients, is also supported by the finding that lower cholesterol levels were associated with better outcomes, underscoring the need for lipid-lowering therapy and lifestyle modifications. This also applies to the nondiabetic group. Moreover, in this cohort, BMI was retained as a determinant in some models, indicating the importance of weight management in this population.

Our findings emphasize the importance of adherence in patients in general but certainly in diabetic patients. Adherence was associated with lower SBP and DBP values and higher odds of achieving BP control. In an analysis of this same pooled data set comparing adherent and nonadherent patients, BP values and BP control rates were consistently better among adherent patients [10]. Interestingly, this analysis revealed that adherence to antihypertensive regimens may be a function of prior treatment-line failure, severity of illness, and patients experiencing (major) health problems related to their hypertension and/or diabetes. Particularly the latter may motivate patients to change their medication behavior. Noteworthy also was the fact that medication adherence tended to be better if the treating GPs were female.

Focusing specifically on our findings for diabetic patients, previous studies have shown that tight BP control in diabetic individuals is associated with better morbidity and mortality outcomes. In the UK Prospective Diabetes Study (UKPDS), diabetic patients with high BP were randomly assigned to receive either tight (<150/85 mm Hg) or less tight blood pressure control (<180/105 mm Hg) for a median follow-up of 8.4 years. Compared to the less intensively treated group and taking into account the fact that these targets are well above current guidelines, tight BP control was associated with a significant reduction in the diabetes endpoint and in the diabetes-related death, stroke, and microvascular endpoints [11, 12]. These findings were supported by a retrospective analysis of the diabetes subgroup ($n = 1501$) of the Hypertension Optimal Treatment (HOT) trial, where DBP ≤ 80 mmHg was associated with a significant reduction in major cardiovascular events compared to those assigned to the goal of ≤90 mmHg [13, 14].

Some of our findings were counter-intuitive; specifically, cardiovascular disease (defined as having had a myocardial infarct or having coronary artery disease) and renal impairment were associated with better BP outcomes. As we have argued before [7], the retention of these variables in the models may be a proxy for greater clinician vigilance in managing hypertension in patients with these conditions. In fact, diabetes itself may trigger greater clinician vigilance. These seemingly counter-intuitive findings may also suggest that clinicians adhere to guidelines and specifically those pertaining to risks associated with comorbidities. However, this needs to be investigated further because some of the studies in our pooled data set have shown that GPs tend not to know guidelines well and do not tend to practice in accordance with these guidelines [7]. Our findings also accentuate the importance of focusing on the hypertension, diabetes, and chronic kidney disease triangle and its consequences rather than each condition separately [15].

BP outcomes are determined, at least in part, by the treating physician, in the case of our data, the GP. The intraclass correlation coefficients confirm that about a quarter of the variation in BP readings at follow-up may be accounted for by a clinician class effect [7]. Further, and this applied in particular to nondiabetic patients, outcomes tended to be relatively poorer if the GP was male and older (as indicated by years in practice) [16]. While older practitioners have the benefit of accumulated experience, they may be less likely to intensify treatment and thus exhibit more therapeutic inertia [17, 18]. On the other hand, a GP's volume of hypertensive patients was associated with better BP outcomes as was the time a GP typically spends with a newly diagnosed hypertensive patient. Lastly, one area that merits clinical consideration concerns the early detection of hypertension. Consistently, higher SBP and DBP at the time the diagnosis of hypertension were associated with poorer BP outcomes. More timely diagnosis, which requires both clinical attention to and screening of patients at risk for hypertension, is indicated.

Our pooled analyses have limitations. All six studies were noncontrolled observational studies, not randomized controlled trials. On the other hand, the fact that the studies shared a nearly identical methodology and yielded a pooled sample in excess of 15,000 patients emphasizes the strength of the observed associations in the diabetic and nondiabetic groups. The groups were unbalanced in size, though they mirrored the distribution of diabetic and nondiabetic patients with hypertension. This could have affected the intercept and other estimates and their relative precision. Although not a guarantee, the large sample and the variation in outcomes observed should have buffered against this, thus foregoing the need to apply corrections to the intercept. We were interested in a comparative analysis of diabetic and nondiabetic patients; hence we did not construct a model that uses diabetic status as a cofactor. Relatively few physician-specific determinants were retained in the models, despite the finding that about a quarter of the variance in BP readings was attributable to a physician class effect. The six constituent studies involved valsartan-centric regimens and the findings may not be generalizable to other regimens. Applicable though not specific to our study, diurnal blood pressure variation could have affected measurements, though this would be difficult to control or account for in observational studies of real-world practice patterns and outcomes. The lack of generally agreed upon goodness-of-fit metrics for hierarchical linear and logistic regressions may have lent some subjectivity to the adoption of models.

5. Conclusion

In both diabetic and nondiabetic patients, the use of valsartan-centric treatment regimens in second- or later-line antihypertensive treatment was associated with significant reductions in SBP and DBP values and with significant increases in SBP, DBP, and combined SBP/DBP control rates. Common and unique patient- and physician-related determinants of these outcomes were identified. These provide guidance to the management of hypertension in diabetic and nondiabetic patients treated with valsartan: the need for timely diagnosis of hypertension; the importance of aggressive treatment and avoiding therapeutic inertia; attention to such factors as BMI, lipid levels, comorbidities, adverse events, and relevant medical history; and assessing and promoting patient adherence. On the clinical side, clinicians are advised to spend more time with diabetic patients when they are first diagnosed with hypertension and to gain extensive clinical experience in managing hypertension. Valsartan proved to be both effective and safe in reducing blood pressure in adults with essential hypertension.

Disclosure

The analysis reported here was performed independently and without external financial support as was the preparation of the manuscript. The six constituent studies were sponsored by Novartis, with certain design, analysis, and dissemination activities contracted to Matrix45.

References

[1] E. Ferrannini and W. C. Cushman, "Diabetes and hypertension: the bad companions," *The Lancet*, vol. 380, no. 9841, pp. 601–610, 2012.

[2] W. B. Kannel, J. D. Neaton, D. Wentworth et al., "Overall and coronary heart disease mortality rates in relation to major risk factors in 325,348 men screened for the MRFIT," *American Heart Journal*, vol. 112, no. 4, pp. 825–836, 1986.

[3] J. Stamler, O. Vaccaro, J. D. Neaton, and D. Wentworth, "Diabetes, other risk factors, and 12-yr cardiovascular mortality for men screened in the multiple risk factor intervention trial," *Diabetes Care*, vol. 16, no. 2, pp. 434–444, 1993.

[4] A. I. Adler, I. M. Stratton, H. A. W. Neil et al., "Association of systolic blood pressure with macrovascular and microvascular complications of type 2 diabetes (UKPDS 36): prospective observational study," *British Medical Journal*, vol. 321, no. 7258, pp. 412–419, 2000.

[5] G. Mancia, R. Fagard, and K. Narkiewicz, "2013 ESH/ESC guidelines for the management of arterial hypertension: the Task Force for the Management of Arterial Hypertension of the European Society of Hypertension (ESH) and of the European Society of Cardiology (ESC)," *European Heart Journal*, vol. 34, pp. 2159–2219, 2013.

[6] P. A. James, S. Oparil, B. L. Carter et al., "2014 Evidence-based guideline for the management of high blood pressure in adults: report from the panel members appointed to the Eighth Joint National Committee (JNC 8)," *Journal of the American Medical Association*, vol. 311, no. 5, pp. 507–520, 2014.

[7] I. Abraham, K. MacDonald, C. Hermans et al., "Real-world effectiveness of valsartan on hypertension and total cardiovascular risk: review and implications of a translational research program," *Vascular Health and Risk Management*, vol. 7, no. 1, pp. 209–235, 2011.

[8] L. Villa, D. Sun, K. Denhaerynck et al., "Predicting blood pressure outcomes using single-item physician-administered measures: a retrospective pooled analysis of observational studies in Belgium," *British Journal of General Practice*, vol. 65, no. 630, pp. e9–e15, 2015.

[9] J. W. R. Twisk, *Applied Multilevel Analysis: A Practical Guide for Medical Researchers*, Practical Guides to Biostatistics and Epidemiology, Cambridge University Press, Cambridge, UK, 1st edition, 2006.

[10] I. Abraham, Y. Van Camp, L. Villa et al., "Hierarchical modeling of patient and physician determinants of blood pressure outcomes in adherent vs nonadherent hypertensive patients: Pooled analysis of 6 studies with 14,646 evaluable patients," *Journal of Clinical Hypertension*, vol. 15, no. 9, pp. 663–673, 2013.

[11] UK Prospective Diabetes Study Group, "Tight blood pressure control and risk of macrovascular and microvascular complications in type 2 diabetes: UKPDS 38," *British Medical Journal*, vol. 318, no. 7175, p. 29, 1999.

[12] . UK Prospective Diabetes Study Group, "Efficacy of atenolol and captopril in reducing risk of macrovascular and microvascular complications in type 2 diabetes: UKPDS 39," *BMJ*, vol. 317, no. 7160, pp. 713–720, 1998.

[13] L. Hansson, A. Zanchetti, S. G. Carruthers et al., "Effects of intensive blood-pressure lowering and low-dose aspirin in patients with hypertension: principal results of the Hypertension Optimal Treatment (HOT) randomised trial," *Lancet*, vol. 351, no. 9118, pp. 1755–1762, 1998.

[14] A. Zanchetti, L. Hansson, D. Clement et al., "Benefits and risks of more intensive blood pressure lowering in hypertensive patients of the HOT study with different risk profiles: does a J-shaped curve exist in smokers?" *Journal of Hypertension*, vol. 21, no. 4, pp. 797–804, 2003.

[15] I. Abraham, S. Kurdi, and K. MacDonald, "The hypertension, diabetes and chronic kidney disease triangle in Arab countries," *Journal of Human Hypertension*, vol. 31, pp. 373–375, 2017.

[16] I. Gouni-Berthold and H. K. Berthold, "Role of physician gender in drug therapy," *Handbook of Experimental Pharmacology*, vol. 214, pp. 183–208, 2012.

[17] G. A. Verpooten, A. Aerts, N. Coen et al., "Antihypertensive effectiveness of aliskiren for the 'real-world' management of hypertension: multilevel modelling of 180-day blood pressure outcomes (the Belgian DRIVER Study)," *International Journal of Clinical Practice*, vol. 65, no. 1, pp. 54–63, 2011.

[18] N. K. Choudhry, R. H. Fletcher, and S. B. Soumerai, "Systematic review: the relationship between clinical experience and quality of health care," *Annals of Internal Medicine*, vol. 142, no. 4, pp. 260–273, 2005.

Permissions

All chapters in this book were first published in IJCD, by Hindawi Publishing Corporation; hereby published with permission under the Creative Commons Attribution License or equivalent. Every chapter published in this book has been scrutinized by our experts. Their significance has been extensively debated. The topics covered herein carry significant findings which will fuel the growth of the discipline. They may even be implemented as practical applications or may be referred to as a beginning point for another development.

The contributors of this book come from diverse backgrounds, making this book a truly international effort. This book will bring forth new frontiers with its revolutionizing research information and detailed analysis of the nascent developments around the world.

We would like to thank all the contributing authors for lending their expertise to make the book truly unique. They have played a crucial role in the development of this book. Without their invaluable contributions this book wouldn't have been possible. They have made vital efforts to compile up to date information on the varied aspects of this subject to make this book a valuable addition to the collection of many professionals and students.

This book was conceptualized with the vision of imparting up-to-date information and advanced data in this field. To ensure the same, a matchless editorial board was set up. Every individual on the board went through rigorous rounds of assessment to prove their worth. After which they invested a large part of their time researching and compiling the most relevant data for our readers.

The editorial board has been involved in producing this book since its inception. They have spent rigorous hours researching and exploring the diverse topics which have resulted in the successful publishing of this book. They have passed on their knowledge of decades through this book. To expedite this challenging task, the publisher supported the team at every step. A small team of assistant editors was also appointed to further simplify the editing procedure and attain best results for the readers.

Apart from the editorial board, the designing team has also invested a significant amount of their time in understanding the subject and creating the most relevant covers. They scrutinized every image to scout for the most suitable representation of the subject and create an appropriate cover for the book.

The publishing team has been an ardent support to the editorial, designing and production team. Their endless efforts to recruit the best for this project, has resulted in the accomplishment of this book. They are a veteran in the field of academics and their pool of knowledge is as vast as their experience in printing. Their expertise and guidance has proved useful at every step. Their uncompromising quality standards have made this book an exceptional effort. Their encouragement from time to time has been an inspiration for everyone.

The publisher and the editorial board hope that this book will prove to be a valuable piece of knowledge for researchers, students, practitioners and scholars across the globe.

List of Contributors

Huda Marzouk, Hala M. Lotfy and Yomna Farag
Department of Pediatrics, Faculty of Medicine, Cairo University, Cairo 11562, Egypt

L. A. Rashed
Department of Medical Biochemistry, Faculty of Medicine, Cairo University, Cairo 11562, Egypt

Kamal El-Garf
Department of Rheumatology, Faculty of Medicine, Cairo University, Cairo 11562, Egypt

Tatsuya Hirose, Ayaka Kuroda, Aya Yoshida, Machiko Mitsuoka, Kouki Mori, Yuki Kawachi, Akihiro Moriya, Kouji Tanaka and Atsuko Takeda
Department of Pharmacy, Ogaki Municipal Hospital, 4-86 Minaminokawa-cho, Ogaki-shi, Gifu 503-8502, Japan

Tadashi Sugiyama
Laboratory of Pharmacy Practice and Social Science, Gifu Pharmaceutical University, 1-25-4 Daigagu-nishi, Gifu-shi 501-1196, Japan

Yasutaka Shinoda and Tomoaki Yoshimura
Department of Pharmacy, Ogaki Municipal Hospital, 4-86 Minaminokawa-cho, Ogaki-shi, Gifu 503-8502, Japan
Laboratory of Pharmacy Practice and Social Science, Gifu Pharmaceutical University, 1-25-4 Daigagu-nishi, Gifu-shi 501-1196, Japan

Xuefeng Liu
Department of Systems Leadership and Effective Science, University of Michigan, Ann Arbor, MI 48109, USA
Institute for Quantitative Biology, East Tennessee State University, Johnson City, TN 37614, USA

Van Minh Hoang
Department of Health Economics and Center for Health System Research, Hanoi Medical University, Hanoi, Vietnam
Institute for Preventive Medicine and Public Health, Hanoi Medical University, Hanoi, Vietnam

Yali Liu
Institute for Quantitative Biology, East Tennessee State University, Johnson City, TN 37614, USA
Department of Mathematics and Statistics, East Tennessee State University, Johnson City, TN 37614, USA

Rachel L. W. Brown
Department of Pharmaceutical Practice, East Tennessee State University, Johnson City, TN 37614, USA

Ali Yildirim, Fatma Keles, Pelin Kosger, Gokmen Ozdemir, Birsen Ucar and Zubeyir Kilic
Department of Pediatric Cardiology, Medical Faculty, Eskisehir Osmangazi University, 26480 Eskisehir, Turkey

Anastasia Bougea, Evangelos Anagnostou, Giatas Konstantinos, Paraskevas George, Nikolaos Triantafyllou and Evangelia Kararizou
1st Department of Neurology, University of Athens Medical School, Eginition Hospital, Athens, Greece

Yusuf Kayar and Orhan Kocaman
Division of Gastroenterology, Internal Medicine Department, Bezmialem Vakif University, Turkey

Özgül Pamukçu, Hatice Eroğlu and Kübra Kalkan Erol
Internal Medicine Department, Şişli Etfal Training and Research Hospital, Turkey

Aysegul Ilhan
Sisli Etfal Hamidiye Education and Research Hospital, Clinics of Internal Medicine, Turkey

Sonu Punia, Sivachidambaram Kulandaivelan and Varun Singh
Department of Physiotherapy, GJUST, Hisar 125001, India

Vandana Punia
Human Resource Development Center, GJUST, Hisar 125001, India

Ulf Brinkjær
Department of Education, University of Aarhus, 2400 Copenhagen, Denmark

Kristian Larsen
Department of Education, Learning and Philosophy, University of Aalborg, 2450 Copenhagen, Denmark

Hanne Konradsen
Gentofte University Hospital, 2900 Gentofte, Denmark

Lone Birgitte Skov Jensen
Department of Education, University of Aarhus, 2400 Copenhagen, Denmark

Respiratory Department, Gentofte University Hospital, 2900 Gentofte, Denmark

Marina Komaroff, Michael A. Joseph and Elizabeth Helzner
School of Public Health, Department of Epidemiology and Biostatistics, State University of New York Downstate Medical Center, Brooklyn, NY, USA

Fasika Tedla
College of Medicine, Department of Medicine, State University of New York Downstate Medical Center, Brooklyn, NY, USA

Carlos Peñaherrera-Oviedo, Daniel Moreno-Zambrano, Michael Palacios, María Carolina Duarte-Martinez, Carlos Cevallos, Ximena Gamboa, María Beatriz Jurado and Rocío Santibañez
Universidad Catolica de Santiago de Guayaquil, 090112 Guayas, Ecuador

Leonardo Tamariz and Ana Palacio
Miller School of Medicine, University of Miami, Miami, FL 33136, USA

Dinesh Kumar, Shyamsundar J. Raithatha and Nikhil Kharod
Pramukhswami Medical College, Karamsad, Gujarat 388325, India

Shanti Gupta and Ravi Raj
Extension Programmes Department, HM Patel Center for Medical Care and Education, Karamsad, Gujarat 388325, India

Fabiola V. Moshi, Elisa B. Vandervort and Stephen M. Kibusi
College of Health Sciences, School of Nursing and Public Health, University of Dodoma, Dodoma, Tanzania

Kapil Gudala, Raju Kanukula and Dipika Bansal
Department of Pharmacy Practice, National Institute of Pharmaceutical Education and Research, SAS Nagar, Punjab 160062, India

Sharad R. Jain, Kaushik Barot and Kamal H. Sharma
Department of Cardiology, U. N. Mehta Institute of Cardiology and Research Center, BJ Medical College and Civil Hospital Campus, Asarwa, Ahmedabad, Gujarat 380 016, India

Komal H. Shah and Himanshu N. Acharya
Department of Research, U. N. Mehta Institute of Cardiology and Research Center, BJ Medical College and Civil Hospital Campus, Asarwa, Ahmedabad, Gujarat 380 016, India

Nora H. Ahmed, Taghrid B. El-Abaseri and Taher I. El-Serafi
Department of Medical Biochemistry, Faculty of Medicine, Suez Canal University, Ismailia 41111, Egypt

Hesham F. El-Sayed
Department of Pediatrics and Unit of Clinical Epidemiology, Faculty of Medicine, Suez Canal University, Ismailia 41511, Egypt

Sibasis Sahoo and Kamal H. Sharma
Department of Cardiology, U. N. Mehta Institute of Cardiology and Research Centre (UNMICRC), Asarwa, Ahmedabad 380016, India

Komal H. Shah and Ashwati R. Konat
Research Department, U. N. Mehta Institute of Cardiology and Research Centre (UNMICRC), Asarwa, Ahmedabad 380016, India

Payal Tripathi
Pathology Department, U. N. Mehta Institute of Cardiology and Research Centre (UNMICRC), Asarwa, Ahmedabad 380016, India

Richard Ofori-Asenso and Akosua Adom Agyeman
Research Unit, Health Policy Consult,Weija, Accra, Ghana

Amos Laar
Department of Population, Family and Reproductive Health, School of Public Health, University of Ghana, Legon, Accra, Ghana

Amos Tambo, Mohsin H. K. Roshan and Nikolai P. Pace
Centre for Molecular Medicine and Biobanking, University of Malta, Msida, Malta

Mahnaz Abbasi
Rheumatology, Metabolic Diseases Research Center, Qazvin University of Medical Sciences, Qazvin, Iran

Mohammadali Zohal
Pulmonary Diseases, Metabolic Diseases Research Center, Qazvin University of Medical Sciences, Qazvin, Iran

Banafsheh Atapour
Metabolic Diseases Research Center, Qazvin University of Medical Sciences, Qazvin, Iran

Zohreh Yazdi
Occupational Medicine, Social Determinants of Health Research Center, Qazvin University of Medical Sciences, Qazvin, Iran

Chintamaneni Raja Lakshmi, Dharmavaram Ayesha Thabusum and Sujana Mulk Bhavana
Department of Oral Medicine and Radiology, Drs. Sudha & Nageswara Rao Siddhartha Institute of Dental Sciences, Gannavaram Mandal, Krishna District, Andhra Pradesh 521286, India

Esme Fuller-Thomson and Rachel S. Chisholm
Factor-Inwentash Faculty of Social Work, University of Toronto, Toronto, ON, Canada

Sarah Brennenstuhl
Lawrence Bloomberg Faculty of Nursing, University of Toronto, Toronto, ON, Canada

Olaf Suess
Zentrum fuer Wirbelsaeulenchirurgie und Neurotraumatologie, DRK Kliniken Berlin Westend, Spandauer Damm 130, 14050 Berlin, Germany

Theodoros Kombos
Neurochirurgische Klinik, Schlosspark Klinik, Heubnerweg 2, 14059 Berlin, Germany

Frank Bode
Neurochirurgische Klinik, Klinikum Darmstadt, Grafenstrasse 9, 64283 Darmstadt, Germany

Bright Addo
University of Ghana School of Public Health, Legon, Accra, Ghana

Sally Sencherey
Komfo Anokye Teaching Hospital (KATH), Kumasi, Ghana

Michael N. K. Babayara
Postgraduate College, 37 Military Hospital, Accra Central, Ghana

Ezra Belay, Abel Abera, Aman Mehari, Gidey Gebremeskel and Asrat Endrias
Department of Medical Biochemistry, College of Health Sciences, Mekelle University, 1871 Mekelle, Ethiopia

Kedir Endris
Department of Nursing, College of Health Sciences, Mekelle University, 1871 Mekelle, Ethiopia

Kedir Endris
Department of Nursing, College of Health Sciences, Mekelle University, 1871 Mekelle, Ethiopia

H. M. M. Herath and T. P.Weerarathna
Department of Medicine, Faculty of Medicine, University of Ruhuna and University Unit, Teaching Hospital, Karapitiya, Galle, Sri Lanka

N. P.Weerasinghe
Department of Microbiology, Faculty of Medicine, University of Ruhuna, Galle, Sri Lanka

A. Amarathunga
Department of Medicine, Faculty of Medicine, University of Ruhuna, Galle, Sri Lanka

Pilar Z.Murphy and Charles Sands
Department of Pharmacy Practice, Samford University McWhorter School of Pharmacy, 800 Lakeshore Drive, Birmingham, AL 35229, USA

Frances Ford
Sowing Seeds of Hope, 1748 S. Washington Street, Marion, AL 36756, USA

Koubaa Afifa and Younes Kawthar
Stah Jabeur Primary Health Center, Monastir Health Group, 5000 Monastir, Tunisia

Sriha Belguith Asma and Soltani Mohamed
Department of Preventive Medicine and Epidemiology, Faculty of Medicine, Monastir, Tunisia

Harzallah Nabil
Primary Health Center, Monastir Health Group, Monastir, Tunisia

Bellaleh Ahlem
Department of Pathology, Monastir, Tunisia

Sahtout Mounira
C2 Primary Health Center, Monastir Health Group, Monastir, Tunisia

Triki Sonia, Hellara Ilhem, Neffati Fadoua and Najjar Fadhel
Biochemistry Laboratory, Faculty of Pharmacy, Monastir, Tunisia

Alex Kojo Anderson
Department of Foods and Nutrition, University of Georgia, Athens, GA 30602, USA

Apexa S. Raithatha and Daxa G. Mishra
KM Patel Institute of Physiotherapy, Shree Krishna Hospital, Gokal Nagar, Karamsad, Gujarat 388325, India

Vitus Sambo Badii, Arnold Donkor Forkuo, Bright Boafo Boamah and Stephen Mensah Arhin
Department of Pharmacology, Faculty of Pharmacy and Pharmaceutical Sciences,
Kwame Nkrumah University of Sciences and Technology, Kumasi, Ghana

Kwame Ohene Buabeng
Department of Pharmacy Practice, Faculty of Pharmacy and Pharmaceutical Sciences,
Kwame Nkrumah University of Sciences and Technology, Kumasi, Ghana

Thomas Agyarko Poku
Suntreso Government Hospital, Kumasi, Ghana

Daniel Edem Kpewou
Department of Biochemistry and Biotechnology, College of Science, Kwame Nkrumah University of Sciences and Technology, Kumasi, Ghana

Rahul Pal,Moiz A. Ansari, Saif Hameed and Zeeshan Fatima
Amity Institute of Biotechnology, Amity University Haryana, Gurgaon, Manesar 122413, India

Gebremedhin Gebremicael, Feyissa Challa, Atsbeha Gebreegziabxier and Desta Kassa
HIV and TB Research Directorate, Ethiopian Public Health Institute (EPHI), Addis Ababa, Ethiopia

Yemane Amare
Institute of Biomedical Science, College of Health Sciences, Mekelle University, Mekele, Ethiopia

Girmay Medhin
Aklilu Lemma Institute of Pathobiology, Addis Ababa University, Addis Ababa, Ethiopia

Mistire Wolde
Department of Medical Laboratory Sciences, Addis Ababa University, Addis Ababa, Ethiopia

James Osei-Yeboah, Sylvester Yao Lokpo, Jones Gyamfi, Emmanuel Alote Allotey and Romeo Asumbasiya Aduko
Department of Medical Laboratory Sciences, School of Allied Health Sciences, University of Health and Allied Sciences, Ho, Ghana

William K. B. A. Owiredu
Department of Molecular Medicine, School of Medical Sciences, Kwame Nkrumah University of Science and Technology, Kumasi, Ghana
Department of Clinical Biochemistry, Diagnostic Directorate, Komfo Anokye Teaching Hospital, Kumasi, Ghana

Gameli Kwame Norgbe
School of Allied Health Sciences, University of Health and Allied Sciences, Ho, Ghana

Mark Noagbe
Laboratory Department, Ho Municipal Hospital, Ghana Health Service, Ho, Volta Region, Ghana

Florence A. Attah
Diabetic Clinic, Ho Municipal Hospital, Ghana Health Service, Ho, Volta Region, Ghana

Noha Ashy
College of Pharmacy, King Abdulaziz University
Center for Health Outcomes and Pharmaco Economic Research, University of Arizona, 1295 N Martin, Tucson, AZ 85721, USA

Thanh-Nga Nguyen
Center for Health Outcomes and Pharmaco Economic Research, University of Arizona, 1295 N Martin, Tucson, AZ 85721, USA
College of Pharmacy, University of Wyoming, 1000 E University Ave, Laramie, WY 82071, USA

Kris Denhaerynck
Matrix45, 6159WSunset Rd, Tucson, AZ, USA
Institute of Nursing Science, University of Basel, Bernoullistrasse 29, 4001 Basel, Switzerland
Cardiovascular Research Institute Basel, University Hospital Basel, Spitalstrasse 2, 4056 Basel, Switzerland

Mahdi Gharaibeh
Center for Health Outcomes and Pharmaco Economic Research, University of Arizona, 1295 N Martin, Tucson, AZ 85721, USA

Abdulaziz Alhossan
Center for Health Outcomes and Pharmaco Economic Research, University of Arizona, 1295 N Martin, Tucson, AZ 85721, USA
College of Pharmacy, King Saud University

Stefaan Vancayzeele and Heidi Brié
Novartis Pharma, Medialaan 40, 1800 Vilvoorde, Belgium

Ann Aerts
Novartis Foundation, Novartis Campus, Forum 1-3.97, 4002 Basel, Switzerland

Karen MacDonald
Matrix45, 6159 W Sunset Rd, Tucson, AZ, USA

Ivo Abraham
Center for Health Outcomes and Pharmaco Economic Research, University of Arizona, 1295 N Martin, Tucson, AZ 85721, USA
Matrix45, 6159 W Sunset Rd, Tucson, AZ, USA
Department of Pharmacy Practice and Science, College of Pharmacy, University of Arizona, 1295 N Martin, Tucson, AZ 85721, USA

Index